GUIDE FOR
HIV/AIDS
Clinical Care

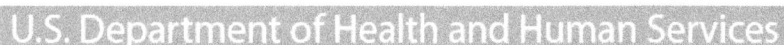

U.S. Department of Health and Human Services

Health Resources and Services Administration

HIV/AIDS Bureau

January 2011

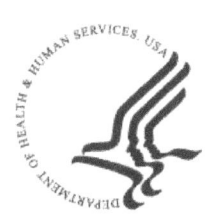

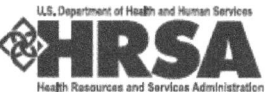

U.S. Department of Health and Human Services
HRSA
Health Resources and Services Administration

This publication was funded by the U.S. Health Resources and Services Administration, HIV/AIDS Bureau, under contract number HHSH231200533009C with WriteProcess, Inc. and the AETC National Resource Center.

U.S. Department of Health and Human Services

Health Resources and Services Administration

HIV/AIDS Bureau

Parklawn Building, Room 7-05

5600 Fishers Lane

Rockville, MD 20857

Table of Contents

Editor

- Susa Coffey, MD

Contributing Authors

- Bruce D. Agins, MD, MPH; *AIDS Institute/New York State Department of Health*
- Oliver Bacon, MD; *University of California San Francisco*
- Kirsten Balano, PharmD; *San Francisco AETC; University of California San Francisco*
- Robin Bidwell, RNC, BSN, CCRC; *Christiana Care Health Services*
- Carolyn K. Burr, EdD, RN; *AETC National Resource Center; University of Medicine and Dentistry of New Jersey*
- Diane L. Casdorph, RPh, PharmD, BCPS, AAHIVE
- Susa Coffey, MD; *AETC National Resource Center; University of California San Francisco*
- Jonathan Allen Cohn, MD, MS, FACP; *Midwest AETC, Michigan Local Performance Site*
- Francine Cournos, MD; *New York/New Jersey AETC*
- Dena Dillon, PharmD; *Midwest AETC*
- Minda Dwyer, ANP-C; *New York/New Jersey AETC, Upstate Local Performance Site and Regional Resource for Corrections; Albany Medical College*

- Douglas G. Fish, MD; *New York/New Jersey AETC, Upstate Local Performance Site and Regional Resource for Corrections; Albany Medical College*
- Rena Fox, MD; *University of California San Francisco*
- Rebecca Fry, MSN, APN; *AETC National Resource Center; University of Medicine and Dentistry of New Jersey*
- Abigail V. Gallucci, BS; *New York/New Jersey AETC, Upstate Local Performance Site and Regional Resource for Corrections; Albany Medical College*
- Marshall Glesby, MD; *New York/New Jersey AETC, Cornell Clinical Trials Unit Local Performance Site*
- Katherine Grieco, MD; *University of California San Francisco*
- Elaine Gross, MS, RN, APNC; *AETC National Resource Center*
- Geeta Gupta, MD; *Pacific AETC*
- Lois Hall, ARNP, MSN; *Florida/Caribbean AETC*
- Marta Kochanska, MD; *University of California San Francisco*
- Jeffery Kwong, MS, MPH, ANP, ACRN; *Mountain Plains AETC*
- Annie Luetkemeyer, MD; *University of California San Francisco*
- Mary Monastesse, NP; *Texas/Oklahoma AETC*

- David Reznik, DDS; *Southeast AETC*
- Susan Richardson, MN, MPH, FNP-BC; *Southeast AETC*
- Suzan Stringari-Murray, RN, MS, ANP; *University of California San Francisco*
- Alfredo Tiu, DO, FACP, FASN; *University of California San Diego*
- Milton Wainberg, MD; *New York/New Jersey AETC*
- Sarah J. Walker, MS; *New York/New Jersey AETC, Upstate Local Performance Site and Regional Resource for Corrections; Albany Medical College*
- Dianne Weyer, RN, MS, CFNP; *Southeast AETC*
- Sophie Wong, MD; *University of California San Francisco; Pangaea Global AIDS Foundation; Asian Health Services*

Clinical review by
National HIV/AIDS Clinicians' Consultation Center:

- Helena Dummler, PharmD
- Lisa Goozé, MD
- Lori Hensic, PharmD
- Megan Mahoney, MD
- Mina Matin, MD
- Patricia Myung, MD
- Nancy Nguyen, PharmD
- Jason Tokumoto, MD

Introduction

HIV/AIDS clinical care has improved dramatically over the decades, given the availability of new medications and a better understanding of how best to use antiretrovirals and deliver primary care to persons living with HIV/AIDS. Positive change on such a massive scale, however, brings with it new demands on clinicians.

Along with innovations in HIV drug therapies, HIV/AIDS care has become more complex than ever before due to increasing comorbidities that are attributable to HIV treatment and the aging of the HIV-infected population in the United States. Patient needs also have expanded across a broad spectrum of medical, psychological, behavioral, and social issues. Notably, significant numbers of infected individuals are identified and enter care late in the course of their HIV disease, confronting clinicians with complex and immediate care challenges.

Since the early days of the epidemic, clinicians have received training in HIV/AIDS clinical care through the AIDS Education and Training Centers (AETCs) Program – the clinical training arm of the Ryan White HIV/AIDS Program that is administered by the Health Resources and Services Administration (HRSA) and its HIV/AIDS Bureau (HAB). The AETC network trains approximately 150,000 health care providers each year during more than 18,000 training events.

The *Guide for HIV/AIDS Clinical Care* is a pillar of the Ryan White HIV/AIDS Program's mission to continuously improve HIV/AIDS clinical care. The *Guide* was first published in 1993 as a collaborative effort of several regional AETCs and was subsequently updated and expanded in 2006. The version before you incorporates many new insights, but the time-tested format has been retained – easy access to crucial facts for a busy clinician.

The developers of the *Guide* strive to be responsive to how HIV/AIDS clinical care is provided today.

- With more routine HIV testing in medical settings, a large number of individuals are entering care via primary care sites that have relatively limited experience managing HIV/AIDS disease.

- A notable proportion of HIV/AIDS primary care in the United States is provided by advanced practice nurses and physician assistants.

- Shortages in the health care work force are worsening. Experienced staff members are aging and retiring, a limited number of new clinicians are entering primary care and specializing in HIV/AIDS care, and fewer clinicians are available in geographic areas with limited resources.

As a result, front line primary care providers may be less familiar with management of HIV/AIDS disease, as outlined in U.S. Department of Health and Human Services treatment guidelines (available at aidsinfo.nih.gov) and clinical practices presented in this *Guide*.

By presenting best practices in the clinical management of HIV/AIDS disease, the *Guide* can help us continue the remarkable advances in HIV/AIDS care that have made the Ryan White HIV/AIDS Program a model for health care delivery for our Nation and for the world.

— Laura W. Cheever, MD, ScM
Deputy Associate Administrator
HIV/AIDS Bureau
U.S. Department of Health
and Human Services
Health Resources and Services
Administration (HRSA)

Abbreviations for Dosing Terminology

BID = twice daily

BIW = twice weekly

IM = intramuscular (injection), intramuscularly

IV = intravenous (injection), intravenously

PO = oral, orally

Q2H, Q4H, etc. = every 2 hours, every 4 hours, etc.

QAM = every morning

QH = every hour

QHS = every night at bedtime

QID = four times daily

QOD = every other day

QPM = every evening

TID = three times daily

TIW = three times weekly

Dosing Abbreviations

Supporting Patients in Care

Robin Bidwell, RNC*

Background

Patients infected with HIV face a complex array of medical, psychological, and social challenges. A strong provider-patient relationship, the assistance of a multidisciplinary care team, and frequent office visits are key aspects of care. Through both the specific services they provide and their overall approach to patients, clinics can have a substantial impact on the quality of care for HIV-infected persons. For example, a patient-centered clinic environment in which education and supportive interventions are emphasized will greatly enhance patients' knowledge about HIV infection. Improving patients' skills in self-management will increase their participation in making health care decisions and provide a stimulus for more active involvement in their own care.

Special Challenges of Caring for HIV-Infected Patients

Providers need to be mindful of several special issues, including the following:

- Many medical, psychological, and social challenges confront persons living with HIV. The delivery of effective care usually requires a strong provider-patient relationship, a multidisciplinary approach, and frequent office visits.

- The stigma associated with HIV/AIDS places a major psychosocial burden on patients. Stigma and discrimination must be addressed through strong confidentiality protections, emotional support, and cultural sensitivity.

- Underserved racial and ethnic groups are overrepresented among people with HIV. Efforts to understand and acknowledge the beliefs of patients from a variety of cultural backgrounds are necessary to establish trust between providers and patients. Cultural competency is imperative in the field of HIV care.

- Providers play a key role in the public health system's HIV prevention strategy. Disease reporting, partner notification, and risk assessment are important aspects of care.

Patients may see this as threatening and may need education and emotional support in order to participate in this process.

- Many patients have inaccurate information about HIV infection that can heighten their anxiety, sabotage treatment adherence, and interfere with prevention behaviors. Patients need assurance that HIV is a treatable disease and that, with successful treatment, they may live indefinitely. They also need to hear explicitly that HIV may be transmitted through sexual contact, injection drug use and other blood contact, and perinatal exposure, and that they can take specific measures to prevent transmission to others.

- Many patients need the support that only a peer can provide. Peer educators should be available to help patients navigate difficult health care systems, medication regimens, and lifestyle changes.

- HIV-infected patients need to have an active voice in their health care. Patient advisory groups can provide valuable program evaluation, which can be used to promote the patient-centered focus of the health care system.

These issues are discussed further in the sections that follow.

*Based on Sheffield and Casale, see "References."

Components of HIV Care and Ways to Enhance Care

Important Components of HIV Care

A first step in ensuring that patients are "engaged in care" is the establishment of systems that include mechanisms for coordination and communication of care.

- Clinics must offer a nonjudgmental and supportive environment, because of the sensitive nature of issues that must be discussed.

- A multidisciplinary approach, utilizing the special skills of nurses, pharmacists, nutritionists, social workers, case managers, and others is highly desirable to help address patient needs regarding housing, medical insurance, emotional support, financial benefits, substance abuse counseling, and legal issues.

- Providers and other clinic staff members should be prepared to conduct appropriate interventions and make timely referrals to community resources and institutions.

- The primary provider should coordinate the various aspects of health care, with close communication among providers across disciplines.

- Individual office visits should be long enough to allow time for thorough evaluation.

- Providers must be able to see patients as frequently as their medical and psychosocial needs require, and clinic scheduling should be flexible so that patients with acute problems can be seen quickly.

- A range of medical resources, including providers with subspecialty and laboratory expertise, needs to be established. Co-locating services within testing and counseling sites or within HIV clinics is an excellent way to enhance patient compliance (see chapter *Clinic Management*).

- Patient education is a vital aspect of care that begins during the initial evaluation and continues throughout the course of care (see chapter *Patient Education*).

Taking Steps to Enhance Care

Providing comprehensive care for HIV-infected patients requires a patient-centered focus, a multidisciplinary team, and a willingness to spend time on building relationships with patients. Providers should do the following:

- Make available self-management education to help patients identify problems, teach decision making techniques, and support patients to take appropriate actions to make necessary changes in their lives.

- Offer care in a patient-centered environment that allows the patient to actively participate in care decisions and provides patient-specific education.

- Encourage patients to learn all they can about their condition.

- Give accurate information regarding prognosis and the real hope that antiretroviral therapy provides.

- Foster an atmosphere of nonjudgment, trust, and openness.

- Anticipate that significant time will be required for patient education.

- Outline the range of clinic operations and state the expectations for provider-patient communication. Outline how appointments are scheduled and how prescription refill requests are managed.

- Arrange to see patients with acute problems quickly. Establish a triage system to provide efficient service delivery.

- Ensure that there are open lines of communication with all patients to receive and answer questions, assess treatment effectiveness, and manage side effects.

Helping Patients Cope with Emotional Issues

Patients coming to terms with HIV infection often experience a range of emotions, including anger, fear, shock, disbelief, sadness, and depression. Loss is a major issue for patients with HIV because health, employment, income, relationships with friends, lovers, and family, and hope all may be threatened. Many patients feel overwhelmed, and even patients who seem to be adjusting reasonably well can find it difficult to keep all of the many appointments that may be scheduled as they initiate care. Providers need to recognize that patients' emotional states affect their ability to solve problems and attend to important medical or social issues. Providers can do the following:

- Assess each patient's emotional state and the availability of friends and family for emotional support. Some patients will need counseling to help them decide whether to disclose their diagnosis to friends, family, or employers as well as support in dealing with HIV infection. Patients often feel hesitant about seeking emotional and practical support.

- Deliver important information in easily understood terms and in small amounts. Reassess patient understanding of crucial information at subsequent visits, and repeat important information as necessary.

- Screen for anxiety, depression (including suicidal ideation), and substance use.

- Refer patients to community resources for crisis counseling, support groups, and, if appropriate, psychiatric treatment to help them achieve emotional stability.

- Assist patients in finding a case manager who can help them learn to navigate the health care system and reduce anxiety about keeping their lives in order.

- Assist patients in linking to social work services to assist with enrollment into medical insurance and to meet other social services needs, such as housing, food, child care, and substance abuse treatment.

Helping Patients Develop Self-Management Skills

Self-management support is defined by the Institute of Medicine as the systematic provision of education and supportive interventions by health care staff to increase patients' skills and confidence in managing their health problems, including regular assessment of progress and setbacks, goal setting, and help with problem solving.

It can be viewed as a portfolio of techniques and tools to help patients choose healthy behaviors, and as a fundamental shift of the provider-patient relationship toward a collaborative partnership.

After patients have come to terms with their HIV infection, they are ready to embark upon the lifelong process of caring for themselves. Patient self-management involves adopting new health behaviors and requires changes that will occur as a progression of motivational skills. Motivation is defined as the "probability" that a person will enter into, continue, and adhere to a specific change strategy. Patients will feel empowered as they gain the skills and confidence to be active participants in their care.

Providers need to do the following:

- Create an atmosphere conducive to learning these self-management skills, including but not limited to the following areas:
  - Problem solving
  - Medication issues
  - Working with the health care team
  - Planning for the future
  - Goal setting
  - Dealing with difficult emotions

- Healthy eating
- Advance directives
- Sex, intimacy, and disclosure
- Adopt a team approach to health care with the patient as the central team player (patient-centered care).
- Incorporate problem-solving skills into all education efforts.
- Allow the patient time to set small obtainable goals as "first steps" in self-management.
- Realize that many appointments with multiple members of the health care team may be necessary before a patient has all the necessary skills.

Helping Patients Make Positive Changes in Health Care Behaviors

Regardless of whether a patient is new to care or has been in care for many years, the burden of a chronic disease is wearing. Positive change in behavior needs to be an ongoing focus of patient-centered care. After patients have self-management skills, they still need help setting action plans for their health care. The provider needs to help patients adopt realistic action plans by:

- Realizing that new health behaviors require motivation and occur as a progression of learned skills
- Bolstering patients' self-confidence by adopting action plans that:
  - Are realistic
  - Are something that patients find of value (i.e., something they *want to do*)
  - Are reasonable (it is better to underestimate and exceed the goal than to overestimate and fail)
  - Are action-specific, with small, obtainable goals

Peer Educators and Patient Advisory Groups

Patients need to be active participants in making decisions regarding their health care. Peer educators and patient advisory groups can help patients become more involved in their care.

In order to best support patients, it is helpful to have peer educators available for them during initial and subsequent visits. This helps to decrease patient anxiety and promotes a patient-centered atmosphere. Providers need to realize that peer educators:

- Are trained, HIV-infected individuals who provide a unique approach to client-centered care
- Attend clinical sessions and provide referrals for one-on-one counseling and support to the patients
- Are "seasoned clients" who have a desire to help patients in their care
- Work under the same confidentiality guidelines as all other staff members

Another valuable tool for patient-centered care is the use of a patient advisory group (PAG). The PAG is the voice of the people that the clinic serves. The HIV program will listen to this group's suggestions and use them to improve patient satisfaction and clinic functionality. The PAG's role could involve identifying clinic problems, recommending changes in the care delivery system, and discussing new treatment approaches. A successful PAG does the following:

- Provides comprehensive, individualized client-based education to all active patients
- Encourages clients to actively participate in treatment decisions and to involve family members and others who comprise their support system
- Designates members who facilitate meetings, promote upcoming meetings, coordinate

speakers, and provide feedback to clinic staff and management

- Allows members to serve as cofacilitators, choose topics of discussion, set meeting guidelines, and invite new members
- Fulfills requirements of grants and other funding streams to have enhanced patient involvement

Stigma and Discrimination

Stigma is founded on fear and misinformation. Theodore de Bruyn observed that stigma is associated with HIV/AIDS because, "It is a life-threatening disease; people are afraid of contracting HIV; it is associated with behaviors that are considered deviant; a belief that HIV/AIDS has been contracted due to unacceptable lifestyle choices; and, some believe it is the result of a moral fault which deserves punishment."

Stigma can adversely affect how patients are perceived by others and how they view themselves. The stigma associated with HIV/AIDS is such that individuals known to be or suspected of being infected with HIV may be excluded from community activities and suffer isolation or abandonment. Some patients may feel ambivalent about seeking medical care if, by doing so, they risk disclosing their condition. Others may have learned from experience to expect rejection and therefore may not trust care providers. It is essential for providers to be supportive of patients who are dealing with the burden of stigma.

Stigma of Fear of Contagion

Unfortunately, patients and their families are often unaware that routine household contact with a person with HIV poses no risk of contagion. They should be educated about that, and also taught what to do in situations that do pose risk, such as when bleeding occurs. Clinic staff members must model behavior in this area. For example, gloves should be worn only as appropriate during physical examinations and as consistent with universal precautions. There should not be separate facilities or special procedures for HIV-infected patients.

Stigma Associated with Being Gay, Lesbian, Bisexual, or Transgender

Demonstrating respect and providing excellent care to patients with various cultural backgrounds, beliefs, and sexual orientations are central to medical professionalism. Providers should approach patients in an open and nonjudgmental fashion and be familiar with medical management issues unique to these populations, such as appropriate screening for sexually transmitted infections for men who have sex with men (MSM) and hormonal treatment for transgender patients. Clinic staff members also must be respectful and supportive; having a staff that is familiar with lesbian, gay, bisexual, and transgender (LGBT) cultures is a natural way to create a welcoming environment. Providers and social workers should be aware of community agencies with resources available to people who are lesbian, gay, or transgender. In addition, providers and clinic staff members should be aware of special legal issues that affect these populations. For example, designating a durable power of attorney for medical decision making can be particularly important in states that do not recognize same-sex partners as legal next of kin.

Other Special Cultural Issues

African-Americans, Hispanics, and some immigrant groups are disproportionately affected by HIV, and many people of color with HIV infection have major socioeconomic problems such as poverty, homelessness, lack of medical insurance, lack of acculturation, and undocumented immigration status. All these obstacles can make accessing health care difficult and attending to health problems less of a priority for the individual. A patient's cultural background influences health-related beliefs and behaviors, and personal or historical adverse experiences may make some patients distrustful of medical care. In addition, some patients' distrust of medical research can impede their willingness to access new drug therapies. Culturally competent communication between provider and patient may substantially affect adherence with therapies. For all these reasons, providers should do the following:

- Carefully explore what each patient believes about his or her health, what would be appropriate treatment, and who should be involved in medical decision making.

- Use professional interpreters to help overcome language barriers.

- Use case managers and peer educators to help bridge social barriers. The team of peer educators should be culturally diverse in order to be effective with all minority groups.

Confidentiality and Disclosure

Confidentiality of medical information is always mandatory, but the stakes are particularly high for patients infected with HIV, who risk losing medical insurance, employment, and the support of friends or family if their diagnosis is disclosed inappropriately. Although people with HIV infection are protected against discrimination under provisions of the Americans with Disabilities Act, discrimination can be difficult to prove, and there are strict time limits after which charges of discrimination can no longer be made.

Protecting Patient Confidentiality

Adherence to the Health Insurance Portability and Accountability Act (HIPAA) regulations is an important aspect of protecting patient confidentiality. Personnel policies should reinforce measures such as requirements that papers and computer screens containing patient-identifying information not be left unattended and should include provisions for documenting whether phone messages can be left for the patient, and if so, with whom.

Helping Patients Disclose Their HIV Status

Patients who have a support network function better than those who are isolated. However, patients' fears of disclosure are often well founded, and providers must find a balance between accepting patients' unwillingness to disclose their HIV status and the need to develop support networks. Patients may find support groups or individual psychotherapy sessions beneficial in deciding when to disclose, and to whom.

The sex and needle-sharing partners of people with HIV need to be informed about their possible exposure to HIV. Local health departments can either assist patients in making these disclosures or provide anonymous partner notification for them.

A patient-centered clinic staff can help patients with disclosure. For example, they could encourage patients to bring their partners to one of their clinic or counselor appointments in order to disclose their HIV serostatus in the context of the clinic visit. This could allow the health care professional to answer the partners' questions and would provide a neutral environment for the disclosure discussion. Risk of intimate-partner violence should be assessed.

Public Health Role of Providers in the HIV Epidemic

Primary care providers must consider their public health role in curbing the spread of HIV. The incidence of HIV remains unacceptably high, and may be increasing in some populations, especially in communities with relaxed adherence to safer sex recommendations.

All AIDS diagnoses and, in some states, all positive HIV test results must be reported to the state health department. State laws vary in reporting requirements and subsequent notification of potentially exposed individuals (see the National HIV/AIDS Clinicians' Consultation Center *Compendium of State HIV Testing Laws* at www.nccc.ucsf.edu/), but the name of the source contact is never divulged to the person being notified. Providers should become familiar with the laws of their jurisdiction by contacting their health department. (The Association of State and Territorial Health Officers provides links to all state health departments at www.astho.org.) Providers are required to do the following:

- Inform patients that their AIDS diagnosis or positive HIV status (depending on individual state requirements) must be reported to the state health department, tell them whether partner notification is required, and explain what they should expect regarding efforts that must be made by the patient, provider, or health department to notify sex partners or individuals who may have been exposed to HIV through their needle sharing. Assure them that their names are always kept confidential and are never given to potentially exposed individuals by the health department.

- Carefully assess patients' risk-taking behaviors, educate them regarding HIV transmission, and perform screening for sexually transmitted infections. (See chapters *Preventing HIV Transmission/ Prevention with Positives*, *Initial History*, *Initial Physical Examination*, and *Initial and Interim Laboratory and Other Tests*.)

- Provide counseling to encourage safer sexual practices and make referrals to drug rehabilitation or needle exchange centers as indicated. (See chapter *Preventing HIV Transmission/Prevention with Positives.*)

- Provide information about the role of antiretroviral therapy in reducing the risk of HIV transmission.

References

- de Bruyn T. *HIV/AIDS and Discrimination: A Discussion Paper.* Montreal: Canadian HIV/AIDS Legal Network and Canadian AIDS Society; 1998. Available at www.aidslaw.ca/publications/.

- Institute of Medicine. *Crossing the Quality Chasm: A New Health System for the 21st Century.* Washington, DC: National Academy Press; 2001. Available at www.nap.edu/openbook.php?isbn=0309072808.

- Rollnick S, Miller WR. *What is motivational interviewing?* Behav Cogn Psychother. 1995;23:325-334.

- Sheffield JVL, Casale GA. *Approach to the Patient.* In: *A Guide to Primary Care of People with HIV/AIDS, 2004 Edition.* Bartlett JG, Cheever LW, Johnson MP, et al., eds. Rockville, MD: U.S. Department of Health and Human Services; 2004:5-11.

Clinic Management

Jonathan A. Cohn, MD

HIV outpatient care is unique in that it combines two very different approaches to patient care: long-term health care for individuals with a chronic condition, and the vital public health service of reducing transmission of an infectious disease. Thus, chronic treatment and retention in care are important for both individuals and public health.

HIV services often are provided to persons who have challenges in regard to participation in their own health because of discrimination, poverty, active substance use, or mental health disorders. The context of HIV care still is one of persistent stigma regarding HIV infection itself and discrimination against racial, ethnic, and sexual minorities who constitute the groups with the highest HIV prevalence and incidence. At the same time, funding streams from federal, state, and local governments create opportunities for treatment of uninsured and underinsured individuals and provide resources for creating innovative, effective programs. Treatment guidelines, operations research data, and technical support are available to assist in designing, operating, and improving service programs.

Patient Recruitment into Clinic

The persons who were easy to recruit and retain in care are already enrolled; the more challenging patients await recruitment. The U.S. Centers for Disease Control and Prevention (CDC) estimates that up to 25% of HIV-infected persons in the United States are not aware of their HIV infection, so there is still much work to be done to diagnose those individuals and link them to care. For newly diagnosed patients, studies show that there often is a substantial delay in attendance at an initial HIV care visit, with only 20-40% of them accessing care within 6 months of diagnosis (Mugavero, 2008). However, for the clinics, the numbers of newly diagnosed patients who present for care is substantial. A recent survey of 15 HIV programs across the country (median of 1,300 active patients each year) showed that a median of 250 (range 60-730) new patients were enrolled in each clinic each year (Yehia, 2008).

To facilitate linkage to care, every HIV clinic should 1) be linked to agencies that provide HIV testing and services for persons with HIV, and 2) make clinic access easy and comfortable for the clients of those outside services. Many HIV clinics establish referral linkages with community HIV counseling and testing services (CTS), AIDS service organizations (ASOs), sexually transmitted infection (STI) treatment facilities, family planning agencies, drug treatment facilities, local health departments, regional HIV/AIDS hotlines, and local hospitals and emergency rooms. Many clinics also offer free confidential or anonymous CTS using state or federal funding. Clinic personnel should build personal relationships with agencies that may provide referrals, invite staff of community agencies to visit the clinic, or hold open houses. Providers from ASOs, such as case managers, can be invited to accompany patients on clinic visits. Referring agencies must know what services the clinic provides and which patients it serves, as well as those it cannot serve.

Various approaches may help facilitate the patient's entry into care. A randomized study showed that using case managers to increase linkage of newly diagnosed persons to care can be effective: 78% of patients who had case management that focused on the initial clinic appointment kept an appointment within 6 months, whereas only 60% of patients without case management kept an appointment in the time frame (Mugavero, 2008).

Frequently, there is a delay of several weeks for a new appointment with an HIV clinician. Model programs have been established nationwide to improve linkage to HIV care. For example, the HIV/AIDS clinic at the University of Alabama at Birmingham offers new patients an orientation visit in the HIV program within 5 days of their request for a new patient appointment. In this clinic, an HIV program staff member initiates a welcoming interaction during the patient's first phone call requesting an appointment and invites the patient to an orientation visit. During that visit, a psychosocial assessment is performed, specimens are taken for baseline laboratory tests, any immediate health issues are addressed, and referrals for mental health or substance use disorder care are initiated, if indicated. The orientation visit is used to give patients information on how to use the clinic effectively, provide other on-site nonmedical services, and start processes to access health insurance or AIDS Drug Assistance Program (ADAP) services as needed. The full initial medical visit is scheduled for a later date. In a nonrandomized comparison, the no-show rate at that clinic dropped from 31% to 19% with that approach (Mugavero, 2008).

Success in linking newly diagnosed persons to care may be enhanced through the participation of HIV-infected consumers as peer advocates (see chapter *Supporting Patients in Care*). Either volunteer or paid peer advocates can meet newly diagnosed patients who have been referred to the clinic, help familiarize them with the clinic services and staff, and help them adjust to both the fact of their HIV infection and their role as a chronic care patient. Groups for newly diagnosed persons co-led by a peer advocate and a professional as well as one-on-one interactions with patients within or outside the clinic (e.g., through a buddy system) can help newly diagnosed persons succeed in the clinic. In clinics that use peers, particular attention must be paid to confidentiality issues. The peers must be trained and supervised (see below), and the patients must agree to participate with peers, either individually or in groups.

Clinics differ in terms of the characteristics of people living in their catchment area and in regard to the levels of expertise of clinic staff members. Some successful clinics target a narrow but underserved population and concentrate on meeting the needs of that population. The environment and services offered by the clinic may be tailored to the patient population. For example, a youth-friendly clinic may differ in these respects from one targeting the working poor.

Retaining Patients in Care

Retaining patients in care is an ongoing challenge (see chapter *Supporting Patients in Care*). Among the 15 surveyed HIV clinics mentioned above, the median no-show rate for appointments was 28% (range 8-40%). For new patients, the range was 5-54% and for returning patients it was 2-40%. Across all the clinics there was a median annual loss-to-follow-up rate of 15% (range 5-25%). A number of approaches may help patients maintain continuous care in the clinic (Yehia, 2008).

- **Respect and cultural competence:** Respecting patients and providing them with effective care builds trust and keeps them coming back. New clinic attendees may have strong feelings related to HIV infection (e.g., fear of death) or how they acquired it (e.g., issues of shame or of secrecy). They may lack trust in medical care (from prior personal experiences or from historic events such as the Tuskegee syphilis experiments) or in current treatments (e.g., "Everyone I knew who took AZT died…"). Some patients believe that HIV was created in government laboratories to target African-Americans and may or may not believe that the clinic staff is part of the conspiracy. It is important that all staff members be trained to anticipate, recognize, and work with issues such as these. Patients may experience obstacles to care when there are cultural differences or language barriers between themselves and the staff members. Diversity among health care staff can further improve the experience of ethnic minority patients.

- **Welcoming staff attitude:** Providers must know the target population and build a system that will make patients feel welcome. Patients always should be made to feel that they came to the right place (even in cases in which they must be referred on to another provider or clinic). Patients should receive understanding and support, even if they arrive at the clinic without the required managed care referral form (at least for the first few visits).

  Many clinics funded through the Ryan White Care Act (RWCA) employ patient advocates, persons from the target community who may or may not be HIV infected. Advocates directly assist patients in navigating the clinical care system and help patients ask questions or make their needs known to the clinic staff. Advocates or peer support persons can be instrumental in helping patients build self-esteem and acquire new habits that will enable them to use health care services in a proactive manner. It is very helpful for patients to be able to forge a personal connection with at least one staff member.

- **Welcoming environment:** Physically comfortable waiting and examination areas, with linguistically and culturally appropriate decoration and reading material, are important for patient retention. A clinic that serves parents or children should make available toys or children's books.

- **Orientation to clinic systems and rules:** New patients need a brief description of clinic staff and services, routine and emergency procedures, prescription refill

procedures, and after-hours follow-up. They must understand requirements for referrals from managed care providers, and new patients may need help with fulfilling such requirements. Patients also must be oriented to what is expected of them (e.g., arriving on time, calling to cancel or reschedule appointments) and the consequences of not fulfilling their responsibilities (e.g., clinic rules regarding late arrivals). A handout or pamphlet with this information can be very helpful. Patients need to know how to determine the insurance coverage and other benefits for which they may qualify, and how to find out their options if their insurance coverage changes.

- **Peer support:** Many programs have HIV-infected staff members who provide specific peer-support services. Patients who have had unpleasant experiences seeking medical care in the past, or those who are not used to engaging in medical care, may get better support from another consumer than from a nonpeer staff member. Youth especially may trust information from peers more so than from adult professional staff members.

  Peer advocates may work in this role part time or full time, as either volunteers or paid staff. Often they work specifically to make new or recently returned patients comfortable in the clinic. Some programs designate consumers as peer navigators, emphasizing their role in helping new patients, or patients returning after being lost to care, in finding their way through the health care system and support systems. Peers are especially helpful when they model good health behaviors, including adherence with appointments and medications and with avoiding unsafe sex or other HIV transmission activities. In some cases, peers have been the basis of a successful program, but in other cases peers model poor health behaviors and themselves become ill. Peers need to adhere to confidentiality rules and good work habits and need to provide accurate information to other clinic staff. Effective selection, training, and supervision of peers are extremely important.

- **Systems to support attendance:** Patients should receive appointment reminders about 48 hours before each appointment. Reminders typically are given by phone or mail, although text messaging or other form of electronic communication may be more useful in some settings. It also may be effective to have a staff member contact patients who have missed appointments to find out what prevented them from attending, offer to reschedule, and try to eliminate barriers to clinic attendance.

Clinic sessions should be scheduled at times that are convenient for the patients. For example, mid-to-late afternoon is best for school-age children, occasional evenings or weekends are good for working people.

For patients with transportation problems, ASOs and other community organizations may have funding available (e.g., door-to-door taxi service for selected patients, van service, vouchers for use on public transportation). Addressing other barriers may require a coordinated effort by the clinic staff, case manager, and others.

Some programs have a policy detailing their interventions following one or more missed visits: usually one or more phone calls comes first, then a letter to the last known address, and as a last measure, some programs will dispatch personnel to visit the last known address in an attempt to reconnect with a patient who is lost to follow-up. These efforts are more successful when patients are asked for current telephone, address, and other contact information at every clinic visit. Staff members must know to whom a patient has disclosed his or her status; in verbal and written correspondence, staff members must

avoid unintended disclosure of the patient's HIV infection.

It is important to document movement of patients to other locations (including correctional facilities) or other care providers whenever the information is known so that these patients are considered transferred rather than lost. Some states provide public lists of incarcerated persons; larger programs may use those lists to find patients who have been missing for some time.

HIV programs can be aggressive in trying to connect with patients who are missing, but also must respect explicit decisions by competent persons to change providers or to forgo medical care.

- **Outreach encounters to promote participation in care:** A study of seven sites across the United States, funded by the U.S. Health Resources and Services Administration (HRSA), found that outreach by health care professionals increased clinic attendance and that frequent outreach by any program staff member increased adherence with antiretroviral therapy (see "References," below). Outreach by medical professionals included efforts by physicians, nurses, or physician assistants to meet patients outside the HIV clinic setting, often in another part of a medical facility such as an inpatient unit. These encounters were the most expensive type of outreach, but the most effective in engaging new patients in care. Encounters with medical professionals did not increase adherence with medications, however. Other types of outreach, either face-to-face or otherwise (by phone, email, or postal service), by professional, nonprofessional, or paraprofessional staff members, increased adherence with medications, but not with clinic attendance. More frequent encounters of this type were associated with greater improvements in adherence. The results of the study suggest that initial face-to-face contact with medical providers is important for establishing trust that enables new patients to engage in care, and that frequent encounters with other staff members is important for maintaining patients on medications.

Special Population: Women of Color

A 2008 report commissioned by HRSA collected data from the published literature, key informant interviews, and a consultation meeting with RWCA-funded providers to provide information on barriers and effective interventions to assist women of color in succeeding with HIV care. Three central themes were extracted from these varied inputs:

1. development of a responsive care environment that incorporates respect, cultural competency, and flexibility to meet women's needs;

2. incorporation of peers into the care system as trained and paid participants in the care teams; and

3. addressing women's needs through care coordination, flexibility, health system navigation, and better coordination and communication between medical and social service providers.

HRSA funded a number of clinical sites to test different methodologies applying these principles through the Special Programs of National Significance mechanism; these projects are ongoing and results are not yet available.

Models of Care

- ### Chronic Care Model

Popular in recent years, the chronic care model refers to a mechanism for providing patient-centered care using a variety of staff personnel and interventions to maximize desired health outcomes. This approach has been most highly developed for diabetes care, but it can apply equally well to a wide range of chronic illnesses. In this model, patient training in self-care is key. In contrast to the tradition of teaching patients the pathophysiology of their health condition in lay terms, with this model, training involves focused skills building so that patients can better monitor their health status, use their discretionary medications, and know when and how to contact the professionals for assistance. Frequent contact between patient and clinical staff, both face-to-face and through other means, both in clinics and in the community, usually are involved. Care is directed toward panels of patients, not just individual patients. Program-wide monitoring of process and outcome variables, such as frequency and results of CD4 cell counts and plasma HIV RNA levels, informs the practice as a whole as well as the quality of care for individuals. These interventions have been shown to improve outcomes, but do not necessarily reduce costs because the staff time required can be substantial.

- ### Medical Home Model

The concepts of the chronic care model have been modified to create the model of the patient's "medical home," which may involve a primary care provider but also may involve a specialist who cares for the most prominent or demanding of a patient's health problems. The chronic care model is limited to treatment of one health condition whereas the medical home model supplements such targeted care (e.g., HIV-specific care) with coordination of the other health services the patient may need. HIV programs often act as the primary care provider, especially for patients who do not have insurance and therefore have limited access to other providers. Many HIV clinics have the capacity to better organize and implement a chronic care approach and to better coordinate services across other specialties and providers in order to be a true medical home.

Clinical Services Needed for HIV Care
Optimal array of services provided by an HIV clinic

At a minimum, HIV medical care providers need to offer confirmation of HIV infection, education, recommendations, and management regarding antiretroviral therapy; prevention, diagnosis, and management of HIV-related opportunistic diseases and treatment-related complications; screening and referral for common comorbidities, and linkages to other general health services. Most patients will need additional primary care and specialty health care and support services; it is often more effective and more convenient when these are available on-site rather than by referral. For health interventions to be successful, many patients will need assistance with health behavior change.

The services ideally provided by the HIV clinic include those on the list that follows. Detailed information on most of these topics is available in other chapters in this manual. These standards are derived from the primary care guidelines of the HIV Medicine Association of the Infectious Disease Society of America (HIVMA/IDSA), the DHHS *Guidelines for the Use of Antiretroviral Agents* in *HIV-1-Infected Adults and Adolescents*, the DHHS *Guidelines for Prevention and Treatment of Opportunistic Infections in HIV-Infected Adults and Adolescents*, the CDC guidelines on prevention services in HIV care programs, as well as U.S. Public Health Service Prevention Task Force and American Cancer Society recommendations (see "References," below).

- Age-appropriate immunizations including HIV-specific indications for some: pneumococcal vaccine, influenza vaccine, hepatitis A and B vaccines, tetanus-adult diphtheria and tetanus-adult diphtheria-acellular pertussuis vaccines, and human papillomavirus vaccine.

- Screening for sexually transmitted infections (syphilis, gonorrhea, chlamydia) at enrollment and periodically.

- Assessment of ongoing sexual or drug-use behaviors associated with HIV transmission, and counseling or other interventions to reduce transmission behaviors. Interventions regarding sexual transmission behaviors should be linked with family planning.

- General health screening for hypertension, diabetes, dyslipidemia, and cardiovascular risks, and cervical, breast, colon, and prostate cancer. The role of screening for anal cancer remains controversial because of limited data on effective management of anal dysplasia.

- Care of common general medical illnesses including hypertension, dyslipidemia, uncomplicated diabetes, obesity, asthma, and chronic obstructive pulmonary disease. Care of a wider range of disorders, such as congestive heart failure and chronic kidney disease will vary by practice.

- Evaluation and care of common comorbidities including hepatitis B and C infection and latent and active tuberculosis (TB). Treatment of active TB, including directly observed therapy, often is provided by public health agencies; treatment of hepatitis may require referral to a specialist.

- Provision or linkage to oral health care, nutritional services, and other medical specialties including ophthalmology, dermatology, oncology, and others.

- Provision or linkage to HIV care for pregnant women, adolescents, and infected or perinatally exposed infants.

- Behavior change for general health issues including smoking cessation and other unhealthy substance use, diet for weight control, and exercise.

- Behavioral health services for adaptation to the illness, mental health disorders, and substance use disorders including unhealthy alcohol use.

- Provision or linkage to social support services, including community-based case management.

- Additionally, clinics should have a system in place to protect the safety of their employees in regard to occupational HIV exposure (see chapter *Occupational Postexposure Prophylaxis*).

Resources required in providing comprehensive HIV care

- **Financial and coverage issues:** Patient access is maximized in clinics that can accept Medicare, Medicaid (including Medicaid managed care), and county insurance programs. Ideally, clinics should have a sliding fee scale. Clinics with access to Ryan White Treatment Extension Act funding should be able to accept patients regardless of health insurance status or ability to pay. Federally qualified health centers also can accept uninsured patients and have an important role in expanding access to care. Every state receives Ryan White Part B funds for an ADAP to pay for antiretroviral agents and often other drugs for the uninsured or other eligible persons with HIV. Details vary by state and are available at each state's HIV hotline (see www.hab.hrsa.gov/findcare/statehotlines. htm for phone numbers). Clinics should assist appropriate patients to enroll in the ADAP, and to access the drug coverage or other clinical services that vary by state.

  Within designated metropolitan areas, Ryan White HIV/AIDS Program Part A funding may be available. Clinics planning to serve a moderate-to-high volume of HIV patients can apply for a Ryan White Part C planning grant. Clinics serving women, pregnant women, youth, and families are eligible to apply for Ryan White Part D funding. Clinics may collaborate with other agencies in seeking Ryan White funding. Smaller programs may become satellites of larger Ryan White-funded programs. Other individual providers or small clinics may be eligible for Part B reimbursement for medical care of uninsured persons, by working with local case management agencies.

- **Personnel:** For patients who are self-sufficient or can access community-based services on their own, a lone provider potentially can deliver comprehensive HIV care. In most circumstances, however, patient care needs are met more effectively when multiple team members are available at the clinical site.

- **Facilities:** In addition to the usual office layout, other facilities are useful. An examination room suitable for gynecologic examinations is important. An apparatus for pulse oximetry is very useful in assessing patients with respiratory symptoms. Easy access to facilities for collecting venous blood, urine, and stool specimens should be available. On-site access to rapid tests that do not require Clinical Laboratory Improvement Amendments (CLIA) certification may be useful, such as urine pregnancy tests, fingerstick blood glucose tests, and perhaps the rapid HIV antibody screening tests. Laboratory certification to perform urine analysis and microscopic examination of vaginal fluid specimens is very useful. Refrigeration to maintain vaccines and material for tuberculin skin testing is necessary. Refrigeration also enables the clinic to provide patients with on-site injection of medications required once a week or less frequently.

- **Training and technical assistance:** Patients look to nontechnical staff to corroborate information given by physicians and midlevel providers. Further, patients expect the same accepting attitude from all staff members. Thus, all clinic personnel need training in both technical and cultural matters. One important resource is the National Resource Center (NRC) (www. aidsetc.org) and the local performance sites of the AIDS Education and Training Centers (AETCs) funded by HRSA to provide training and technical assistance to clinics. The NRC, local AETCs, and the website of the National HIV/AIDS Clinicians' Consultation Center (www. nccc.ucsf.edu) provide detailed and patient-specific education to assist clinicians in making treatment decisions. Written educational materials for staff, such as national and regional treatment guidelines, are available free of charge on the Internet and are updated regularly. Many regional and national meetings provide training in both clinical care and prevention. Assistance with enhancing and implementing systems of care, including instituting a quality management program, also is available from the AETCs. See chapter *Web-Based Resources* for other resources for training and information. The National HIV/AIDS Clinicians' Consultation Center's Warmline provides expert clinical advice on HIV/AIDS management for health care providers. This telephone consultation service is available Monday through Friday, 8 AM to 8 PM eastern time, at 800-933-3413.

Implementing interdisciplinary care in the clinic

It is not enough to have staff members from many disciplines on the payroll; rather, systems that allow staff members to function as a team must be created. Training with follow-up by supervisors is essential. Specific tasks for each staff member need to be assigned (see Table 1). Ideally, members of the staff can meet for a few minutes prior to each clinic session to anticipate special needs and allocate personnel resources. Some clinics place a checklist on each chart at each visit to indicate which team members a patient is meant to see that day and to confirm that all intended interactions have occurred.

The team's potential can be best utilized if there is a regular opportunity to meet and discuss patients outside clinic sessions, in multidisciplinary team meetings. When all members participate, the discussions can range from the selection of antiretroviral regimens for a patient to addressing the patient's adherence issues or chronic mental illness. Services for infected and affected family members also can be coordinated at these meetings.

Table 1. Clinic Personnel Responsibilities

Tasks prior to a clinic visit
- Remind every patient of appointments via phone call or mail.
- Review charts to list items to address during the visit.

Tasks during a clinic visit
- Verify patient's current contact information and current insurance status.
- Orient new patients.
- Assist with insurance gaps (e.g., teaching about need for referrals, help with insurance application or ADAP).
- Assess other barriers to care and psychosocial needs.
- Assess medication adherence.
- Teach and provide behavior change counseling about medications and self-care.
- Assess ongoing transmission behaviors.
- Teach and provide behavior change counseling about transmission behaviors.
- Educate about clinical trial opportunities (if applicable).
- Make referrals for psychosocial services.
- Make referrals/appointments for medical, dental, mental health care.

Tasks following clinic sessions
- Make follow-up calls regarding new medication regimens or referrals.
- Call or mail correspondence to patients who missed their visits.
- Help patients overcome barriers to clinic attendance.
- Extract patient data and enter it into the information system (not necessary with electronic medical records).

Support Services and Linkages Needed for HIV Care

Case management and support services enhance clinical care

It is a rare clinic that has the funding, personnel, and expertise to address all of its patients' psychosocial issues. Most patients need services from an array of agencies. Case managers assist patients in accessing the range of services and entitlements that can help them succeed in treatment. This may include helping patients apply for insurance; access support groups; access supplemental food, housing, homemaker and other concrete services; and access mental health and substance abuse services. Excellent case managers also help motivate patients.

Case managers should perform periodic assessments of clients' needs and update their comprehensive care plans at least every 6 months. Home visits can be very useful as part of the assessment. Some case managers or their agencies will provide certain direct services themselves; these may include short-term counseling, transportation for clinic visits, accompanying patients to clinic visits, and providing financial assistance for specific emergencies.

Close coordination between clinic staff and case management is important for avoiding duplication of efforts and services. Periodic case conferences between clinic staff and case managers are ideal. Written communication, for example, when sharing case management care plans, can be useful. Case management agencies and clinical sites need to obtain written consent from patients to share the information that allows coordination.

Creating useful linkages with community-based services

Clinics can develop relationships with community-based case managers or directly with providers of specific services, such as mental health, substance abuse, or housing services. Personal contact between staff members of clinics and outside agencies is important for establishing the relationship, and ongoing contacts are necessary for coordination. Community organizations often are pleased to give in-service education to clinic staff personnel in order to streamline the referral process. Clinics should make their expectations clear to community-based agencies. Clinics can function as advocates to ensure that their patients receive the attention and services for which they were referred. Periodic interdisciplinary meetings of clinic staff with representatives of community-based agencies, including case managers, are very useful.

Consumer involvement in HIV clinical care

Many clinics have created patient (consumer) advisory groups to participate in planning and quality management. The role these groups take depends on the specific clinic; some advisory boards educate themselves about clinic issues and provide expert input to clinic processes. Other boards act more as social event or support groups. See chapter *Supporting Patients in Care* for further information.

Enhancements to increase the HIV clinic's effectiveness: information and support

Clinics can enable patients to better care for themselves by providing them with information about HIV and by helping to build a community among them.

Much information is available for patients, including publications on medications, side effects, and adherence. Many clinics display HIV-related education materials, including information on safer sex practices and birth control; many also provide male and female condoms with instructions about their use. In some clinics, a separate area for educational materials may help clients maintain

confidentiality. Free educational materials are available from federal and state HIV websites, and the pharmaceutical industry also produces some excellent materials.

Many ASOs and clinics host support groups for interested patients. Participation must be voluntary, and only patients who are comfortable with revealing their status to other patients will be willing to participate. Some support groups target specific populations. Groups may be more effective if an experienced counselor or mental health provider leads them.

Some clinics hold classes on HIV and adherence. Other clinics provide periodic symposia to keep patients up-to-date on treatment advances. Clinics serving pregnant women and parents may include classes on birth preparation and parenting. For clinics that have a community advisory board, the board can be the organizing force for these community updates. Both public grants and funds from the pharmaceutical industry may be used to support these events.

Some youth-oriented clinics arrange social events and outings for their patients. Programs for children or mothers may provide support services for both infected and affected children, ranging from formal psychological care to supportive recreational activities after school or during school breaks.

Medical Information Systems: Tools for Enhancing Care

Medical information systems may include Practice Management Software (PMS), Electronic Medical Records (EMR), and Personal Health Records (PHR). The phrase Electronic Health Records (EHR) sometimes is used to describe the combination of the latter two. These three types of software may be available as a suite or as separate products that can be linked, although the linkage of separate products sometimes is challenging. Software products may be designed to run on one desktop computer in a small practice or on a computer server that can be accessed by many users simultaneously, or they may be based on the Internet and managed by the vendor. In all instances, backup of the data and maintenance of confidentiality and compliance with *Health Insurance Portability and Accountability Act* (HIPAA) rules and other laws are necessary.

PMS refers to software used principally for scheduling and billing; it includes information on patient demographics, insurance or payer, attendance with appointments, diagnoses, and sometimes other information. This is very useful in tracking clinic productivity and patient adherence with visits, and in developing an overview of a patient population and understanding the finances of a practice. PMS software can provide data regarding some quality measures, because services such as vaccinations and procedures performed within the practice can be tracked easily.

EMR refers to software used for clinical care, as a substitute for or supplement to a paper medical record. Providers enter their notes into these systems, and clinic staff document procedures and interventions performed in the office. With many systems, prescriptions may be written within the system and sent to pharmacies electronically or by fax, diagnostic tests may be ordered, and test results may be sent electronically into the EMR for clinician review and action. Paper documents often can be scanned into the system so that hard copies of outside reports can be included in the medical record. EMRs that substitute for paper records can reduce issues of storage, retrieval, and access to paper charts once the transition is complete.

EHR refers to software that the patients can access to see part or all of their medical record. These systems are designed to empower patients as members of their health care team, to provide detailed information to them, and to promote interaction between the consumer and provider.

Potential advantages of EMR, PHR, and EHR

In an era of transformation of the U.S. health care system, much is said about the potential of these software products to increase efficiency and reduce errors. While this potential is real, substantial effort and investment is required to deploy and maintain systems that are useful to clinicians, administrators, and payers. An EMR for a small office or one that is deployed only in an HIV program can be managed fairly easily, and some products developed specifically for HIV care are available. An EMR for a large organization, such as a multispecialty group, is more complex and requires much more planning, training, maintenance, and sometimes customization to meet the needs of all the users. Success in EMR implementation is greater when the users are involved in the selection and implementation of the system, although it will never be possible to satisfy all users with one product. Commercially available systems run on servers for large organizations may provide options for customization; however, customization greatly increases the cost and complexity of installing the software updates that are likely to be required.

EMRs may be text based (such as the system used by the Veterans Health Administration) or data based. Text-based systems are often quicker to learn; however data-based systems may provide more information for quality and program management and reporting needs and may be more useful for billing functions. Some EMR software packages are available at no cost (such as the Veterans Health Administration system and other open-source software) whereas others are available commercially and are maintained by vendors.

Once fully implemented, EMRs are expected to improve quality by improving communication and coordination among clinicians, reminding clinicians about standards of care and the timing of health maintenance or monitoring, avoiding errors associated with handwritten notes or prescriptions, documenting prescriptions, and providing warnings on potential drug interactions or hazards associated with specific diagnoses. EMRs are expected to lower costs by reducing the expense of maintaining paper records and by reducing duplication by sharing prescriptions, test orders, and test results among all users. EMRs can provide both process and outcome data for quality improvement activities (see chapter *Quality Improvement*), and data for Ryan White grantee reports. They also may make it easier for practices to fulfill and document adherence with the standards of payers.

Medicare and other payers are currently offering incentives for specific uses of EMRs, for example when at least 75% of prescriptions are sent electronically (because this is thought to reduce prescription errors) and for other types of "meaningful use" that are thought to improve the organization of care and adherence with clinical care standards.

Cautions regarding EMR, PHR, and EHR

These software packages are complex entities that require substantial staff time and effort, hardware purchase and maintenance, training, and modifications in workflow. EMRs are not simply replacements for paper records; effective use involves changes in the work habits of clinicians. Successful implementation of an EMR system requires working with the end users as the system is developed so that reasonable compromises and accommodations can be made. Choices must be made regarding both the software and the hardware to be used (e.g., a laptop computer used by a single clinician in multiple examination rooms versus a fixed desktop computer in each room). An EMR system that must share data with another system such as a hospital EMR or a laboratory reporting system can be very complex and require substantial investment of time and money, even when the different software

systems use compatible data standards. Effective implementation often occurs over the course of years. Implementation of EMR systems is not a panacea and will not solve all health care system problems, but use of EMRs is likely to be a necessity for functioning in the evolving systems of health care finance and reimbursement.

Ensuring that patients receive necessary services at clinics without EMRs

At clinics in which paper charts are in use, forms, checklists, and flow sheets can be designed to remind providers of care standards, simplify data collection, and serve other purposes as well. Sample forms for initial and follow-up visits are posted on the HRSA HIV/AIDS Bureau (HAB) website (www.hab.hrsa.gov). They include reminders regarding clinical standards, reminders of services required for billing levels, checklists built around definitions used by Ryan White HIV/AIDS Program grantees for reporting to HRSA, and other data for quality management. These instruments often can be used to generate reports to individual providers. Staff members may find it challenging to adjust to using new forms; however, using checklists often saves time by listing required elements of the visit and by reducing the amount of writing. Including representatives from clinical, data, and quality management staffs in the process of designing forms increases the acceptability of new forms or procedures.

Effective Management of HIV Programs

Managing a program with all the components described in this chapter is challenging. To enhance communication and advance the clinic's objectives, staff meetings are important. Smaller organizations may include the entire staff at monthly meetings, whereas larger organizations may have staff meetings less often, such as on a quarterly basis. Some larger organizations find it useful to have a monthly interdisciplinary meeting of program leadership, with representation of the different disciplines or program components, such as nursing or clinical care, psychosocial support, data and quality management, behavioral health, research, finance, administration, satellite services, and consumers. These coordinating meetings provide an opportunity for personnel from each discipline to update others on current activities, challenges, successes, and initiatives. They also provide a regular forum for updates on fulfilling grant-related work plan tasks and reviews of financial reports. Minutes of the meetings, which include decisions taken and assignments made, should be prepared and circulated to participants; minutes should be reviewed at the subsequent meeting and reports on assigned tasks should be delivered.

These larger organizations also may have monthly meetings by discipline, for example, comprising the nursing or clinical staff, to transmit information from the larger meeting and to coordinate the discipline-specific activities. In smaller programs, quality management may be part of staff monthly meetings whereas in larger programs it is more practical to have a separate quality management committee (see chapter *Quality Improvement*).

HIV programs often are contained within larger health organizations, and may be outliers with regard to the patients they serve and other features. It is important for program leadership to build and maintain support within the host institution. Where applicable, this may involve reminding the host institution of the grant or other funding the program generates. HIV programs often are on the forefront of innovative health care delivery, for example, in adopting quality management approaches and using other data to assist program management, incorporating EMR and PHR systems, implementing interdisciplinary care that integrates medical care with behavioral health, using a chronic care model or providing a medical home

for patients, and linking with community-based programs. An important task for HIV program leadership is making the host institution feel proud and supportive of the HIV program itself.

Suggested Resources

- National Resource Center of the AIDS Education and Training Centers (*www.aids-ed.org/*)

- National HIV/AIDS Clinicians' Consultation Center (*www.nccc.ucsf.edu/*) (free and confidential advice from a multidisciplinary team):

    - **National HIV/AIDS Telephone Consultation Service (Warmline):** 800-933-3413 (*Monday-Friday, 8 AM to 8 PM eastern time*)

    - **National Clinicians' Post-Exposure Prophylaxis Hotline (PEPline):** 888-448-4911 (*24 hours a day/7 days a week*)*

    - **National Perinatal HIV Consultation and Referral Service (Perinatal Hotline):** 888-448-8765 (24 hours a day/7 days a week)*

    * May be subject to temporary reduction in 24-hour service availability.

- New York State AIDS Institute guidelines (*www.hivguidelines.org/*)

References

- Aberg JA, Kaplan J, Libman H; et al.; *HIV Medicine Association of the Infectious Disease Society of America. Primary care guidelines for the management of persons infected with human immunodeficiency virus: 2009 update by the HIV medicine Association of the Infectious Diseases Society of America.* Clin Infect Dis. 2009 Sep 1;49(5):651-81.

- Branson BM, Handsfield HH, Lampe MA, et al.; Centers for Disease Control and Prevention. *Revised recommendations for HIV testing of adults, adolescents, and pregnant women in health-care settings.* MMWR Recomm Rep. 2006 Sep 22;55(RR-14):1-17.

- Centers for Disease Control and Prevention. *Guidelines for Prevention and Treatment of Opportunistic Infections in HIV-Infected Adults and Adolescents: Recommendations from CDC, the National Institutes of Health, and the HIV Medicine Association of the Infectious Diseases Society of America.* April 10, 2009. Available at *www.aidsinfo.nih.gov/guidelines/.*

- Centers for Disease Control and Prevention. *Incorporating HIV prevention into the medical care of persons living with HIV: Recommendations from CDC, the Health Resources and Services Administration, the National Institutes of Health, and the HIV Medicine Association of the Infectious Disease Society of America.* MMWR 2003;52:(RR-12)1-17. Available at aidsinfo.nih.gov/contentfiles/HIVPreventionInMedCare_TB.pdf.

- Mugavero MJ. *Improving engagement in HIV care: what can we do?* Top HIV Med. 2008 Dec;16(5):156-61.

- Naar-King S, Outlaw A, Green-Jones M, et al. *Motivational interviewing by peer outreach workers: a pilot randomized clinical trial to retain adolescents and young adults in HIV care.* AIDS Care. 2009 Jul;21(7):868-73.

- Naar-King S, Parsons JT, Murphy DA, et al. *Improving health outcomes for youth living with the human immunodeficiency virus: a multisite randomized trial of a motivational intervention targeting multiple risk behaviors.* Arch Pediatr Adolesc Med. 2009 Dec;163(12):1092-8.

- Outlaw AY, Naar-King S, Parsons JT, et al. *Using motivational interviewing in HIV field outreach with young African American men who have sex with men: a randomized clinical trial.* Am J Public Health. 2010 Apr 1;100 Suppl 1:S146-51.

- Rollnick S, Miller WR, Butler CC. *Motivational Interviewing in Health Care: Helping Patients Change Behavior.* New York: Guilford Press; 2008.

- U.S. Department of Health and Human Services. *Guidelines for the Use of Antiretroviral Agents in HIV-1-Infected Adults and Adolescents.* January 10, 2011. Available at www.aidsinfo.nih.gov/guidelines/.

- U.S Department of Health and Human Resources, Health Resources and Services Administration, HIV/AIDS Bureau. *The Utilization and Role of Peers in HIV Interdisciplinary Teams. Consultation Meeting Proceedings.* October 2009. Available at hab.hrsa.gov/publications/PeersMeetingSummary.pdf. Accessed June 30, 2010.

- U.S. Department of Health and Human Services, Health Resources and Services Administration, HIV/AIDS Bureau, Special Projects of National Significance. *The Costs and Effects of Outreach Strategies That Engage and Retain People with HIV in Medical Care.* March 2010. Available at hab.hrsa.gov/special/outreach.pdf. Accessed June 30, 2010.

- Yehia BR, Gebo KA, Hicks PB, et al.; HIV Research Network. *Structures of care in the clinics of the HIV Research Network.* AIDS Patient Care STDS. 2008 Dec;22(12):1007-13.

Quality Improvement

Bruce D. Agins, MD, MPH

Quality Improvement: Raising the Bar

Quality improvement (QI) has become a standard of practice for HIV programs in the United States. Quality management is included in contractual requirements for Ryan White-funded programs and has been integrated into training programs. Many clinicians have learned the basics of quality management, and may be participating in or even leading improvement efforts in their clinics. Moving beyond the basics, however, remains a challenge for clinicians who have limited time to participate in activities not related to direct patient care. Yet, focusing on quality can reveal important phenomena in the clinic of which the leadership is unaware or may point out factors that explain why problems have not been easily resolved.

> "Quality of care is the degree to which health services for individuals and populations increase the likelihood of desired health outcomes and are consistent with current professional knowledge."
>
> *(Institute of Medicine, 1990)*
>
> "All health care organizations, professional groups, and private and public purchasers should pursue six major aims; specifically, health care should be safe, effective, patient-centered, timely, efficient, and equitable."
>
> *(Institute of Medicine, 2001)*

Increasingly, QI work in the HIV field is associated with important health outcomes such as HIV viral load suppression, retention in care, and reductions in costly service utilization such as hospitalizations and emergency department visits. Simple subanalyses of basic performance data may reveal disparities in how care is being provided to different patient groups in the clinic, for example, according to age, gender, or race/ethnicity. At the same time, advances in health information technology have made it easier to generate data for performance measurement, and for performing the simple analyses that can be used for improvement activities.

This chapter will quickly review the basics of QI; an appendix at the end of the chapter illustrates concepts with examples of more advanced improvement work. Chapter *Health Resources and Services Administration HIV/AIDS Bureau Performance Measures* in this manual presents a national quality initiative developed by the U.S. Health Resources and Services Administration (HRSA) HIV/AIDS Bureau (HAB) for Ryan White HIV/AIDS Program-funded clinics; HRSA's Performance Measures can be incorporated into the quality improvement programs of local clinics, and establishment of an HIV-specific quality management program is itself a HRSA performance measure.

The fundamental concepts of QI have evolved over the past century to include the following:

- QI provides an opportunity to solve problems that are part of the system and not dependent on one individual.

- Improving problematic processes within the health care delivery system will lead to improvements in outcomes.

- Focusing on performance measurement and improvement usually stimulates employees to maximize their performance.

- Leadership is key to the success of improvement work, and clinicians have the opportunity to provide this leadership through championing best outcomes for patient care.

- Team-based problem-solving techniques lead to better care and promote a positive working environment.
- Consumers play a pivotal role in providing the "end-user" perception of the quality of the services delivered; their active participation in the quality management program strengthens improvement work and leads to better results.

In addition, documentation of QI activities helps to demonstrate institution-wide compliance with accreditation responsibilities and funding requirements, while often giving the clinic or institution an advantage when competing for alliances with purchasers. Data generated from the clinic's QI program showing improvements over time demonstrate to constituents that the program is successful and help to justify its funding.

Finally, monitoring systems that are dependent on single individuals will not last when these key players leave the clinic or are absent for long periods, whereas a fully functioning QI program that involves staff working in teams with a clearly defined infrastructure will keep going when even the most dynamic individuals depart.

This chapter will articulate the core principles and describe activities that easily can be adapted into the HIV ambulatory care setting to implement a sustainable QI program.

Introduction to Quality Improvement

QI includes regular measurement of care processes and outcomes to analyze the performance of the system of care. It involves the implementation of solutions to improve care and the monitoring of their effectiveness, with the goal of achieving optimal health outcomes for patients. Ongoing cycles of change and remeasurement are implemented to test and try different ideas to determine which practices result in improved care. QI activities in clinics can range from a single team focusing on improving one aspect of care to a comprehensive QI program with many teams working on a wide variety of improvement projects, with a well-established plan and an oversight committee.

The methods of QI are based on core principles that are readily translated into a practical approach and integrated into the clinical care delivery system (see Table 1). Successful implementation of QI involves actions at two levels: the QI activities and the HIV program processes that provide the structural backbone for them.

Table 1. Core Principles of Quality Improvement
• **Focus on the customer:** improvement activities result in improved patient health
• **Measurement:** collect and use data to improve care
• **Emphasis on systems of care:** improve processes that link to desired outcomes
• **Involvement of participants:** encourage direct participation in teams by those individuals who implement the processes being evaluated

Measurement and Management Are Not Sufficient

Although it is the bedrock for improving care, measurement alone is not sufficient to improve quality. A common pitfall in implementing QI programs is to rely solely upon performance data, the medical or program director's interpretation of it, and one person's decisions about how to make changes. Successful improvements occur most often when staff members from the systems being assessed work together in teams. When they are engaged in the process, staff members are more likely to generate ideas for improvement and to accept changes. Staff review of improvement charts (see Figure 1, below) generates pride and a sense of accomplishment based on members' participation in the QI work. These charts may be posted on bulletin boards in common areas of clinics so that everyone can view them.

Key Components of a Quality Plan

The key elements of a quality plan include a quality statement that describes the purpose, priorities, and goals of the QI program; a description of the organizational systems needed to implement the program, including committee structure and functions, definitions of accountability, roles and responsibilities, the process for obtaining consumer input, core measures, and data collection processes; and a description of how the plan will be evaluated. For further information, see New York State Department of Health AIDS Institute HIVQUAL Group Learning Guide (see "References," below).

QI Personnel

The size of the clinic will determine who participates in quality-of-care activities. In small HIV clinics with a primary care provider, case manager, nurse, and support staff, most of the staff members are involved in all aspects of QI work. Larger institutions usually establish an HIV Quality Committee that includes senior management of the HIV clinic, designated QI staff if there are any, and other key players who work in the clinic. A member of this committee represents the group in the agency-wide QI committee. The Quality Committee identifies the priorities for improvement or agrees to pursue the priorities identified by staff members or patients in the clinic. The Quality Committee also charters improvement teams and identifies potential members who are key stakeholders in the process under investigation. In a small clinic that has only a handful of staff members, all clinic personnel may participate in the quality management program and in QI activities, although perhaps in a less formal way than in larger clinics.

Team Membership and Responsibilities

Teams are formed to address the specific care processes or systems that are targeted for improvement. Team members should be selected to represent the different functions involved in these processes or to represent the components of the system under focus. The size of a team varies according to the size of the clinic and the process under study. In small clinics, the few dedicated HIV program staff members may constitute the project teams, with added representation from different departments as needed (such as from the laboratory, or from other medical disciplines). In larger clinics, teams often include 6-10 members. Membership should include representatives from the different groups in the clinic who are involved in the care process. In addition to the clinical and case management staff, scheduling clerks and medical records personnel often are important participants, especially when follow-up appointments and documentation are important components of the care process or have been identified as areas that need to be improved.

Involving consumers in QI project teams enhances the work of the team. Consumers who are involved in the clinic's community advisory board often are natural leaders and have a good grasp of clinic processes. Their feedback on the experience of care delivery can reveal areas that need improvement. They know the bottlenecks and can inform the staff how long a clinic visit lasts, whether assessments truly occurred, and whether behavioral interventions are effective. Their ideas about what improves care often diverge significantly from those generated by providers and may not even be recognized unless they participate directly in discussions about the system.

Teams are expected to analyze clinical processes, identify areas of change, implement tests of the changes, review data assessing the change, and ultimately make recommendations about which improvements should be adopted in the clinic.

As the project team conducts its work and gains experience, it will become more independent and assume more responsibility for ongoing measurement, data collection, and implementation of steps toward improvement. It should disband when implementation has resulted in sustainable results.

Data Collection

Selecting Indicators

Indicators are measurable aspects of care that can help to evaluate the extent to which a facility provides a certain element of care. Indicators should be based on standards or guidelines, meet the primary goals of QI, and reflect priorities specific to the community and the clinic. In addition, they should represent processes where changes are feasible. For example, in HIV clinics where the population consists of a large number of women, indicators may include rates of routine cervical cancer screening, rates of preconception

counseling, or other aspects of care specific to women. In clinics that care for a high volume of patients who have been treated with antiretroviral therapy (ART) for a long time, indicators may focus on rates of virologic suppression, screening for adverse effects of antiretroviral medications, and resistance testing. Some indicators should be selected by soliciting input from patients who attend the clinic (see Table 2). Staff members also often know what aspects of care would benefit from being measured and improved, and they should be consulted to determine priorities. If routine data collection systems already exist in the clinic, data should be reviewed to determine which components of care would be prime candidates for improvement. On a national level, the HRSA HIV/AIDS Bureau (HAB) has developed HIV/AIDS Core Clinical Performance Measures for Adults and Adolescents for monitoring the quality of care provided in Ryan White HIV/AIDS Program-funded clinics. These can be used as a starting point if local priorities have not been established. See chapter *Health Resources and Services Administration HIV/AIDS Bureau Performance Measures* for these.

Table 2. Methods for Obtaining Input from Patients
• Suggestion box
• Surveys
• Focus groups
• Consumer advisory board

Ideally, a balanced set of measures should be selected. Different ways to categorize measures might include the following:

- Structure/process/outcome

- Treatment/care (non-ART)/prevention/ nonclinical service

- Provider/consumer/funder driven

- Aspects representing overutilization, underutilization, or misutilization of services

Developing and Measuring Indicators

Three major activities constitute the process of indicator development:

- Defining the measurement population
- Defining the measures
- Developing the data collection plan

The measurement population is defined by determining factors such as the location of care being studied, whether both men and women are eligible, the applicability of the indicator to various age groups, whether any clinical conditions are necessary to determine whether the indicator is applicable, and whether the patient must have been in treatment or visited the clinic more than once.

After the population is defined, the measure needs to be defined. The measure should be objective and should address specific aspects of quality care. It also should have a straightforward, dichotomous answer. For each measure, specific criteria must be developed to define the "yes" response and the "no" response (see Table 3). This often involves deciding the time period during which an activity has been performed. For example, an indicator that measures viral load monitoring must include the frequency with which that test should be performed. One simple way to construct this measure would be to ask, "Was viral load measured within the past 6 months?"

Table 3. Examples of Specific Measures with Definitions of Responses		
Measure	**Definition of Measure**	**Yes/No Response**
Pneumocystis jiroveci pneumonia (PCP) prophylaxis	Did the patient whose CD4 count was <200 cells/µL during the review period receive PCP prophylaxis?	**Yes:** The patient received PCP prophylaxis **No:** The patient did not receive PCP prophylaxis
Latent TB infection (LTBI) screening (eligibility: HIV-infected patients without a history of previous TB disease or a history of a test for LTBI)	Was a test for LTBI performed (tuberculin skin test or interferon-gamma release assay) and were results documented in the past 12 months?	**Yes:** LTBI testing was performed **No:** LTBI testing was not performed (or the test was done but results were not documented)

Several indicators should be measured simultaneously, whether abstracted from medical records or analyzed through administrative databases. Indicators reflecting different aspects of patient management should be selected, as should those involving different populations. Indicators also should be selected to evaluate various components of the health care system, such as the components of the chronic disease model.

The data collection plan includes determining the source of information (e.g., whether medical records or an electronic database will be used), how the data will be recorded, who will record the data, and how a data sample will be selected. A representative sample will allow inferences to be made about the overall clinic population based on observations of the smaller sample. Some form of random sampling should be used, either by using a random numbers table or by selecting every nth record from the list of eligible patients.

A common pitfall at this point is to think of the measurement sample as a research project. For the purposes of QI, a sample needs only to be current, representative, and readily obtained (i.e., sample size calculations and the achievement of statistically significant results are not necessary).

Analyzing and Displaying Data

Data should be reviewed and distributed to all members of the team and others involved in the care process under evaluation. When possible, data should be displayed in graphic format. After data from multiple time periods have been collected (e.g., percentage of patients

Identifying Targets and Implementing Improvements

After the project team has reviewed the data, it must decide where opportunities for improvement exist. The first step in this process is to investigate the care process in greater detail. Several techniques are used to accomplish this goal. The simplest is brainstorming, in which key stakeholders offer their suggestions as to which processes are the best candidates for change. Another easy method is flowcharting, in which the group breaks down the process into its components to identify how it is coordinated and how its parts fit together. A fishbone diagram, or cause-and-effect diagram, may aid in exploring and displaying the causes of a particular problem (Figures 2 and 3). It often helps for staff members to consider factors potentially influencing a process that are not obvious, and to help sort out those factors that are external to the clinic and those that are internal. Then, the areas that would be most likely to benefit from improvement are selected for change (see Figure 4) and tested in the Plan-Do-Study-Act (PDSA) cycle (see Figure 5). See "Appendix," below, for examples of QI projects conducted in HIV clinics.

Figure 1. Percentage of Patients Screened for Latent TB, by Month

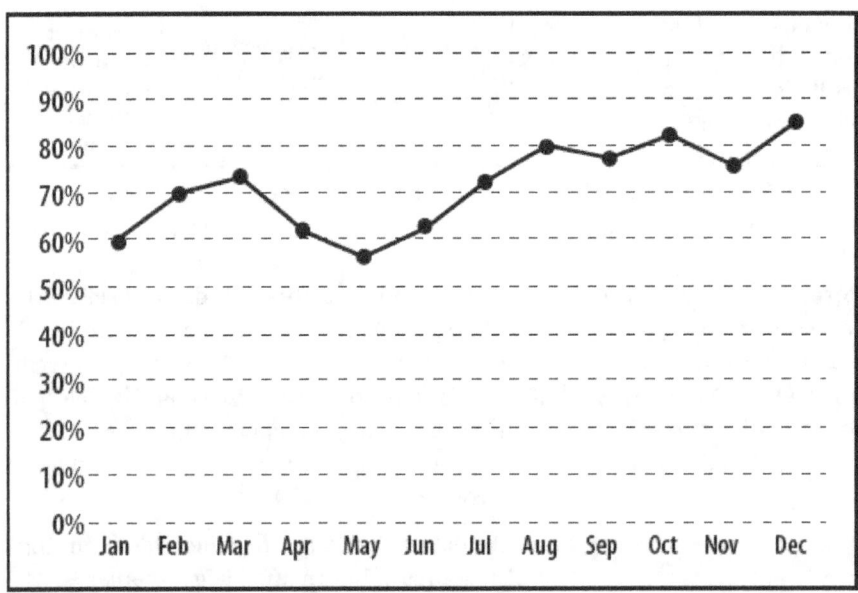

Adapted from *Measuring Clinical Performance: A Guide for HIV Health Care Providers.* New York: New York State Department of Health AIDS Institute. April 2002.

screened for latent TB), a simple line graph (run chart) can be constructed with each point representing a performance rate (percentage) for a given period of time. This usually is the simplest and most effective way to show performance data (see Figure 1).

Figure 2. Sample Fishbone Diagram

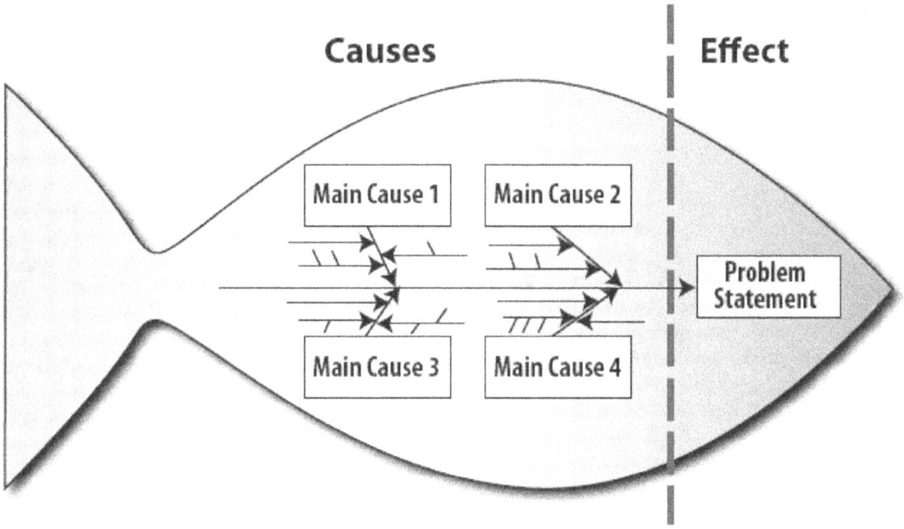

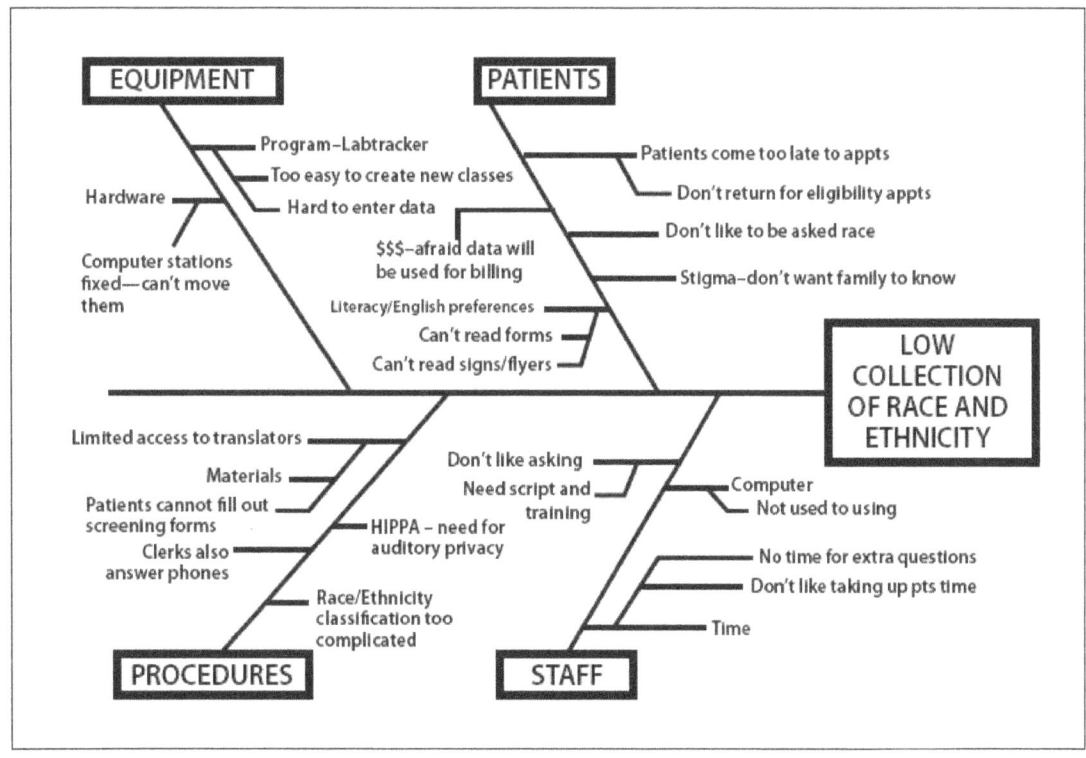

Figure 3. Fishbone Diagram: Low Collection Rates of Race and Ethnicity Patient Data

Used with permission from Kathleen A. Clanon, MD; Alameda County Medical Center.

Figure 4. Sample Flow Chart

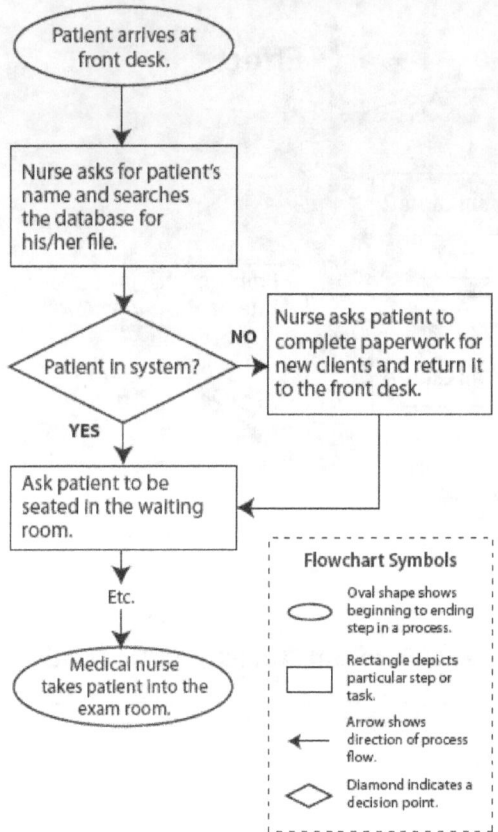

Source: U.S. Department of Health and Human Services, Health Resources and Services Administration, HIV/AIDS Bureau. *A Guide to Primary Care of People with HIV/AIDS.* Bartlett JG, Cheever LW, Johnson MP, Paauw DS, eds. Rockville, MD: U.S. Department of Health and Human Services; 2004:145.

Figure 5. Plan-Do-Study-Act Cycle

Plan: Plan the change and collect baseline data

Do: Test the change and collect data

Study: Analyze the data

Act: If the change did not improve the process, try another idea. If the change resulted in improvement, adopt the change, monitor the process periodically, and spread the change throughout the clinic

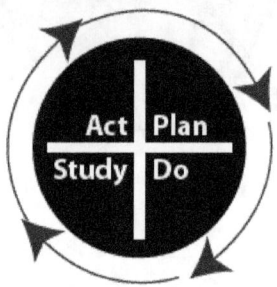

Source: U.S. Department of Health and Human Services, Health Resources and Services Administration, HIV/AIDS Bureau. *A Guide to Primary Care of People with HIV/AIDS.* Bartlett JG, Cheever LW, Johnson MP, Paauw DS, eds. Rockville, MD: U.S. Department of Health and Human Services; 2004:145.

After a change to a particular step of the process has been selected, a test of the change can be quickly implemented and evaluated. A limited implementation of the proposed change can be tested — perhaps with just a few subsequent patients, or those attending on the following day, or those seen by a particular clinician. If the small change does not work, another change can be selected and implemented quickly. If the change is feasible and improvement is noted, it can be adopted more widely, before formal remeasurement occurs, and a regular period of remeasurement can be adopted. If the change was not successful, then another one can be chosen and tested. Occasionally, multiple changes may be tested simultaneously or on different days of the week.

Often teams become caught up in following a rigid series of steps. Many different approaches to QI exist and can be implemented successfully. However, sometimes just stepping back to refocus on the three basic questions of the model for improvement presented by Langley et al. (see "Suggested Resources," below) can effectively guide QI activities. These are as follows:

- What do we want to accomplish?

- How do we know that a change will result in an improvement — in other words what measure will we use to demonstrate whether our improvements worked?

- What kinds of changes can we test that will result in an improvement?

Establishing Systems to Support QI

The key to sustaining QI in the clinic is development of an infrastructure that supports ongoing QI activities. The central components of this infrastructure include the following:

- A QI plan with goals and a process to prioritize these goals

- A work plan that clearly defines steps, sets timeframes for completion, and identifies responsible parties

- An organizational framework that displays clear lines of accountability for QI in the organization

- Commitment of senior management staff to support the program, allocate resources, and celebrate its successes

- Creation of a culture that supports quality in the program and that values the activities of QI as part of the regular work of the clinic (see Table 4)

- Patient participation, to share experiential knowledge and inform QI program development

- Establishment of a formal QI committee to oversee quality activities, monitor the quality plan, and evaluate its effectiveness

Table 4. Tips for Promoting a Culture of Quality Improvement: Integration of Quality into the Regular Work of the Clinic
• Educate staff members about QI and provide them with the skills to participate in QI activities
• Consistently articulate the values of QI in staff meetings
• Display QI data and storyboards (simple statements and visual representations that describe a problem, the evaluation process, the proposed changes and their implementation, and display the results)
• Celebrate successes
• Provide opportunities for all staff to participate in QI teams
• Reward staff members through performance evaluation for their contributions to the QI program

The regular, ongoing work of the QI committee, supported by the clinic leadership, constitutes the backbone of the infrastructure that supports ongoing QI activities. The committee oversees the dynamic process of planning, implementation, and evaluation that involves the following:

- Analysis of data from the QI projects

- Solicitation of feedback from participating staff and from patients

- Decision-making based on the information from its analysis

These contribute to sustaining the QI program and its activities in the clinic.

Sustaining Improvements

Sustainability is probably the biggest challenge that clinics face in the field of QI. All too often, improvements do not last after initial projects are completed, because the structure and culture to support QI is not present or is not supported. The challenge of sustainability therefore is twofold: to maintain the successes of QI work and its clinical outcomes, and to maintain the systems of QI and to keep the QI program vital. By asking questions about how care systems can be improved and how QI activities are progressing, clinicians play an important role in both catalyzing and supporting QI activities.

Appendix: Case Examples of Quality Management Initiatives

Using QI to Improve ART Management and Virologic Suppression

In one community health center, nearly 10% of patients on antiretroviral therapy (ART) were not virologically suppressed. The clinic had adopted a strategy of developing a specific ART management plan for each patient being treated. Review of the charts of the 45 patients not suppressed showed that only 40% had a plan in the chart. Only 20% had a plan that was executed. Improvement goals were set for each step, to increase from 40% to 90% for documentation and from 20% to 75% for execution. Over the course of a 4-month period, clinicians and support staff were educated about the plan and decision-support tools were created, including an algorithm showing key decision points for plan development and execution with corresponding prompts in the clinic database. Visit forms were revised to incorporate data fields specific to the ART plans. Reminders

also were created. All changes were implemented through small tests of change with formal indicator remeasurement in 6 months; this showed that 100% of patients had a plan in their charts and that 71% of them had it executed. Continued monitoring showed a dip in performance 4 months later to 88% and 60%, respectively, but with gains restored 3 months subsequently to 100% and 65%, respectively. Vigilance and reaffirmation of the main steps have been keys to maintaining performance. The fields are now being added to the new clinic electronic medical record (EMR) system with automatic prompts based on changes in viral load values.

Another clinic focused QI efforts directly on improving rates of virologic suppression. Data on the HIV viral loads of each specific provider were generated to show comparative rates as a stimulus for improved performance on the part of individual providers. ART regimens were reviewed for their appropriateness, and renewed education about antiretroviral drug combinations and resistance monitoring was introduced. The clinicians reviewed their own patient lists each day. Patients who were not virologically controlled were contacted by phone by the clinician or a nurse. Nurses eventually were assigned directly to the primary care team to facilitate communication with patients and ensure that specific issues raised during phone conversations were addressed during clinic visits. Adherence problems were particularly common, and were addressed through these multiple contacts. Reasons for adherence lapses were identified, which allowed for more effective targeting of service interventions with specific patients, including substance use and mental health service referrals, regimen switching, and targeted adherence interventions. The individual providers improved their patients' rates of virologic suppression from 45% to 62%. Review of suppression rates also showed that a subset of patients remained controlled and did not require quarterly monitoring. A decrease in visit frequency was possible for this group, reducing overutilization of services and unnecessary costs.

Using QI to Eliminate Disparities

The quality committee in another clinic wanted to determine whether the clinic's performance was consistent across all patient groups and arranged to have the clinic's patient data sorted by race, ethnicity, and primary language spoken. This revealed that data about race, ethnicity, and language spoken were not recorded in a high proportion of patient records. The team invited patients from their community advisory board to attend a staff meeting where a fishbone diagram was developed to identify potential causes of the poor collection rates of these patient data. Potential reasons were identified in all categories: equipment, patients, procedures, and staff (see Figure 3). A flow chart was developed to identify the sequential steps of data collection. A training program for intake staff was developed, resulting in an improvement in collection of these data to 85%.

Subsequent analysis showed that only 54% of African-American patients and 68% of Latino patients had suppressed HIV RNA whereas white patients had a suppression rate of 75%. A focus group with Spanish-speaking patients revealed that these patients were not getting enough information about medication and its side effects. The QI team decided to aim for an improvement in virologic suppression rates to 75%. A number of changes were implemented and tested throughout the clinic including the addition of peer adherence counseling, using teach-back by non-physician staff to facilitate adherence problem-solving, along with medication reconciliation. With these new interventions, virologic suppression rates improved to 71% for African-Americans, 80% for Latinos, and 81% for whites. With ongoing QI activities, suppression rates have subsequently increased for all groups and the gap has narrowed. Ongoing changes aim to narrow the gap even further.

Suggested Resources

- Langley GJ, Nolan KM, Norman CL, et al. *The Improvement Guide: A Practical Approach to Enhancing Organizational Performance.* San Francisco: Jossey-Bass; 1996.

- McGlynn EA, Asch SM. *Developing a clinical performance measure.* Am J Prev Med. 1998 Apr;14(3 Suppl):14-21.

- New York State Department of Health AIDS Institute. *HIVQUAL Group Learning Guide: Interactive Quality Improvement Exercises for HIV Healthcare Providers.* Available at www.hivguidelines.org/quality-of-care/quality-improvement-resources/. Accessed June 30, 2010.

- Scholtes PR, Joiner BL, Streibel BJ. *The Team Handbook (3rd Edition).* Madison, WI: Oriel; 2003.

Websites

HIV-Specific Examples

- hab.hrsa.gov/special/qualitycare.htm
- hab.hrsa.gov/tools/QM
- www.hivguidelines.org Quality of Care Section
- www.qualityhealthcare.org/QHC/Topics/HIVAIDS
- www.ihi.org/collaboratives/breakthroughseries/hiv
- www.qaproject.org

General QI Websites

- www.qualityhealthcare.org/qhc
- www.ihi.org (Institute for Healthcare Improvement)
- www.isqua.org.au (International Society for Quality in Health Care)
- www.asq.org (American Society for Quality)
- www.mytapestry.com (contains many links to other websites)
- www.ahrq.gov (Agency for Healthcare Research and Quality)
- www.jcaho.org (Joint Commission on Accreditation of Healthcare Organizations)
- www.nahq.org (National Association of Healthcare Quality)
- www.musc.edu/fm_ruralclerkship/ (Family Medicine/Rural Clerkship CQI)

References

- Institute for Healthcare Improvement. *HIV/AIDS Bureau Collaborations: Improving Care for People Living with HIV/AIDS Disease.* Boston: Institute for Healthcare Improvement; 2002.
- Institute of Medicine. *Medicare: A Strategy for Quality Assurance, Volume 1.* Washington: National Academies Press; 1990.
- Institute of Medicine. *Crossing the Quality Chasm.* Washington: National Academies Press; 2001.
- Institute of Medicine. *Measuring What Matters: Allocation, Planning, and Quality Assessment for the Ryan White CARE Act.* Washington: National Academies Press; 2004.
- New York State Department of Health AIDS Institute. *HIVQUAL Group Learning Guide: Interactive Quality Improvement Exercises for HIV Healthcare Providers.* May 2002, revised 2006. Available at www.hivguidelines.org/quality-of-care/quality-improvement-resources/. Accessed June 30, 2010.
- New York State Department of Health AIDS Institute. *HIVQUAL Workbook.* September 2006. Available at www.hivguidelines.org/quality-of-care/quality-improvement-resources/hivqual-workbook/. Accessed June 30, 2010.
- U.S. Department of Health and Human Services, Health Resources and Services Administration, HIV/AIDS Bureau. *Case Studies in QI in 9 Community Health Centers.* Rockville, MD: U.S. Department of Health and Human Services; year of publication unknown.

Health Resources and Services Administration HIV/AIDS Bureau Performance Measures

Overview*

Based on input from key stakeholders, the U.S. Health Resources and Services Administration (HRSA) HIV/AIDS Bureau (HAB) has created and released six sets of performance measures to be used to monitor quality of care. These measures can be used as defined or can be further modified by the grantee to meet that agency's individual needs. Grantees are encouraged to select measures that are most important to their agencies and the populations they serve. The measures can be used by the Ryan White HIV/AIDS Program, either at the provider or system level. A brief overview of the performance measures is provided below.

The **Core Clinical Performance Measures for Adults and Adolescents** are offered as a set of indicators for use in monitoring the quality of care provided. Grantees are encouraged to include the core clinical performance measures in their quality management plans. The clinical performance measures are categorized into three groups.

- **Group 1** measures provide an excellent start and can serve as a foundation on which to build, especially if a clinical program has no performance measures.

- **Group 2** measures are important measures for a robust clinical management program and should be seriously considered.

- **Group 3** measures represent areas of care that are considered "best practice," but may lack written clinical guidelines or rely on data that are difficult to collect.

The **Medical Case Management Performance Measures** target all clients, and focus on two key issues: care plans and medical visits. Medical case management programs are encouraged to utilize the core clinical performance measures as appropriate.

The **Oral Health Performance Measures** target all clients. The measures are intended for use by programs providing direct oral health services.

The **AIDS Drug Assistance Program (ADAP) Measures** are intended for use by the ADAP. Four measures are included and target all clients, regardless of age.

The **Systems-Level Performance Measures** address aspects of access and entry to care and may be utilized by any system or network.

The **Pediatric Performance Measures** (not reproduced here) address a range of clinical, social, and system issues for programs that serve pediatric clients.

* Taken from The HIV/AIDS Program: HAB Performance Measures, on the U.S. Department of Health and Human Services (HRSA) HIV/AIDS Program website (hab.hrsa.gov/special/habmeasures.htm).

Core Clinical Performance Measures for Adults and Adolescents

GROUP 1	
Antiretroviral Therapy for Pregnant Women#	Percentage of pregnant women with HIV infection who were prescribed antiretroviral therapy (ART)
CD4 T-Cell Count#	Percentage of clients with HIV infection who had two or more CD4 T-cell counts performed in the measurement year
Antiretroviral Therapy#	Percentage of clients with AIDS who were prescribed ART
Medical Visits#	Percentage of clients with HIV infection who had two or more medical visits in an HIV care setting in the measurement year
Pneumocystis jiroveci Pneumonia (PCP) Prophylaxis#	Percentage of clients with HIV infection and a CD4 count below 200 cells/μL who were prescribed PCP prophylaxis
GROUP 2	
Adherence: Assessment and Counseling#	Percentage of clients with HIV infection on ARVs who were assessed and counseled for adherence two or more times in the measurement year
Cervical Cancer Screening#	Percentage of women with HIV infection who had a Papanicolaou screening in the measurement year
Hepatitis B Vaccination#	Percentage of clients with HIV infection who completed the vaccination series for hepatitis B
Hepatitis C Screening#	Percentage of clients for whom hepatitis C screening was performed at least once since the diagnosis of HIV infection
HIV Risk Counseling	Percentage of clients with HIV infection who received HIV risk counselling within the measurement year
Lipid Screening	Percentage of clients with HIV infection on ART who had a fasting lipid panel in the measurement year
Oral Examination#	Percentage of clients with HIV infection who received an oral examination by a dentist at least once in the measurement year
Syphilis Screening#	Percentage of adult clients with HIV infection who had a test for syphilis performed in the measurement year
Tuberculosis Screening	Percentage of clients with HIV infection who received testing with results documented for latent tuberculosis infection since HIV diagnosis
GROUP 3	
Chlamydia Screening	Percentage of clients with HIV infection at risk of sexually transmitted infections who had a test for chlamydia in the measurement year
Gonorrhea Screening	Percentage of clients with HIV infection at risk of sexually transmitted infections who had a test for gonorrhea in the measurement year
Hepatitis B Screening#	Percentage of clients with HIV infection who have been screened for hepatitis B virus infection status
Hepatitis/HIV Alcohol Counseling	Percentage of clients with HIV and hepatitis B or hepatitis C infection who received alcohol counseling in the measurement year
Influenza Vaccination	Percentage of clients with HIV infection who have received influenza vaccination in the measurement period

GROUP 3 *continued*	
MAC Prophylaxis	Percentage of clients with HIV infection with CD4 count of <50 cells/μL who were prescribed *Mycobacterium avium* complex prophylaxis in the measurement year
Mental Health Screening[#]	Percentage of new clients with HIV infection who have had a mental health screening
Pneumococcal Vaccination	Percentage of clients with HIV infection who ever received pneumococcal vaccine
Substance Use Screening[#]	Percentage of new clients with HIV infection who have been screened for substance use (alcohol and drugs) in the measurement year
Tobacco Cessation Counseling	Percentage of clients with HIV infection who received tobacco cessation counseling in the measurement year
Toxoplasma Screening	Percentage of clients with HIV infection for whom *Toxoplasma* screening was performed at least once since the diagnosis of HIV infection

[#] Indicates that the HRSA Office of Performance Review (OPR) has selected a performance measure that is similar or the same for use during its site visits (performance reviews) to programs that receive funding from HRSA. The absence of a pound sign indicates that the OPR does not have a corresponding measure. Additional information about the OPR site visit process and list of performance measures can be located at hab.hrsa.gov/special/habmeasures.htm .

Medical Case Management Performance Measures

Care Plan	Percentage of HIV-infected medical case management clients who had a medical case management care plan developed and/or updated two or more times in the measurement year
Medical Visits	Percentage of HIV-infected medical case management clients who had two or more medical visits in an HIV care setting in the measurement year

Oral Health Services Performance Measures

Dental and Medical History	Percentage of HIV-infected oral health patients who had a dental and medical health history (initial or updated) at least once in the measurement year
Dental Treatment Plan	Percentage of HIV-infected oral health patients who had a dental treatment plan developed and/or updated at least once in the measurement year
Oral Health Education	Percentage of HIV-infected oral health patients who received oral health education at least once in the measurement year
Periodontal Screening or Examination	Percentage of HIV-infected oral health patients who had a periodontal screen or examination at least once in the measurement year
Phase 1 Treatment Plan Completion	Percentage of HIV-infected oral health patients with a Phase 1 treatment plan that is completed within 12 months

AIDS Drug Assistance Program Performance Measures

Application Determination	Percent of ADAP applications approved or denied for new ADAP enrollment within 14 days (2 weeks) of ADAP receiving a complete application in the measurement year
Eligibility Recertification	Percentage of ADAP enrollees who are reviewed for continued ADAP eligibility two or more times in the measurement year
Formulary	Percentage of new anti-retroviral classes that are included in the ADAP formulary within 90 days of the date of inclusion of new anti-retroviral classes in the DHHS *Guidelines for the Use of Antiretroviral Agents in HIV-1-infected Adults and Adolescents* in the measurement year
Inappropriate Antiretroviral Regimen Components Resolved by ADAP	Percent of identified inappropriate antiretroviral (ARV) regimen components prescriptions that are resolved by the ADAP program in the measurement year

Systems-Level Performance Measures

Waiting time for initial access to outpatient/ambulatory medical care	Percentage of Ryan White Program-funded outpatient/ambulatory care organizations in the system/network with a waiting time of 15 or fewer business days for a Ryan White Program-eligible patient to receive an appointment to enroll in outpatient/ambulatory medical care
HIV test results for PLWHA	Percentage of individuals who test positive for HIV who are given their HIV-antibody test results in the measurement year
Disease status at time of entry into care	Percentage of individuals with an AIDS diagnosis at time of initial outpatient/ambulatory medical care visit in the measurement year
Quality management program	Percentage of Ryan White Program-funded clinical organizations with an HIV-specific quality management program in the measurement year
System-level performance	Rate of achievement (percentage of patients) of the performance measurement of interest in the system/network in the measurement year

References

- U.S. Department of Health and Human Services HRSA HIV/AIDS Program. *The HIV/AIDS Program: HAB Performance Measures.* July 2008. Available at hab.hrsa.gov/special/habmeasures.htm. Accessed October 30, 2010.

HIV Care in Correctional Settings

Minda Dwyer, ANP-C; Douglas G. Fish, MD; Abigail V. Gallucci, BS; Sarah J. Walker, MS

Background

Caring for HIV-infected patients who are incarcerated is a complex and challenging task. For many of these patients, the prison health service provides their first opportunity for access to consistent health care. This chapter will discuss some of the issues relevant to the HIV-infected population in correctional settings.

Jail vs. Prison Settings

It is important to note the distinction between "jail" and "prison" custodial settings. These terms are often used interchangeably, but doing so can create confusion for health care providers, as the services that an inmate receives while incarcerated may differ greatly according to the type of facility (NYSDOH, 2008).

Jails are locally operated, or managed, institutions that detain individuals who typically are serving short sentences of 1 year or less. They also hold individuals who are awaiting arraignment, trial, or sentencing, or those who have violated terms of their parole (Harrison and Beck, 2006). Because inmates who are detained in jail settings have shorter confinement terms, providers often face time constraints in establishing longer-term treatment plans for chronic conditions such as HIV/AIDS, and for substance use and mental health problems. Opportunities for inmate education also may be more limited. In addition, because jail inmates often are released within days, weeks, or months after initial confinement, establishing continuity of health care may be challenging for providers and administrators (Okie, 2007).

Prisons, in contrast, are operated by state governments or the Federal Bureau of Prisons. Prisons generally detain people who have been convicted of state or federal felonies and are sentenced to terms of longer than 1 year (Harrison and Beck, 2006). The nature of a person's crime, namely a state

or federal offense, will dictate the type of prison in which he or she will be detained. The length of sentences for inmates in state or federal custody is longer than those for persons serving time in jail, and prison inmates typically have a firm release date in advance. As a result, HIV-infected inmates released from prison may be more likely to have treatment and discharge plans in place (NYSDOH, 2008).

Note that these characteristics may differ from prison to prison and jail to jail.

Epidemiology

Inmates continue to be disproportionately affected by the epidemic, with the estimated overall rate of AIDS among prison inmates at more than 2.5 times the rate in the United States general population. In 2006, there were 21,980 HIV-infected inmates in prisons, according to the latest report from the Bureau of Justice Statistics, and there are many more in jails. With the advent of effective combination antiretroviral therapy (ART), AIDS-related mortality as a percent of total deaths in state prisons decreased significantly between 1995 and 2006, from 34.2% to 4.6% (Maruschak, 2006).

Often, behaviors that lead to incarceration also put inmates at high risk of becoming infected with HIV, hepatitis C virus (HCV), and other infectious pathogens. These risk factors may include unsafe substance use behaviors, such as sharing syringes and other injection equipment, and high-risk sexual practices, such as having multiple sex partners or unprotected sex. Many inmates also may have conditions that increase the risk of HIV transmission or acquisition, such as untreated sexually transmitted infections (STIs).

The prevalences of chronic viral hepatitis and tuberculosis are much higher among incarcerated persons than among the general public. Depending on the prison system, 13% to 54% of inmates are infected with HCV (Cassidy, 2003). The incidence is 10 times higher among inmates than among non-inmates and is 33% higher among women than among men (Nerenberg et al., 2002). The Centers for Disease Control and Prevention (CDC) recommends that all incoming inmates be screened for HCV, and those who are infected should be evaluated for liver damage and the need for treatment (Cassidy, 2003). Chronic hepatitis B virus (HBV) infection and tuberculosis also are substantially more common among the incarcerated population than among the general public. The presence of any of these conditions should prompt HIV testing (Nicodemus and Paris, 2002).

Incarcerated Women

Women account for almost 7% of the prison population in the United States (West and Sobol, 2009). The HIV epidemic in the United States increasingly affects women of color, and this trend is reflected in HIV rates among the incarcerated. In terms of total numbers, there are more males than females with HIV/AIDS in state and federal prisons nationally (19,809 and 2,135, respectively). However, the percentage of female inmates with known HIV infection in these settings is higher than that for incarcerated males (2.4% and 1.6 percent, respectively) (Maruschak, 2006).

In many cases, incarcerated women are low-income and have limited education and sporadic employment histories. Compared with men, they are less likely to be incarcerated for a violent crime, and more likely to be

incarcerated for a drug or property offense. Women's property crimes often are the result of poverty and substance-use histories (National Institute of Corrections, 2003). Numerous studies have shown that the behaviors that lead to incarceration also put women at increased risk of HIV infection. Risk factors that are present in abundance among female inmates include the following:

- History of childhood sexual abuse and neglect
- History of sex work, with increased frequency of forced, unprotected sex
- High rates of STIs
- High rates of mental illness
- History of injection drug use (IDU) or sex partners with IDU history
- Poverty

Among all women entering a correctional facility, 10% are pregnant (De Groot and Cu Uvin, 2005). These women should be offered HIV testing, and HIV-infected pregnant women should be offered combination ART immediately to prevent perinatal HIV transmission. Many incarcerated women will receive their first gynecologic care in prison. Because the incidence of cervical cancer is higher among women with HIV, referrals for colposcopy should be made for any HIV-infected woman with an abnormal Papanicolaou test result.

Testing and Prevention

The correctional facility is an ideal location for identifying individuals already infected with HIV, HCV, or HBV, and for education interventions that are geared to prevent infection among those at highest risk of these acquiring diseases. For many adults, the prison or jail setting is a rare potential point of contact with the health care system, making it an important avenue for HIV testing and linkage to care.

Inmates commonly are hesitant to be tested for HIV because they fear a positive diagnosis and because of the potential stigma involved. They often lack accurate information about HIV, including awareness of behaviors that may have put them at risk and knowledge of means for protecting themselves from becoming infected. Health care providers in correctional settings are in a key position to evaluate inmates for HIV risk factors, to offer HIV testing, and to educate and counsel this high-risk group about HIV.

HIV testing policies in correctional facilities vary from state to state and among local, state, and federal penal institutions. Depending on the setting, policies may require testing of inmates upon entry, upon release, or both, but more than 50% of state prison systems do not require HIV testing at any point. Some prisons may do HIV testing based on clinical indication or risk exposure during incarceration, and this may be voluntary or mandatory. Most prison systems do provide HIV testing for inmates who request it. See Table 1 for an overview of the circumstances under which inmates in state prisons were tested for HIV in 2006 (Maruschak, 2006).

In high-risk settings such as correctional facilities, routine, voluntary HIV testing has been shown to be cost-effective and clinically advantageous (Paltiel et al., 2005). The CDC supports universal opt-out HIV screening in prisons and jails and has produced the *HIV Testing Implementation Guidance for Correctional Settings* (www.cdc. gov/correctionalhealth/default.htm). This document serves as a guide for individual institutions in determining and establishing the most appropriate testing strategy for their settings, presents the components of such a testing program, and explains obstacles that may be encountered in the implementation process. It also provides information regarding the following:

- Background statistics on HIV in correctional facilities
- Inmate privacy and confidentiality
- Opt-out HIV screening in correctional medical clinics
- HIV testing procedures
- HIV case reporting

Testing inmates for HIV prior to their release is a critical aspect not only of individuals' own health care needs but also of preventing transmission of HIV to others. Knowledge of their HIV status affects people's HIV risk behaviors: Studies have shown that, after learning they are infected with HIV, many persons take measures to reduce the risk of transmitting HIV to others.

Risk-Reduction Education

Given the high HIV seroprevalence among inmates, the reentry of inmates into the community presents a danger of spreading HIV and other infectious diseases, and it is a public health concern. Thus, inmates need adequate HIV prevention counseling before release, both to protect themselves and to decrease the likelihood of infecting others in their communities with HIV (Gaiter and Doll, 1996). The World Health Organization (WHO) has stated: "All inmates and correctional staff and officers should be provided with education concerning transmission, prevention, treatment, and management of HIV infection. For inmates, this information should be provided at intake and updated regularly thereafter."

Risk-reduction counseling addresses specific ways the inmate can reduce the risk of becoming infected with HIV. If an inmate is already HIV infected, the goal of counseling is to reduce the risk of infecting others or becoming infected with a drug-resistant strain of HIV.

Education should focus on the use of latex barriers with all sexual activity. Condoms and dental dams are not available in most jails and prisons; nonetheless, the inmate should receive education regarding their proper use. The state prisons systems that provide condoms to inmates are those of Vermont and Mississippi. The larger metropolitan jails in New York City, such as Riker's Island, as well as those in Los Angeles, San Francisco, Philadelphia, and Washington, also provide condoms. Within the systems that allow condoms, inmates' ability to obtain them may be restricted (e.g., limited to one per week or available only via medical prescriptions or dispensing machines) (Sylla, 2007); see chapter *Preventing HIV Transmission/Prevention with Positives*.

No correctional system in the United States provides clean injection needles as a part of a prevention program (Sylla, 2007). However, inmates with a history of IDU should be educated about the risks of sharing needles and injection equipment, specifically the high risk of transmitting or acquiring HIV, HCV, and HBV. Inmates also should be counseled about the risks of sharing needles and other "sharps," such as those used for tattooing or body piercing. Substance abuse treatment should be provided when appropriate. Recovery from addiction often is a chronic process and relapses are common. In addition to substance abuse treatment, risk-reduction strategies should include planning for support after release from the correctional setting. For example, prior to release, inmates should be provided with information about needle exchange or clean needle access programs in their communities. These programs have proved to be quite effective in decreasing the rate of parenteral HIV transmission (CDC, 1999).

Furthermore, overdose prevention should be discussed with inmates leaving correctional systems. Using heroin after a period of abstinence, such as during incarceration, hospitalization, or drug treatment, is a major risk factor for overdose. Former inmates are at highest risk of overdose within the first 2 weeks after release (NYSDOH, 2008). Overdose risk is heightened when someone has a significant medical condition, such as HIV infection (Catania, 2007). The literature documents an increased number of correctional systems that consider including naloxone (Narcan) prescriptions in prerelease planning for inmates with a history of opiate addiction (Wakeman et al., 2009). Naloxone is a prescription medicine that reverses an overdose by blocking heroin (or other opioids) in the brain for 30-90 minutes (NYSDOH, 2008).

Antiretroviral Therapy in Correctional Facilities

In correctional facilities, as in any setting, a consideration of HIV treatment must begin with educating the patient about the risks and benefits of treatment and the need to fully adhere to the entire regimen, and with an assessment of the patient's motivation to take ART (see chapter *Antiretroviral Therapy*).

Correctional facilities have two main methodologies for dispensing medications to those who are on ART. Each has advantages and disadvantages that can impact treatment adherence. These are directly observed therapy (DOT) and keep-on-person (KOP).

Directly Observed Therapy

DOT is the system in which the inmate goes to the medical unit or pharmacy for all medication doses ; dosing is observed by staff members. This system offers the advantage of more frequent interaction between the patient and the health care team, allowing for earlier identification of side effects and other issues. In general, patients have better medication adherence in this system, resulting in better control of HIV. For some inmates, however, the need for frequent visits to the medical unit or pharmacy may be a barrier to receiving proper treatment, particularly if they are housed at a distance from the medical unit. Another disadvantage of DOT is the potential loss of confidentiality, as many inmates feel that the frequency of dosing and the large number of pills they may take will reveal clues that they are HIV infected. In addition, this system puts inmates in a passive role in terms of medication treatment and does not foster self-sufficiency.

Keep-on-Person

KOP is the system that allows inmates to keep their medications in their cells and take them independently. Monthly supplies are obtained at the medical unit or pharmacy. This system offers greater privacy and confidentiality regarding HIV status. It also allows inmates to develop self-sufficiency in managing medications, which may facilitate improved adherence upon release. However, as the KOP system involves less interaction with medical staff, problems with adherence can be more difficult to identify (Ruby, 2000). Problems with refills also can occur. For example, inmates usually must initiate the process for obtaining a refill. They may be told that a refill request was made too early or too late, which can result in delays in dispensing medications, and ultimately, treatment interruptions. In addition, many facilities do not have on-site pharmacies, but rely on local pharmacies, or a regional or central pharmacy in the state; this may further delay refills (NYSDOH, 2008).

In a study comparing DOT in HIV-infected inmates with KOP in nonincarcerated HIV-infected patients receiving ART as part of a clinical trial, a higher percentage of DOT patients achieved undetectable viral loads compared with the KOP patients (85% vs. 50%) over a 48-week period (Fischl, 2001).

Adherence

Adherence is one of the most important factors in determining the success or failure of ART. For the HIV-infected inmate

starting ART, a number of issues can affect medication adherence. These include patient-related factors, factors related to systems of care (including the medication dispensing systems described above), and medication-related factors. The following are suggestions for supporting adherence to ART. (Also see chapter *Adherence*.)

Patient-Related Factors

- Correct misconceptions about HIV and ART that are common among inmates and could affect adherence adversely. Inmates should be educated about the disease process and the role of the medications, along with the risks and benefits of taking ART.

- Use teaching tools that are appropriate in terms of language and reading level. Illiteracy and low-level reading ability are common among inmates. Diagrams and videos may be more effective than reading-intensive material in some cases. Basic HIV education prior to initiation of ART should include the following topics:

  - How the medications work

  - Consequences of nonadherence

  - Names and dosages of all medications

  - Potential side effects and strategies for managing them

- Encourage participation in peer support groups. These can be effective ways to foster self-esteem, empower inmates to come to terms with a positive diagnosis, allay fears and correct misconceptions about HIV disease, and aid adherence. Upon release, telephone hotlines may be available to provide follow-up support and linkages to community services. To the extent possible, family and friends should be included in the education process.

- Provide alcohol and substance abuse treatment before, or while, initiating ART. Without appropriate treatment during incarceration, linkages to supports, and follow-up treatment upon discharge, inmates are more likely to resume high-risk behaviors that may interfere with adherence to ART. In 2004, nearly one third of inmates in state facilities and one fourth of inmates in the federal system committed their offenses under the influence of drugs (Mumola and Karberg, 2006).

- Use mental health consultation to identify inmates with psychiatric needs. Treatment for underlying mental health disorders should precede or take place concurrently with the initiation of ART to ensure successful adherence. Depression and other psychiatric illnesses are more prevalent among inmates than among the general population (James and Glaze, 2006).

Factors Related to Systems of Care

- Educate the facility's security staff about the importance of timely medication dosing, and communicate with other facilities in advance of a transfer; this can eliminate or reduce the frequency of missed doses.

- Schedule frequent follow-up medical visits in the early weeks after ART is initiated; these can make the difference in whether or not patients "stay the course."

- Consult with an HIV specialist, if possible. If a facility's medical provider lacks experience in treating patients with HIV, the results may be undertreatment of side effects or errors in prescribing medications. Because caring for HIV-infected patients is complicated, HIV specialists can provide assurance that patients are receiving proper care. Of particular concern are patients whose current ART regimens are failing, those who are declining clinically, and those who are coinfected with other diseases such as tuberculosis, HCV, and HBV.

Medication-Related Factors

- Aggressively monitor and treat side effects. The most common barrier to proper adherence to ART is side effects from the medications. Inmates should be educated in advance about potential adverse events and urged to observe and report them. In the first weeks after starting a new ART regimen, patients should be assessed frequently for side effects. For treating gastrointestinal toxicities, antiemetics and antidiarrheals should be available on an as-needed basis. As with all patients on ART, inmates should have appropriate laboratory monitoring.

- Be aware of food requirements. Various food requirements must be considered carefully when administering ART. That can be especially challenging in the correctional environment, particularly in facilities that do not allow inmates to self-administer medications. Make arrangements with prison authorities to provide food when inmates are taking medications that require administration with food.

- Avoid complex regimens and regimens with large pill burdens, if possible. Simple regimens with fewer pills appear to help improve adherence.

- Avoid drug-drug interactions. Some antiretroviral medications have clinically significant interactions with other drugs (e.g., methadone, oral contraceptives, cardiac medications, antacids). These interactions may cause failure of either the antiretroviral drug or the other medication, or they may cause additional toxicity. Consult an HIV specialist or pharmacist for information on drug interactions.

- Question patients about medication adherence at each appointment.

- ART regimens need to fit into each patient's schedule and lifestyle. This becomes a bigger issue when an inmate is close to release. Education about HIV management, including ART adherence, should begin well before the inmate is discharged back to the community.

Transition to Community Care

It is estimated that 630,000 individuals are released from jails and prisons in the United States each year (Bonczar, 2003; Travis, 2005), and many of these individuals are HIV infected. Many will have difficulty managing even the most basic elements for successful reintegration into their communities. Inmates living with HIV face many challenges when reentering the community, such as finding stable housing, employment, adequate medication supply, follow-up medical care, and psychiatric and substance use treatment services (Hammett et al., 1997).

Ideally, the discharge process at the correctional facility will maximize the likelihood that the releasee will have continuous medical care. At the time of discharge from the correctional facility, all HIV-infected inmates should have a discharge plan that addresses the following:

- Housing
- Health insurance
- 30-day supply of HIV medications
- Follow-up appointments for medical care and, if necessary, psychiatric and substance abuse care

As discussed, inmates in prisons generally serve longer sentences than do those incarcerated in jails, and they have a release date that is known in advance. Thus, HIV-infected inmates in prisons may be more likely than HIV-infected inmates in jails to have treatment and discharge plans in place before their release. However, because the extent of discharge planning resources varies among correctional systems of care, it is important for care providers to discuss the scope of services

their clients received while incarcerated to learn of any service gaps upon reentry to the community (NYSDOH, 2008).

The need to find housing often is the greatest challenge for an HIV-infected inmate leaving a correctional facility. In many correctional systems, inmates must document a physical address at which they intend to reside in order to be released. However, problems with housing availability, stability, and location can create significant stressors for an HIV-infected releasee and can compromise the likelihood that he or she will access HIV health care and adhere to an HIV medication regimen (NYSDOH, 2008).

Medication Continuity Issues

HIV-infected individuals leaving correctional settings have a variety of experiences with ARV medication continuity. A short confinement period, for example, can prevent the development of a solid transitional plan. Jail inmates may be released without their medications and have no choice but to call or walk into community health centers or clinics for their medications and ongoing care. Being released from jail after business hours, such as on a Friday night, can result in treatment interruptions over the weekend (NYSDOH, 2008). Depending on the state system, HIV-infected inmates leaving prison are more likely than jail releasees to have a medication supply in hand when they reenter the community. For example, in the New York State Department of Correctional Services, inmates will leave prison with a 30-day supply of HIV medications as well as a prescription for another 30-day supply (NYSDOH, 2008).

For some individuals, interruptions in treatment occur during their time in jail or prison. For example, many inmates choose not to disclose their HIV infection while they are incarcerated. Particularly if the sentence is short, an inmate may feel it better not to mention HIV status and instead plan to resume taking medications upon release. Such treatment interruptions can result in adverse health outcomes (NYSDOH, 2008).

It is important that clinic staff and community-based organizations develop the capacity to work with clients in real time as they present for care in order to help them maintain continuity with their medications.

Strategies for Supporting Inmates upon Release

- A clear way to support clients is to intervene immediately and directly upon their release, such as by meeting them as they step off a bus or exit a facility.

- Engage clients by:

  - Hearing their stories; listening to concerns, wishes, history, perceptions, feelings, and so forth

  - Asking open-end questions, affirming strengths, listening reflectively, and summarizing discussions and plans

  - Understanding their backgrounds, goals, and motivations (understand "where they are coming from")

  - Avoiding getting caught up in issues about the crimes they committed

  - Identifying perceived needs by asking how services can be beneficial to them

  - Acting honestly by providing a full disclosure of one's role as a provider (e.g., what you can or cannot do)

- Provide material assistance by giving clients something tangible such as a meal ticket, condoms, bleach kit, or hygiene kit.

- Provide information and referrals to short-term and survival services for clients to help improve their immediate situation.

- If possible, accompany clients to support them in obtaining short-term and survival services such as health care, food, shelter, and clothing.

- Respond to emergency situations.

- Support clients in meeting parole or probation requirements to avoid reincarceration. Based on their individual histories, anticipate circumstances that may result in them breaking parole. For example, if a client confides that he or she has anxiety regarding meeting the parole officer, initiate and practice role plays to better prepare the client for this encounter.

- Be culturally competent.

- Link to services (e.g., medical care, mental health, substance use, domestic violence).

- Diversify clinic staffing, and use a multidisciplinary approach, including peer support.

- Think outside the box! (NYSDOH, 2008)

A number of HIV education resources for inmates and correctional health care providers are cited on the Albany Medical College website at www.amc.edu/patient/hiv/index.htm (go to the section on correctional education).

Table 1. HIV Testing in Prisons: Circumstances Under Which Prison Inmates Were Tested for HIV (by Jurisdiction)

Jurisdiction	All Inmates			Random	High-risk	Inmate request	Court order	Clinical indication	Involvement in incident	Other
	Entering	In Custody	Upon Release							
Federal					X	X	X	X	X	
Northeast										
Connecticut					X	X	X	X	X	
Maine						X	X	X		
Massachusetts						X			X	
New Hampshire	X						X	X		
New Jersey						X	X	X	X	
New York				X	X	X	X	X	X	
Pennsylvania						X	X	X	X	
Rhode Island	X					X	X	X	X	
Vermont						X		X	X	
Midwest										
Illinois					X	X	X	X	X	X
Indiana	X				X	X	X	X	X	
Iowa	X	X				X	X	X	X	
Kansas					X	X	X	X	X	X
Michigan	X					X	X		X	
Minnesota	X					X	X	X	X	
Missouri	X	X	X		X		X	X	X	
Nebraska	X					X	X	X	X	
North Dakota	X	X				X	X	X	X	
Ohio	X					X	X	X	X	
South Dakota						X	X	X	X	X
Wisconsin					X	X	X	X	X	

Section 1: The HIV Clinic: Providing Quality Care

Jurisdiction	All Inmates			Random	High-risk	Inmate request	Court order	Clinical indication	Involvement in incident	Other
	Entering	In Custody	Upon Release							
South										
Alabama	X		X	X		X	X	X	X	X
Arkansas	X		X	X	X	X	X	X	X	X
Delaware						X	X	X	X	
Florida			X			X	X	X	X	
Georgia	X					X	X		X	
Kentucky					X			X	X	
Louisiana						X	X	X	X	
Maryland					X	X	X	X	X	X
Mississippi	X				X	X	X	X	X	
North Carolina						X	X	X		X
Oklahoma	X					X	X	X	X	X
South Carolina	X					X	X	X	X	X
Tennessee					X	X	X	X	X	
Texas	X		X		X	X	X	X	X	
Virginia						X	X	X	X	X
West Virginia						X				
West										
Alaska					X	X		X	X	
Arizona					X	X	X	X		
California						X	X	X	X	
Colorado	X					X	X	X	X	
Hawaii						X		X	X	
Idaho	X	X			X	X	X	X	X	
Montana						X	X	X	X	
Nevada	X	X	X			X	X	X	X	
New Mexico						X		X		
Oregon						X	X			
Utah	X				X			X	X	
Washington	X				X	X	X	X	X	
Wyoming	X					X		X		

Adapted from Maruschak L. *HIV in Prisons, 2006. Bureau of Justice Statistics Bulletin*. Washington: U.S. Department of Justice, Office of Justice Programs; revised April 2008. Publication NCJ 222179. Available at bjs.ojp.usdoj.gov/content/pub/pdf/hivp08.pdf. Accessed June 30, 2010.

References

- Bartlett J, Rappaport E, Ruby W, et al. *HIV in Corrections, Correctional Medical Institute.* Available at www.cm-institute.org/hivin.htm. Accessed June 30, 2010.

- Bloom B, Owen B, Covington S. *Gender Responsive Strategies: Research, Practice, and Guiding Principles for Women Offenders.* Washington: National Institute of Corrections; 2003. Available at www.nicic.org/Library/018017. Accessed June 30, 2010.

- Bonczar TP. *Prevalence of Imprisonment in the U.S. Population, 1974-2001.* Bureau of Justice Statistics special report. Washington: U.S. Department of Justice, Office of Justice Programs; 2003.

- Cassidy W. *Hepatitis C Infection in Prisons.* Available at www.hcvadvocate.org/hcsp/articles/cassidy-1.html. Accessed June 30, 2010.

- Catania H. *Drug Dependence Treatment in Prison and upon Release.* Presented at the 18th International Conference to Reduce Drug-Related Harm (Satellite on HIV/AIDS in Prison Settings); May 13, 2007; Warsaw.

- Centers for Disease Control and Prevention. *Drug Use, HIV, and the Criminal Justice System.* Available at www.cdc.gov/idu/facts/druguse.htm. Accessed June 30, 2010.

- Centers for Disease Control and Prevention. *HIV Testing Implementation Guidance for Correctional Settings.* January 2009. Available at www.cdc.gov/correctionalhealth/rec-guide.html. Accessed June 30, 2010.

- De Groot A, Cu Uvin S. *HIV Infection among Women in Prison: Considerations for Care. Infectious Diseases in Corrections Report.* Vol. 8, Issues 5 & 6; 2005. Available at www.idcronline.org/archives/mayjune05/article.html. Accessed June 30, 2010.

- Fischl M, Castro J, Monroid R, et al. *Impact of directly observed therapy on long-term outcomes in HIV clinical trials.* In: Program and abstracts of the 8th Conference on Retroviruses and Opportunistic Infections; February 4-8, 2001; Chicago, IL. Abstract 528.

- Gaiter J, Doll LS. *Improving HIV/AIDS prevention in prisons is good public health policy.* Am J Public Health. 1996 Sep;86(9):1201-3.

- Hammett TM, Harmon MP, Rhodes W. *The burden of infectious disease among inmates of and releasees from US correctional facilities, 1997.* Am J Public Health. 2002;92:1789-1794.

- Harrison P, Beck A. *Prison and Jail Inmates at Midyear 2005.* Bureau of Justice Statistics Bulletin. Washington: U.S. Department of Justice, Office of Justice Programs; May 2006. Publication NCJ213133. Available at www.ojp.usdoj.gov/bjs/pub/pdf/pjim05.pdf. Accessed June 30, 2010.

- James D, Glaze L. *Mental Health Problems of Prison and Jail Inmates.* Bureau of Justice Statistics Bulletin. Washington: U.S. Department of Justice, Office of Justice Programs; September 2006. Publication NCJ 213600. Available at www.ojp.usdoj.gov/bjs/pub/pdf/mhppji.pdf. Accessed June 30, 2010.

- Maruschak L. *HIV in Prisons, 2006.* Bureau of Justice Statistics Bulletin. Washington: U.S. Department of Justice, Office of Justice Programs; revised April 2008. Publication NCJ 222179. Available at www.ojp.usdoj.gov/bjs/pub/html/hivp/2006/hivp06.htm. Accessed June 30, 2010.

- Mumola J, Karberg J. *Drug Use and Dependence, State and Federal Prisoners. Bureau of Justice Statistics Bulletin.* Washington: U.S. Department of Justice, Office of Justice Programs; October 2006. Publication NCJ 213530. Available at www.ojp.usdoj.gov/bjs/pub/pdf/dudsfp04.pdf. Accessed June 30, 2010.

- Nerenberg R, Wong M, DeGroot A. *HCV in corrections: Front line or backwater?* HEPP News. Vol 5 (4); 2002. Available at www.idcronline.org/archives/april02/. Accessed June 30, 2010.

- New York State Department of Health AIDS Institute HIV Education and Training Programs, Office of the Medical Director and Bureau of Community Based Services, Division of HIV Prevention. *Improving Health Outcomes for HIV-Positive Individuals Transitioning from Correctional Settings to the Community (Trainer Manual).* March 2008.

- Nicodemus M, Paris P. *Bridging the Communicable Disease Gap: Identifying, Treating and Counseling High Risk Inmates.* HIV Education Prison Project; August/September 2001.

- Okie S. *Sex, drugs, prisons and HIV.* N Engl J Med. 2007 Jan 11;356(2):105-8.

- Paltiel AD, Weinstein MC, Kimmel AD, et al. *Expanded screening for HIV in the United States — an analysis of cost-effectiveness.* N Engl J Med. 2005 Feb 10;352(6):586-95.

- Ruby W, Tripoli L, Bartlett J, et al. *HIV in Corrections.* In: *Medical Management of HIV Infection.* Philadelphia: Lippincott, Williams & Wilkins; 2000.

- Sylla, M. *Prevention in Practice: Prisoner Access to Condoms — The California Experience.* Infectious Disease in Corrections Report (IDCR); 2007 Oct/Nov 9;20:2-3.

- Travis J. *But They All Come Back: Facing the Challenges of Prisoner Reentry.* Washington: Urban Institute Press, 2005: 21-38.

- Wakeman SE, Bowman SE, McKenzie, M, et al. *Preventing death among the recently incarcerated: an argument for naloxone prescription before release.* J Addict Dis. 2009;28(2):124-9.

- West H, Sabol W. Prison *Inmates at Midyear 2008—Statistical Tables.* Bureau of Justice Statistics Bulletin. Washington: U.S. Department of Justice, Office of Justice Programs; March 2009. Publication NCJ 225619. Available at www.ojp.usdoj.gov/bjs/pub/pdf/pim08st.pdf. Accessed June 30, 2010.

Patient Education

Background

Informed and empowered patients are better able to achieve healthy outcomes as a result of improved communication and development of trust with their care providers. HIV patient education provides patients with knowledge about HIV infection, including prevention, treatment, and other aspects of care, along with tools that enable them to participate more actively in decisions regarding their medical care. Given the complexity and the rapid evolution of HIV information, education and skills-building should be an ongoing activity and a key aspect of the clinical care of HIV patients. This chapter provides a brief review of the areas that should be addressed in patient education and discusses some strategies for integrating patient education into HIV care; additional information on patient education is found in many other chapters, particularly *Supporting Patients in Care, Preventing HIV Transmission/Prevention with Positives, Smoking Cessation,* and *Adherence,* as well as in the "Patient Education" sections found at the end of most of the clinical chapters.

S: Subjective

A newly diagnosed patient presents to clinic after being referred from a testing center in the community. The patient received the positive HIV test results more than a year ago, but has not been ready to seek care until now. The patient feared hearing that he/she was "going to die." Now, he/she is ready to consider facing this "terminal" illness. The patient received some information about HIV infection at the testing center, but that was months ago.

O: Objective

See chapters *Initial History, Initial Physical Examination,* and *Initial and Interim Laboratory and Other Tests* for information on the initial clinic evaluation.

A/P: Assessment and Plan

The patient will need extensive information and education about HIV infection in general, his/her individual health status and prognosis, and the support and care systems that are available. Below are some suggestions about specific areas to review with a new patient.

Topics for Patient Education

Patient education should cover the following topics:

- What is HIV?
- How is HIV transmitted?
- Progression of HIV; prognosis
- Interpretation of laboratory results
- Treatment information
  - Indications for treatment, goals of treatment
  - General information regarding the benefits of treatment
  - General information regarding potential side effects and risks of treatment
  - Access to medication
  - Insurance information
- Treatment options
- Prevention for positives
- Support services and support groups available to the patient

Patient Educators

In most clinics, a number of different personnel may take on the responsibilities of providing health education to patients. They may include primary care providers, nurses, social workers, case managers, and pharmacists. Some clinics have designated health educators whose role is to provide this type of support for patients. Even when a formal health educator is available, a collaborative, multidisciplinary approach to patient education serves both patients and providers optimally. However, it is important to ensure that patient education messages are coordinated and that patients are receiving consistent information.

Patient education must be provided in a language and at a literacy level appropriate for the patient. Patient education should be conducted in the patient's primary language, if possible; otherwise, skilled medical interpreters should be involved.

Conducting Patient Education

Rarely are patients able to absorb all of the necessary information in a single session. Attention and comprehension levels are optimal during the first 15-20 minutes of a visit, after which an individual's ability to absorb and retain information declines. Therefore, clinics should consider strategies to integrate brief patient education messages throughout the course of patient care and to engage patients in this process. Support groups, case managers, and peer educators can be invaluable in this process of engagement.

It is important to keep the medical information specific to the patient. Although there are some areas of education that should be considered for all patients (see above), patients should not be required to have a high level of understanding in each area. Patients should be given the opportunity to learn as much about an area as they would like, and should be encouraged to gain a working knowledge of the information that is necessary to keep them healthy and safe. Patients vary widely in terms of their interest level in mastering the details of their illness. For example, in the area of "What is HIV?" there may be some patients who want to know details about the basic science and immunologic impact of HIV. With this information, these patients might then want to take the lead in making treatment and care decisions for themselves, in consultation with their care providers. Other patients, however, would feel overwhelmed by this volume of information and involvement and may be best engaged in participating in their care by knowing how HIV is transmitted, how to keep themselves healthy, and how to access more information if they want it. Some patients would prefer for their care providers to "just tell them what to do" rather than take the lead in making their own treatment decisions.

There are a number of websites that provide HIV information for patients (see chapter *Web-Based Resources*). Many patients may prefer this form of self-education. Encourage patients to convey any information they discover to their care providers for further discussion. Reminding patients that they can be teachers as well as students can be a useful strategy for engaging patients in this process. In addition, patients may learn of novel tools and information sources that could be useful to others.

The following are some useful suggestions that providers can convey to their patients:

- Define your goals for each visit; please let your provider know your concerns and what you hope to learn in the course of the visit.

- Write down questions and concerns as they arise, and take that list with you to your appointments.

- Meet all the members of your care team and learn their areas of expertise and what they might be able to offer you.

- Ask about support groups and other peer groups that might be able to provide support/education.

- Review brochures and websites that provide additional information.

- Ask supportive friends or family members to accompany you to clinic visits. They may be able to obtain information that is helpful for their role in supporting your health or reminding you of information discussed at visits.

Initial History

Background

Conducting a thorough initial history and physical examination is important even if previous medical records are available. This is the best opportunity to get a complete picture of the patient's HIV disease status, comorbid conditions, and his or her physical and emotional condition, as well as to establish the basis for an ongoing relationship with the patient. Many of the conditions that put immunocompromised patients at risk of disease can be detected early, by means of a thorough assessment.

The information gathered through the initial history and physical examination will provide a comprehensive standardized database for the assessment and treatment of HIV-related problems, including acute intervention and ongoing supportive care.

This chapter includes essential topics to cover during the clinic intake and examples of questions that can be used to elicit important information (the questions should be tailored to the individual patient). This can be completed during the initial visit or divided over the course of two or three early visits. For essential aspects of the physical examination to cover in an initial clinic intake visit, see chapter *Initial Physical Examination*.

HRSA HAB Core Clinical Performance Measures

Percentage of clients with HIV infection who had **two or more medical visits in an HIV care setting** in the measurement year

(Group 1 measure)

Percentage of clients with HIV infection who received **HIV risk counseling** within the measurement year

(Group 2 measure)

Percentage of new clients with HIV infection who have been **screened for substance use** (alcohol and drugs) in the measurement year

(Group 3 measure)

Percentage of new clients with HIV infection who have had a **mental health screening**

(Group 3 measure)

S: Subjective

Initial History	
Category / Topics to Cover	Sample Questions
History of Present Illness	
HIV Testing	• What was the date of your first positive HIV test? • Did you have a previous HIV test? If so, when was the last negative result?
Treatment Status	• Where do you usually receive your health care? • Have you ever received care for HIV? • What was the date of your last HIV care visit? • What is your current CD4 (T-cell) count? • Do you know what your first CD4 count was? • What was your lowest CD4 count? • What was your highest CD4 count? • Do you know what your first viral load count was? • What is your current viral load count? • Have you participated in any research protocols? What studies, and when? • Would you be interested in participating in research studies (if available)?

HIV-Related Illnesses	• What opportunistic infection(s) have you had, if any? (PCP, MAC, cryptococcal meningitis, TB, etc.) • What year(s) were you diagnosed with these infections? • Have you had cancer(s)? • What other HIV-related illnesses have you had? Have you had zoster (shingles), oral thrush, pneumonia?
Active TB and TB Testing History	• Have you ever had tuberculosis (TB)? • When was your last TB test? • Was it a TB skin test (TST) or interferon-gamma release assay (IGRA)? • What were the results of this test? • Have you ever had a positive TB result? • What year and what health care setting? • What medications did you take and for how long?
Antiretroviral Therapy (ART) History	• Are you taking HIV medications now? • If so, please name them or describe them, and tell me how many times a day you take them. • How many doses have you missed in the past 3 days? The past week? The past month? • What side effects, if any, do you have now? In the past? • What HIV medicines have you taken in the past (names or descriptions)? • When did you start and stop taking them (dates)? • Do you know why you stopped taking these medications? • Do you know what your HIV viral load or your CD4 counts were while you were taking your medications? • Have you ever had a resistance test? • Did you have any side effects to past ARVs?
Past Medical and Surgical History	
Chronic Diseases	Do you have any chronic conditions, such as the following? • Diabetes • High blood pressure • Heart disease • Cholesterol problems • Asthma or emphysema • Sickle cell disease • Ulcers, acid reflux, or irritable bowel syndrome • Thyroid disorders • Kidney or liver problems • Mental health disorders If so, do you receive medical care for these conditions?
Previous Illnesses	• Have you had any hospitalizations? Where, when, and for what reason? • Have you had any surgeries? When and where? • Have you had any major illnesses, including mental health conditions?
Hepatitis	• Have you ever had hepatitis? What type (A, B, C)? • Do you have chronic hepatitis? • Do you know whether you are immune to hepatitis A or hepatitis B? Have you been vaccinated?

Gynecologic and Women's Health	• When was your last cervical Papanicolaou (Pap) test? • What were the results? • Have you ever had an abnormal Pap test? • When was your last menstrual period? • What is the usual length of your cycle? Is it regular or irregular? • Have you noticed changes in your menstrual cycle? • When was your most recent breast examination? • Have you had a mammogram? When? • Have you ever had an abnormal breast examination or mammogram? • Do you get yeast infections? How often? • Do you get urinary infections? • Have you ever had kidney stones?
Obstetric	• How many pregnancies have you had? • How many live births? Ages of children now? • How many miscarriages or therapeutic abortions? • Were you tested for HIV during any pregnancy? What year? • Did you deliver an infant while you were HIV infected? • Was HIV medication given during pregnancy and delivery? • Do you have children? What is their HIV status? • Do you intend to become pregnant?
Anorectal History	• Have you ever had an anal Pap test? • What were the results? • Have you had anal warts? Other abnormalities?
Urologic History	Have you ever had: • Kidney stones • Urinary tract Infections • Prostate infection or enlargement • Have you had a prostate-specific antigen (PSA) test? (What were the results?)
Sexually Transmitted Infections	Have you ever had any of the following infections? • Syphilis • Chlamydia • Vaginitis • Genital warts (HPV) • Genital herpes • Proctitis • Nongonococcal urethritis (NGU) • Pelvic inflammatory disease (PID) • Gonorrhea
Dental/Oral Care	• When was your last oral health examination? • Do you have all your natural teeth? • Do you have partials or dentures?
Eye Care	• When was your last vision examination? • When was your last dilated retinal examination? • Do you wear glasses or corrective lenses?
Medications	• What (non-ARV) medications do you take? • What herbs, vitamins, nutritional supplements, or over-the-counter (OTC) medications, do you take?

Allergies; Medication Intolerance	• Have you had an allergic reaction to any medications? What type of reaction, how severe? • Have you had allergic reactions to other types of exposures? • Have you had severe side effects from any medications?
Immunizations	When was your last vaccination for the following: • Streptococcal pneumonia (Pneumovax) • Tetanus/Pertussis (Tdap) • Influenza • H1N1 • Hepatitis A • Hepatitis B Did you have chickenpox as a child, or were you vaccinated against chickenpox? What about measles, mumps, and rubella?
Health-Related Behaviors	**Tobacco use:** • Do you smoke? How many cigarettes per day? How long have you smoked? How much have you have smoked in the past? • Besides tobacco, what do you smoke? • Do you chew tobacco? **Alcohol use:** • How often do you have a drink containing alcohol? How many drinks do you have on a typical day? • Have you ever had a problem fulfilling work, social, or school obligations because of alcohol use? **Drug use:** • Do you use any street drugs we haven't covered in earlier questions, or drugs not prescribed to you? • If so, what drugs and how do you use them (inject, smoke, inhale, etc.)? • How often do you use substances? • Have you shared your drug-use equipment with another person? • What pain relievers do you use on a regular basis? • Are you interested in treatment for alcohol or drug use? **Exercise:** • What kind of exercise do you participate in? How frequently? **Diet:** • What do you eat during a typical day? • Do you consume raw (unpasteurized) milk, raw eggs, raw or rare meat, deli meats, soft cheeses, or raw fish? • How much water do you drink during a typical day? • What is your source of water? • How much caffeine do you drink during a typical day?
Sensitive Sexual and Gender History Questions	
Gender Identity	• Do you consider yourself male or female? • Have you had or considered treatment for sex change? • Are you presently taking hormone therapy? • Have you had hormone therapy in the past? • Have you had any gender confirmation (sex reassignment) surgery?

General Sexual	• Do you have sex with men, women, or both? • In the past, have you had sex with men, women, or both?
Sexual Practices	• Do you have anal sex? Vaginal? Oral? • How do you protect yourself from sexually transmitted infections, or HIV reinfection? • **For men who have sex with men:** Are you the receptive or insertive partner, or both? • How often do you use alcohol or drugs before or during sex?
HIV Prevention	• Do you know the HIV status of your partner(s)? • How do you protect your partners from HIV? • In what situations do you or your partner use condoms or some other barrier? • Are there situations in which you do not use barrier protection?
Sex Trading	• Have you ever exchanged sex for food, shelter, drugs, or money?
Contraception	• What birth control measures do you use, if any? • How often do you use condoms or other latex barriers? • Do you have plans for you or your partner to become pregnant?
Family History	
	Do you have a family history of: • Heart disease? Heart attacks or strokes? • Cholesterol problems? Diabetes? • Cancer? • Mental health conditions (e.g., depression, bipolar disorder, anxiety, phobias)? • Addictions? Which family member(s) and what is their health status currently?
Social History	
Relationship Situation	• What is your relationship status (single, married, partnered, divorced, widowed)? Do you have children?
Living Situation	• Do you live alone or with others? With whom?
Support System	• Who knows about your HIV status? • Which individual has been the most supportive since your HIV diagnosis? • Who has been the least supportive? • Have you used any community services such as support groups?
Employment	• Are you currently employed? • Where do you work? • Describe your job task(s). • What setting do you work in on a daily basis? • Does your employer provide health insurance? • Does your employer know of your HIV status? • If on disability: How long have you been on disability? • What medical condition has made you disabled?
Incarceration History	• Have you ever been incarcerated? When was the last time?

Pets	• What kind of pets do you have, and who cleans up after them?
Travel	• Where have you traveled outside the United States? • When did travel take place?
Mental Health	
Coping	• How do you handle your problems/stresses? • What do you do to relax?
History	• Have ever been diagnosed with depression, anxiety, panic, bipolar disorder, schizophrenia, etc.? • Have you taken or are you taking any medications for these conditions? • Are you seeing a therapist or mental health professional? • Have you had any previous counseling or mental health problems? • Have you ever been hospitalized for a psychiatric condition? • Have you ever thought about hurting yourself? (If yes, probe for previous suicide attempts: Are you feeling that way now?) (See chapter *Suicide Risk* and prepare for immediate referral if necessary.)
Violence	• Have you ever been sexually abused, assaulted, or raped? • Has an intimate partner ever forced you to do something you did not want to do? • Has a partner, family member, or other person ever physically hurt you? • Have you lived in any situation with physical violence or intimidation? • When has this occurred? • Are you afraid for your safety now? • (If yes) Did you seek legal help, therapy, or other type of assistance?
Childhood Trauma	• Was there any alcoholism or drug abuse in your household when you were a child? • Did you experience or observe violence; physical, sexual, or emotional abuse; or neglect?

Review of Systems

For each positive answer, ask about location, characteristics, duration of symptoms, exacerbating and alleviating factors, previous diagnostic workup, and treatments tried.	
General	• Do you ever wake up feeling tired?
Fever	• Do you have fevers? How high, and for how long? How often?
Night Sweats	• Do you ever sweat so much at night that it soaks your sheets and nightclothes?
Anorexia	• How is your appetite?
Weight	• What was your weight 1 year ago? • What is a normal weight for you? • Have you lost or gained weight unintentionally?
Body Changes	• Have you noticed any changes in the shape of your body (describe)? For example, has there been an increase in your waist, collar, or breast size or a decrease in your arm, leg, or buttocks size? • Have you noticed increased visibility of veins in your arms and legs? • Have you noticed thinning of your face, especially around the cheeks?
Head, Ears, Eyes, Nose, and Throat	
Vision	• Have you noticed any changes in your vision, especially blurred vision or vision loss, double vision, new "floaters" or flashes of light? • Have you noticed this problem in one or both eyes? • When did you first notice these changes?
Mouth, Ears, Nose, Throat	• Have you noticed any white spots in your mouth or a white coating on your tongue (thrush, oral hairy leukoplakia)? • Do you ever get sores in your mouth or the back of your throat? Gum problems? • Any nosebleeds? • Do you ever experience hearing loss, ringing in your ears, or ear pain?
Cardiovascular	
Cardiac	• Any chest pain or pressure? Palpitations? • Any shortness of breath during activities or while you are lying down? • How far can you walk or run before you get short of breath? • Any swelling in your feet or legs?
Pulmonary	
Cough	• Do you have a cough? • Can you describe it? Dry or productive, amount, color, odor, presence of blood in sputum? When is it the worst?
Dyspnea	• Do you ever feel short of breath? • Does that happen when you are sitting still, lying down, or moving around? • How severe is your shortness of breath? • What does it prevent you from doing? • Do you ever wheeze?

Gastrointestinal	
Dysphagia	• Do you have any problems with food sticking in your throat or being difficult to swallow? • Do you gag or get nauseated when trying to eat? • Do you notice it is easier to swallow liquids or solids? • Do you have difficulty swallowing pills?
Odynophagia	• Do you have pain in your throat, esophagus, or behind your breastbone when you swallow?
Dyspepsia/Reflux	• Do you ever have heartburn (or a burning feeling rising from the stomach to behind the breastbone)? • When does it happen — after eating, lying down, on an empty stomach? • Do you get the taste of stomach acid in your mouth?
Nausea/Vomiting	• Do you have nausea or vomiting? • When? Are there specific things that cause this?
Diarrhea	• Do you have diarrhea, or more than 3-5 unformed stools a day? • Stool characteristics: bloody, pus, mucus? • Pain or cramping with diarrhea? Tenesmus?
Bowel Habits	• How frequently do you have bowel movements? • Do you have problems with constipation, blood in the stools, or other? • Do you have problems with flatulence or belching after eating?
Genitourinary	
Genital	• Do you have any lesions or sores on your genital area now, or have you in the past? • Have you ever had genital herpes? If yes, how often do you have outbreaks? • When was the most recent outbreak?
Women	• Have you had any lower abdominal pain? • Have you noticed a vaginal discharge or odor? • Do you have any burning or pain on urination? • Frequent urination? • Do you lose control of your urine or have problems getting to the bathroom before you start to urinate?
Men	• Have you noticed any swelling or testicular pain? • Do you have difficulty starting your stream of urine? • Are you getting up at night to urinate? • Have you had burning or pain on urination? • Do you lose control of your urine or have problems getting to the bathroom before you start to urinate? • Do you have any difficulty developing or maintaining an erection? • Any discharge from your penis?

Musculoskeletal	
	• Do you have any muscle aches or pains? Joint pain or swelling?
	• Back pain?
	• Have you ever broken any bones?
	• Do you have chronic pain?
	• Describe the pain — location, duration, rating (scale of 1-10), alleviating factors.

Skin	
Skin Lesions	• Have you noticed any rash or skin problems? If so, where?
	• Have you noticed any new moles, bruises, or bumps on your skin?
	• Do you have any moles that have changed shape, size, or color?
Tinea	• Do you have fungal infections on your skin, especially groin, fingernails, toenails, or feet?
Folliculitis	• Do you have any itchy bumps on your face, back, or chest?
Seborrhea	• Do you have flaking or itching on your skin or scalp?

Neurologic	
Headache	• How often do you get headaches?
	• Describe the headaches — location, timing, duration, alleviating or aggravating factors.
	• Do they cause nausea or vomiting?
	• Does sensitivity to light lead to headaches?
Neuropathy	• Do you have any numbness, tingling, burning, or pain in your hands or feet?
Weakness	• Do you have or have you had any weakness in your arms or legs?
Gait	• Have you noticed any changes in the way you walk?
Memory	• Do you have difficulty with your memory or ability to concentrate? If so, describe.
Seizures	• Have you ever had a seizure or "fit"?
	• If so, describe the seizure — When? How long did it last? Did you experience loss of consciousness? Did you receive medical care?

Endocrine	
Diabetes	• Have you had any increase in thirst, hunger, or urination?
Thyroid	• Have you noticed changes in your energy level?
	• Do you have intolerance to heat or cold?
	• Have you noticed changes in your hair (thinning, coarse texture)?
Sex Steroids	• Have you noticed any changes in your libido? In your energy level, mood?

Hematologic/Lymphatic	
Adenopathy	• Do you have swollen glands?
	• If so, describe — location, pain, size.
Bruising or Bleeding	• Have you noticed easy bruising or prolonged bleeding after injury?
	• Nosebleeds or bleeding gums?

Psychiatric	
Mood	• Depression screening: Have you experienced a decrease in your interest or pleasure in your activities? Have you felt depressed, down, or hopeless? • Do you feel more angry, sad, depressed, numb, irritable, or anxious than usual? • Have any major life events have occurred to cause you to feel sad or depressed? • When did these events occur?
Sleep	• How is your sleep? • How many hours do you sleep each night? • What is your sleeping schedule — time to bed and time to rise? • Do you take naps?

O: Objective

• Conduct a physical examination, focusing on subjective findings elicited in the history. (See chapter *Initial Physical Examination*.) Note: If significant time has elapsed between the review of symptoms (ROS) and the physical examination, perform another ROS.

A/P: Assessment and Plan

• Arrange for baseline/intake laboratory work. (See chapter *Initial and Interim Laboratory and Other Tests*.)

• Compose a problem list. Initiate a medication list (if appropriate).

• Refer the patient to social services, mental health care, community and other resources, or other clinic services as needed.

During the current visit or a future visit:

• Perform tuberculosis testing (TST or IGRA) if not done in the past year or if the previous result was negative. The patient will need to return to have the TST read. See chapter *Latent Tuberculosis Infection*.

• Perform immunizations for pneumonia (Pneumovax), influenza (as appropriate), and other immunizations as indicated. (See chapter *Immunizations for HIV-Infected Adults and Adolescents*.)

• Provide counseling on prevention of HIV transmission (e.g., safer sex and injection practices), as appropriate. See chapter *Preventing HIV Transmission/Prevention with Positives*.

References

- Aberg JA, Kaplan JE, Libman H, et al.; HIV Medicine Association of the Infectious Diseases Society of America. *Primary care guidelines for the management of persons infected with human immunodeficiency virus: 2009 update by the HIV medicine Association of the Infectious Diseases Society of America.* Clin Infect Dis. 2009 Sep 1;49(5):651-81.

- Hollander H. *Initiating Routine Care for the HIV-Infected Adult.* In: Sande MA, Volberding PA, eds. *The Medical Management of AIDS, 5th Edition.* Philadelphia: WB Saunders; 1997:107-112.

- Kaplan JE, Benson C, Holmes KH, et al; Centers for Disease Control and Prevention (CDC); National Institutes of Health; HIV Medicine Association of the Infectious Diseases Society of America. *Guidelines for prevention and treatment of opportunistic infections in HIV-infected adults and adolescents: recommendations from CDC, the National Institutes of Health, and the HIV Medicine Association of the Infectious Diseases Society of America.* MMWR Recomm Rep. 2009 Apr 10;58(RR-4):1-207.

- U.S. Department of Health and Human Services. *Guide to Clinical Preventive Services, 2009: Recommendations of the U.S. Preventive Services Task Force.* Available at www.ahrq.gov/clinic/pocketgd.htm.

- U.S. Department of Health and Human Services. *Guidelines for the Use of Antiretroviral Agents in HIV-1-Infected Adults and Adolescents.* January 10, 2011. Available at www.aidsinfo.nih.gov/guidelines/.

Initial Physical Examination

Background

Many of the conditions that put immunocompromised patients at risk of disease can be detected early, by means of a thorough history and physical evaluation.

HRSA HAB Core Clinical Performance Measures

Percentage of women with HIV infection who have a **Pap screening** in the measurement year

(Group 2 measure)

S: Subjective

See chapter *Initial History.*

O: Objective

Assess the patient's general appearance, affect, demeanor in answering questions, body language, and other relevant characteristics. Measure vital signs; perform a physical examination.

Vital Signs	
(These measurements establish a baseline against which future measurements can be compared.)	
Vital Sign	**Recommendation/Notes**
• Height	• Should be measured once.
• Weight	• Record at each visit.
• Temperature	• Record at each visit.
• Blood pressure	• Record at each visit. The BP cuff size should be appropriate for the patient's arm circumference.
• Heart rate	• Record at each visit.
• Respiratory rate	• Record at each visit.
• Oxygen saturation	• Record at each visit.
• Waist, hip circumferences	• Waist and hip circumference should be measured for comparison in case the patient later develops obesity or lipoaccumulation related to antiretroviral therapy (ART). **Abdominal circumference:** >102 cm (39") in men = abdominal obesity >88 cm (35") in women = abdominal obesity **Waist-hip ratios:** >0.95 in men = increased risk of coronary heart disease (CHD) >0.85 in women = increased risk of CHD

Body mass index (BMI)	BMI can be helpful in assessing underweight or overweight conditions, HIV/AIDS-related weight loss, and ART-related weight gain. Perform at baseline and upon changes in weight. **BMI calculation:** $$\frac{(weight\ in\ pounds)}{(height\ in\ inches) \times (height\ in\ inches)} \times 703$$ or, $$\frac{(weight\ in\ kilograms)}{(height\ in\ meters) \times (height\ in\ meters)}$$ **BMI:** <18.5 = underweight 25-29.9 = overweight 18.5-24.9 = normal range ≥30 = obese

Physical Examination

General

- State of nourishment, well or ill appearing

Eyes

- Examine visual acuity by Snellen chart, visual fields by confrontation.
- Test extraocular movements and pupillary size and reactivity.
- Perform funduscopic examination, with or without mydriatics. Note any retinal lesions, white or yellow retinal discoloration, infiltrates, or hemorrhages (could indicate cytomegalovirus retinitis, retinal necrosis, or ocular toxoplasmosis).
- Referral to ophthalmologist for retinal examination every 6 months if the CD4 count is <50 cells/μL.
- Refer immediately if the patient has retinal lesions or new visual disturbances.

Ears/Nose

- Examine ear canals and tympanic membranes.
- Visualize nasal turbinates.
- Palpate frontal and maxillary facial sinuses.

Oral Cavity

- Good lighting is essential for this examination.
- Examine:
  - Gingiva and teeth (note loss of teeth, decay, inflammation)
  - Mucosal surfaces (with dentures removed) (note any lesions or discolorations)
  - Posterior tongue
  - Tonsils (note absence or presence; any abnormality in tonsil size)
  - Pharynx (note lesions, exudate)
- Refer to oral health specialist for examination.

Endocrine

- Check thyroid for enlargement, tenderness, nodules, and asymmetry.

Lymph Nodes

- Document site and characteristics of each palpable node.

  Node Sites :

  - Posterior cervical chain
  - Anterior cervical chain
  - Submandibular
  - Supraclavicular
  - Submental
  - Axillary
  - Epitrochlear
  - Inguinal
  - Femoral

  Characteristics:

  - Size (two dimensions, in millimeters)
  - Consistency (hard, fluctuant, soft)
  - Tenderness
  - Mobility
  - Definition (discrete, matted)
  - Symmetry

Lungs

- Inspect, auscultate, and percuss.
- Note any abnormal sounds including crackles or wheezes (e.g., signs of infections, asthma, congestive heart failure).
- Note any absence of air movement (e.g., pneumothorax, pleural effusion).

Heart

- Examine for jugular venous distention (JVD).
- Palpate for point of maximal impulse (PMI).
- Note rate and rhythm, heart sounds, murmurs, extra heart sounds.

Breasts

- Palpate for breast masses in both men and women.
- Check for symmetry, nipple discharge, dimpling, and masses.

Abdomen

- View: examine for distention, obesity, undernutrition, vascular prominence, petechiae.
- Auscultate; note bowel sounds.
- Percuss; record liver size.
- Palpate for hepatomegaly, splenomegaly, masses, tenderness or rebound tenderness.

Genitals/Rectum

- Inspect the genitalia and perirectal area; note lesions, warts, etc.
- Look for discharges, ulcerative lesions, vesicles, or crusted lesions; take samples for diagnostic studies (e.g., for chlamydia, gonorrhea, herpes simplex virus, syphilis, chancroid, as appropriate).

Female Patients

- Perform speculum examination; note any lesions on vaginal walls or cervix.
- Obtain a Papanicolaou (Pap) test.
- Obtain endocervical swab for gonorrhea and chlamydia, and a posterior pool swab for wet mount evaluation for trichomoniasis, candidiasis, and bacterial vaginosis.
- Consider anal Pap test, especially if the patient has a history of an abnormal cervical Pap test or genital warts (perform before introduction of lubricant).*
- Bimanual examination; note size of uterus and ovaries, shape, and any tenderness or pelvic pain.
- Rectal examination (e.g., for anorectal lesions, warts) and evaluation of posterior uterine abnormalities.

Male Patients

- Examine external genitalia; note whether patient is circumcised; note any lesions, discharge, or other abnormalities, as above. Perform testicular examination for masses, tenderness.
- Consider anal Pap test (perform before introduction of lubricant).*
- Digital rectal examination to evaluate rectal tone, discharge or tenderness, masses, or lesions; perform prostate examination if appropriate.

* Anal Pap test: Consider this test if follow-up evaluation of an abnormal Pap test result is available. Rates of anal dysplasia and anal cancer are higher in HIV- infected women and men than in HIV-uninfected individuals; see chapter *Anal Dysplasia*.

Extremities/Musculoskeletal

- Joints; note any enlargement, swelling, or tenderness.
- Muscles; for the major muscle groups, evaluate muscle bulk (normal or decreased), tenderness, or weakness.
- Look for evidence of peripheral fat atrophy.
- Consider measuring baseline arm, thigh, and chest circumferences for later comparison.
- Note nail changes (clubbing, cyanosis, thickening, discoloration).
- Assess for pedal or leg edema.

Habitus

- Look carefully for signs of lipoatrophy or lipohypertrophy, wasting, or obesity.
- Subcutaneous fat loss (face, extremities, buttocks).
- Central fat accumulation (neck, dorsocervical area, breasts, abdomen).

Skin

- Examine the entire body, including scalp, axillae, palms, soles of feet, and pubic and perianal areas.
- Describe all lesions (e.g., size, borders, color, symmetry/asymmetry, distribution, raised/flat, induration, and encrustation).
- Note evidence of folliculitis, seborrheic dermatitis, psoriasis, Kaposi sarcoma, fungal infections, prurigo nodularis, etc.
- Note any tattoos and or body piercings.

Neurologic

- Assess the following:
  - Mental status, including orientation, registration, recent and remote memory, and ability to calculate (serial subtraction)
  - Cranial nerves
  - Peripheral sensory examination, including pinprick, temperature, and vibratory stimuli
  - Extremity strength and gait to discern myopathy, neuropathy, and cerebellar disease
  - Fine motor skills such as rapid alternating movements (often abnormal in dementia)
  - Deep tendon and plantar reflexes

Psychiatric

- Assess the patient's general mood (e.g., depressed, anxious, hypertalkative).
- Note verbal content (e.g., whether the patient answers questions appropriately; unusual or odd content).
- Note inappropriate or unusual behavior, such as extremes of denial, hostility, or compulsiveness.
- See section *Neuropsychiatric Disorders* for more complete information on common pathologies.
- If the possibility of an emergency situation exists (e.g., potential suicide or violence), refer to crisis mental health services for immediate evaluation.

A/P: Assessment and Plan

After completing the initial history and physical examination, do the following:

- Enter the information garnered through the history and physical examination into the patient's chart or database.

- Continue to develop the problem list, assessment, and plan for patient care.

- Complete follow-up or laboratory studies suggested by the history and physical examination. (See chapter *Initial and Interim Laboratory and Other Tests*.)

- Prescribe opportunistic infection prophylaxis as appropriate. (See chapter *Opportunistic Infection Prophylaxis*.)

- Arrange for any appropriate vaccinations. (See chapter *Immunizations for HIV-Infected Adults and Adolescents*.)

- Refer for dental, nutrition, and social services, as well as case management and mental health care, as appropriate.

- Refer for any additional specialty care needs identified in the history or physical examination.

- Make follow-up appointment with health care provider.

- Answer the patient's questions.

Patient Education

A very important aspect of caring for HIV-infected individuals is educating patients about HIV infection, including goals of care and ways of achieving those goals.

Review the following with each patient:

HIV disease
- Disease course
- Significance of CD4 cell count and HIV viral load
- Possible treatment approaches
- Disclosure (e.g., whom the patient may need to tell about HIV status, relevant legal requirements, approaches to disclosure)

HIV transmission prevention and risk reduction for HIV-positive individuals
(see chapter *Preventing HIV Transmission/ Prevention with Positives*)

- Strategies to prevent transmission of HIV to uninfected partners and to prevent acquisition of sexually transmitted infections, hepatitis, and other infections

- Safer-sex approaches, including the use of condoms or other latex barriers during sexual contacts

- Safer use of recreational drugs

Nutrition
- Maintaining a healthy weight
- Nutritional support resources, if appropriate
- Importance of including a nutritionist in medical care

Mental health
- Stress reduction
- Rest and exercise to enhance a healthy mental state

Adherence
- Importance of keeping medical appointments
- Need for adhering to any medication regimen and the consequences of missed HIV medication doses

References

- Aberg JA, Kaplan JE, Libman H, et al.; HIV Medicine Association of the Infectious Diseases Society of America. *Primary care guidelines for the management of persons infected with human immunodeficiency virus: 2009 update by the HIV medicine Association of the Infectious Diseases Society of America.* Clin Infect Dis. 2009 Sep 1;49(5):651-81.

- Hollander H. *Initiating Routine Care for the HIV-Infected Adult.* In: Sande MA, Volberding PA, eds. *The Medical Management of AIDS, 5th Edition.* Philadelphia: WB Saunders; 1997:107-112.

- Kaplan JE, Benson C, Holmes KH, et al; Centers for Disease Control and Prevention (CDC); National Institutes of Health; HIV Medicine Association of the Infectious Diseases Society of America. *Guidelines for prevention and treatment of opportunistic infections in HIV-infected adults and adolescents: recommendations from CDC, the National Institutes of Health, and the HIV Medicine Association of the Infectious Diseases Society of America.* MMWR Recomm Rep. 2009 Apr 10;58(RR-4):1-207.

- U.S. Department of Health and Human Services. *Guidelines for the Use of Antiretroviral Agents in HIV-1-Infected Adults and Adolescents.* January 10, 2011. Available at www.aidsinfo.nih.gov/guidelines/.

Initial and Interim Laboratory and Other Tests

Background

This chapter discusses the laboratory tests and other monitoring that should be performed for HIV-infected individuals. This involves testing for staging HIV infection, screening for comorbidities, establishing baselines before treatment with antiretroviral (ARV) medications, and monitoring responses to ARV therapy (ART).

HRSA HAB Core Clinical Performance Measures

Percentage of clients with HIV infection who had two or more **CD4 T-cell counts** performed in the measurement year

(Group 1 measure)

Percentage of clients for whom **hepatitis C** screening was performed at least once since the diagnosis of HIV infection

(Group 2 measure)

Percentage of clients with HIV infection on ART who had a fasting **lipid panel** within the measurement year

(Group 2 measure)

Percentage of adult clients with HIV infection who had a test for **syphilis** performed within the measurement year

(Group 2 measure)

Number of clients who received documented testing for **latent tuberculosis** infection with any approved test (tuberculin skin test or interferon gamma release assay) since HIV diagnosis

(Group 2 measure)

Percentage of women with HIV infection who have a **Pap screening** within the measurement year

(Group 2 measure)

Percentage of clients with HIV infection who have been screened for **hepatitis B** virus infection status

(Group 3 measure)

Percentage of clients with HIV infection at risk of sexually transmitted infections who had a test for **chlamydia** within the measurement year

(Group 3 measure)

Percentage of clients with HIV infection at risk of sexually transmitted infections who had a test for **gonorrhea** within the measurement year

(Group 3 measure)

Percentage of clients with HIV infection for whom *Toxoplasma* **screening** was performed at least once since the diagnosis of HIV infection

(Group 3 measure)

Note that documentation of a positive HIV serologic test result is essential for each patient, and it should be included in the patient's chart.

O: Objective

Laboratory Evaluations for HIV-Infected Patients

Test	Rationale	Result	Frequency and Comments
HIV Staging and ART Monitoring			
CD4 Count	• For HIV staging and prognosis • Helps guide initiation of ART • Indicates risk of opportunistic illnesses and guides initiation of prophylaxis against opportunistic infections • Used to monitor immune reconstitution during ART	• Reported in cells/µL	• Perform at baseline (twice). • Repeat every 3-6 months for stable patients on or off ART. • Repeat if results are inconsistent with the clinical picture or with previous trends. • See chapter *CD4 and Viral Load Monitoring*.
CD4 Percentage	• Used in addition to the absolute CD4 count for monitoring trends; may be discrepant with absolute CD4 • *Pneumocystis* pneumonia prophylaxis is indicated for CD4 percentage <14% regardless of absolute count	CD4 Count (cells/µL): >500 — Expected CD4 Percentage: >29% 200-500 — 14-28% <200 — <14%	• Usually obtained with absolute CD4 count.
Quantitative Plasma HIV RNA (HIV Viral Load)	• Estimates level of HIV replication • Used to monitor effect of ART • May be used to identify acute HIV infection; has high sensitivity in setting of acute infection, when antibody may be negative; must be confirmed by positive result on HIV antibody test (one viral load test is FDA approved for diagnosis of HIV)	• Reported in copies/mL • In untreated patients, detectable (with rare exceptions) and measured to the upper limit of detection (usually >500,000 copies/mL) • For patients taking ART, ideally suppressed to undetectable levels (usually <50 or <75 copies/mL)	• Perform at baseline (twice). • For patients on new or modified ART regimen: perform 2-8 weeks after initiation or change in ART, then every 4-8 weeks until viral load is suppressed. • For patients on stable ART: perform every 3-4 months (if stable and viral load suppressed >2-3 years, consider every 6 months). • For patients not taking ART: perform every 3-6 months; more frequently if CD4 count is low. *Factors that may temporarily increase viral load:* • Immunizations • Active infections

Predicting Safety and Efficacy of ARVs		
Drug Resistance Testing (Genotype, Phenotype)	• To assess whether the patient's HIV virus is likely to be resistant to specific ARV medications	• Genotype: detects specific mutations to ARV medications • Phenotype: measures HIV viral replication in the presence of ARVs	• Genotype is recommended for all ARV-naive patients. For greatest accuracy, should be done as early as possible in the course of HIV infection. • Acute or primary infection: recommended (genotype). • Chronic infection and treatment naive: recommended before initiation of ART (genotype). If resistance test was performed at entry, consider repeat testing. • Pregnancy: recommended before initiation of ART or for patients with detectable HIV RNA while taking ART. • Virologic failure: recommended. • Consider genotype for integrase mutations if integrase inhibitor resistance is a concern. (See chapter *Resistance Testing* for more information.)
Coreceptor Tropism Test	• Determine coreceptor tropism	• If CXCR4-tropic (or dual/mixed tropic) virus is detected, CCR5 antagonist is not likely to be effective and should be avoided	• Test before making decision to treat with CCR5 antagonist, or if virologic failure occurs while on a CCR5 antagonist. • For standard assay, HIV RNA must be >1,000 copies/mL (a proviral DNA test is available for samples with HIV RNA below limits of detection; has not been clinically validated).
HLA-B*5701	• Establish risk of hypersensitivity reaction to abacavir	• If positive, high risk of abacavir hypersensitivity reaction; abacavir should not be used	• Test before starting treatment with abacavir.

Baseline and Subsequent Hematologic, Renal, Hepatic, and Metabolic Screening			
Complete Blood Count (CBC) with Differential and Platelets	• Detects anemia, thrombocytopenia, leukopenia	• Normal	• Perform at baseline. • Repeat every 3-6 months.
		• Abnormal	• Requires follow-up evaluation as indicated; may influence choice of ARVs. • Repeat more frequently if the patient's results are abnormal or if the patient is taking bone marrow suppressive drugs.
Chemistry Profile **Electrolytes, Creatinine, eGFR (Estimated Glomerular Filtration Rate), Blood Urea Nitrogen** **Liver Transaminases, Bilirubin (Total and Direct)**	• Detects electrolyte abnormalities, kidney disease, liver disease	• Normal/abnormal	• Perform at baseline; before starting ART. • Repeat every 3-6 months, and as needed. • May influence ARV selection. • May be useful in monitoring drug toxicities. • Abnormalities should prompt evaluation of cause.
Urinalysis with Urine Protein and Creatinine	• Used to screen for kidney disease	• Normal/abnormal	• Screen at baseline and before initiation or change of ART regimen. • Repeat every 6 months in patients with HIV-associated nephropathy. • Repeat every 12 months (for patients on tenofovir, every 6 months); more frequently if indicated. • Abnormalities should prompt evaluation of cause. See chapter *Renal Disease*.

Lipid Profile (Total Cholesterol, LDL, HDL, Triglycerides); fasting	• Detects dyslipidemia, identifies risk factors for cardiovascular disease	• Normal/abnormal	• Baseline; before starting ART. • Repeat ≤3 months after starting or changing ART, annually if normal (on or off ART), or more frequently (every 3-6 months) if abnormal or risk of cardiovascular disease. • May influence ARV selection. • May be useful in monitoring drug toxicities. See chapter *Dyslipidemia.*
Glucose (preferably fasting)	• Detects diabetes and hyperglycemia	• Normal/abnormal	Baseline; before starting ART. • Repeat every 3 months if abnormal, every 6 months if normal. • May influence ARV selection. • May be useful in monitoring drug toxicities. See chapter *Insulin Resistance, Hyperglycemia, and Diabetes on Antiretroviral Therapy.*
Hepatitis A, B, and C Screening			
Hepatitis A Serology			
Hepatitis A Antibody (HAV IgG)	• Screen for immunity to hepatitis A; vaccinate those not immune	• Negative	• Offer hepatitis A vaccine if indicated. (See chapter *Immunizations for HIV-Infected Adults and Adolescents.*)
		• Positive	• Immune; no vaccine necessary.
Hepatitis B Serology. See chapter *Hepatitis B Infection.*			
Hepatitis B Surface Antigen (HBsAg)	• Indicates active hepatitis B	• sAg negative	• Most likely, no chronic infection (may be falsely negative). • Vaccinate if HBsAb negative (not immune).
		• sAg positive	• Indicates chronic or acute hepatitis B infection; requires further evaluation (check HBV DNA). (See chapter *Hepatitis B Infection.*)

Hepatitis B Core Antibody (Anti-HBc, IgG)	• Indicates past infection or ongoing infection	• Anti-HBc negative	• The patient most likely has not been infected with hepatitis B; consider vaccination if HBsAb negative and HBsAg negative.
		• Anti-HBc positive	• The patient most likely has been infected with hepatitis B; this test alone does not distinguish past exposure and active infection. • In rare cases, may be falsely negative in some patients with chronic infection. • If sAb negative and sAg negative, check HBV DNA to rule out active infection. • If sAb is positive, patient is immune.
Hepatitis B Surface Antibody (Anti-HBs)	• Indicates immunity status	• Anti-HBs negative	• The patient is not immune to hepatitis B; consider vaccination, unless patient has active hepatitis (sAg positive or HBV DNA positive).
		• Anti-HBs positive	• The patient is immune to hepatitis B either by previous infection or by immunization; may be negative in acute hepatitis B infection.
Hepatitis C Serology			
Hepatitis C Antibody (HCV IgG)	• Hepatitis C status	• HCV negative	• Patient is not infected with hepatitis C. • Consider annual screening for high-risk patients.
		• HCV positive	• Patient has chronic hepatitis C infection or past infection with spontaneous clearance (no protective immunity); confirm positive results with HCV RNA.

Other Opportunistic Infection Screening Tests			
Toxoplasma gondii IgG	• Detects past exposure; if positive, patient has increased risk of developing CNS toxoplasmosis if CD4 count <100 cells/μL	• Negative	• Repeat if patient becomes symptomatic or when CD4 count drops to ≤100 cells/μL.
		• Positive	• Note as baseline information. • Start toxoplasmosis prophylaxis when CD4 count drops to ≤100 cells/μL.
Tuberculosis (TB) Screening TST (Tuberculin Skin Test) or IGRA (Interferon-Gamma Release Assay) (if no history of TB or positive TB screening test in the past)	• Detects latent TB infection (LTBI)	• Normal	• Repeat every 6-12 months. • Repeat TST if CD4 count was <200 cells/μL on initial TST but increases to >200 cells/μL.
		• Abnormal (TST induration ≥5 mm or positive IGRA)	• Evaluate for active TB. (See chapter *Latent Tuberculosis*.)
Chest X Ray (if pulmonary symptoms are present or positive LTBI test)	• Detects latent or active diseases	• Normal	• Repeat as indicated for pulmonary symptoms or positive LTBI test.
		• Abnormal	• Evaluate for TB, PCP, or other pathology.
Papanicolaou Test (cervical for women; consider anal for women and men)	• Detects abnormal cell changes, dysplasia	• Normal	• Cervical: Repeat in 6 months; then annually if negative on two tests and no ongoing risk factors. • Anal: Follow-up interval has not been determined; consider same as in cervical Pap screening.
		• Abnormal	• Perform workup, treat (see chapters *Cervical Dysplasia* and *Anal Dysplasia*) and follow up more frequently as indicated by condition.

Pregnancy Screening			
Pregnancy Test	• Indicates pregnancy status	• Positive/negative	• Perform before starting efavirenz (given risk for teratogenicity). • If positive, consider ART initiation; avoid efavirenz (see chapters *Reducing Maternal-Infant HIV Transmission* and *Care of HIV-Infected Pregnant Women*).
Sexually Transmitted Infection Testing **(identify STIs in any patient at risk)**			
Serum VDRL (Venereal Disease Research Laboratory) or RPR (Rapid Plasma Reagin)	• Syphilis screening	• Negative/nonreactive	• Repeat every 3-12 months, depending on risk factors.
		• Positive/reactive: confirm with treponemal test	• Treat patient; refer partner(s) of previous 60 days for evaluation and treatment; counsel about safer sex. • Perform serial testing if monitoring active disease. (See chapter *Syphilis*.)
Women			
Gonorrhea (GC) and Chlamydia (CT) Testing	Screen for STIs in sexually active women at risk; screen all at baseline; frequency of subsequent testing depends on risk factors Screen all sites of possible exposures: • Pharynx (recommended for GC screening) • Cervix/vagina • Urethra • Rectum	• Negative	• Counsel about safer sex and avoiding STIs. • Repeat every 6-12 months; more frequently if at high risk.
		• Positive	• Treat patient; refer partner(s) of previous 60 days for evaluation and treatment; counsel about safer sex.
Trichomoniasis Testing	• Wet mount or culture of vaginal secretions	• Negative	• Counsel about safer sex and avoiding STIs.
		• Positive	• Treat patient; refer partner(s) for evaluation and treatment; counsel about safer sex.

Men			
Gonorrhea (GC) and Chlamydia (CT) Testing	Screen for STIs in sexually active men who are at risk, especially men who have sex with men (MSM) Screen all at baseline; frequency of subsequent testing depends on risk factors Screen sites of possible exposures: • Pharynx (recommended for GC screening) • Rectum • Urethra (consider for MSM with history of unprotected insertive intercourse in preceding year)	• Negative	• Retest every 3-6 months for patients with risk factors.
		• Positive	• Treat; refer partner(s) of previous 60 days for evaluation and treatment; counsel about safer sex.
Consider/Optional			
G6PD Level	Prevent hemolytic reactions to certain medications by screening higher-risk patients (African, Mediterranean, Asian, Sephardic Jewish descent); some would recommend screening all patients	• Normal range	• No intervention is necessary beyond documentation.
		• Abnormal range	• Avoid oxidant drugs such as dapsone, primaquine, and sulfonamides, if possible.
Cytomegalo-virus (CMV) Antibody (anti-CMV IgG) **(for those at low risk of CMV, especially those who are not MSM or injection drug users)**	• Detects exposure; may reveal future disease risk	• Negative	• Avoid exposure by practicing safer sex. • If blood transfusion is required, use CMV-negative or leukocyte-reduced blood.
		• Positive	• Be aware of disease risk in advanced HIV infection, when CD4 count is <50 cells/µL.
Varicella zoster (Varicella IgG) for those without history of chickenpox or shingles	• Detects exposure	• Negative	• Consider vaccination, if CD4 count is >200 cells/µL.
		• Positive	• No intervention is necessary.
Dilated Retinal Examination	• Detects CMV, ophthalmic toxoplasmosis, or HIV retinopathy	• Normal	• If CD4 count is >100 cells/µL, repeat annually. • If CD4 count is <50 cells/µL or symptoms of retinal changes are present, repeat every 6 months.
		• Abnormal	• Follow up immediately with ophthalmologist.

Patient Education

- Discuss safer sex (review specifics appropriate to the patient's sexual practices and infections) to prevent the patient's exposure to herpes, hepatitis B, hepatitis C, and other STIs, and to prevent the patient from exposing others to HIV or other pathogens. In addition, remind the patient that safer sex practices will limit the risk of reinfection with HIV. (See chapters *Preventing HIV Transmission/Prevention with Positives* and *Preventing Exposure to Opportunistic and Other Infections*.)

- If *Toxoplasma* IgG test result is negative, see chapter *Preventing Exposure to Opportunistic and Other Infections.*

- If CMV test result is negative, counsel the patient that CMV is shed in semen, vaginal and cervical secretions, saliva, and urine of infected people. Latex condoms will help reduce risk. For women considering childbearing, CMV should be avoided assiduously to prevent severe disease and even death of the neonate. (See chapter *Preventing Exposure to Opportunistic and Other Infections*.)

- For patients who are hepatitis C negative and are using injection drugs, offer referral to a drug treatment program or a clean needle exchange program. (See chapters *Preventing HIV Transmission/Prevention with Positives* and *Preventing Exposure to Opportunistic and Other Infections*.)

References

- Aberg JA, Kaplan JE, Libman H, et al.; HIV Medicine Association of the Infectious Diseases Society of America. *Primary care guidelines for the management of persons infected with human immunodeficiency virus: 2009 update by the HIV Medicine Association of the Infectious Diseases Society of America.* Clin Infect Dis. 2009 Sep 1;49(5):651-81.

- Bartlett JG, Cheever L. *A Guide to Primary Care of People with HIV/AIDS, 2004 Edition.* Rockville, MD: Department of Health and Human Services, HIV/AIDS Bureau. 2004. Available at hab.hrsa.gov/tools/primarycareguide/.

- Centers for Disease Control and Prevention. *Sexually Transmitted Diseases Treatment Guidelines*, 2010. MMWR 2010 Dec 17; 59 (No. RR- 12):1-110. Available at www.cdc.gov/STD/treatment/2010.

- Feinberg J, Maenza J. *Primary Medical Care.* In: Anderson JR, ed. *A Guide to the Clinical Care of Women with HIV.* Rockville, MD: Health Services and Resources Administration; 2001:354-359. Available at hab.hrsa.gov/publications/womencare05/.

- Kaplan JE, Benson C, Holmes KH, et al.; Centers for Disease Control and Prevention (CDC); National Institutes of Health; HIV Medicine Association of the Infectious Diseases Society of America. *Guidelines for prevention and treatment of opportunistic infections in HIV-infected adults and adolescents: recommendations from CDC, the National Institutes of Health, and the HIV Medicine Association of the Infectious Diseases Society of America.* MMWR Recomm Rep. 2009 Apr 10;58(RR-4):1-207.

- U.S. Department of Health and Human Services. *Guidelines for the Use of Antiretroviral Agents in HIV-1-Infected Adults and Adolescents.* January 10, 2011. Available at www.aidsinfo.nih.gov/guidelines/.

Interim History and Physical Examination

Background

This chapter shows the suggested frequency and follow-up intervals of the history and physical examination for monitoring HIV-infected patients, as well as specific areas to assess in an ongoing manner. With this information, the clinician can track disease progression and formulate and maintain an appropriate care plan. Note that information gathered in the history or physical examination may call for additional directed explorations.

It is important to document new or ongoing symptoms and functional limitations at each visit. This information is particularly useful when outside agencies must determine the patient's disability status. (See chapter *Karnofsky Performance Scale*.)

HRSA HAB Core Clinical Performance Measures

Percentage of clients with HIV infection who had **two or more medical visits in an HIV care setting** in the measurement year.

(Group 1 measure)

Percentage of women with HIV infection who have a **Pap screening** in the measurement year.

(Group 2 measure)

Percentage of clients with HIV infection who received **HIV risk counseling** within the measurement year

(Group 2 measure)

Percentage of new clients with HIV infection who have been **screened for substance use** (alcohol and drugs) in the measurement year

(Group 3 measure)

Percentage of new clients with HIV infection who have had a **mental health screening**

(Group 3 measure)

Table 1. History and Physical Examinations

History	Physical Examination
Every visit (at least every 3-4 months)	

• New symptoms
• Medications
  • HIV-related medications
  • Medications for other conditions
  • Over-the-counter medications
  • Herbs or vitamins
• Adherence to medications and clinical care visits
• Antiretroviral (ARV) doses missed in the past 3 days, in the past month
• Knowledge of HIV regimen
• Risk reduction; prevention with positives
• Mood
• Alcohol and recreational drug use
• Tobacco use
• Allergies
• Pain
• Social supports
• Housing
• Insurance
• Intimate partner violence
	• Vital signs (temperature, blood pressure, heart rate, respiratory rate, oxygen saturation)
	• Weight
	• General appearance, body habitus (including evaluation for lipodystrophy)
	• Skin
	• Oropharynx
	• Lymph nodes
	• Heart and lungs
	• Abdomen
	• Neurologic
	• Psychiatric — mood, affect

Every 6 months	
As above	As above, plus: • Vision and funduscopic examination (if CD4 count <100 cells/μL) • Ears/nose • Screening for chlamydia, gonorrhea, and syphilis in all patients at risk of these infections
Every 6 months (twice), and, if both are normal, annually thereafter (see chapters *Cervical Dysplasia* and *Anal Dysplasia*)	
As above	Women: cervical Papanicolaou (Pap) test, pelvic examination; consider anal Pap test Men: consider anal Pap test
Annually	
Update initial history: HIV-related symptoms, hospitalizations, major illnesses, family history	Complete physical to include: • Genitorectal examination • Testicular examination • Prostate examination • Breast examination

References

- Aberg JA, Kaplan JE, Libman H, et al.; HIV Medicine Association of the Infectious Diseases Society of America. *Primary care guidelines for the management of persons infected with human immunodeficiency virus: 2009 update by the HIV medicine Association of the Infectious Diseases Society of America.* Clin Infect Dis. 2009 Sep 1;49(5):651-81.

- Hecht F, Soloway B. *The physical exam in HIV infection.* AIDS Clin Care. 1991:3(1):4-5.

- Hollander H. *Initiating Routine Care for the HIV-Infected Adult.* In: Sande MA, Volberding PA, eds. *The Medical Management of AIDS, 5th Edition.* Philadelphia: WB Saunders; 1997:107-112.

- Kaplan JE, Benson C, Holmes KH, et al; Centers for Disease Control and Prevention (CDC); National Institutes of Health; HIV Medicine Association of the Infectious Diseases Society of America. *Guidelines for prevention and treatment of opportunistic infections in HIV-infected adults and adolescents: recommendations from CDC, the National Institutes of Health, and the HIV Medicine Association of the Infectious Diseases Society of America.* MMWR Recomm Rep. 2009 Apr 10;58(RR-4):1-207.

HIV Classification: CDC and WHO Staging Systems

Background

HIV disease staging and classification systems are critical tools for tracking and monitoring the HIV epidemic and for providing clinicians and patients with important information about HIV disease stage and clinical management. Two major classification systems currently are in use: the U.S. Centers for Disease Control and Prevention (CDC) classification system and the World Health Organization (WHO) Clinical Staging and Disease Classification System.

The CDC disease staging system (most recently revised in 1993) assesses the severity of HIV disease by CD4 cell counts and by the presence of specific HIV-related conditions. The definition of AIDS includes all HIV-infected individuals with CD4 counts of <200 cells/μL (or CD4 percentage <14%) as well as those with certain HIV-related conditions and symptoms. Although the fine points of the classification system rarely are used in the routine clinical management of HIV-infected patients, a working knowledge of the staging criteria (in particular, the definition of AIDS) is useful in patient care. In addition, the CDC system is used in clinical and epidemiologic research.

In contrast to the CDC system, the WHO Clinical Staging and Disease Classification System (revised in 2007) can be used readily in resource-constrained settings without access to CD4 cell count measurements or other diagnostic and laboratory testing methods. The WHO system classifies HIV disease on the basis of clinical manifestations that can be recognized and treated by clinicians in diverse settings, including resource-constrained settings, and by clinicians with varying levels of HIV expertise and training.

S: Subjective

When a patient presents with a diagnosis of HIV infection, review the patient's history to elicit and document any HIV-related illnesses or symptoms (see chapter *Initial History*).

O: Objective

Perform a complete physical examination and appropriate laboratory studies (see chapters *Initial Physical Examination* and *Initial and Interim Laboratory and Other Tests*).

A: Assessment

Confirm HIV infection and perform staging.

P: Plan

Evaluate symptoms, history, physical examination results, and laboratory results, and make a staging classification according to the CDC or WHO criteria (see below).

CDC Classification System for HIV Infection

The CDC categorization of HIV/AIDS is based on the lowest documented CD4 cell count and on previously diagnosed HIV-related conditions (see Table 1). For example, if a patient had a condition that once met the criteria for category B but now is asymptomatic, the patient would remain in category B. Additionally, categorization is based on specific conditions, as indicated below. Patients in categories A3, B3, and C1-C3 are considered to have AIDS.

Table 1. CDC Classification System for HIV-Infected Adults and Adolescents

CD4 Cell Categories	Clinical Categories		
	A Asymptomatic, Acute HIV, or PGL	**B*** Symptomatic Conditions, not A or C	**C#** AIDS-Indicator Conditions
(1) ≥500 cells/µL	A1	B1	C1
(2) 200-499 cells/µL	A2	B2	C2
(3) <200 cells/µL	A3	B3	C3

Abbreviations: PGL = persistent generalized lymphadenopathy

* Category B Symptomatic Conditions

Category B symptomatic conditions are defined as symptomatic conditions occurring in an HIV-infected adolescent or adult that meet at least one of the following criteria:

- They are attributed to HIV infection or indicate a defect in cell-mediated immunity.
- They are considered to have a clinical course or management that is complicated by HIV infection.

Examples include, but are not limited to, the following:

- Bacillary angiomatosis
- Oropharyngeal candidiasis (thrush)
- Vulvovaginal candidiasis, persistent or resistant
- Pelvic inflammatory disease (PID)
- Cervical dysplasia (moderate or severe)/ cervical carcinoma in situ
- Hairy leukoplakia, oral
- Herpes zoster (shingles), involving two or more episodes or at least one dermatome
- Idiopathic thrombocytopenic purpura
- Constitutional symptoms, such as fever (>38.5°C) or diarrhea lasting >1 month
- Peripheral neuropathy

Category C AIDS-Indicator Conditions

- Bacterial pneumonia, recurrent (two or more episodes in 12 months)
- Candidiasis of the bronchi, trachea, or lungs
- Candidiasis, esophageal
- Cervical carcinoma, invasive, confirmed by biopsy
- Coccidioidomycosis, disseminated or extrapulmonary
- Cryptococcosis, extrapulmonary
- Cryptosporidiosis, chronic intestinal (>1 month in duration)
- Cytomegalovirus disease (other than liver, spleen, or nodes)
- Encephalopathy, HIV-related
- Herpes simplex: chronic ulcers (>1-month in duration), or bronchitis, pneumonitis, or esophagitis
- Histoplasmosis, disseminated or extrapulmonary
- Isosporiasis, chronic intestinal (>1-month duration)
- Kaposi sarcoma
- Lymphoma, Burkitt, immunoblastic, or primary central nervous system
- *Mycobacterium avium* complex (MAC) or *Mycobacterium kansasii*, disseminated or extrapulmonary
- *Mycobacterium tuberculosis*, pulmonary or extrapulmonary

- *Mycobacterium*, other species or unidentified species, disseminated or extrapulmonary
- *Pneumocystis jiroveci* (formerly *carinii*) pneumonia (PCP)
- Progressive multifocal leukoencephalopathy (PML)
- *Salmonella* septicemia, recurrent (nontyphoid)
- Toxoplasmosis of brain
- Wasting syndrome caused by HIV (involuntary weight loss >10% of baseline body weight) associated with either chronic diarrhea (two or more loose stools per day for ≥1 month) or chronic weakness and documented fever for ≥1 month

WHO Clinical Staging of HIV/AIDS and Case Definition

The clinical staging and case definition of HIV for resource-constrained settings were developed by the WHO in 1990 and revised in 2007. Staging is based on clinical findings that guide the diagnosis, evaluation, and management of HIV/AIDS, and it does not require a CD4 cell count. This staging system is used in many countries to determine eligibility for antiretroviral therapy, particularly in settings in which CD4 testing is not available. Clinical stages are categorized as 1 through 4, progressing from primary HIV infection to advanced HIV/AIDS (see Table 2). These stages are defined by specific clinical conditions or symptoms. For the purpose of the WHO staging system, adolescents and adults are defined as individuals aged ≥15 years.

Table 2. WHO Clinical Staging of HIV/AIDS for Adults and Adolescents

Primary HIV Infection	
• Asymptomatic	• Acute retroviral syndrome

Clinical Stage 1	
• Asymptomatic	• Persistent generalized lymphadenopathy

Clinical Stage 2	
• Moderate unexplained weight loss (<10% of presumed or measured body weight) • Recurrent respiratory infections (sinusitis, tonsillitis, otitis media, and pharyngitis) • Herpes zoster	• Angular cheilitis • Recurrent oral ulceration • Papular pruritic eruptions • Seborrheic dermatitis • Fungal nail infections

Clinical Stage 3	
• Unexplained severe weight loss (>10% of presumed or measured body weight) • Unexplained chronic diarrhea for >1 month • Unexplained persistent fever for >1 month (>37.6°C, intermittent or constant) • Persistent oral candidiasis (thrush) • Oral hairy leukoplakia • Pulmonary tuberculosis (current)	• Severe presumed bacterial infections (e.g., pneumonia, empyema, pyomyositis, bone or joint infection, meningitis, bacteremia) • Acute necrotizing ulcerative stomatitis, gingivitis, or periodontitis • Unexplained anemia (hemoglobin <8 g/dL) • Neutropenia (neutrophils <500 cells/μL) • Chronic thrombocytopenia (platelets <50,000 cells/μL)

Clinical Stage 4	
• HIV wasting syndrome, as defined by the CDC (see Table 1, above) • *Pneumocystis* pneumonia • Recurrent severe bacterial pneumonia • Chronic herpes simplex infection (orolabial, genital, or anorectal site for >1 month or visceral herpes at any site) • Esophageal candidiasis (or candidiasis of trachea, bronchi, or lungs) • Extrapulmonary tuberculosis • Kaposi sarcoma • Cytomegalovirus infection (retinitis or infection of other organs) • Central nervous system toxoplasmosis • HIV encephalopathy • Cryptococcosis, extrapulmonary (including meningitis)	• Disseminated nontuberculosis mycobacteria infection • Progressive multifocal leukoencephalopathy • Candida of the trachea, bronchi, or lungs • Chronic cryptosporidiosis (with diarrhea) • Chronic isosporiasis • Disseminated mycosis (e.g., histoplasmosis, coccidioidomycosis, penicilliosis) • Recurrent nontyphoidal *Salmonella* bacteremia • Lymphoma (cerebral or B-cell non-Hodgkin) • Invasive cervical carcinoma • Atypical disseminated leishmaniasis • Symptomatic HIV-associated nephropathy • Symptomatic HIV-associated cardiomyopathy • Reactivation of American trypanosomiasis (meningoencephalitis or myocarditis)

References

• Centers for Disease Control and Prevention. *1993 revised classification system for HIV infection and expanded surveillance case definition for AIDS among adolescents and adults.* MMWR Recomm Rep. 1992 Dec 18;41(RR-17):1-19. Available at www.cdc.gov/mmwr/preview/mmwrhtml/00018871.htm.

• Centers for Disease Control and Prevention. *Guidelines for national human immunodeficiency virus case surveillance, including monitoring for human immunodeficiency virus infection and acquired immunodeficiency syndrome.* MMWR Recomm Rep. 1999 Dec 10;48(RR-13):1-27, 29-31. Available at www.cdc.gov/mmwr/preview/mmwrhtml/rr4813a1.htm.

• World Health Organization. *WHO Case Definitions of HIV for Surveillance and Revised Clinical Staging and Immunological Classification of HIV-Related Disease in Adults and Children; 2007.* Available at www.who.int/hiv/pub/guidelines/HIVstaging150307.pdf.

CD4 and Viral Load Monitoring

Background

The CD4 cell count and HIV viral load (RNA level) are closely linked to HIV-related illness and mortality. They give prognostic information on HIV progression and on response to therapy.

HRSA HAB Core Clinical Performance Measures

Percentage of clients with HIV infection who had **two or more CD4 T-cell counts** performed within the measurement year

(Group 1 measure)

CD4 Monitoring

CD4 lymphocyte cells (also called T-cells or T-helper cells) are the primary targets of HIV. The CD4 count and the CD4 percentage mark the degree of immunocompromise. The CD4 count is the number of CD4 cells per microliter (µL) of blood. It is used to stage the patient's disease, determine the risk of opportunistic illnesses, assess prognosis, and guide decisions about when to start antiretroviral therapy (ART) (see chapters *Risk of HIV Progression/Indications for ART* and *Antiretroviral Therapy*).

The CD4 percentage is the percentage of the lymphocyte population that is CD4+; it is measured directly by flow cytometry. A CD4 percentage of <14% is considered to correspond to the same degree of immunosuppression as an absolute CD4 count of <200 cells/µL. The absolute CD4 count is calculated from the CD4 cell percentage and the total white blood cell count. The normal values for CD4 count vary considerably among different laboratories. The mean normal value for most laboratories is approximately 500-1,300 cells/µL. This calculated value is subject to more fluctuations than the CD4 cell percentage. Illness, vaccination, diurnal variation, laboratory error, and some medications can result in transient CD4 cell count changes, whereas the CD4 percentage remains more stable. Because CD4 counts may vary, treatment decisions generally should not be made on the basis of a single CD4 value. When results are inconsistent with previous trends, tests should

be repeated, and treatment decisions usually should be based on two or more similar values. A change between two test results is considered significant if it is a 30% change in absolute CD4 count or 3 percentage point change in CD4 percentage.

In persons with untreated HIV infection, the CD4 count declines by approximately 50-80 cells/µL per year, on average. The pattern of decline may be slow and steady, or the CD4 count may level off for an extended period of time (as in long-term nonprogressors) and then decrease. Although it takes an average of 10 years for a newly infected person to progress to AIDS, there is great variation among patients. For some patients, disease progression occurs within a couple of years. For others, it takes more than 20 years, and a small number of patients appear to maintain high CD4 counts and undetectable HIV RNA levels without ART (aviremic or "elite" controllers).

Among asymptomatic individuals, the CD4 count typically is the major factor that guides the decision to initiate therapy, though the trend in recent years has been to treat willing individuals even at very high CD4 levels. Clinical status, viral load, pregnancy, comorbidities, and patient adherence to medications are among the other factors that should be taken into consideration (see chapters *Risk of HIV Progression/Indications for ART* and *Antiretroviral Therapy*).

Prophylaxis against opportunistic infections is based on CD4 count, and sometimes on

CD4 percentage. For example, a CD4 count of <200 cells/μL or a CD4 percentage of <14% is an indication for prophylaxis against *Pneumocystis jiroveci* pneumonia; a CD4 count of <50 cells/μL is an indication for prophylaxis against *Mycobacterium avium* complex. (See chapters *Opportunistic Infection Prophylaxis* and *Risk of HIV Progression/ Indications for ART.*) The CD4 count also guides decision making in determining when to stop prophylaxis against opportunistic infections with patients whose CD4 counts rise in response to ART.

Effective ART typically results in CD4 count increases of >50 cells/μL within weeks after viral suppression, and increases of 50-100 cells/μL per year thereafter. For some patients, CD4 counts may not increase this quickly or steadily, even with durable viral load suppression. Patients who are older (age >50 years) and those with lower baseline CD4 cell counts are more likely to have blunted CD4 count responses. For monitoring purposes, the CD4 count should be repeated approximately every 3-6 months both in stable untreated patients and in patients on ART (for patients on ART with persistently suppressed HIV RNA and CD4 counts solidly above thresholds for opportunistic infection risk, current guidelines suggest monitoring every 6-12 months). The CD4 count should be checked more frequently if clinically indicated (e.g., switching therapy, ART failure, rapidly declining CD4 count) (see Table 1).

Viral Load Monitoring

The HIV-1 viral load measurement indicates the number of copies of HIV-1 RNA per milliliter of plasma. Although HIV ultimately resides within cells, the plasma measurement is an accurate reflection of the burden of infection and the magnitude of viral replication. It is used to assess the risk of disease progression and can help guide initiation of therapy. It is critical in monitoring virologic response to ART.

There are several commercially available HIV-1 viral load assays and numerous institution-specific assays. The range of detectable virus differs somewhat with each test, but the lowest level of detection generally is 40-75 copies/ mL. A viral load below this "undetectable" level indicates the inability of the assay to detect HIV in the plasma, but does not indicate absence or clearance of the virus from the body. The highest levels of detection of the viral load assays typically are between 500,000 copies/mL and 750,000 copies/mL. Viral loads higher than these levels are reported, for example, as >500,000 copies/mL. Note that commercially available assays may not detect HIV-2, and they do not accurately quantify it.

After initial infection with HIV, the viral load quickly peaks to very high levels, usually >100,000 copies/mL (see chapter *Primary HIV Infection*). During the period of acute infection, when HIV antibody testing may indicate negative results, the viral load test may be used to detect HIV infection (however, most viral load assays are not diagnostic tests, so the HIV antibody assay should be repeated in 4-6 weeks to confirm the HIV diagnosis). Generally, 3-6 months after primary infection, the viral load declines and then levels off, remaining in a steady state. Among patients who are not taking ARV medications, a small number maintain a low or even undetectable viral load (aviremic or "elite" controllers), but the vast majority of those patients have relatively high HIV RNA levels.

Higher plasma viral loads are associated with increased risk of progression to symptomatic disease and AIDS; they also are associated with higher risk of HIV transmission (see chapter *Risk of HIV Progression/Indications for ART*). Although the CD4 cell count is more predictive of clinical disease progression than the HIV RNA level, and is the major factor in determining when to initiate ART for asymptomatic patients, the viral load can play a role (for example, if the viral load is very high).

Once a patient has started ART, the viral load is used to monitor the response to therapy. A key goal of ART is to achieve a viral load that is below the level of detection (e.g., <40 copies/

mL). Because CD4 and clinical responses may lag behind changes in viral load, viral load testing is essential for detecting virologic failure in a timely manner. With an effective ARV regimen, a 10-fold decline (1 logarithm) is expected within the first month, and suppression to undetectable levels should be achieved within 3-6 months after initiation of therapy. Isolated low-level elevations (typically <400 copies/mL) in viral load may occur in patients on ART; these "blips" generally do not predict subsequent virologic failure. (Additionally, some viral load assays appear to produce low-level positive results (<200 copies/mL) more commonly than others; as with blips, these do not appear to increase the risk of virologic failure.) To avoid confusing virologic failure with blips or test variability, current guidelines define virologic failure as repeated HIV RNA levels >200 copies/mL. If the viral load does not reduce to an undetectable level (or at least <200 copies/mL), or if it rebounds after suppression, virologic failure has occurred, and possible causes should be investigated (e.g., poor ARV adherence, resistance to ARVs, or reduced drug exposure).

The HIV viral load should be checked at least twice at baseline, before the patient starts an ART regimen. Follow-up viral load measurement should be performed at regular intervals, depending on the patient's clinical situation (see Table 1). For stable patients, viral load usually should be monitored every 3-4 months; for highly adherent and stable patients with suppressed viral loads for at least several years, some experts monitor every 6 months. With new therapy or changes in therapy, significant change in viral load or CD4 count, or declining clinical status, the viral load should be measured at more frequent intervals.

Viral loads, like CD4 counts, are affected by laboratory variation, assay fluctuations, and patient variables such as acute illness and recent vaccinations. Variations of <0.5 $\log_{10}$ copies/mL (threefold) usually are not clinically significant. Viral load results that are inconsistent with previous trends should be repeated, and treatment decisions usually should be based on two or more similar values. Recent illnesses or vaccinations can transiently increase viral load. If a patient has had a recent illness or vaccination, the viral load measurement should be deferred for 4 weeks, if possible.

Table 1. CD4 and HIV Viral Load Monitoring Schedule

	Baseline	Follow-Up Before ART Initiation	At ART Initiation or Switch	After ART Initiation or Switch	Follow-Up on Effective ART	Treatment Failure or Clinical Indications
CD4 Count	√	Every 3-6 months	√	1-3 months	Every 3-6 months*	√
HIV Viral Load	√	Every 3-4 months	√	2-8 weeks, then every 4-8 weeks until HIV RNA is undetectable	Every 3-4 months**	√

* Patients on a stable ART regimen with sustained viral suppression for >2-3 years may be monitored every 6-12 months.

** Adherent patients on stable ART with sustained viral suppression and stable clinical and immunologic status for >2-3 years: some experts may monitor every 6 months.

Adapted from U.S. Department of Health and Human Services. *Guidelines for the Use of Antiretroviral Agents in HIV-1-Infected Adults and Adolescents*; Table 3. January 10, 2011. Available at www.aidsinfo.nih.gov/guidelines/.

Patient Education

- The CD4 cell count is the best indicator for gauging the strength of the immune system and for determining whether a person is at risk of infection with certain organisms. The higher the CD4 count, the stronger the immune system.

- CD4 counts are variable. Caution patients not to pin emotions and hopes to a single laboratory result. A change of <30% may not be significant.

- The HIV viral load is the best indicator of the level of HIV activity in the patient's body.

- The CD4 count and HIV viral load are used to help determine when to initiate therapy.

- The goal of therapy is to suppress the viral load to below the level of detectability by laboratory tests. An undetectable viral load does not mean HIV has been completely eradicated or that the patient is not infectious to others.

- For most patients on effective ART, the CD4 count will rise as the virus is suppressed. This indicates an improvement in the immune system.

- In stable patients, the CD4 count and HIV viral load usually should be monitored every 3-4 months.

References

- Centers for Disease Control and Prevention. *Guidelines for Prevention and Treatment of Opportunistic Infections in HIV-Infected Adults and Adolescents: Recommendations from CDC, the National Institutes of Health, and the HIV Medicine Association of the Infectious Diseases Society of America.* April 10, 2009. Available at www.aidsinfo.nih.gov/guidelines/.

- Hogg RS, Yip B, Chan KJ, et al. *Rates of disease progression by baseline CD4 cell count and viral load after initiating triple-drug therapy.* JAMA. 2001 Nov 28;286(20):2568-77.

- Palella FJ, Deloria-Knoll M, Chmiel JS, et al. *Survival benefit of initiating antiretroviral therapy in HIV-infected persons in different CD4+ cell strata.* Ann Intern Med. 2003 Apr 15;138(8):620-6.

- Schacker TW, Hughes JP, Shea T, et al. *Biological and virologic characteristics of primary HIV infection.* Ann Intern Med. 1998 Apr 15; 128(8):613-20.

- U.S. Department of Health and Human Services. *Guidelines for the Use of Antiretroviral Agents in HIV-1-Infected Adults and Adolescents.* January 10, 2011. Available at www.aidsinfo.nih.gov/guidelines/.

Risk of HIV Progression/ Indications for ART

Background

The CD4 cell count and HIV viral load (RNA level) are closely linked to HIV-related illness and mortality, and are the laboratory measures that are followed in clinical practice. They are the primary markers that give prognostic information on disease progression and on response to antiretroviral therapy (ART) (see chapter *CD4 and Viral Load Monitoring*). However, it is increasingly recognized that a number of other factors are involved in HIV disease progression. These include individual HIV-specific immune responses, immune activation, viral factors, host genetics, and age. The role of these factors and their interplay are complex and incompletely understood.

CD4 Count

The CD4 count (and CD4 percentage) marks the degree of immunocompromise. The CD4 count is used to stage the patient's disease progression, determine the risk of opportunistic illnesses, and assess prognosis (see chapter *CD4 Monitoring and Viral Load Testing*). The CD4 count also guides decision making about the timing of ART initiation, helps in determining the need for prophylaxis against opportunistic infections, and helps in formulating differential diagnoses for symptomatic patients (see Table 1, Figure 1, and chapters *CD4 and Viral Load Monitoring* and *Opportunistic Infection Prophylaxis*).

Persons with HIV infection are at increased risk of complications at lower CD4 counts. A CD4 count of <200 cells/μL (or CD4 percentage of <14%) indicates severe immunosuppression, and is an AIDS-defining condition. Persons with CD4 counts below this level are at greater risk of a number of opportunistic illnesses and death, increasingly so at lower CD4 counts (see Table 1).

Table 1. Correlation Between CD4 Cell Counts and Complications of HIV Infection

CD4 Count* (cells/μL)	Infectious Complications	Noninfectious Complications#
>500	• Acute retroviral syndrome • Candidal vaginitis	• Persistent generalized lymphadenopathy (PGL) • Guillain-Barré syndrome • Myopathy • Aseptic meningitis
200-500	• Pneumococcal and other bacterial pneumonias • Pulmonary tuberculosis • Herpes zoster • Oropharyngeal candidiasis (thrush) • Cryptosporidiosis (self-limited) • Kaposi sarcoma (cutaneous) • Oral hairy leukoplakia • Herpes simplex (oral/genital)	• Cervical intraepithelial neoplasia • Cervical cancer • B-cell lymphoma • Anemia • Mononeuropathy multiplex • Idiopathic thrombocytopenic purpura • Hodgkin lymphoma • Lymphocytic interstitial pneumonitis • Fatigue
<200	• *Pneumocystis jiroveci* pneumonia (PCP) • Disseminated histoplasmosis and coccidioidomycosis • Miliary/extrapulmonary tuberculosis • Progressive multifocal leukoencephalopathy (PML)	• Wasting • Peripheral neuropathy • HIV-associated dementia • Cardiomyopathy • Vacuolar myelopathy • Progressive polyradiculopathy • Non-Hodgkin lymphoma
<100	• Disseminated herpes simplex virus • Toxoplasmosis • Cryptococcosis • Cryptosporidiosis, chronic • Microsporidiosis • Candidal esophagitis • Kaposi sarcoma (visceral/pulmonary)	
<50	• Disseminated cytomegalovirus (CMV) • Disseminated *Mycobacterium avium* complex (MAC)	• Central nervous system (CNS) lymphoma

* Most complications occur with increasing frequency at lower CD4 cell counts.

Some conditions listed as "noninfectious" are associated with transmissible microbes. Examples include lymphoma (Epstein-Barr virus) and anal and cervical cancers (human papillomavirus).

Adapted from Bartlett JG, Gallant JE, Pham P. *Medical Management of HIV Infection.* Baltimore: Johns Hopkins University School of Medicine; 2009-2010. Used with permission.

Increasing evidence suggests that the risk of complications from HIV infection occur across a broad spectrum of CD4 counts, and that patients with relatively high CD4 counts (those with counts of >350 cells/μL and even those with counts of >500 cells/μL) also have increased rates of morbidities compared with HIV-uninfected persons. The complications in persons with higher CD4 counts typically are not the classic AIDS-related opportunistic illnesses but are "non-AIDS" illnesses such as cardiovascular disease, neurocognitive decline, and non-AIDS-associated cancers.

In asymptomatic individuals, CD4 count has typically been the main indicator of need for ART. It is well established that ART is extremely effective at reducing HIV-related illness in persons with lower CD4 counts. In recent years, accumulating data have suggested that ART may be beneficial even for persons with higher pretreatment CD4 counts.

Randomized trials have shown that starting ART for asymptomatic patients with pretreatment CD4 counts of 200-350 cells/µL results in decreased morbidity and mortality compared with starting therapy for persons with CD4 counts of <200 cells/µL. For patients with pretreatment CD4 counts of >350 cells/µL, data from randomized controlled studies showing benefit of ART are not available, but several cohort studies have found decreased rates of complications and death among persons who initiated ART at CD4 counts of 350-500 cells/µL, compared with persons who initiated treatment at lower CD4 counts. Additionally, some (though not all) observational evidence suggests a mortality benefit of ART even among persons with

pretreatment CD4 counts of >500 cells/µL. These cohort studies are complemented by a number of investigations that demonstrate ongoing and adverse effects of HIV and associated inflammation on various organ systems.

These lines of evidence, along with the demonstrations of the impact of ART in decreasing HIV transmission, and the availability of ARVs that generally are safe, tolerable, and effective, support the rationale for earlier initiation of treatment. Many experts favor treatment of all HIV-infected individuals, regardless of CD4 count. The current U.S. Department of Health and Human Services (DHHS) adult and adolescent treatment guidelines recommend starting ART for all willing asymptomatic patients whose CD4 counts are <500 cells/µL. Additionally, the guidelines emphasize that half of its panel members favor initiating ART for patients with CD4 counts of >500 cells/µL, whereas the other half consider ART for those patients to be optional (see Table 2 and chapter *Antiretroviral Therapy*).

Table 2. DHHS Recommendations on Initiation of Antiretroviral Therapy

Symptomatic Disease
- Antiretroviral therapy is strongly recommended

CD4 Count <350 Cells/µL
- Antiretroviral therapy is strongly recommended

Pregnancy, HIV-Associated Nephropathy, Hepatitis B Coinfection (if treatment for hepatitis B is indicated)
- Antiretroviral therapy is strongly recommended

CD4 Count <500 Cells/µL
- Antiretroviral therapy is moderately to strongly recommended (more urgent at lower CD4 levels)

CD4 Count >500 Cells/µL
- 50% of the expert panel recommended treatment, 50% considered it optional

Considerations
- Patients should be willing to commit to lifelong therapy and should understand the importance of adherence
- Patients or providers may elect, on an individualized basis, to defer therapy based on clinical or psychosocial factors

HIV Viral Load

Whereas the CD4 count is an indicator of immune system function, the HIV viral load (RNA level) gives prognostic information on how quickly the CD4 count is likely to decline and, consequently, the risk of disease progression. Patients with high HIV viral loads generally demonstrate a faster decline in CD4 count and progression to AIDS-related illnesses, whereas those with low viral loads will usually have higher CD4 counts and remain asymptomatic for prolonged periods. A small percentage of persons with HIV infection may have very low or undetectable viral loads for extended periods of time.

By themselves, CD4 count and HIV viral load are useful, albeit rough, prognostic indicators. When considered together, they constitute a finer tool to estimate the risk of progression (see Figure 1).

Figure 1. Prognosis According to CD4 Cell Count and Viral Load in the Pre-ART and ART Eras: Kaplan-Meier Estimates of the Probability of AIDS at 3 Years

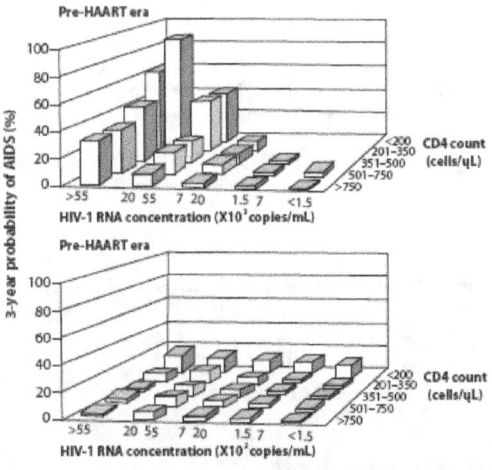

Abbreviations: HAART = highly active antiretroviral therapy
Egger M, May M, Chene G, Phillips AN, Ledergerber B, Dabis F, Costagliola D, D'Arminio Monforte A, de Wolf F, Reiss P, Lundgren JD, Justice AC, Staszewski S, Leport C, Hogg RS, Sabin CA, Gill MJ, Salzberger B, Sterne JA; ART Cohort Collaboration. *Prognosis of HIV-1-infected patients starting highly active antiretroviral therapy: a collaborative analysis of prospective studies.* Lancet. 2002 Jul 13;360(9327):119-29. Reprinted with permission from Elsevier.

Other Factors Associated with HIV Progression

Although the CD4 count and HIV viral load are the most important predictors of HIV progression, it is increasingly recognized that a number of other factors, and likely others that remain unknown, contribute to disease progression in HIV infection.

Viral factors

Variations in the HIV genome have been associated with an altered rate of disease progression. For example, deletions in the *nef* gene have been associated with a slow rate of progression. On the other hand, virus that uses the CXCR4 protein as a coreceptor for entry (termed X4 virus or syncytia-inducing virus) has been associated with accelerated progression. As another example, drug-resistance mutations may affect how efficiently the virus replicates (viral fitness). Patients who have virus with decreased fitness have slower immune deterioration than those with wild-type virus.

Host immune factors

Host genetic factors have been shown to alter the rate of HIV progression. Various human leukocyte antigen (HLA) alleles have been associated with faster or slower progression rates. Genetic polymorphisms also play a role. For example, CCR5 is a chemokine receptor that can serve as a coreceptor for HIV entry into the CD4 cell. A naturally occurring variant allele for CCR5 has a 32 base pair deletion. Individuals who are heterozygous for this allele have slower progression of HIV disease.

Increased immune activation and elevated markers of inflammation, such as IL-6 and D-dimer, also have been associated with risk of disease progression and death. They also may be involved in the ongoing damage seen in a number of end organs. Although T-cell activation and levels of inflammation decrease with ART, they often do not return to normal.

Age

Several studies have shown a higher risk of morbidity and mortality in older patients. When followed from seroconversion, older patients demonstrate faster disease progression compared with younger patients (see Table 2). Older patients also are found to have a less robust increase in the CD4 count in response to ART. These observations have led to the recommendation to consider age as a factor in determining when to initiate therapy in the European AIDS Clinical Society (EACS) guidelines.

Table 2. Median Survival and Time to AIDS by Age at Seroconversion

Age at Seroconversion (years)	Median (95% CI) Survival (years)	Median (95% CI) Time to AIDS (years)
15-24	12.5 (12.1-12.9)	11.0 (10.7-11.7)
25-34	10.9 (10.6-11.3)	9.8 (9.5-10.1)
35-44	9.1 (8.7-9.5)	8.6 (8.2-9.0)
45-54	7.9 (7.4-8.5)	7.7 (7.1-8.6)
55-64	6.1 (5.5-7.0)	6.3 (5.5-7.2)
≥65	4.0 (3.4-4.6)	5.0 (4.0-6.2)

Adapted from Concerted Action on SeroConversion to AIDS and Death in Europe. *Time from HIV-1 seroconversion to AIDS and death before widespread use of highly-active antiretroviral therapy: a collaborative re-analysis. Collaborative Group on AIDS Incubation and HIV Survival including the CASCADE EU Concerted Action.* Lancet. 2000 Apr 1;355(9210):1131-7.

Patient Education

- The CD4 cell count and HIV viral load are the two markers that provide information on the degree of current immunocompromise and the risk of disease progression.

- The lower the CD4 count, the higher the risk of AIDS-related illness.

- In asymptomatic persons, CD4 count is the major indicator for initiation of antiretroviral therapy.

- A low HIV viral load is associated with slower immune deterioration; a high viral load is associated with quicker immune deterioration.

- Older individuals may have a poorer response to therapy; earlier initiation of therapy may be considered for older patients.

References

- Collaboration of Observational HIV Epidemiological Research Europe (COHERE) Study Group. *Response to combination antiretroviral therapy: variation by age.* AIDS. 2008 Jul 31;22(12):1463-73.

- Collins KL, Nabel GJ. *Naturally attenuated HIV: lessons for AIDS vaccines and treatment.* N Engl J Med. 1999 Jun 3;340(22):1756-7.

- Concerted Action on SeroConversion to AIDS and Death in Europe. *Time from HIV-1 seroconversion to AIDS and death before widespread use of highly-active antiretroviral therapy: a collaborative re-analysis. Collaborative Group on AIDS Incubation and HIV Survival including the CASCADE EU Concerted Action.* Lancet. 2000 Apr 1;355(9210):1131-7.

- Connor RI, Sheridan KE, Ceradini D, et al. *Change in coreceptor use coreceptor use correlates with disease progression in HIV-1-infected individuals.* J Exp Med. 1997 Feb 17;185(4):621-8.

- Deeks SG, Barbour JD, Martin, JN, et al. *Sustained CD4+ T cell response after virologic failure of protease inhibitor-based regimens in patients with human immunodeficiency virus infection.* J Infect Dis. 2000 Mar;181(3):946-53.

- Deeks SG, Wrin T, Liegler T, et al. *Virologic and immunologic consequences of discontinuing combination antiretroviral-drug therapy in HIV-infected patients with detectable viremia.* N Engl J Med. 2001 Feb 15;344(7):472-80.

- Egger M, May M, Chene G, et al. *Prognosis of HIV-1-infected patients starting highly active antiretroviral therapy: a collaborative analysis of prospective studies.* Lancet. 2002 Jul 13;360(9327):119-29.

- European AIDS Clinical Society. *Clinical Management and Treatment of HIV-Infected Adults in Europe. English Version 5; November 2009.* Available at www.europeanaidsclinicalsociety.org/guidelines.asp.

- Kirchhoff F, Greenough TC, Brettler DB, et al. *Brief report: absence of intact nef sequences in a long-term survivor with nonprogressive HIV-1 infection.* N Engl J Med. 1995 Jan 26;332(4):228-32.

- Kuller L, SMART Study Group. *Elevated levels of interleukin-6 and D-dimer are associated with an increased risk of death in patients with HIV.* In: Program and Abstracts of the 15th Conference on Retroviruses and Opportunistic Infections; Boston; February 3-6, 2008. Abstract 139.

- Lederman MM, Rodriquez B, Sieg S. *Immunopathogenesis of HIV Infection.* In: Coffey S, Volberding PA, eds. *HIV InSite Knowledge Base* [online textbook]. San Francisco: UCSF Center for HIV Information; January 2006.

- Mellors JW, Rinaldo CR Jr, Gupta P, et al. *Prognosis in HIV-1 infection predicted by the quantity of virus in plasma.* Science. 1996;272:1167-70.

- Rodríguez B, Sethi AK, Cheruvu VK, et al. *Predictive value of plasma HIV RNA level on rate of CD4 T-cell decline in untreated HIV infection.* JAMA. 2006 Sep 27;296(12):1498-506.

- Sterne JA, May M, Costagliola D, et al; When to Start Consortium. *Timing of initiation of antiretroviral therapy in AIDS-free HIV-1-infected patients: a collaborative analysis of 18 HIV cohort studies.* Lancet. 2009 Apr 18;373(9672):1352-63.

- U.S. Department of Health and Human Services. *Guidelines for the Use of Antiretroviral Agents in HIV-1-Infected Adults and Adolescents.* January 10, 2011. Available at www.aidsinfo.nih.gov/guidelines/.

Primary HIV Infection

Background

Primary HIV infection refers to the very early stages of HIV infection, or the interval from initial infection to the time that antibody to HIV is detectable. During this stage of HIV infection, patients typically have symptoms of acute HIV seroconversion illness, very high HIV RNA levels (>100,000 copies/mL), and negative or indeterminate HIV antibody test results.

Diagnosing patients with primary HIV infection is a clinical challenge. The symptoms of primary HIV are nonspecific, and although many patients seek medical care for symptoms of HIV seroconversion illness, the diagnosis commonly is missed at initial presentation. The difficulties involve recognizing the clinical presentation of acute HIV infection and testing patients appropriately. In HIV treatment facilities, clinicians generally do not see patients with primary HIV infection unless they are referred with the diagnosis already established. In other health care settings, clinicians may not be familiar with the signs and symptoms of acute HIV infection and often do not consider this diagnosis. Despite the difficulties, recognizing primary HIV infection in symptomatic patients is essential. Early diagnosis provides an opportunity for early linkage to HIV care and may decrease future HIV transmission by newly identified patients, who are particularly infectious during early untreated HIV infection.

After infection with HIV, it takes a median of 25 days before the HIV antibody test indicates positive results; in some individuals, it may be several months before seroconversion occurs. Persons with known exposures to HIV, whether occupational or not, should be monitored closely beginning at about 3 weeks after exposure (routine monitoring at 6 weeks, 3 months, and 6 months after exposure to HIV is likely to result in delayed diagnosis of HIV infection). For information on postexposure prophylaxis, see chapters *Nonoccupational Postexposure Prophylaxis* and *Occupational Postexposure Prophylaxis*.

S: Subjective

Approximately two thirds of patients infected with HIV develop symptoms of acute HIV infection, a condition known as acute retroviral syndrome. Symptoms typically appear 2-6 weeks after exposure to HIV and generally include several of the following:

- Fever (present in 80-90%)
- Rash, often erythematous and maculopapular
- Fatigue
- Pharyngitis (with or without exudate)
- Generalized lymphadenopathy
- Urticaria
- Myalgia/arthralgia
- Anorexia
- Mucocutaneous ulceration
- Headache, retroorbital pain
- Neurologic symptoms (e.g., aseptic meningitis, radiculitis, myelitis, cranial nerve palsies)

This symptomatic phase usually persists for 2-4 weeks or less, although lymphadenopathy may last longer. Symptoms and signs are similar to those of many other illnesses, including other viral syndromes, influenza, and mononucleosis. However, generalized lymphadenopathy, rash, thrush, and mucosal ulceration are sufficiently uncommon in most adult febrile illnesses that, when present, they should trigger suspicion of acute HIV infection. It is important to obtain a history of recent risk behaviors from all patients who present with symptoms consistent with acute HIV infection and to have a low threshold for testing for acute HIV infection. Common laboratory findings include leukopenia, thrombocytopenia, and mild transaminase elevations.

O: Objective

HIV antibody tests usually show positive results within 4 weeks after an infection occurs. However, during the symptomatic phase of HIV seroconversion, these HIV antibody tests may still indicate negative or indeterminate serostatus. For patients who have symptoms consistent with seroconversion illness and a recent risk history for HIV exposure, an HIV RNA (viral load) test should be performed, in addition to the HIV antibody test, as part of the evaluation. Patients with negative antibody test results but high HIV viral loads (>100,000 copies/mL) can be considered to be infected with HIV, although the antibody test should be repeated later to confirm seroconversion. False-positive HIV viral loads have been reported in approximately 5% of cases involving patients who were tested after HIV exposures. A low viral load (<1,000 copies/mL) usually indicates a false-positive result at this stage, because viral loads typically run very high (i.e., >100,000 copies/mL and, often, millions of copies/mL) during the acute infection stage. Patients who have indeterminate HIV antibody test results, low HIV viral loads, and no clear HIV risk factors or symptoms of primary HIV infection should undergo repeat antibody testing in 4-6 weeks, without other interventions. For patients without significant risk factors, indeterminate antibody results rarely indicate evolving seroconversion.

A/P: Assessment and Plan

Patients with primary HIV infection will need additional medical evaluation, baseline laboratory testing, and intensive support, counseling, and education about HIV infection. See chapters *Initial History, Initial Physical Examination,* and *Initial and Interim Laboratory and Other Tests* for detailed information on the initial evaluation of HIV-infected patients.

Laboratory

The initial laboratory work should include the following:

- CD4 cell count and HIV viral load.

- A baseline HIV genotype test for all patients with primary HIV infection, even those who do not choose to start antiretroviral treatment (ART). In some cities in the United States and Europe, 6-16% of infected individuals have acquired HIV virus strains with mutations that confer resistance to antiretroviral medications. These resistance mutations may be identified by early resistance testing, but may not be detectable later. (See chapter *Resistance Testing.*)

- Patients diagnosed on the basis of HIV RNA should have an HIV antibody test repeated in 4-6 weeks to confirm seroconversion and HIV infection.

Treatment

It is reasonable to consider starting ART for patients with acute HIV infection, because some limited evidence suggests that treatment initiated during primary HIV infection may preserve HIV-specific immune function that would otherwise be lost as the infection progresses. However, it is not clear whether initiating early treatment yields long-term immunologic, virologic, or clinical benefits. The potential advantages of ART for primary infection must be weighed against the possibility of short- and long-term toxicities, the possibility of developing drug resistance, and the adherence challenges associated with starting ART quickly for newly diagnosed patients. These issues are complex, and consultation with an HIV expert or referral to a clinical trial is recommended. Issues concerning the possible treatment of primary HIV infection are reviewed in the U.S. Department of Health and Human Services *Guidelines for the Use of Antiretroviral Agents in HIV-1-Infected Adults and Adolescents.*

For pregnant women with acute or recent HIV, the risk of perinatal HIV transmission is very high; thus, ART should be started as early as possible to try to prevent infection of the infant (see chapter *Reducing Maternal-Infant HIV Transmission*).

For patients who opt to start therapy during primary HIV infection, the choice of agents and the recommendations for monitoring are the same as those for the treatment of patients with chronic HIV infection (see chapter *Antiretroviral Therapy*). The initial goal of therapy in primary HIV infection is to suppress the HIV viral load to undetectable levels.

Patient Education

- Patients with primary HIV infection need support and counseling, as do all newly diagnosed patients.

- Intensive education about HIV infection, the course of disease progression, prognosis, and the risks and benefits of ART must be undertaken.

- Counseling patients about safer sex and drug injection techniques, as indicated, is especially important because these patients may have ongoing high-risk behaviors for HIV transmission and because they may

be highly infectious during the primary infection period. (See chapter *Preventing HIV Transmission/Prevention with Positives* for more information about patient support and counseling in these areas.)

References

- Kassutto S, Rosenberg ES. *Primary HIV type 1 infection.* Clin Infect Dis. 2004 May 15;38(10):1447-53.

- Pilcher CD, Tien HC, Eron JJ Jr, et al.; Quest Study; Duke-UNC-Emory Acute HIV Consortium. *Brief but efficient: acute HIV infection and the sexual transmission of HIV.* J Infect Dis. 2004 May 15;189(10):1785-92.

- Schacker T, Collier AC, Hughes J, et al. *Clinical and epidemiologic features of primary HIV infection.* Ann Intern Med. 1996 Aug 15;125(4):257-64.

- U.S. Department of Health and Human Services. *Guidelines for the Use of Antiretroviral Agents in HIV-1-Infected Adults and Adolescents.* January 10, 2011. Available at www.aidsinfo.nih.gov/guidelines/.

- Zetola NM, Pilcher CD. *Diagnosis and management of acute HIV infection.* Infect Dis Clin North Am. 2007 Mar;21(1):19-48, vii.

Rapid HIV Testing

Background

About 1.5 million people are thought to be living with HIV in the United States, and it has been estimated that about 20% of these individuals are unaware of their HIV serostatus. Almost 56,000 new HIV infections occur in the United States each year. It is important to identify persons who are infected with HIV, in order both to link them to health care services and to reduce the risk that they will unknowingly transmit HIV to others.

The U.S. Centers for Disease Control and Prevention recommends routine voluntary HIV screening for all adults, adolescents, and pregnant women. Nevertheless, many people are reluctant to be tested. Rapid HIV testing is one tool that makes it much easier for individuals to be tested for HIV and to obtain their test results promptly and reliably. Results of standard HIV tests typically are not available until about 1 week after the test, and clients are required to return for a second visit in order to obtain their results. Because of this, many people do not return to learn their results. With rapid HIV testing, clients can be tested and receive their results during a single visit. Rapid testing can allow immediate referrals to engage patients in medical care; it also makes possible referrals for urgent treatment, such as for pregnant women, and allows quick decisions to be made in a number of clinical situations, such as assessment for postexposure prophylaxis.

Clients and Settings for Rapid Testing

Rapid HIV testing is recommended for use in settings in which the availability of rapid HIV test results would influence medical care immediately, or as a routine screening tool in settings where HIV prevalence is high or clients are not likely to return for the results of HIV tests. These settings include labor and delivery facilities (to allow intervention to reduce the risk of perinatal HIV transmission in women with undocumented or unknown HIV status), prenatal care facilities for women who present late in pregnancy, hospital emergency departments, urgent care and acute care clinics, sexually transmitted infection clinics, drug treatment clinics, hospitals, and other clinical care or testing sites. Rapid HIV testing is being implemented in employee health departments at hospitals as part of evaluation for and provision of postexposure prophylaxis. In addition, rapid testing is becoming common in nonclinical settings in high-risk jurisdictions such as jails and mobile health service vans, and in community outreach programs.

Rapid HIV Tests

The U.S. Food and Drug Administration (FDA) has approved six rapid tests for use in the United States (Table 1). Federal regulations under the Clinical Laboratory Improvement Amendments (CLIA) program categorize tests as waived, moderate complexity, or high complexity. Four rapid tests are approved as CLIA-waived tests, meaning that they may be performed at the point of care after appropriate staff training and with procedures in place to insure quality control. These tests use whole blood or oral fluid and require a few simple steps to perform. Other rapid tests are "nonwaived" tests and must be performed in laboratories. Results for rapid tests performed at the point of care are available in less than 30 minutes; results for those done in a laboratory should be available within 1 hour.

Table 1. FDA-Approved Rapid HIV Antibody Screening Tests

Test	Specimen Type	CLIA Category	Sensitivity (95% CI*)	Specificity (95% CI*)	Manufacturer	Approved for HIV-2 Detection
OraQuick Advance Rapid HIV-1/2 Antibody Test	Oral fluid	Waived	99.3% (98.4-99.7)	99.8% (99.6-99.9)	OraSure Technologies (www.orasure.com)	Yes
	Whole blood (fingerstick or venipuncture)	Waived	99.6% (98.5-99.9)	100% (99.7-100)		
	Plasma	Moderate complexity	99.6% (98.9-99.8)	99.9% (99.6-99.9)		
Uni-Gold Recombigen HIV	Whole blood (fingerstick or venipuncture)	Waived	100% (99.5-100)	99.7% (99.0-100)	Trinity Biotech (www.unigoldhiv.com)	No
	Serum/plasma	Moderate complexity	100% (99.5-100)	99.8% (99.3-100)		
Reveal G-3 Rapid HIV-1 Antibody Test	Serum	Moderate complexity	99.8% (99.2-100)	99.1% (98.8-99.4)	MedMira (www.medmira.com)	No
	Plasma		99.8% (99.0-100)	98.6% (98.4-98.8)		
MultiSpot HIV-1/HIV-2 Rapid Test	Serum	Moderate complexity	100% (99.9-100)	99.9% (99.8-100)	BioRad Laboratories (www.biorad.com)	Yes, differentiates HIV-1 and HIV-2
	Plasma					
Clearview HIV 1/2 STAT-PAK	Whole blood (fingerstick or venipuncture)	Waived	99.7% (98.9-100)	99.9% (99.6-100)	Inverness Medical Professional Diagnostics (www.invernessmedicalpd.com)	Yes
	Serum, plasma	Nonwaived	99.7% (98.9-100)	99.9% (99.6-100)		
Clearview COMPLETE HIV 1/2	Whole blood (fingerstick or venipuncture)	Waived	99.7% (98.9-100)	99.9% (99.6-100)	Inverness Medical Professional Diagnostics (www.invernessmedicalpd.com)	Yes
	Serum, plasma	Nonwaived				

* CI = confidence interval

Adapted from CDC and Health Research and Education Trust (HRET), FDA-Approved Rapid HIV Antibody Screening Tests, February 4, 2008. Available at www.cdc.gov/hiv/topics/testing/rapid/rt-comparison.htm.

Interpreting Rapid Test Results

All FDA-approved rapid tests are highly sensitive and specific, as shown in Table 1, and are as accurate as a standard enzyme-linked immunosorbent assay (ELISA). The negative predictive value of all rapid HIV tests is close to 100%. This means that a client who receives a negative rapid test result almost assuredly is not infected, barring recent exposures (e.g., sexual contact or needle sharing with an infected person within the past 3 months). A client with a history of recent HIV risk behaviors or possible exposures should repeat the HIV test in the near future, because it may take up to 3 months for HIV antibodies to be detectable after infection with HIV.

The positive predictive value of a single positive rapid HIV test result depends on the specificity of the test and the HIV prevalence in the community. The high specificity of the rapid tests (Table 1) means that, if a test result is positive, the likelihood that a client is truly HIV infected depends on the local HIV prevalence. In a population with a high HIV prevalence, a positive rapid test result is likely a true positive, but in a population with a low HIV prevalence, that result has a greater chance of being a false positive. For this reason, every positive rapid HIV test result is considered a preliminary result and must be confirmed by either Western blot or immunofluorescence assay (IFA), just as a positive standard ELISA result must be confirmed in this way.

Information for the Client

Educating the Client Before Testing

It is important to offer rapid HIV testing as part of a health screening, to educate clients about HIV infection and about the test, and to give them an opportunity to ask questions and to decline testing. The provider should reassure clients that the rapid HIV test is just as accurate as the standard HIV test. The provider should emphasize that a second test always is performed in order to confirm a positive rapid test result. When possible, rapid testing should be made available during a regular office visit so that clients do not face additional waiting time.

Giving Reactive (Preliminary Positive) Rapid Test Results

Example of simple language to use outside labor and delivery settings

The following wording is suggested when the client's rapid test result is positive:

"Your preliminary test result was positive, but we won't know for sure if you are infected with HIV until we get the results from your confirmatory test. In the meantime, you should take precautions to avoid transmitting the virus. This means protecting sex partners from possible exposure (using condoms, for example), not sharing injection drug needles or syringes, and so forth."

Emphasize the importance of a confirmatory test, arrange for the confirmatory test to be performed as soon as possible, and schedule a return visit for the patient to receive the test result.

Language to use in labor and delivery settings

The following wording is suggested when the client's rapid test result is positive:

"Your preliminary HIV screening result was positive. You may have HIV infection. We need to do a second (or confirmatory) test, but it is important to start medication to reduce the risk of passing HIV to your baby while we wait for the result. It is important to delay breast-feeding until we have the second test result."

Follow-Up for Results of Confirmatory Tests

Clinical sites that offer rapid HIV testing should have a protocol for conveying the results of confirmatory HIV tests to clients. Rapid testing sites should either provide this service in-house or have mechanisms in place for referring clients to community-based HIV services. For example, when women have preliminary positive results on tests done during labor and delivery, confirmatory test results may be sent to their obstetrician, but often may be sent to the local health department. These women should be given appointments specifically for receiving their confirmatory test results. Clinicians should be familiar with community resources for referring clients with positive rapid test results. All clients with confirmed positive HIV test results should be referred for HIV care; testing sites should establish reliable referral pathways to qualified HIV care providers.

Section 2: Testing and Assessment

Patient Education

In general settings and in situations not involving labor and delivery, advise patients of the following:

- Rapid HIV testing is an important component of health screening. Learning early that they have HIV infection can help patients better maintain their health.

- Knowing that they have HIV infection can help patients take precautions to prevent transmission of HIV to others.

- Patients can refuse an HIV test, and it will not affect the care they receive.

- The results from the rapid tests are available at the same visit, usually in less than 1 hour.

- The rapid test is very accurate — as accurate as the standard HIV test.

- If the rapid test result is positive, a second, confirmatory test always is done in order to provide assurance that the rapid test result was accurate.

- It is important that patients return for the results of the confirmatory test.

- If a patient's rapid test result is negative, that patient almost certainly does not have HIV infection, but the test may not detect recent infection.

- Test results are kept confidential. However, if a confirmatory test result is positive, most state laws require that information to be reported to the health department.

- There are clinics and other resources to help patients obtain more information as well as counseling, care, or treatment. The provider should provide specific referrals to these.

References

- Beckwith CG, Atunah-Jay A, Cohen J, et al. *Feasibility and acceptability of rapid HIV testing in jail.* AIDS Patient Care STDS. 2007 Jan;21(1):41-7.

- Centers for Disease Control and Prevention. *Rapid HIV Testing.* Available at www.cdc.gov/hiv/topics/testing/rapid. Accessed June 30, 2010.

- Centers for Disease Control and Prevention. *Rapid HIV testing in emergency departments—three U.S. sites, January 2005-March 2006.* MMWR Morb Mortal Wkly Rep. 2007 Jun 22;56(24):597-601.

- Colfax GN, Buchbinder SP, Cornelisse PG, et al. *Sexual risk behaviors and implications for secondary HIV transmission during and after HIV seroconversion.* AIDS. 2002 Jul 26;16(11):1529-35.

- Hall HI, Song R, Rhodes P, et al.; HIV Incidence Surveillance Group. *Estimation of HIV incidence in the United States.* JAMA. 2008 Aug 6;300(5):520-9.

- Hutchinson AB, Corbie-Smith G, Thomas SR, et al. *Understanding the patient's perspective on rapid and routine HIV testing in an inner-city urgent care center.* AIDS Educ Prev. 2004 Apr;16(2):101-14.

- Lubelchek R, Kroc K, Hota B, et al. *The role of rapid vs conventional human immunodeficiency virus testing for inpatients: effects on quality of care.* Arch Intern Med. 2005 Sep 26;165(17):1956-60.

- Marks G, Crepaz N, Senterfitt JW, et al. *Meta-analysis of high-risk sexual behavior in persons aware and unaware they are infected with HIV in the United States: implications for HIV prevention programs.* J Acquir Immune Defic Syndr. 2005 Aug 1;39(4):446-53.

- U.S. Preventive Services Task Force. *Screening for HIV: recommendation statement.* Am Fam Physician. 2005 Dec 1;72(11):2287-92.

Resistance Testing

Background

Genotype and phenotype testing for resistance currently is commercially available for all nucleoside reverse transcriptase inhibitors (NRTIs), nonnucleoside reverse transcriptase inhibitors (NNRTIs), and protease inhibitors (PIs) that have been approved by the U.S. Food and Drug Administration (FDA). In addition, standardized genotype testing is commercially available for raltegravir (an integrase inhibitor) and enfuvirtide (a fusion inhibitor). Resistance tests for CCR5 antagonists are not commercially available.

Neither genotype nor phenotype predicts which antiretroviral (ARV) drugs will be active in a particular patient, only ARVs that are not likely to be active. Nevertheless, studies comparing the use of resistance testing with expert opinion alone have shown that resistance testing can improve virologic control of HIV. Resistance testing is used to guide subsequent treatment for patients whose antiretroviral therapy (ART) is failing and for those whose viral load is not completely suppressed after starting therapy. It also is used to select an initial regimen that is likely to be effective for patients who have never been treated, and it is recommended for all patients with HIV infection (both acute and chronic) upon entry into care, whether or not ART is to be initiated. In addition, resistance testing is recommended for pregnant women who are not on ART and for those who are on ART but have a detectable HIV viral load.

Genotype Tests

Genotype testing works by amplifying and sequencing HIV taken from a patient to look for mutations in the HIV reverse transcriptase, protease, integrase, or envelope genes that are known to correlate with clinical resistance to ARV drugs. Genotype tests generally can detect mutations in plasma samples with HIV RNA levels of >1,000 copies/mL, but sometimes are successful with viral loads of 500-1,000 copies/mL. Species representing 20% or more of the amplified product usually can be detected by current techniques, but minor species may not be detected. Resistance mutations that developed in the past during treatment with certain ARV medications may be archived as minor species and become invisible to genotype testing (as early as 4-6 weeks) after the drug is discontinued. These resistance mutations may reemerge and cause drug failure, however, if the previous drug is used again. By contrast, mutations acquired at the time of infection (from a transmitted virus that was already resistant) appear to persist for years, although the duration is not known

precisely and may vary by mutation.

A genotype test takes 1-2 weeks to complete. The results are reported as a list of the mutations detected; most reports also include an interpretation that indicates the drug resistance likely to be conferred by those mutations (see "Modifying Factors," below, for a discussion of the limitations of resistance testing).

Note that the standard genotype tests detect mutations that may affect reverse transcriptase inhibitors and PIs; a specific genotype for the integrase inhibitor (or fusion inhibitor) class must be ordered if there is concern for resistance to this class. Also, there are no commercially available tests for resistance to CCR5 antagonists. For patients with virologic failure while taking a CCR5 antagonist, a coreceptor tropism assay should be considered (though the result does not rule out the possibility of resistance to CCR5 antagonists).

Genotype results must be interpreted carefully. Because mutations can become invisible to the genotype testing process when the selective pressure of a drug is removed, a thorough

ARV history, a review of any past resistance tests, and expert clinical assessment are necessary to put the results of a genotype test in proper perspective and to identify options for further treatment (see "Limits of Resistance Testing," below). A compilation of the most common HIV mutations selected by the three classes of antiretroviral agents is available at hiv-web.lanl.gov. Other resources useful in understanding resistance testing and interpreting test results include the information complied by International AIDS Society — USA (www.iasusa.org/resistance_mutations/index.html), and the Stanford University HIV Drug Resistance Database (hivdb.stanford.edu).

A "virtual phenotype" is a genotype that is compared with a databank of patient samples that have been analyzed by paired genotype and phenotype testing. The patient's genotype is matched to a banked genotype, and the patient's phenotype is then predicted on the basis of the phenotypes paired to the banked genotype. A virtual phenotype can be completed in the same amount of time as a genotype. Results are reported as a genotype (listing the mutations detected) as well as a predicted fold change in the 50% inhibitory concentration (IC50) of each drug to the patient's virus (see "Phenotype Tests," below). The predicted susceptibility of the patient's virus to each drug is then reported, based on biologic and clinical cutoffs.

Phenotype Tests

Phenotype testing works by splicing the HIV reverse transcriptase and HIV protease genes from a patient's virus into a standardized laboratory strain, which is then grown in the presence of escalating concentrations of ARV drugs. The test measures the IC50 of each drug against the virus in vitro. Results are reported as fold change in IC50, as compared with a drug-susceptible control strain or with a previous test of the same patient's blood. The predicted susceptibility of the patient's virus to each drug is then reported, based on what is known about the correlation between

fold change in IC50 of that drug and clinical resistance. As with genotype testing, the phenotype may not be able to detect resistance if the HIV RNA is low (<1,000 copies/mL) and may not detect minor species Therefore, a thorough history of ARV use and resistance tests, as well as expert interpretation, are essential for determining the significance of the results (see "Limits of Resistance Testing," below). A phenotype takes 2-3 weeks to complete.

Choosing Between Genotype and Phenotype

Genotype testing is faster and cheaper than phenotype testing, and it can detect emerging resistance, that is, virus with a mixture of strains of which some may be sensitive and some may be resistant to a given drug, as long as they are present in sufficient quantity. It is therefore generally recommended (including by the U.S. Department of Health and Human Services [DHHS]) for ART-naive patients and for patients whose first or second ART regimens are failing. The DHHS recommends adding phenotype testing when patients are suspected of having complicated or multidrug resistance patterns (for example, in the setting of extensive prior ART), or when patients are found to have such patterns on genotype testing (especially resistance to PIs).

Using Genotype and Phenotype Tests at the Same Time

Genotype and phenotype tests have a few complementary properties that may, in some circumstances, make it desirable to use both tests at the same time. This strategy is especially advantageous when trying to devise a regimen for patients who have been exposed to many ARV agents and have few remaining treatment options, and for whom the development of additional resistance could be particularly dangerous. For example, early mutations may appear on a genotype before increases in inhibitory concentrations are detectable on a phenotype. Phenotype testing can detect loss or gain of drug efficacy caused by complex interactions of mutations that, by themselves, would not be predictive. In some cases, results of the genotype and the phenotype may be discordant; in these cases consultation with an expert is recommended.

Recommendations for Resistance Testing

An overview of when genotype and phenotype testing is and is not recommended is presented in Table 1.

Table 1. Resistance Testing Recommendations

Clinical Setting/Recommendation	Rationale
Recommended	
Acute or primary HIV infection • Genotype	• Determine whether drug-resistant virus was transmitted, to help design an initial regimen or to change a regimen accordingly. • If ART is deferred, consider repeating genotype at the time of ART initiation.
Chronic HIV infection before starting ART • Genotype	• Determine whether drug-resistant virus was transmitted to help design an initial regimen. • Perform upon entry to care (as close to the time of infection as possible), because transmitted drug-resistant virus is more likely to be detected earlier in the course of HIV infection. • If ART is deferred, consider repeating genotype at the time of ART initiation. • Consider integrase genotypic resistance assay if integrase inhibitor resistance is a concern.
Virologic failure during ART • Genotype if failure of 1st or 2nd regimen • Both phenotype and genotype if multiple prior regimens, suspicion of mutations to multiple ARVs (especially PIs), or if evidence of such mutations on genotype	• Determine the role of resistance in drug failure and optimize the selection of active drugs for the new regimen, if indicated. • Perform while patient is taking ARVs, or ≤4 weeks after discontinuing ARVs. • If virologic failure on integrase inhibitor or fusion inhibitor, obtain specific genotypic testing for resistance to these to determine whether to continue them.
Suboptimal suppression or viral load	• Determine role of resistance: identify active drugs for new regimen.
Pregnant women • Genotype or phenotype, depending on treatment history (as above)	• Before initiation of ART or prophylaxis. • For all on ART with detectable HIV RNA levels. • Optimize the selection of active drugs for ARV regimen.
Not Usually Recommended	
After discontinuation (>4 weeks) of ARVs	• Assist in selecting optimal regimen to achieve maximal viral suppression.
	• Drug-resistance mutations may decrease in number and become undetectable on assays.
Plasma viral load <500 HIV RNA copies/mL	• Resistance assays are likely to be unsuccessful in patients with HIV RNA <500 copies/mL, because of the low number of RNA copies. In those with levels >500 but <1,000 copies/mL, testing may fail but can be considered.

Adapted from U.S. Department of Health and Human Services. *Guidelines for the Use of Antiretroviral Agents in HIV-1-Infected Adults and Adolescents;* Table 4. January 10, 2011.

Antiretroviral-Naive Patients

With treatment-naive patients, resistance testing may reveal resistance mutations that were acquired at the time of infection, through infection with a strain of HIV that had already developed ARV resistance. Current guidelines recommend genotype testing for recently infected patients and for ARV-naive, chronically infected patients before initiation of therapy. It is important to test as early as possible in the course of HIV infection, to increase the likelihood of detecting transmitted mutations. The rationale for resistance testing in ARV-naive patients is twofold: 1) The prevalence of primary resistance is substantial, particularly in locations with a high prevalence of persons taking ART; and 2) Unknowingly starting a patient on ARV medications to which his or her virus is already resistant may risk failure of the initial regimen, rapid acquisition of additional resistance mutations, and curtailment of future treatment options.

Limits of Resistance Testing

As discussed above, drug-resistant HIV evolves in response to selective pressure applied by the ARV drugs in the patient's system. Specific resistance mutations develop in response to the pressure exerted by specific drugs (M184V, for example, evolves in response to lamivudine or emtricitabine). The presence of viral resistance suggests that a particular drug (and drugs with similar resistance patterns, or cross-resistance) is unlikely to be successful in suppressing viral replication.

In contrast, the absence of resistance to a drug on a genotype or phenotype test does not necessarily indicate that the drug will be effective, particularly if that drug (or drugs sharing cross-resistance) has been used previously. If a particular drug is discontinued, the viral strains harboring the mutations that confer resistance to that drug may decrease below the threshold of detection by the resistance assay, so the resistance test may not reveal certain resistance mutations. In such situations, minority populations of resistant viruses may exist in reservoirs and may emerge rapidly under selective pressure if that drug is restarted, or if drugs with similar or overlapping resistance patterns are used. The implications of archived mutations are twofold: 1) Resistance tests are most reliable while the patient is still taking the failing regimen; and 2) Resistance testing should be interpreted in the context of both the drugs that the patient was taking at the time of the test and the drugs that the patient had been exposed to previously (i.e., the patient's ARV history). In addition, it is important to review any previous resistance tests, which may show resistance mutations that were not revealed on subsequent testing.

Resistance Testing in Patients with Virologic Failure

As discussed in the chapter *Antiretroviral Therapy*, factors other than resistance may cause failure of ART; these include nonadherence, drug-drug interactions, and malabsorption. Therefore, before assuming drug failure, it is important to assess the causes of ARV regimen failure. If resistance is suspected, resistance testing should be done while the patient is taking the failing regimen, for the reasons noted above.

Patient Education

- Advise patients of the following:

  - Resistance testing can improve the likelihood of virologic control of HIV.

  - Most treatment guidelines recommend resistance testing in certain circumstances.

  - Both genotype and phenotype testing can detect resistance only if it exists in at least 20% of the viral species present in a patient (known as the dominant species). Minor species may harbor resistance that remains undetected by either test.

  - In general, a patient's viral load must be at least 1,000 copies/mL for either test to be reliable, although samples with >500 copies/mL sometimes can be analyzed.

  - Resistance tests are most reliable when performed while a patient is still taking a failing regimen, or within 4 weeks after stopping.

  - Neither test predicts which drugs will be active in a particular patient, only drugs that are not likely to be active.

References

- Bartlett JG, Gallant JE. *2009-2010 Medical Management of HIV Infection.* Baltimore: Johns Hopkins University Division of Infectious Diseases; 2009. Available at www.hopkins-aids.edu/publications/. Accessed June 30, 2010. [Registration required.]

- Shafer RW. *Genotypic Testing for HIV-1 Drug Resistance.* In: Coffey S, Volberding PA, eds. *HIV InSite Knowledge Base* [textbook online]; San Francisco: UCSF Center for HIV Information; April 2004. Available at hivinsite.ucsf.edu/InSite?page=kb-03-02-07. Accessed June 30, 2010.

- U.S. Department of Health and Human Services. *Guidelines for the Use of Antiretroviral Agents in HIV-1-Infected Adults and Adolescents.* January 10, 2011. Available at www.aidsinfo.nih.gov/guidelines/.

Karnofsky Performance Scale

Background

The Karnofsky Performance Scale is an assessment tool intended to assist clinicians and caretakers in gauging a patient's functional status and ability to carry out activities of daily living.

It is important to assess a patient's performance on a regular basis, especially as the effects of HIV progress. Documentation of Karnofsky scores over time may be very useful in following a patient's course of illness, and can help a disabled patient in his/her application for disability benefits. It also is used for some research applications.

Table 1. The Karnofsky Performance Scale

Description	Percent (%)
Normal; no complaints; no evidence of disease	100
Able to carry on normal activity; minor signs or symptoms of disease	90
Normal activity with effort; some signs or symptoms of disease	80
Cares for self; unable to carry on normal activity or do work	70
Requires occasional assistance, but is able to care for most personal needs	60
Requires considerable assistance and frequent medical care	50
Disabled; requires special care and assistance	40
Severely disabled; hospitalization indicated although death not imminent	30
Very sick; hospitalization necessary; requires active support treatment	20
Moribund; fatal processes progressing rapidly	10
Dead	0

Occupational Postexposure Prophylaxis

Background

Health care workers (HCWs) and other employees in medical, public safety, sanitation, and laboratory settings are at risk of occupational exposure to HIV. Although avoiding exposure to HIV is the only reliable way of preventing HIV infection, postexposure prophylaxis (PEP), can reduce the risk of HIV infection in exposed HCWs. PEP is defined as antiretroviral (ARV) therapy that is initiated soon after exposure to HIV with the intention of preventing HIV infection.

This chapter examines the general issues involved with PEP in occupational settings. The information is based on the U.S. Public Health Service (USPHS) guidelines for PEP (see "References," below). For information on PEP for nonoccupational HIV exposures (such as sexual exposure), see chapter *Nonoccupational Postexposure Prophylaxis*. Note that other bloodborne pathogens, particularly hepatitis B virus (HBV) and hepatitis C virus (HCV), also may be transmitted through occupational exposure; it is important to consider these potential infections when assessing occupational exposures. For information on the management of occupational exposures to HBV and HCV, refer to the 2001 USPHS PEP guidelines (see "References," below). In addition, the National Clinicians' Post-Exposure Prophylaxis Hotline (PEPline) is available for telephone consultation at 888-HIV-4911 (888-448-4911).

The risk of HIV infection after exposure depends on several factors that are related to the exposure itself and to the source patient (see below). To make sound PEP recommendations, the clinician must assess the risk of HIV infection from the particular exposure. After this assessment, the clinician and the exposed worker must discuss the possible benefit of PEP (given the risk of HIV transmission from the injury) in relation to the willingness of the exposed worker to adhere to a 28-day course of ARV medicines, the potential toxicity of the regimen, and drug interactions. HCWs who are pregnant at the time of their exposure must weigh the risk of fetal exposure to HIV against the potential teratogenic and other risks of the ARV drugs (it should be noted that pregnancy is not a contraindication to PEP, and that a number of ARVs are recommended for use during pregnancy, based on safety and efficacy data (see chapter *Reducing Maternal-Infant HIV Transmission*). The efficacy of PEP is related to the specific PEP regimen, the timing of PEP, and the exposed worker's level of adherence to the PEP regimen. PEP is most likely to be effective if it is started within hours of an exposure, and outcomes may be compromised as the time from exposure increases. Nevertheless, it may be reasonable to offer PEP up to 72 hours after exposure. Although the optimal duration of PEP is not known; studies support ARV treatment for 28 days.

In the work setting, HIV infection may occur through percutaneous injuries (e.g., needlesticks) or mucocutaneous exposures (e.g., mucous membrane or nonintact skin exposure to blood or other potentially infectious body fluids). The risk of HIV seroconversion after occupational exposure with an HIV-contaminated hollow-bore needle is best described as 0.3%, on average. Another way of describing this to an exposed HCW is that, without PEP, HIV transmission occurs about once in 300 instances of needlestick from a known HIV-infected source patient. In a retrospective case-control study of HCWs with percutaneous exposure to HIV, the following exposure and source patient factors were associated with an increased risk of HIV transmission:

Section 3: Health Maintenance and Disease Prevention

- Large-gauge (<18-gauge) hollow-bore needle
- Deep injury
- Visible blood on the device
- Procedure with needle in a blood vessel
- Terminal AIDS in the source patient

The factor described as "terminal AIDS in the source patient" is considered a surrogate for a source patient with a high HIV viral load (this study was done prior to the routine use of HIV viral load assays); high HIV viral load is known to be a substantial risk factor for HIV transmission.

Compared with percutaneous injury, exposure of infectious body fluids to mucous membranes (e.g., eye or mouth) or to skin with an obvious impairment of integrity (e.g., abrasion or wound) typically involves a lower risk of HIV transmission (the transmission risk for mucous membrane exposure to HIV is approximately 1 in 1,000, and less than 1 in 1,000 for cutaneous exposure). However, mucocutaneous exposures that involve large volumes of blood or other infectious fluid from an HIV-infected patient with a high HIV RNA level or prolonged duration of contact are considered increased-risk exposures.

S: Subjective

An HCW reports possible exposure to HIV through a needlestick injury or mucocutaneous exposure.

Ideally, the HCW immediately decontaminated the injured or exposed skin with soap and water, or flushed the exposed mucous membranes with copious amounts of water or saline. The HCW should report the exposure immediately to appropriate authorities in the health care institution (e.g., the institution's needlestick hotline).

Take a thorough history of the specific exposure, including the type of exposure, the type and amount of body fluid involved, the point of entry or exposure, the time it occurred, the HIV status of the source patient (if known), and HIV risk factors of the source patient (if HIV status is not known).

A: Assessment

Assess potential exposure to HIV (and to HBV and HCV). Consider the HIV status of the source and the characteristics of the exposure to estimate the risk of HIV infection. The decision about whether to offer PEP should be based on the estimated risk of HIV exposure. See Table 1 (percutaneous exposures) and Table 2 (mucocutaneous exposures) for recommendations about PEP.

Table 1. Recommended HIV Postexposure Prophylaxis After Percutaneous Injuries

Exposure Type	HIV Negative	HIV Positive (Class 1)	HIV Positive (Class 2)	Unknown HIV Status	Unknown Source
Infection Status of Source*					
Less Severe (e.g., solid needle, superficial injury)	No PEP warranted	Recommend basic 2-drug PEP	Recommend expanded ≥3-drug PEP	Generally, no PEP warranted; however, consider basic 2-drug PEP for source with HIV risk factors# §	Generally, no PEP warranted; however, consider basic 2-drug PEP if exposure to HIV-infected persons is likely#
More Severe (e.g., large-bore hollow needle, deep puncture, visible blood on device, needle used in patient's artery or vein)	No PEP warranted	Recommend expanded ≥3-drug PEP	Recommend expanded ≥3-drug PEP	Generally, no PEP warranted; however, consider basic 2-drug PEP for source with HIV risk factors# §	Generally, no PEP warranted; however, consider basic 2-drug PEP if exposure to HIV-infected persons is likely# §

* HIV positive (class 1): asymptomatic HIV infection or known low HIV RNA viral load (e.g., <1,500 copies/mL); HIV positive (class 2): symptomatic HIV infection, AIDS, acute seroconversion, or known high viral load; unknown HIV status: for example, a deceased source person with no samples available for HIV testing; unknown source: for example, a needle from a sharps disposal container.

The recommendation "consider PEP" indicates that PEP is optional; a decision to initiate PEP should be based on a discussion between the exposed person and the clinician regarding the risks versus benefits of PEP.

§ If PEP is offered and administered, and the source is later determined to be HIV negative, PEP should be discontinued.

Adapted from U.S. Department of Health and Human Services. *Updated U.S. Public Health Service Guidelines for the Management of Occupational Exposures to HIV and Recommendations for Postexposure Prophylaxis.* MMWR Recomm Rep. 2005 Sep 30; 54(RR09); 1-24. Available at www.aidsinfo.nih.gov/guidelines/.

Table 2. Recommended HIV Postexposure Prophylaxis After Mucous Membrane Exposures and Nonintact Skin Exposures*

Exposure Type	HIV Negative	HIV Positive (Class 1)	HIV Positive (Class 2)	Unknown HIV Status	Unknown Source
Infection Status of Source#					
Small Volume (e.g., a few drops)	No PEP warranted	Consider basic 2-drug PEP§	Recommend basic 2-drug PEP	Generally, no PEP warranted**	Generally, no PEP warranted
Large Volume (e.g., a major blood splash)	No PEP warranted	Recommend basic 2-drug PEP	Recommend expanded ≥3-drug PEP	Generally, no PEP warranted; however, consider basic 2-drug PEP for source with HIV risk factors**§	Generally, no PEP warranted; however, consider basic 2-drug PEP if exposure to HIV-infected persons is likely §

* For skin exposures, follow-up is indicated only if evidence exists of compromised skin integrity (e.g., dermatitis, abrasion, or open wound).

HIV positive (class 1): asymptomatic HIV infection or known low HIV RNA viral load (e.g., <1,500 copies/mL); HIV positive (class 2): symptomatic HIV infection, AIDS, acute seroconversion, or known high viral load; unknown HIV status: for example, a deceased source person with no samples available for HIV testing; unknown source: for example, a needle from a sharps disposal container

§ The recommendation "consider PEP" indicates that PEP is optional; a decision to initiate PEP should be based on a discussion between the exposed person and the clinician regarding the risks versus benefits of PEP.

** If PEP is offered and administered, and the source is later determined to be HIV negative, PEP should be discontinued.

Adapted from U.S. Department of Health and Human Services. *Updated U.S. Public Health Service Guidelines for the Management of Occupational Exposures to HIV and Recommendations for Postexposure Prophylaxis.* MMWR Recomm Rep. 2005 Sep 30; 54(RR09); 1-24. Available at www.aidsinfo.nih.gov/guidelines/.

Section 3: Health Maintenance and Disease Prevention

P: Plan

Laboratory Testing (for the exposed HCW)

- Perform a baseline HIV antibody test.

- Test for other infections transmitted through occupational exposure, particularly hepatitis B (HBV surface antigen, surface antibody, core antibody), and hepatitis C (HCV antibody).

- Obtain complete blood count (CBC), creatinine and estimated glomerular filtration rate (GFR), and hepatic transaminases at baseline, before treatment with ARV medications.

- For women who may be pregnant, perform a pregnancy test.

(The institution should perform appropriate testing of the source patient testing for bloodborne pathogens [e.g., HIV, HBV, and HCV] if the patient's status is unknown.)

Treatment

Consult Table 1 or Table 2 to determine whether the HCW should be offered PEP medications. For occupational exposures to infectious body fluids from an HIV-infected source patient, the USPHS guidelines state that PEP should be either recommended (in most cases) or considered (in the small-volume mucocutaneous exposures), depending on the assessed risk. The assessed risk also helps to determine whether a "basic" two-drug regimen or an "expanded" regimen consisting of three or more drugs should be selected. Other considerations in choosing the medications for a PEP regimen include:

- The likelihood that the source patient's virus is resistant to ARV medication(s)

- Possible drug toxicities for the exposed HCW

- Drug-drug interactions with other medications the HCW may be taking

If the HCW is a candidate for PEP, provide counseling about the potential risks and benefits of PEP. If the HCW elects to start therapy, consider potential regimens (Table 3). **Note that these recommendations are drawn from the 2005 guidelines for occupational PEP but have been adapted to reflect more recent PEP strategies, the availability of newer ARVs, and current DHHS adult treatment guidelines.**

Select a regimen that is likely to be effective but tolerable; consider the potential adverse effects of ARVs. Certain ARVs are not recommended for PEP, including abacavir, delavirdine, nevirapine, and the combination of didanosine + stavudine. The 2005 guidelines list lopinavir/ritonavir as the preferred third agent for the expanded PEP regimen, and it continues to be a commonly used agent. Newer protease inhibitors (i.e., atazanavir, darunavir) or the integrase inhibitor raltegravir may be appropriate for individual HCWs, and should be considered particularly if HCW factors (e.g., comorbidities or interacting drugs) or source patient factors (e.g., concern for resistance) make therapy with lopinavir/ritonavir problematic. Although the 2005 guidelines list it as an alternative agent, efavirenz may have a higher rate of significant adverse effects than other listed agents. Additionally, efavirenz should not be used with pregnant women, because of possible teratogenicity. Refer to the appendix in the updated USPHS guidelines and to the DHHS adult ARV treatment guidelines for more complete information on the dosing, advantages, and disadvantages of the various ARV agents available for PEP. Consider consultation with experts (see "Expert Consultation," below).

Table 3. ARV Options for Occupational Postexposure Prophylaxis of HIV Infection

Basic Regimens with Two Nonnucleoside Reverse Transcriptase Inhibitors
Preferred   • Tenofovir 300 mg once daily + emtricitabine 200 mg once daily (available as Truvada, 1 tablet once daily)   • Zidovudine 300 mg BID + lamivudine 150 mg BID (available as Combivir, 1 tablet BID)
Expanded Regimens (one of the following may be added to a basic regimen)
Protease Inhibitors
Preferred   • Lopinavir/ritonavir (Kaletra) 400/100 mg BID   **Alternative**   • Atazanavir 300 mg once daily + ritonavir 100 mg once daily   • Darunavir 800 mg once daily + ritonavir 100 mg once daily   • Atazanavir 400 mg once daily*
Integrase Inhibitors
Alternative   • Raltegravir 400 mg BID
* Unboosted atazanavir cannot be coadministered with tenofovir (use atazanavir + ritonavir).   Adapted from U.S. Department of Health and Human Services. *Updated U.S. Public Health Service Guidelines for the Management of Occupational Exposures to HIV and Recommendations for Postexposure Prophylaxis.* MMWR Recomm Rep. 2005 Sep 30; 54(RR09); 1-24; and U.S. Department of Health and Human Services. *Guidelines for the Use of Antiretroviral Agents in HIV-1-Infected Adults and Adolescents.* January 10, 2011. Available at www.aidsinfo.nih.gov/guidelines/.

Section 3: Health Maintenance and Disease Prevention

If the HIV status of the source patient is unknown, a rapid HIV test may help in determining the need for PEP (see chapter *Rapid HIV Testing*). Although a positive rapid test result requires confirmation before the individual is diagnosed as HIV infected, for the purposes of PEP, it should be considered a true positive until proven otherwise, and the exposed worker should be counseled accordingly. If, upon further testing, the source patient is determined to be HIV uninfected, PEP can be discontinued. A negative rapid test result is considered reliable unless the source reports recent high-risk HIV exposure or symptoms of primary HIV (see chapters *Rapid HIV Testing* and *Primary HIV Infection*). If a rapid test is not available, PEP is considered "generally not warranted" for exposures involving source patients whose HIV status is unknown. However, PEP can be considered if the source patient has risk factors for HIV infection. PEP should not be delayed (beyond 1-2 hours) while awaiting information about the source patient. PEP is not recommended for exposures to HIV-seronegative source patients.

If the source patient is known or suspected to have infection with HIV that is resistant to ARV medications, seek expert consultation in selecting an appropriate PEP regimen. However, PEP should not be delayed while consultation is being solicited, and it is possible to adjust regimens based on expert advice. Begin ARV prophylaxis as soon as possible after the exposure occurs, preferably within a few hours and no later than 72 hours postexposure. Treatment should be continued for 28 days unless the source person is determined to be HIV uninfected.

Provide counseling about the efficacy of PEP, including the importance of protection against future HIV exposures, timely initiation of PEP medications, adherence to these medications for 28 days, and management of common adverse effects. Counsel exposed workers to use latex barriers with their sex partners until transmission of HIV infection has been ruled out.

Follow-Up

Exposed workers should be evaluated at 1 week for review of all test results. For patients taking PEP, adherence assessment and evaluation of any side effects should be included. At 2 weeks, blood testing (e.g., CBC, creatinine, liver function tests) should be done for patients on a 28-day PEP regimen to monitor for PEP toxicity, as indicated by the particular ARV regimen. PEP is discontinued at 4 weeks, and laboratory studies generally should not be repeated unless there is a need to recheck an abnormal result. Follow-up HIV antibody testing should be done at 6 weeks, 3 months, and 6 months after the exposure. In addition to health education counseling, many exposed workers need emotional support during their follow-up visits.

Symptoms of primary HIV infection such as fever, rash, and lymphadenopathy (see chapter *Primary HIV Infection*) may occur in HCWs who have been infected with HIV through occupational exposure. Exposed HCWs should be counseled about the symptoms of primary HIV infection and instructed to return for reevaluation as soon as possible if symptoms develop. If symptoms consistent with primary HIV appear within 4-6 weeks after an occupational exposure, the HCW should be evaluated immediately (and an HIV RNA test should be obtained if acute HIV infection is suspected). If an HCW is found to be infected with HIV, that individual should be referred immediately to an HIV specialist for further evaluation and care.

Expert Consultation

For consultation on the treatment of occupational exposures to HIV and other bloodborne pathogens, the clinician managing the exposed person can call the National Clinicians' Post-Exposure Prophylaxis Hotline (PEPline) at 888-HIV-4911 (888-448-4911). This service is available 7 days a week, at no charge. (additional information is available at www.nccc.ucsf.edu). PEPline support may be especially useful in challenging situations, such as when drug-resistant HIV strains are suspected to be involved in the exposure or when the HCW is pregnant.

Prophylaxis Against HBV and HCV

Prophylaxis against HBV is recommended for patients with potential exposure to HBV who do not have immunity against HBV. Give hepatitis B immune globulin (HBIG) as a 0.06 mL/kg intramuscular injection and initiate the vaccination series. For patients who received the vaccination series but did not develop protective antibodies (HBV sAb+), give HBIG at the time of the postexposure workup and initiate revaccination; consider repeat of HBIG in 1 month. For patients with immunity to HBV, no treatment is indicated.

For HCV, no prophylactic treatments are recommended. After potential exposure, conduct a baseline HCV antibody test. If the source is known to have HCV infection, consider alanine aminotransferase (ALT) and HCV viral load testing at 4-6 weeks. HCV antibody testing should be repeated at 4-6 months. If HCV seroconversion occurs (indicated by ALT elevation, detectable HCV viral load, or confirmed positive HCV antibody test result), refer the patient to a hepatologist because early treatment of HCV may be indicated.

Addendum: Workplace Obligations

- The health care institution has certain obligations to an exposed employee.* The institution should do the following:

- Evaluate the circumstances of the exposure, the type of fluid, and possible entry points.

- Evaluate the source patient.

- Perform baseline HIV antibody testing of the exposed HCW.

- Counsel the exposed HCW about the possible risks and benefits of PEP.

- Offer or recommend PEP as soon as possible after the exposure, preferably within the first several hours.

- Counsel the HCW about avoiding secondary transmission to others (safer sex and other risk-reduction practices, as indicated).

- Support and maintain the confidentiality of the HCW.

- For an HCW who is taking PEP, monitor for medication toxicity and adherence, and check for drug-drug interactions with other medications the HCW may be taking.

- Repeat HIV testing at 6 weeks, 3 months, and 6 months.

- Report the exposure as required by federal and state regulations (including U.S. Occupational Safety and Health Administration requirements).

* Legal issues vary from state to state. In many states, institutions and clinics have no obligation toward non-employees or students who are exposed to HIV in their settings. In such situations, clinical supervisors or school or university officials often are the first contact for notification. However, everyone working in a health care setting should be familiar with the procedures and financial responsibility for HIV exposure management to avoid delays in HIV PEP treatment.

Patient Education

- Persons who have possible exposures to HIV in the work setting should contact the PEP service of their employer or a qualified medical provider as soon as possible after the exposure, or they should go to an emergency department. Although PEP may be effective if it is started within 72 hours of exposure, the sooner medications are initiated, the better the chance for preventing HIV transmission.

- PEP medications should be taken as directed for the full 28-day course. Adherence to PEP medications is essential for successful treatment.

- PEP recipients should be advised to contact their providers if they experience uncomfortable side effects. Providers may prescribe medications to alleviate the side effects, or they may prescribe different PEP medications.

- Until HIV infection has been ruled out, exposed workers should be advised to use latex barriers to prevent transmission of HIV to their sex partners.

- Exposed HCWs should be counseled about the symptoms of primary HIV infection and instructed to contact their care providers immediately if symptoms develop.

Section 3: Health Maintenance and Disease Prevention

References

- Bassett IV, Freedberg KA, Walensky RP. *Two drugs or three? Balancing efficacy, toxicity, and resistance in postexposure prophylaxis for occupational exposure to HIV.* Clin Infect Dis. 2004 Aug 1;39(3):395-401.

- Cardo DM, Culver DH, Ciesielski CA, et al.; Centers for Disease Control and Prevention Needlestick Surveillance Group. *A case-control study of HIV seroconversion in health care workers after percutaneous exposure.* N Engl J Med. 1997 Nov 20;337(21):1485-90.

- Do AN, Ciesielski CA, Metler RP, et al. *Occupationally acquired human immunodeficiency virus (HIV) infection: national case surveillance data during 20 years of the HIV epidemic in the United States.* Infect Control Hosp Epidemiol. 2003 Feb;24(2):86-96.

- Gerberding JL. *Clinical practice. Occupational exposure to HIV in health care settings.* N Engl J Med. 2003 Feb 27;348(9):826-33.

- Gupta A, Anand S, Sastry J, et al. *High risk for occupational exposure to HIV and utilization of post-exposure prophylaxis in a teaching hospital in Pune, India.* BMC Infect Dis. 2008 Oct 21;8:142.

- Puro V, Francisci D, Sighinolfi L, et al. *Benefits of a rapid HIV test for evaluation of the source patient after occupational exposure of healthcare workers.* J Hosp Infect. 2004 Jun;57(2):179-82.

- U.S. Department of Health and Human Services. *Updated U.S. Public Health Service Guidelines for the Management of Occupational Exposures to HBV, HCV, and HIV and Recommendations for Postexposure Prophylaxis.* MMWR Recomm Rep. 2001 Jun 29;50(RR11);1-42. Available at www.aidsinfo.nih.gov/guidelines/.

- U.S. Department of Health and Human Services. *Updated U.S. Public Health Service Guidelines for the Management of Occupational Exposures to HIV and Recommendations for Postexposure Prophylaxis.* MMWR Recomm Rep. 2005 Sep 30; 54(RR09); 1-24. Available at www.aidsinfo.nih.gov/guidelines/.

- Wang SA, Panlilio AL, Doi PA, et al. *Experience of healthcare workers taking postexposure prophylaxis after occupational HIV exposures: findings of the HIV Postexposure Prophylaxis Registry.* Infect Control Hosp Epidemiol. 2000 Dec;21(12):780-5.

- Zenner D, Tomkins S, Charlett A, et al. *HIV prone occupational exposures: epidemiology and factors associated with initiation of post-exposure prophylaxis.* J Epidemiol Community Health. 2009 May;63(5):373-8.

Nonoccupational Postexposure Prophylaxis

Background

Although avoiding exposure to HIV is the only reliable way of preventing HIV infection, postexposure prophylaxis (PEP) can decrease the risk of infection after exposure to HIV. Antiretroviral (ARV) therapy is an important prophylactic intervention for appropriate persons with nonoccupational exposures (e.g., sexual contact; sharing of injection drug needles or other equipment) as well as those with occupational exposures (e.g., needlesticks). The U.S. Department of Health and Human Services (DHHS) has developed recommendations for nonoccupational PEP (nPEP) based on data from animal models, perinatal clinical trials, and observational studies. Efficacy of nPEP remains hypothetical, and randomized clinical trials are not possible, but nPEP appears to be safe.

Overall, nPEP is more likely to be effective when the exposure is a single episode and nPEP is initiated in a timely manner. It is not appropriate for cases of multiple sexual exposures or injection drug use (IDU) exposures over time or for exposures that occurred >72 hours before starting nPEP treatment (see Figure 1).

The model for nPEP is derived in part from protocols for occupational PEP (e.g., in terms of risk stratification, pretreatment testing, timing of treatment, treatment regimens, and duration of treatment). However, the recommendations for PEP and nPEP are distinct and should not be confused. (For information on occupational PEP, see chapter *Occupational Postexposure Prophylaxis*.) One significant difference between the protocols is that nPEP protocols should include interventions to reduce the risk of HIV transmission. Although exposed individuals usually seek care because they are interested specifically in antiretroviral prophylaxis, the nPEP model takes advantage of a critical opportunity to provide risk-reduction counseling and education.

See chapter *Occupational Postexposure Prophylaxis* for further discussion of evaluating possible benefits and risks of PEP.

S: Subjective

The patient reports potential exposure to HIV through a sexual encounter or the sharing of needles or other equipment for IDU.

Take a thorough history of the specific sexual or drug-use activities, the time the exposure occurred, the HIV status of the source person (if known), and HIV risk factors of the source person (if HIV status is not known). In cases of sexual assault, evidence collection and specific paperwork may be required as well.

O: Objective

Examine for trauma and for signs or symptoms of sexually transmitted infections (STIs), which may increase the risk of HIV transmission. In injection drug users, examine for abscesses and signs or symptoms of infection. For women who may be pregnant, perform a pregnancy test.

A: Assessment

Assess for potential exposures to HIV and other bloodborne pathogens and for the presence of other STIs. The risk of HIV infection depends on the HIV status of the source and on the characteristics of the source (e.g., HIV viral load) and of the exposure (see Figure 1). The estimated risk of HIV exposure will determine whether nPEP should be offered. An algorithm for risk evaluation and treatment decisions is presented in Figure 1.

P: Plan
Laboratory Testing

- Perform a baseline HIV antibody test.

- Evaluate and test for other infections transmitted through sexual or IDU exposures, including chlamydia, gonorrhea, syphilis, herpes simplex virus infection, hepatitis B (HBV surface antigen, surface antibody, and core antibody), and hepatitis C (HCV antibody).

- Obtain complete blood count (CBC), liver function tests (LFTs), and creatinine and estimated glomerular filtration rate (GFR) at baseline before treatment with ARV medications.

Treatment

Follow the algorithm in Figure 1 to determine whether the patient should be offered nPEP medications. If the patient is a candidate for treatment, provide counseling about the potential risks and benefits of nPEP. Note that the current DHHS nPEP guidelines were last updated in 2005 and do not reflect current practice. **The recommendations presented here are drawn from the 2005 nPEP guidelines but have been adapted to reflect more recent nPEP strategies, the availability of newer ARVs, and current DHHS adult treatment guidelines** (see Table 1). A number of alternatives are available; consult with an expert. Note that, although these regimens

are effective in treating HIV infection, their efficacy as prophylaxis has not been demonstrated.

If the source person is known or suspected to have infection with HIV that is resistant to ARV medications, seek expert consultation in selecting an appropriate nPEP regimen.

In general, the recommendations for nPEP involve three-drug combination therapy and are more aggressive than the occupational PEP recommendations. However, if the HIV status of the source person is unknown and the exposure is thought to be of relatively low risk, consider two-drug nPEP (e.g., tenofovir + emtricitabine) to minimize toxicity.

Select a regimen that is likely to be effective but tolerable; consider the potential adverse effects of ARV agents. Certain ARVs are not recommended for PEP, including abacavir,

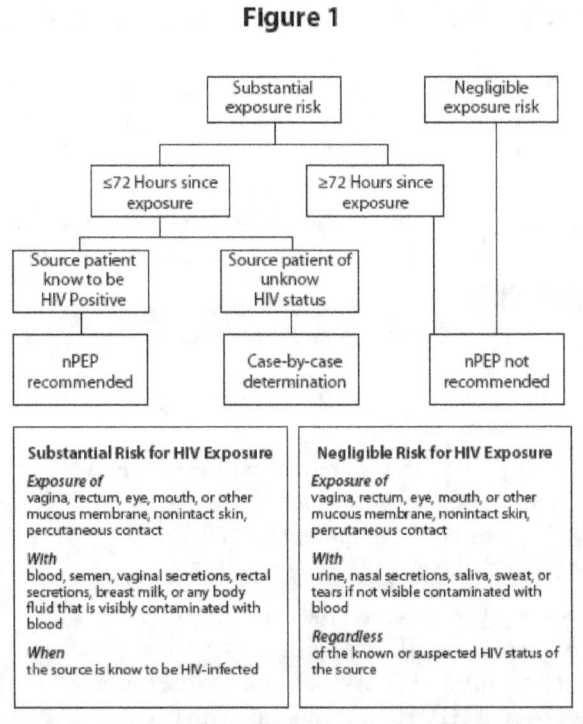

Figure 1

Source: U.S. Department of Health and Human Services. *Antiretroviral Postexposure Prophylaxis After Sexual, Injection-Drug Use, or Other Nonoccupational Exposure to HIV in the United States – January 21, 2005.* Available at www.aidsinfo.nih.gov/guidelines/.

delavirdine, nevirapine, and the combination of didanosine + stavudine. The 2005 DHHS guidelines list lopinavir/ritonavir as the preferred third agent for the expanded PEP regimen, and it still is commonly used. Newer protease inhibitors (i.e., atazanavir, darunavir) or the integrase inhibitor raltegravir may be appropriate for certain individuals, and should particularly be considered if exposure factors (e.g., comorbidities or interacting drugs) or source patient factors (e.g., concern for resistance) make therapy with lopinavir/

ritonavir problematic. Although the 2005 guidelines designate it as a preferred agent, efavirenz may have a higher rate of significant adverse effects than other listed agents. Additionally, efavirenz should not be used with pregnant women, because of possible teratogenicity. Refer to the appendix in the updated DHHS adult treatment guidelines for more complete information on the dosing, advantages, and disadvantages of the various ARV agents. Consider consultation with experts (see "Expert Consultation," below).

Table 1. Antiretroviral Regimens for Nonoccupational Postexposure Prophylaxis of HIV Infection

Preferred Regimens	
PI based	Lopinavir/ritonavir (Kaletra) 400/100 mg BID + 2-NRTI combination (see below)
Alternative Regimens	
PI based	Atazanavir 300 mg once daily + ritonavir 100 mg once daily + 2-NRTI combination (see below)
	Darunavir 800 mg once daily + ritonavir 100 mg once daily + 2-NRTI combination (see below)
	Atazanavir 400 mg once daily*
Integrase inhibitor based	Raltegravir 400 mg BID + tenofovir/emtricitabine 1 tablet once daily
NRTI combinations (to be used with Preferred or Alternative third agents listed above)	
	Tenofovir 300 mg once daily + emtricitabine 200 mg once daily (available as Truvada, 1 tablet once daily)
	Zidovudine 300 mg BID + lamivudine 150 mg BID (available as Combivir, 1 tablet BID)

* Unboosted atazanavir cannot be coadministered with tenofovir (use atazanavir + ritonavir)
Abbreviations: NNRTI = nonnucleoside reverse transcriptase inhibitor; NRTI = nucleoside analogue reverse transcriptase inhibitor; PI = protease inhibitor

Adapted from U.S. Department of Health and Human Services. *Guidelines for the Use of Antiretroviral Agents in HIV-1-Infected Adults and Adolescents.* January 10, 2011. (available at www.aidsinfo.nih.gov/guidelines/) and U.S. Department of Health and Human Services. *Antiretroviral Postexposure Prophylaxis After Sexual, Injection-Drug Use, or Other Nonoccupational Exposure to HIV in the United States – January 21, 2005.* Available at www.aidsinfo.nih.gov/guidelines/.

Once the decision is made to institute nPEP, do the following:

Begin ARV prophylaxis as soon as possible after the exposure, but always within 72 hours. Treatment should be continued for 28 days, unless the source person is determined to be HIV negative.

Provide counseling about the efficacy of nPEP, including the importance of protection against future HIV exposures, timely initiation of

nPEP medications, and adherence to these medications for 28 days.

Counsel exposed patients to use latex barriers with their sexual partners until transmission of HIV infection has been ruled out.

Counsel patients, as appropriate, about ways to reduce risks of future exposure to HIV.

In cases of sexual assault, refer the patient to a rape counselor.

Follow-Up

Patients should be evaluated at 1 week for review of all test results and further risk reduction counseling. For patients taking nPEP, this follow-up should include adherence assessment and evaluation of any adverse effects. A 2-week blood screening (CBC, LFTs, and creatinine) should be checked for patients on the 28-day nPEP regimen to monitor for nPEP toxicity. Follow-up testing for HIV antibody in patients with a negative baseline HIV antibody test should be done at 6 weeks, 3 months, and 6 months after the exposure.

Patients need health education and risk-reduction counseling and emotional support during their follow-up visits. Nonoccupational PEP programs should focus efforts on risk reduction counseling rather than the continued use of medicines for prevention. To this end, many programs have case managers, social workers and health educators as the key providers of follow-up and counseling after an exposure, with referral to clinicians as needed.

If patients develop acute HIV infection or are discovered to be HIV seropositive at follow-up testing, refer to an HIV specialist for evaluation and care (see chapter *Primary HIV Infection*).

Expert Consultation

For consultation on the treatment of exposures to HIV (and HBV and HCV), the clinician managing the exposed person can call the National HIV/AIDS Clinicians' Post-Exposure Prophylaxis Hotline (PEPline) at 888-HIV-4911 (888-448-4911). This service is available 24 hours a day at no charge. (However, 24-hour availability may be temporarily interrupted. Additional information on the Internet is available at www.nccc.ucsf.edu.) PEPline support may be especially useful in challenging situations, such as when drug-resistant HIV strains are suspected to be involved in the exposure or when the exposed person is pregnant.

Prophylaxis Against HBV and HCV

Prophylaxis against HBV is recommended for patients with potential exposure to HBV who do not have not have immunity against HBV. Give HBV immune globulin (HBIG) as a 0.06 mL/kg IM injection and initiate the vaccination series. For patients who received the vaccine series but did not develop protective antibody (HBV sAb+), give HBIG at the time of the postexposure workup and initiate revaccination; consider repeat of HBIG in 1 month. For patients with immunity to HBV (HBV sAb+), no treatment is indicated.

For HCV, no prophylactic treatments are recommended. After potential exposure, conduct a baseline HCV antibody test. If the source is known to have HCV infection, consider alanine aminotransferase (ALT) and HCV viral load testing at 4-6 weeks. HCV antibody testing should be repeated at 4-6 months. If HCV seroconversion occurs (indicated by ALT elevation, detectable HCV viral load, or confirmed positive HCV antibody test result), refer the patient to a hepatologist because early treatment of acute HCV may be indicated.

Note on Preexposure Prophylaxis

A number of investigations have been undertaken to evaluate the efficacy of ARV medications as preexposure prophylaxis (PrEP) – that is, oral ARVs taken by at-risk HIV-uninfected individuals with the goal of preventing HIV infection. Other studies are examining ARV-based microbicides, topical preparations applied before HIV exposure, with the same goal. Two recent studies have shown that these approaches can reduce the risk of sexual acquisition of HIV. In one, oral tenofovir + emtricitabine (Truvada), taken daily, reduced the risk of HIV acquisition in high-risk MSM and transgender women who have sex with men. In another, tenofovir vaginal gel (available only through research studies), used before and after vaginal intercourse, reduced the rate of HIV infection in high-risk heterosexual women in South

Africa. In both studies, the ARV prophylaxis was given *in conjunction with* other risk-reduction interventions, including counseling, condom provision, and STI testing and treatment. This and other studies will explore the efficacy and safety, and possible effects on risk of various types of PrEP and microbicides in different populations. The CDC has issued interim guidelines on the use of oral tenofovir-emtricitabine as PrEP in MSM (see "References," below); until more data are available, alternative approaches to PrEP should not be undertaken.

Patient Education

- Persons who have possible exposures to HIV should contact a medical provider or go to an emergency room as soon as possible after the potential exposure has occurred. PEP may be effective if it is started within 72 hours of exposure, but the sooner medications are initiated, the better the chance for preventing HIV transmission.

- PEP medications should be taken as directed for a full 28-day course. Adherence to PEP medications is essential for successful treatment.

- If patients are experiencing uncomfortable adverse effects, they should contact their care provider. Providers may prescribe medications to alleviate the adverse effects or select other PEP medications.

- Until HIV infection has been ruled out, exposed persons should be advised to use latex barriers to prevent transmission of HIV to their sex partners.

- Exposed persons should be counseled about the symptoms of primary HIV infection and instructed to contact their care provider immediately if symptoms develop.

- The most effective way to prevent HIV infection is to prevent exposure to HIV by practicing safer sex and safer IDU techniques. Using condoms and avoidance of needle sharing are successful preventive measures. If patients have questions about access to condoms or clean needles, they should contact their care provider for assistance.

References

- Bryant J, Baxter L, Hird S. *Non-occupational postexposure prophylaxis for HIV: a systematic review.* Health Technol Assess. 2009 Feb;13(14):iii, ix-x, 1-60.

- Centers for Disease Control and Prevention. *Interim Guidance: Preexposure Prophylaxis for the Prevention of HIV Infection in Men Who Have Sex with Men.* MMWR Recomm Rep. 2011 Jan 28;60(RR-3):65-69. Available at www.cdc.gov/mmwr/PDF/wk/mm6003.pdf.

- Panlilio AL, Cardo DM, Grohskopf LA, et al; U.S. Public Health Service. *Updated U.S. Public Health Service guidelines for the management of occupational exposures to HIV and recommendations for postexposure prophylaxis.* MMWR Recomm Rep. 2005 Sep 30;54(RR-9):1-17. Available at www.aidsinfo.nih.gov/guidelines/.

- U.S. Department of Health and Human Services. *Antiretroviral postexposure prophylaxis after sexual, injection-drug use, or other nonoccupational exposure to HIV in the United States.* MMWR Recomm Rep. 2005 Jan 21;54(RR02);1-20. Available at www.aidsinfo.nih.gov/guidelines/.

- U.S. Department of Health and Human Services. *Guidelines for the Use of Antiretroviral Agents in HIV-1-Infected Adults and Adolescents.* January 10, 2011. Available at www.aidsinfo.nih.gov/guidelines/.

- U.S. Department of Health and Human Services. *Updated U.S. Public Health Service Guidelines for the Management of Occupational Exposures to HBV, HCV, and HIV and Recommendations for Postexposure Prophylaxis.* MMWR Recomm Rep. 2001 Jun 29;50(RR11). Available at www.aidsinfo.nih.gov/guidelines/.

Preventing HIV Transmission/ Prevention with Positives

Background

Helping patients to reduce the risk of transmitting HIV to others is an important aspect of medical care for HIV-infected individuals. Most people with HIV infection want to prevent others from being infected with HIV, but they may practice sexual or injection drug behaviors that put others at risk of infection. Most HIV-infected patients also want to protect themselves from acquiring sexually transmitted infections (STIs) or bloodborne infections. This chapter offers recommendations for discussing HIV transmission and prevention with HIV-infected patients, with the goal of reducing HIV transmission. This aspect of care is often referred to as "prevention with positives" (PWP).

HRSA HAB Core Clinical Performance Measures

Percentage of clients with HIV infection who received **HIV risk counseling** within the measurement year

(Group 2 measure)

Taking responsibility for preventing HIV transmission is an important concern for most people with HIV, as well as for their health care providers. Multiple studies have shown that one third to three fourths of HIV medical providers do not ask their patients about sexual behavior or drug use. However, many HIV-infected individuals report that they want to discuss prevention with their health care providers. Each patient visit presents an opportunity to provide effective prevention interventions, even in busy clinical settings.

It is clear that information alone, especially on subjects such as sexual activity and drug use, cannot be expected to change patients' behavior. However, health care providers can help patients understand the transmission risk of certain types of behavior and help patients establish personal prevention strategies (sometimes based on a harm-reduction approach) for themselves and their partners. Some patients may have difficulty adhering to their safer sex goals. In these cases, referrals to mental health clinicians or other professional resources such as prevention case management may be helpful.

Patient-education needs are variable and must be customized. Providers must assess the individual patient's current level of knowledge as part of developing a prevention plan. All the information that a patient needs cannot be covered during a single visit. A patient's prevention strategy should be reinforced and refined at each visit with the clinician. Clinicians also should ask patients questions to determine life changes (e.g., a new relationship, a breakup, or loss of a job) that may affect the patient's sexual or substance use practices. If the patient can read well, printed material can be given to reinforce education in key areas, but it cannot replace a direct conversation with the clinician.

Techniques for Brief, Effective Interventions by Providers

A number of strategies have been shown to be more effective than providing information alone. Effective and brief provider-initiated interventions include the following elements:

- **Establish rapport** and provide services in an understanding, nonjudgmental manner. Patient educators, nurses, peer counselors, social workers, and mental health providers may be effective in discussing prevention strategies with patients.

- **Conduct a quick, detailed behavioral risk assessment:**

  1. See the key areas of risk assessment and intervention listed in Table 1, below.

  2. Assess where the patient's risk behavior lies along the risk continuum (described in chapter *Smoking Cessation*).

  3. Correct misinformation and answer questions.

  4. Assess the patient's readiness for behavior change (see "Stages of Change model," below).

  5. Screen for and treat STIs.

  6. Supply medications, condoms, and lubricant as needed.

- **Assess the patient's readiness for change** and approach any high-risk behavior in a step-wise manner, recognizing when the patient is ready for next steps. Such interventions may be carried out for 5-10 minutes per visit over a series of visits. The "Stages of Change" model and appropriate strategies include the following:

  1. **Precontemplation:** The patient is not ready to change; reassess at subsequent visits.

  2. **Contemplation:** The patient is considering a change in the future; discuss and help the patient to identify concrete next steps, such as a date for initiating change.

  3. **Preparation:** The patient is ready to change soon; discuss a concrete action plan and connect the patient with appropriate resources as needed.

  4. **Action:** The patient is actively engaged in changing behavior; continue to discuss and address challenges; offer encouragement.

  5. **Maintenance:** The patient has made behavioral changes; continue to discuss and address challenges, offer encouragement and congratulations.

  6. **(Relapse):** The patient has relapsed to previous risky behaviors; recognize the triggers and difficulties the patient had with maintenance and offer support and encouragement to try again when the patient is ready.

- **Customize messages**, as each individual patient's needs are variable.

- **Understand** that patients often have **competing priorities and pressures** involving mental health needs, relationships, finances, housing, employment, and other issues that may result in risky sexual and drug-use behaviors.

Examples of Prevention Intervention Programs with Demonstrated Efficacy in Treatment Settings

The U.S. Centers for Disease Control and Prevention (CDC) has identified a number of prevention interventions on individual, group, and community levels that meet criteria for efficacy and scientific rigor. A summary of these interventions can be accessed online at www.cdc.gov/hiv/topics/research/prs/promising-evidence-interventions.htm. Training and educational materials for effective intervention models can be found on the CDC-supported Diffusion of Effective Behavioral Interventions (DEBI) website (www.effectiveinterventions.org/). The following three approaches have demonstrated efficacy in treatment settings:

- **Options/Opciones Program:** The program features brief, 5-10 minute patient-centered discussions between patients and providers at each clinic visit using motivational interviewing techniques. Providers evaluate sexual and drug-use behaviors, assess the patient's readiness to change, and elicit methods from the patient on moving toward and maintaining safer behaviors. The provider and the patient develop an individually tailored plan, which the provider writes out on a prescription pad and gives to the patient.

- **Partnership for Health:** This intervention involves brief, 3-5 minute, one-on-one counseling sessions between the provider and the patient on self-protection, partner-protection, and disclosure. The approach fea-tures loss-framed messages that emphasize the risks or negative consequences of risky behavior. The provider then helps the patient develop a plan for risk reduction.

- **Positive Choice — Interactive Video Doctor:** This program involves an approximately 24-minute session during which HIV-infected patients complete the Positive Choice risk assessment on a laptop computer while waiting for scheduled visits with their providers. Based on the risk-assessment results, a video clip appears with the actor-portrayed Video Doctor who delivers interactive risk-reduction messages that are tailored to the patient's gender, risk profile, and readiness to change. The messages are delivered with motivational interviewing principles, using a patient-centered, empathetic and nonjudgmental approach. After the video session, the computer prints out an individualized educational sheet for the patient and an assessment sheet for the provider to use for follow-up.

Summary of Prevention with Positives: Key Areas of Intervention

More detailed discussions of topics follow this table.

Table 1. Key Areas of Risk Assessment and Intervention

Topic	Questions, Assessment, and Plan
General Risk Assessment	Subjective/objective questions to ask: 1. What do you know about HIV transmission? 2. What, if anything, are you doing that could result in transmitting HIV to another person? Assessment and plan: • Use this as an opportunity to help educate the patient on HIV transmission and to correct misinformation. • Place the patient's behaviors on a risk spectrum and try to prioritize the behaviors that are riskiest or the behaviors that the patient is most willing to address.

Sexual Practices	**Subjective/objective questions to ask:** 1. Tell me about any sexual activity since your last clinic visit. 2. What do you know about the HIV status of each sex partner? 3. Tell me about condom use during any sexual activity. 4. What has made it more difficult for you to use condoms during this sexual encounter or with this partner? 5. Do your sex practices differ with HIV-infected versus HIV-uninfected partners ("sexual positioning")? See below for more on partner notification. **Other information to collect:** • Number of sex partners in the past 6 months • Gender of each partner • Type of relationship with each partner (main, casual, anonymous) • Type of sexual activity engaged with each partner • Safer and less-safe sexual practices with each partner • Substance use, including alcohol, associated with sex • Circumstances of risky sex behaviors (e.g., bars/clubs, anonymous partners, intoxication) **Assessment and plan:** • Assess the patient's level of risk for sexual transmission. • Assess the patient's willingness and ability to use condoms during each sexual encounter, particularly with partners who are HIV uninfected or of unknown HIV serostatus. • Assess the patient's ability to use condoms (male and/or female) and correct any misinformation. See information on how to use condoms below. • Supply the patient with condoms and lubricant. • If the patient is unwilling to use condoms, counsel that risk of transmission can be reduced by screening for and treating STIs, using abundant amounts of lubrication, avoiding concurrent drug use, avoiding the use of spermicides and douching, and by choosing less risky sexual activities. Additionally, advise that serosorting, in which HIV-infected persons have sex only with other HIV-infected individuals, is effective in preventing transmission to uninfected persons.
Partner Notification	**Subjective/objective questions to ask:** 1. What are your thoughts and experiences talking with your partner(s) about your HIV-infection? This may be one of the hardest things you have to do. 2. (If the patient has not disclosed to main partner[s]): How might you approach this? 3. Are you afraid for your safety if you tell your partner(s)? **Assessment and plan: ways to offer help for disclosure** • Local health departments may have programs that help conduct partner tracing and contact in a confidential manner. • Providers and support staff can help disclose to partners with the patient present. • Providers and support staff can help disclose to partners without the patient present.

STI Screening	• The presence of an STI suggests behaviors that can increase HIV transmission, and it is detrimental to the patient's health.
	• Screen all patients at baseline and regularly afterward, depending on their risk factors. For example, screen every 3-6 months for a patient with new sex partners or new drug-injecting partners.
	• Routinely ask patients if they have symptoms of an STI.
	• Depending on risk, it is recommended to screen for the following STIs:
	• **Syphilis:** Serologic test (e.g., RPR, VDRL)
	• **Gonorrhea:** For pharyngeal infections, use nucleic acid amplification test (NAAT) or culture of oral swab*; for rectal infections, use NAAT or culture of rectal swab*; for urethral or cervical infections, use first-catch urine or urethral (male) or cervical (female) specimen for NAAT, or culture of urethra/cervical specimen
	• **Chlamydia:** For pharyngeal infections, use NAAT or culture of oral swab*; for rectal infections, use NAAT or culture of rectal swab*; for urethral or cervical infections use first-catch urine or urethral (men) or cervical (women) specimen for NAAT
	• **Trichomonas:** Wet mount or culture on vaginal secretion
	• **Herpes simplex virus (HSV):** Type-specific HSV-2 antibody testing
	Additionally, **hepatitis B** and **hepatitis C** are not known to increase the risk of HIV infection, they may be transmitted sexually, and persons with risk factors (particularly men who have sex with men [MSM] with risky sexual practices) should be screened regularly (see chapter *Initial and Interim Laboratory and Other Tests*).
	* NAAT is not yet approved for this indication by the U.S. Food and Drug Administration (FDA), though there is evidence that NAAT can accurately diagnose pharyngeal and rectal gonorrhea and chlamydia infections. Many local public health departments and other laboratories have received Clinical Laboratory Improvement Amendments (CLIA) waivers to perform these tests.
Drug and Alcohol Risk Assessment	**Subjective/objective questions to ask:**
	1. Tell me about any drug or alcohol use since your last clinic visit.
	2. How do you think your drug or alcohol use affects your sexual behaviors?
	3. What are your thoughts about quitting or cutting down on drug and alcohol use, and about separating it from sex?
	See below for follow-up on needle-sharing practices.
	Assessment and plan:
	• Assess the patient's level and circumstances of risk to target your intervention.
	• Emphasize that nasal straws or sniffers (e.g., for cocaine) should not be shared.
	• Assess the patient's readiness to quit or cut down on drug and alcohol use, and to separate it from sex.
	• Deliver messages tailored to the patient's readiness; for example, educate on the risks of harming oneself or other, facilitate a plan for harm reduction, or refer to rehabilitation/detoxification programs and centers.

Needle-Use Practices	**Subjective/objective question to ask:**
	• Tell me about any needle sharing since your last clinic visit.
	Assessment and plan:
	• After assessing the patient's risks and readiness, and if the patient is not ready for treatment (e.g., referral to detoxification programs or to buprenorphine and methadone programs for heroin users), the following messages for harm reduction can be offered:
	  • Use only sterile needles from pharmacies or needle exchange programs. (Provide informations about local needle exchange programs. Some are listed here: www.nasen.org.)
	  • Never reuse or share needles, syringes, or drug preparation equipment because it leads not only to transmission of HIV, hepatitis B, and hepatitis C, but also to bacterial infections and abscesses.
	  • Use new or disinfected cookers and new cotton filters to prepare drugs.
	  • Clean the skin with a new alcohol swab before injecting.
	  • If equipment must be reused, it should be cleaned properly with bleach or water.
	  • Safely dispose of syringes in a sharps container (which can be a clean detergent or other container), then take them to a needle exchange program or pharmacy for disposal.

Mental Health Assessment	Mental illnesses such as bipolar disorder, depression, and posttraumatic stress disorder can increase the chances of risky sexual and drug-use behaviors. Ask about mental health illnesses directly and pay attention to any symptoms that may indicate a psychiatric illness (e.g., manic episodes, depressive episodes, hallucinations). **Subjective/objective questions to ask:** 1. Tell me about any previous diagnoses or hospitalizations for mental health illnesses. 2. Have you taken any medications for mental health illnesses? 3. Perform a depression screen: see chapter *Depression*. **Assessment and plan:** See section *Neuropsychiatric Disorders* for more information.
Pregnancy Screening	<div align="center">**Subjective/objective questions to ask:**</div>**For women of childbearing potential:** 1. Are you currently pregnant or wanting to become pregnant at some point in the future? 2. Have you missed any periods recently? Are you having any symptoms of pregnancy? 3. What are your thoughts and plans about birth control? **For men with female sex partners:** 1. What are your thoughts on having a baby with your partner? What are your thoughts about fathering? 2. What are your thoughts on using birth control with your partner? **Assessment and plan:** See chapter *Health Care of HIV-Infected Women Through the Life Cycle*.
Antiretroviral Therapy (ART)	Lower levels of HIV in the blood (in particular, complete suppression of the HIV RNA through effective ART) have been associated with lower levels of HIV virus in genital secretions and with reductions in the rate of HIV transmission among serodiscordant couples. Effective ART with virologic suppression appears to sharply reduce the risk of HIV transmission and is one important means of HIV prevention. However, it does not eliminate transmission risk. In some individuals, there can be substantial discrepancies between HIV RNA levels in the serum and the sexual fluids. Be watchful for attitude shifts away from safer sexual and needle-sharing behaviors among patients who believe that ART protects them from transmitting HIV.

Sexual Transmission and Prevention of HIV

Begin the education process by learning what the patient and his or her immediate family members (if the family is aware of the patient's HIV status) believe about HIV transmission. Also be sure the patient understands how the virus is not transmitted (e.g., via sharing plates and eating utensils or using the same bathrooms) to allay any unnecessary fear.

Advise the patient not to share toothbrushes, razors, douche equipment, or sex toys to avoid transmitting HIV via blood or sexual secretions. This also will help prevent the transmission of other bloodborne or sexually transmitted infections, including hepatitis C, from co-infected patients. The patient should not donate blood, plasma, tissue, organs, or semen because these can transmit HIV to the recipient.

There is no reason why a person with HIV cannot have an active, fulfilling, and intimate sex life. However, the patient must be counseled properly about the risk of transmission. This discussion between the provider and patient should be client centered. This means that the provider should let the patient guide the discussion, starting from the patient's current point of knowledge and practice, always addressing any presenting concerns the patient may have prior to proceeding with a discussion about sexual transmission and risk. The provider should ask open-end questions, in a nonjudgmental manner, to elicit information about the patient's relationships, sexual behaviors, and current means of reducing transmission risk.

It is important to recognize that not every patient seeks the complete elimination of risk (e.g., via abstinence) but rather a reduction in risk, chosen after the options are discussed with the provider. The clinician may help the patient select and practice behaviors that are likely to be less risky. There are many methods for reducing risk, including the following:

- Disclosing HIV status

- Reducing the number of sex partners
- Using condoms, particularly for anal or vaginal intercourse (insertive or receptive)
- Having sex only with other HIV-infected partners (serosorting)
- Maintaining maximal suppression of HIV through ART
- Avoiding drug use in conjunction with sex
- Using adequate lubrication to avoid trauma to genital or rectal mucosa

If the patient requires more extensive counseling to support behavioral changes, the provider should refer the patient to support groups or prevention case management to meet those needs. Certainly, if the patient is dealing with a dual or triple diagnosis (including substance abuse or mental illness), a referral to address those needs is indicated.

Partner Notification

A good way to begin a discussion about HIV prevention and transmission is with an inquiry about any previous experiences disclosing to partners. The provider then can ask whether the patient currently has a need to disclose to one or more partners and whether he or she is ready and motivated to share information about HIV status. The provider should prompt patients to consider several questions about disclosure, including how they might approach the discussion, how their partners might react, what information they might offer their partners, whether partners are likely to keep their status confidential, and whether they have any concerns about personal safety (e.g., owing to fear of a violent reaction). If patients fear violence or retaliation or are not ready to share their status but want their partners to know, the provider may offer assistance with partner notification, for example through the local health department, in a confidential manner. As an alternative, patients may want the provider to talk with their partners, and that option can be offered as well. See the

U.S. Department of Veterans Affairs HIV website (www.hiv.va.gov/vahiv?page=sex-01-00) for a patient-oriented discussion of partner notification.

Helping Patients Reduce the Risk of Sexual Transmission

Standard Condom Use

Make sure that the patient understands how HIV is transmitted and which types of sexual acts are more and less risky than others. For vaginal or anal sex, correct use of latex or polyurethane condoms reduces the risk of HIV transmission considerably. Patients should be encouraged to use condoms as much as possible. For HIV-infected individuals, condom use is effective in reducing the risk of contracting another illness (such as hepatitis C or another STI) and the (apparently low) risk of becoming reinfected with another strain of HIV. It should be noted that condoms are less effective in reducing the transmission of organisms such as human papillomavirus (HPV) and HSV, which may result from viral shedding from skin. In the event of allergy to latex or other difficulty with latex condoms, polyurethane male or female condoms may be substituted. "Natural skin" or "lambskin" condoms are not recommended for HIV prevention.

Of course, condoms must be used correctly to be highly effective in preventing HIV transmission. Be sure that the patient knows exactly how to use a condom. Table 2 provides instructions for condom use.

Table 2. Instructions for Use of Standard Condoms
• Use a new latex or polyurethane condom with each act of sex (oral, anal, or vaginal). Make sure that the condom is undamaged, and that its expiration date has not passed.
• Carefully handle the condom to avoid damage (e.g., from fingernails, teeth).
• Being sure that the condom roll faces out, unroll the condom onto the erect penis before any genital contact with partner.
• Ensure that the tip of the condom is pinched when applying it to the top of the penis, to eliminate air in the tip that could cause breakage during ejaculation.
• Use only water-based lubricants with latex condoms. Oil-based lubricants (such as mineral oil, cooking oil, massage oil, body lotion, and petroleum jelly) can weaken latex or cause it to break, although they are fine with the use of polyurethane condoms. Adequate lubrication during intercourse helps reduce the risk of condom breakage.

Advise patients to avoid using nonoxynol-9 (N-9) spermicides. Data suggest that N-9 may increase risk of HIV transmission during vaginal intercourse and can damage the rectal lining. N-9 never should be used for anal intercourse.

For patients who complain about lack of sensitivity with condom use, the following techniques may help:

- Apply a drop of lubricant inside the condom (not more, because it increases the risk that the condom will come off).

- Use polyurethane condoms instead of latex because they conduct heat and may feel more natural.

- Use insertive (female) condoms, which are not as restrictive to the penis.

- Use specially designed condoms that do not restrict the top of the penis (e.g., Inspiral, Xtra Pleasure).

For patients who are unable or unwilling to use condoms, the following suggestions may help reduce HIV transmission risk:

- Use plenty of lubricant to reduce friction and microtrauma, which create portals of entry for the virus.

- Avoid spermicides that damage the vaginal or anorectal linings.

- Avoid douching products.

- Avoid recreational drugs, especially methamphetamine, that impair the ability to maintain "safer" sexual behaviors.
- Avoid the use of drugs such as nitrates (poppers) that enhance blood flow to the genitals.

Insertive (Female) Condom Use

The insertive "female" condom may be used for vaginal or anal intercourse. It is a thin polyurethane pouch with a flexible ring at the opening, and another unattached flexible ring that sits inside the pouch to keep it in position in the vagina (for use in the anus, the inner ring must be removed and discarded). The female condom may be an option for women whose male partners will not use male condoms or for couples who do not like standard condoms. Female condoms are more expensive than male condoms, but may be procured at a lower cost at some health departments or Planned Parenthood clinics. They generally are less well known to patients and may be unacceptable to some women whose culture or religion prohibits or discourages touching one's own genitals. Note that the female condom cannot be used at the same time as a male condom.

Be sure the patient knows how to use the insertive condom before she or he needs it; after teaching, encourage practice when alone at home and unhurried. Women who have used the diaphragm, cervical cap, or contraceptive sponge may find it easy to use the female condom. Illustrated directions are included in each box of insertive condoms. Instructions on the use of insertive condoms are provided in Table 3.

Table 3. Instructions for Use of Insertive (Female) Condoms

Vaginal Intercourse
• Open the pouch by tearing at notched edge of packet, and take out the female condom. Be sure that the lubricant is evenly distributed on the inside by rubbing the outsides together.
• Find a comfortable position, such as standing with one foot on a chair, sitting with knees apart, or squatting. Be sure the inner ring is inside, at the closed end of the pouch.
• Hold the pouch with the open end hanging down. While holding the outside of the pouch, squeeze the inner ring with your thumb and middle finger. Still squeezing, spread the labia with your other hand and insert the closed end of the pouch into the vagina.
• Now, put your fingers into the pouch itself, which should be inside the vagina, and push the inner ring and the pouch the rest of the way up into the vagina with your index finger. Check to see that the front side of the inner ring is just past the pubic bone. The back part of the inner ring should be up behind the cervix. The outer ring and about an inch of the pouch will be hanging outside the vagina.
• Until you and your partner become comfortable using the female condom, use your hand to guide the penis into the vagina, keeping it inside the pouch. If, during intercourse, the outer ring is pushed inside the vagina, stop, remove the female condom, and start over with a new one. Extra lubricant on the penis or the inside of the female condom may help keep this from happening.
• After intercourse, take out the condom by squeezing and twisting the outer ring to keep the semen inside the pouch. Throw away in a trash can; do not flush. Do not reuse.
• More information is available on the Planned Parenthood website (www.plannedparenthood.com).
Anal Intercourse
• Remove the inner ring and discard it. Put the female condom on the penis of the insertive partner and insert the condom with the penis, being careful not to push the outer ring into the rectum. The outer ring remains outside the anus, for ease of removal after ejaculation.

Prevention with Positives and Oral Sex

Although there is evidence that some people have become infected through receptive oral sex, the risk of HIV transmission via oral sex, in general, is much lower than the risk of transmission by vaginal or anal sex. Thus, most public health and prevention specialists focus their attention on riskier sexual and drug-use behaviors. However, because HIV transmission can occur with oral sex, clinicians should address this issue with patients and help them make informed decisions about risk reduction. Sores or lesions in or around the mouth or on the genitals may increase the risk of HIV transmission, as may a concurrent STI. Patients (and their partners) should avoid oral-genital contact if they have these conditions. Similarly, patients and partners can further reduce risk by not brushing or flossing teeth before oral sex. Individuals who wish to further reduce the risk of HIV transmission during oral sex may use barriers such as condoms, dental dams, and flexible plastic kitchen wrap.

Individuals who smoke crack cocaine often develop open burns, cracked lips, or damaged mucous membranes inside the mouth and thus may be at elevated risk of HIV transmission via oral sex. HIV-infected crack users should be counseled about the risk of transmitting HIV to uninfected partners through those portals of entry during oral sex and should receive risk-reduction counseling. In addition, they (or their partners) may benefit from techniques such as insulating the end of the crack pipe to reduce burns while smoking (e.g., with a rubber band or spark plug cap) and avoiding the brittle or sharp-edged copper scrubbing pads used as screens in the crack pipe.

Influence of Substance Use on Sexual Behavior

Alcohol and drug use can contribute significantly to the risk of sexual transmission of HIV, because of behavioral disinhibition. While intoxicated, substance users may, for example, forgo condom use, practice riskier sexual behaviors, have multiple partners, or use erectile dysfunction agents to sustain sexual activity. Addressing substance use issues is an important aspect of PWP. Patients should be assessed for HIV transmission risks associated with alcohol and injection or noninjection drug use, including crystal methamphetamine, in the context of their sexual behaviors (for injection drug use, see below). As always, it is important to approach the patient in a nonjudgmental manner. If alcohol or other drugs are posing barriers to practicing safer behaviors, the provider should counsel the patient to reduce or avoid substance use before engaging in sex, or refer the patient to prevention case management for more specialized risk reduction. Often, the provider can help the patient identify methods for reducing HIV transmission risk, including means that do not require abstaining from alcohol and drug use.

Injection Drug Use and Prevention of HIV

Clinicians should discuss substance use, including steroid use, and reinforce the patient's understanding of the adverse effects that these drugs can have on the body and the immune system. Assess whether referral for treatment is appropriate, and be knowledgeable about referral resources and mechanisms. If the patient is using injection drugs, emphasize the fact that HIV is readily transmitted by sharing needles and other injection equipment and that reusing or sharing needles and syringes can cause additional infections (e.g., endocarditis, hepatitis C). Assess the patient's readiness to change his or her drug injection practices, and refer to drug treatment programs as appropriate. Refer to an addiction counselor for motivational interviewing or other interventions, if available. After completion of substance abuse treatment, relapse prevention programs and ongoing support will be needed.

If the patient continues to use needles, discuss safer needle-use practices (Table 1) and refer to a needle-exchange program, if one is available, so that syringes and needles are not reused. A partial listing of needle exchange sites may be found at www.nasen.org, although many states either do not have facilities or are prohibited from listing them. Local harm-reduction activists may be aware of specific programs for obtaining clean needles and syringes. Patient-education flyers on safer injection practices, safer stimulant use, overdose prevention, and other topics are available on the Midwest AIDS Education and Training Center website (www.uic.edu/depts/matec/resource.html).

Noninjection Drug Use and Prevention of HIV Transmission

Exposure to HIV through contaminated blood may occur with the use of noninjection drugs; for example, by sharing cocaine straws or sniffers through which cocaine is inhaled. These straws easily can penetrate fragile nasal mucosa and become contaminated with blood from one user before being used by another individual, who may then experience mucous membrane exposure or even a cut or break in the mucous membrane from the bloody object. Straws or sniffers should not be shared.

Tattoo, Piercing, and Acupuncture Equipment

Patients should be aware of the risk of contamination of tattoo equipment, inks, and piercing equipment, and they should avoid situations wherein they might either transmit HIV or pick up other bloodborne pathogens.

Acupuncturists generally use sterile needles, but clients should verify that before using their services.

Maternal-Infant HIV Transmission

HIV-infected women can have healthy pregnancies, with good health outcomes for both mother and baby. For this to occur, women must know their HIV status as early as possible, preferably before becoming pregnant, and must receive effective ART. Although intervention to reduce the risk of perinatal infection is most effective if begun early in pregnancy, or preferably before pregnancy, it may be beneficial at any point in the pregnancy, even as late as during labor. For further information, see chapter *Reducing Maternal-Infant HIV Transmission.*

Preexposure Prophylaxis (PrEP)

A number of investigations have been undertaken to evaluate the efficacy of ARV medications as preexposure prophylaxis (PrEP) – that is, oral ARVs taken by at-risk HIV-uninfected individuals with the goal of preventing HIV infection. Other studies are examining ARV-based microbicides, topical preparations applied before HIV exposure, with the same goal. Two recent randomized trials have shown that ARV chemoprophylaxis can reduce the risk of sexual acquisition of HIV. In one, oral tenofovir + emtricitabine (Truvada), taken daily, reduced the risk of HIV acquisition in high-risk MSM and transgender women who have sex with men. In another, tenofovir vaginal gel (available only through research studies), used before and after vaginal intercourse, reduced the risk of HIV infection in high-risk heterosexual women in South Africa. In both studies, the ARV prophylaxis was given *in conjunction with* other risk-reduction interventions, including counseling, condom provision, and STI testing and treatment, and in both, effectiveness appeared to correlate with adherence to the prophylactic medication. Studies of various types of biomedical prevention in various populations are ongoing. The efficacy and safety of preexposure prophylaxis in "real world" settings need to be explored, and will help determine the role of PrEP in HIV prevention in the United States and elsewhere. It appears that PrEP may be particularly useful in populations and countries in which the risk of HIV infection is high and the availability or uptake of other prevention methods (e.g., condoms) is low. The CDC has issued interim guidelines on the use of oral tenofovir-emtricitabine as PrEP in MSM (see "References," below); until more data are available, alternative approaches to PrEP should not be undertaken.

Postexposure Prophylaxis for Nonoccupational HIV Exposure

Postexposure prophylaxis (PEP) may be considered for certain sexual exposures, sexual assaults, and other nonoccupational exposures to HIV. As with occupational PEP, a risk assessment must be completed and ART, if indicated, must be started as soon after exposure as possible. The risks and toxicities of antiretroviral drugs must be weighed against potential benefits, and the client's informed consent must be obtained. For further information, see chapter *Nonoccupational Postexposure Prophylaxis*.

References

- Centers for Disease Control and Prevention. *2009 Compendium of Evidence-Based HIV Prevention Interventions.* Atlanta: Center for Disease Control and Prevention; 2009. Available at www.cdc.gov/hiv/topics/research/prs/evidence-based-interventions.htm.

- Centers for Disease Control and Prevention. *Incorporating HIV prevention into the medical care of persons living with HIV: recommendations of CDC, the Health Resources and Services Administration, the National Institutes of Health, and the HIV Medicine Association of the Infectious Diseases Society of America.* MMWR Recomm Rep. 2003;52(No. RR-12):1-24. Available at aidsinfo.nih.gov/Guidelines.

- Centers for Disease Control and Prevention. *Interim Guidance: Preexposure Prophylaxis for the Prevention of HIV Infection in Men Who Have Sex with Men.* MMWR Recomm Rep. 2011 Jan 28;60(RR-3):65-69. Available at www.cdc.gov/mmwr/PDF/wk/mm6003.pdf.

- Centers for Disease Control and Prevention. *Sexually Transmitted Diseases Treatment Guidelines, 2010.* MMWR 2010 Dec 17; 59 (No. RR- 12):1-110. Available at www.cdc.gov/STD/treatment/2010.

- Richardson JL, Milam J, McCutchan A, et al. *Effect of brief safer-sex counseling by medical providers to HIV-1 seropositive patients: a multi-clinic assessment.* AIDS. 2004 May 21;18(8):1179-86.

- U.S. Department of Health and Human Services, Health Resources and Services Administration. *A Guide to Primary Care for People with HIV/AIDS, 2004 edition.* Washington: U.S. Department of Health and Human Services; 2004. Available at hab.hrsa.gov/tools/primarycareguide/PCGchap4.htm.

- U.S. Department of Health and Human Services. *Guidelines for the Use of Antiretroviral Agents in HIV-1-Infected Adults and Adolescents.* January 10, 2011.

- U.S. Department of Veterans Affairs. *Prevention for Positives.* In: *Primary Care of Veterans with HIV.* April 2009. Available at www.hiv.va.gov/vahiv?page=pcm-104_prevent. Accessed June 30, 2010.

Immunizations for HIV-Infected Adults and Adolescents

Background

Immunocompromised individuals are at higher risk of acquiring many types of infections compared with immunocompetent people. Although HIV-infected persons could benefit greatly from immunization against preventable infections, little specific research on the effectiveness of immunizations in this population has been completed. In general, vaccines have better efficacy in HIV-infected patients when immune function is relatively well preserved, notably when the CD4 count is >200 cells/μL. Persons with advanced immunodeficiency may have an impaired humoral response, and may not respond to vaccines, or they may require supplemental doses to develop serologic evidence of protection. If possible, vaccines should be administered before the CD4 count decreases to <200 cells/μL; if given when the CD4 count is <200 cells/μL, consideration should be given to repeating the vaccination when the CD4 count increases to >200-300 cells/μL (unless there is evidence of immunity).

Live vaccines generally should not be administered to individuals with HIV infection, particularly those with advanced immunodeficiency, unless the anticipated benefits of vaccination clearly outweigh the risks.

Administration of vaccines can be associated with a transient rise in plasma HIV RNA.

Recommendations about vaccination for patients with HIV infection are presented in Table 1.

HRSA HAB Core Clinical Performance Measures

Percentage of clients with HIV infection who completed the **vaccination series for hepatitis B**

(Group 2 measure)

Percentage of clients with HIV infection who ever received **pneumococcal vaccine**

(Group 3 measure)

Percentage of clients with HIV infection who have received **influenza vaccination** in the measurement period

(Group 3 measure)

Table 1. Vaccine Recommendations

Vaccine Type	Recommendation
Pneumococcal (polysaccharide)	• Recommended for all; consider revaccination 5 years after initial vaccination; some experts recommend vaccination every 5 years. • If CD4 count is <200 cells/μL, may be less effective; consider revaccination when CD4 count increases in response to ART.
Hepatitis A Virus (HAV)	• Recommended, for persons with chronic liver disease, injection drug users, men who have sex with men, international travelers, and hemophiliacs. Consider for all, unless there is serologic evidence of previous disease. • Serologic response (HAV IgG Ab) should be checked 1 month after completion of series, and nonresponders should be revaccinated. • Two doses (0, 6-12 months).

Vaccine Type	Recommendation
Hepatitis B Virus (HBV)	• Recommended for all, unless there is evidence of immunity (HBV surface Ab+) or active HBV infection (HBV surface Ag+, or HBV core Ab+ and evidence of HBV activity). • Many experts recommend giving a high dose of HBV vaccine (40 mcg), as is standard for hemodialysis patients; this may improve immunologic response in HIV-infected patients. • Most HIV-infected patients with isolated HBV core Ab+ (without HBV viremia) are not immune and should receive a complete series of HBV vaccine. • Anti-HBV surface Ab titers should be checked 1 month after completion of vaccine series. Patients whose titer level is ≤10 IU/mL should be revaccinated. • Standard dosing schedule is three doses (0, 1, and 6 months). If 40 mcg is given, the recommended schedule is three doses of Recombivax HB at 0, 1, and 6 months or four doses of Engerix-B at 0, 1, 2, and 6 months.
Influenza (inactivated vaccine)	• Recommended (yearly). • Vaccination is most effective among persons with CD4 counts of >100 cells/μL and HIV RNA of <30,000 copies/mL. • In patients with advanced disease and low CD4 cell counts, inactivated vaccine may not produce protective antibodies. A second dose of vaccine does not improve response in these patients. • Live, attenuated cold-adapted vaccine (LAIV, FluMist) is contraindicated for use in patients with HIV infection. • Close contacts of severely immunocompromised persons (including household members and health care personnel) should not receive live, attenuated influenza vaccine.
H1N1 Influenza (inactivated vaccine)	• Recommended (inactivated vaccine), though not thoroughly studied in HIV-infected persons (see Centers for Disease Control and Prevention [CDC] guidelines for up-to-date recommendations). • The live, attenuated nasal vaccine is not recommended.
Tetanus, Diphtheria (Td); Tetanus, Diphtheria, Pertussis (Tdap)	• Recommended (booster is recommended every 10 years in adults; or, if potential exposure [wound], after 5 years). • To protect against pertussis, substitute single dose of Tdap for Td booster in all patients aged 19-65 who have not received Tdap previously.
Measles, Mumps, Rubella (MMR)	• Live vaccine is contraindicated for use in patients with severe immunosuppression (CD4 count of <200 cells/μL). • Recommended for all nonimmune persons with CD4 counts ≥200 cells/μL.
Varicella-Zoster (VZV)	• Live vaccine is contraindicated for use in patients with severe immunosuppression (CD4 count of <200 cells/μL). • Consider for HIV-infected, VZV-seronegative persons with CD4 counts ≥200 cells/μL. • If vaccination results in infection with attenuated virus, treat with acyclovir. • Susceptible household contacts of susceptible HIV-infected individuals should be vaccinated. • Avoid exposure to VZV, if possible. If someone without immunity to VZV is exposed to VZV, administer varicella-zoster immune globulin (VZIG) as soon as possible (but within 96 hours). • Two doses (0, 3 months).

Vaccine Type	Recommendation

Human Papillomavirus (HPV)	• Two vaccines:
	  • Gardisil includes HPV strains 16 and 18 (oncogenic) and 6 and11 (wart causing)
	  • Cervarix: includes HPV strains 16 and 18
	• Recommended for females aged 9-26.
	• Gardasil vaccine approved for males aged 9-26.
	• Not contraindicated for use in HIV-infected individuals, though no data are available regarding use in this group.
	• No data on efficacy in preventing anal dysplasia.

Meningococcal	• Recommended if risk factor is present (e.g., college freshmen living in dormitory, military recruits, asplenia, complement component deficiency, travel to or residence in endemic area, occupational exposure).

Abbreviations: Ab = antibody; Ag = antigen; ART = antiretroviral therapy

Immunizations for HIV-Infected Patients Traveling to Developing Countries

Routine vaccinations should be reviewed and updated before travel. All patients traveling to other countries should be evaluated for both routine and destination-specific immunizations and prophylaxes. Inactivated (killed) and recombinant vaccines (e.g., diphtheria-tetanus, rabies, hepatitis A, hepatitis B, Japanese encephalitis) should be used for HIV-infected persons just as they would be used for HIV-uninfected persons anticipating travel. For further information, see the U.S. Centers for Disease Control and Prevention (CDC) webpage (www.cdc.gov/travel/). Recommendations specific to HIV-infected travelers are located in "The Immunocompromised Traveler" under the section called "Special Needs Travelers." Select the "Traveler's Health" option for regional travel documents and information on outbreaks.

Decision making about immunization for the HIV-infected traveler should take into consideration the traveler's current CD4 cell count, history of an AIDS-defining illness, and clinical manifestations of symptomatic HIV. In the CDC recommendations, asymptomatic HIV-infected persons with CD4 counts of 200-500 cells/μL are considered to have limited immune deficits, whereas patients with CD4 counts of >500 cells/μL are considered to have no immunologic compromise. For patients taking antiretroviral therapy, current CD4 counts rather than nadir counts should be used in deciding about immunizations. The CDC recommends that newly diagnosed, treatment-naive patients with CD4 counts of <200 cells/μL delay travel until after immunologic reconstitution with antiretrovirals to minimize risk of infection and immune reconstitution illness during travel.

The following should be noted about specific vaccinations:

• Inactivated (killed), enhanced-potency polio and typhoid vaccines should be given instead of the live, attenuated forms. In adults aged >18, vaccinate 8 weeks before travel to allow time for the initial two doses of polio vaccine.

• Measles or measles, mumps, and rubella (MMR; omit if patient has evidence of immunity) should not be given to severely immunocompromised patients. Instead, immune globulin should be given to measles-susceptible, severely immunocompromised persons traveling to measles-endemic countries.

- Yellow fever vaccine is a live-virus vaccine with uncertain safety and efficacy for HIV-infected persons, and it should be avoided if possible. Travelers with asymptomatic HIV infection and relatively high CD4 counts who cannot avoid potential exposure to yellow fever should be offered the choice of vaccination. If travel to a zone with yellow fever is necessary and vaccination is not administered, patients should be advised about the risk of yellow fever, instructed about avoiding the bites of vector mosquitoes, and provided with a vaccination waiver letter (though travelers should be warned that not all countries accept waiver letters).

- The influenza season in the Southern Hemisphere is April through September, but in the tropics, influenza is a year-round infection. Immunocompromised patients should be protected on the basis of influenza risk at the destination. HIV-infected patients should not be given live intranasal influenza vaccine.

References

- Advisory Committee on Immunization Practices. *Recommended adult immunization schedule: United States, 2010.* Ann Intern Med. 2010 Jan 5;152(1):36-9.

- Centers for Disease Control and Prevention. *Guidelines for Prevention and Treatment of Opportunistic Infections in HIV-Infected Adults and Adolescents: Recommendations from CDC, the National Institutes of Health, and the HIV Medicine Association of the Infectious Diseases Society of America.* April 10, 2009. Available at www.aidsinfo.nih.gov/guidelines/.

- Centers for Disease Control and Prevention. *The Immunocompromised Traveler. In: CDC Health Information for International Travel 2010. Atlanta: U.S. Department of Health and Human Services, Public Health Service; 2009.* Available at wwwnc.cdc.gov/travel/. Accessed June 30, 2010.

- Fiore AE, Shay DK, Broder K, et al.; Centers for Disease Control and Prevention. *Prevention and Control of Seasonal Influenza with Vaccines: Recommendations of the Advisory Committee on Immunization Practices (ACIP), 2009.* MMWR Recomm Rep. 2009 Jul 31;58(RR-8):1-52.

- Kroon FP, van Dissel JT, de Jong JC, et al. *Antibody response after influenza vaccination in HIV-infected individuals: a consecutive 3-year study.* Vaccine. 2000 Jul 1;18(26):3040-9.

- National Center for Immunization and Respiratory Diseases, Centers for Disease Control and Prevention. *Use of Influenza A (H1N1) 2009 Monovalent Vaccine Recommendations of the Advisory Committee on Immunization Practices (ACIP), 2009.* MMWR Recomm Rep. 2009 Aug 28;58(RR-10):1-8.

Preventing Exposure to Opportunistic and Other Infections

Background

Persons with HIV infection are more susceptible than others to certain infections. HIV-infected persons may come into contact with opportunistic pathogens in the course of various aspects of their daily activities. Pets, children, personal and sexual contacts, and food and water, as well as involvement in occupational tasks, recreation, hobbies, and other activities all potentially can expose an HIV-infected person to opportunistic pathogens, some of which are ubiquitous and cannot be avoided. Among the ubiquitous pathogens are *Candida*, *Mycobacterium avium* complex, *Pneumocystis jiroveci* pneumonia, and human herpesvirus 6 and 7. Exposure to other opportunistic pathogens may be minimized if patients are aware of the risks.

The following tables group opportunistic pathogens by type of exposure. Mechanisms of transmission and recommendations for avoidance are outlined. Note that a number of infections can be transmitted by several of these modes.

For information about vaccinations, see chapter *Immunizations for HIV-Infected Adults and Adolescents*; for opportunistic infection (OI) prophylaxis, see chapter *Opportunistic Infection Prophylaxis*.

Topics:

- Water related
- Food associated
- Environmental
- Respiratory and bodily contact
- Associated with sexual contact
- Injection drug use associated
- Other bloodborne related
- Pet and animal related
- Contact with children
- Travel related

Water Related	
Pathogens	• Hepatitis A (HAV) • *Amoeba* • *Cryptosporidium* • *Giardia* • *Shigella* • *Isospora* • *Campylobacter* • Microsporidia
Transmission	• Infection occurs through drinking contaminated water or eating produce or other food that has been washed in contaminated water. • Water ingested accidentally during recreation also can make people sick.

Recommended avoidance measures	• To decrease exposure from water in developing countries, take the following precautions:
	  • Do not drink tap water or use it to brush teeth.
	  • Avoid ice that is not made from bottled water.
	  • Avoid raw fruits or vegetables, as they may have been washed in tap water.
	  • Bring tap water to a rolling boil for at least 1 minute before consuming. If this is not possible, treatment with iodine or chlorine, especially if in conjunction with filtering, reduces risk of infection.
	• Additional recommendations, include the following:
	  • Avoid drinking untreated water.
	  • When choosing a home water filter, especially for filtering untreated water, be aware that not all filters remove the pathogens listed above.
	  • Do not drink water from lakes or rivers.
	  • Avoid swimming in water that may be contaminated with stool.
	  • Avoid swallowing water during recreational activities (lakes, rivers, saltwater beaches, pools, hot tubs, and ornamental fountains may be contaminated with *Cryptosporidium*).
	  • In the event of a cryptosporidiosis outbreak in the municipal water supply, boil tap water for at least 1 minute to eliminate risk of infection.
	  • *Cryptosporidium* may be present in municipal water outside outbreak settings, though the magnitude of this risk is unknown. Some HIV-infected patients may chose to take precautions to decrease risk.
	  • Be aware that bottled water may be contaminated with *Cryptosporidium*.
	  • See the discussion of travel-related topics, below.

Food Associated		
Pathogens	• *Toxoplasma* • *Salmonella, Shigella, Campylobacter* (enteric infections)	• *Listeria* • *Cryptosporidium* • Other enteric pathogens
Transmission	• Exposure may occur through eating or handling contaminated food.	

Recommended avoidance measures	• Always wash hands before preparing and consuming food.
	• Wash hands, cutting boards, counters and utensils thoroughly after contact with uncooked foods.
	• Do not allow raw meat or eggs to come into contact with other foods.
	• Wash produce thoroughly.
	• Cook meat and poultry to an internal temperature of 165-170°F. It is safest to confirm temperature with a thermometer. Meat that is no longer pink inside likely has reached a temperature of 165°F.
	• Avoid raw or unpasteurized milk, including goat milk, and foods that contain unpasteurized milk or milk products.
	• Avoid foods that might contain raw egg (e.g., Hollandaise sauce, Caesar salad dressing, some mayonnaises, uncooked cake and cookie batter, eggnog, homemade ice cream). Pasteurized eggs can be used safely in recipes that call for raw egg.
	• Avoid eating raw or lightly steamed shellfish.
	• Avoid eating raw seed sprouts, as these may be contaminated with enteric pathogens.
	• Avoid foods from street vendors, especially in developing countries.
	• Be aware that unpasteurized juices may be contaminated with *Cryptosporidium*.
	• Rates of infection with *Listeria* are low, but HIV-infected people who are severely immunocompromised are at increased risk.
	• HIV-infected persons who wish to decrease their risk of listeriosis should take the following precautions:
	  • Avoid soft cheeses including feta, brie, camembert, blue-veined, and Mexican-style cheeses such as queso fresco unless they are clearly labeled as pasteurized. Hard cheeses, processed cheeses, cream cheese, cottage cheese, and yogurt generally are safe.
	  • Before eating leftover foods or ready-to-eat foods, such as hot dogs, cook them until they are steaming hot.
	  • Avoid foods from deli counters, such as prepared meats, salads, and cheeses, or heat these foods until steaming hot before eating them.
	  • Avoid refrigerated pâté, or heat until steaming hot. Canned or shelf-stable pâté generally is safe.
	  • Avoid refrigerated smoked seafood, unless it is part of a cooked dish. Canned or shelf-stable smoked seafood generally is safe.
	• Also see information on travel-related infections, below.		

Environmental		
Pathogens	• *Toxoplasma gondii* • *Cryptosporidium* • *Coccidioides*	• *Histoplasma capsulatum* • *Cryptococcus neoformans* • *Aspergillus*
Transmission	• *Cryptosporidium* and *Toxoplasma* may be present in soil and sands, and infection can occur through handling soil during gardening or playing in or cleaning sandboxes. • Infection with *Coccidioides* and *Histoplasma* occurs with inhalation of fungal spores that become airborne owing to disturbance of contaminated soil.	

Environmental	

Recommended avoidance measures	• Wash hands thoroughly after contact with soil or sand.
	• Endemic fungi cannot be completely avoided in certain geographic areas; however, avoiding high-risk activities can decrease risk of infection.
	• In endemic coccidioidomycosis areas, avoid exposure to soil disturbance such as that which occurs during dust storms and at excavation and construction sites.
	• Risk of *Aspergillus* infection also may be decreased by avoidance of dusty environments.
	• Patients with CD4 counts of <150 cells/µL should avoid activities that put them at increased risk of exposure to *Histoplasma* in endemic areas, such as:
	  • Cleaning, remodeling or demolishing old buildings
	  • Disturbing soil beneath bird roosting sites
	  • Cave exploration
	  • Other contact with bird or bat droppings
	• Limiting exposure to bird droppings may also decrease risk of infection with *C. neoformans*.

Respiratory and Bodily Contact	
Pathogens	• *Mycobacterium tuberculosis* • Influenza • Enteric pathogens • Varicella-zoster virus (VZV)
Transmission	• Tuberculosis (TB) is transmitted when a person with pulmonary or laryngeal TB coughs, sneezes, shouts, or sings, generating infected droplets that are inhaled by a susceptible person. • HIV-infected persons working or residing in certain environments, such as hospitals, nursing homes, homeless shelters, and correctional institutions, may become exposed to TB. • Influenza virus is spread by exposure to infected respiratory droplets or contaminated surfaces. • VZV is transmitted through contact with aerosolized respiratory droplets or by contact with skin lesions. • Many respiratory and enteric pathogens may be spread by contact with contaminated fomites.

Recommended avoidance measures	• HIV-infected persons should be aware of the increased risk of TB infection associated with certain environments. The following measures decrease risk of infection:
	  • In settings with a high risk of TB transmission, patients with known or suspected TB should be physically separated from others.
	  • All HIV-infected persons should be tested for latent TB infection.
	  • All HIV-infected patients with latent TB infection (LTBI) should receive a complete course of LTBI treatment.
	  • HIV-infected persons with a history of significant TB exposure should be treated presumptively for LTBI regardless of the results of LTBI testing, once active infection has been ruled out.
	  • Bacillus Calmette-Guérin (BCG) vaccine is not recommended in the United States, and it is contraindicated for HIV-infected persons.
	• People susceptible to VZV should avoid persons with active chickenpox or herpes zoster (shingles).
	• VZV-susceptible, HIV-negative household contacts should be vaccinated against VZV.
	• Frequent handwashing can reduce risk of diarrhea in HIV-infected persons.

Associated with Sexual Contact		
Pathogens	• HIV • Hepatitis B virus (HBV) • Hepatitis C virus (HCV) • Hepatitis A virus (HAV) • Human papillomavirus (HPV) • Cytomegalovirus (CMV) • Herpes simplex virus (HSV) • Syphilis • *Chlamydia* • *Gonorrhea* • *Trichomonas*	• Lymphogranuloma venereum (LGV) serovars of *C. trachomatis* • *Cryptosporidium* • *Shigella* • *Campylobacter* • *Amoeba* • *Giardia* • *Isospora* • Microsporidia
Transmission	• Depending on the pathogen, infection may be transmitted by exchange of body fluids, by skin-skin contact, or by oral-fecal contact. • Sexually transmitted infections (STIs) can occur at genitals, rectum, or mouth, depending on sexual practices. • A number of enteric pathogens can be transmitted during sex (by oral-fecal contact).	

Recommended avoidance measures	• Male latex condoms, when used consistently and correctly:
	  • Are highly effective in preventing sexual transmission of HIV and many other STIs, including syphilis, chlamydia, gonorrhea, and trichomoniasis.
	  • Decrease risk of acquiring HSV-2, HPV, CMV, HBV, and HCV.
	  • Do not prevent enteric pathogen exposure (which is via fecal-oral contact).
	• HIV-infected persons should be screened for STIs at least annually. Those with high-risk partners or sexual practices should be screened more frequently.
	• To avoid infection with HSV, HIV-infected persons should avoid sexual contact when a partner has an overt herpetic lesion (genital or oral-labial), though HSV transmission also can occur during asymptomatic shedding.
	• The use of suppressive antiviral therapy by persons with genital herpes reduces HSV-2 transmission to susceptible partners, though the effectiveness of this approach in HIV-infected patients has not been evaluated.
	• The safety and effectiveness of the HPV vaccine in HIV-infected women and in men is being studied.
	• Patients who are CMV seronegative should be advised that CMV can be sexually transmitted.
	• To decrease risk of exposure to enteric pathogens during sex, patients can:
	  • Use barriers such as dental dams during oral-anal contact
	  • Change condoms after anal sex
	  • Wear latex gloves during digital-anal contact
	  • Wash hands after sex	

Injection Drug Use Associated		
Pathogens	• HIV • HCV • HBV • CMV • *Staphylococcus aureus*, including MRSA • *Pseudomonas aeruginosa*	• *Streptococcus* • *Clostridium* • Enteric bacteria and oral anaerobes • *Leishmania* • Fungi
Transmission	• Injection drug users are at risk of a host of infections, including viral hepatitis, skin and soft-tissue infections, infective endocarditis, and pulmonary infections. • Injection drug use also may put users at risk of acquiring TB and STIs. • Infection may occur from contaminated drug-injection equipment (needles, syringes, water, and other preparation equipment). • Infection also may occur from the user's own skin or mouth bacteria, which can enter the bloodstream. • The drug itself, or an adulterating substance, may be contaminated.	

Recommended avoidance measures	• Injection drug users should be advised not to share needles or drug preparation equipment, and should be educated about needle exchange programs.
	• If receptive, injection drug users should be referred to substance abuse treatment programs.
	• Injection drug users should be educated about methods of reducing risk, including the following:
	  • If equipment is being reused, clean with bleach and water.
	  • Avoid dangerous injection sites such as groin and neck.
	  • Do not crush capsules or tablets in the mouth prior to injecting, as this may introduce harmful oral bacteria into the bloodstream.
	  • Do not lick injection needles or syringes.
	  • Use boiled water for preparing drugs for injection; if not available, use tap water.
	  • Boil the drug before injecting.
	  • Use a new or disinfected "cooker," and a new filter to prepare drugs for injection.
	  • Always clean injection sites with alcohol before injecting.
	  • Be aware that black tar heroin may be contaminated with *Clostridium* spores, which are not killed by heating the drug prior to use.	

Other Bloodborne		
Pathogens	• HIV • HCV	• HBV • CMV
Transmission	• Tattooing and body piercing • Reuse of medical equipment and transfusion of infected blood (primarily outside the United States) • Occupational exposures (e.g., needlesticks) of health care workers	
Recommended avoidance measures	• Persons considering tattooing or piercing should be educated about the potential risk of bloodborne pathogen transmission if proper infection control procedures are not followed. • When receiving a transfusion, HIV-infected patients who are seronegative for CMV should be administered only CMV antibody-negative or leukocyte-reduced cellular blood products in nonemergency situations. • Universal precautions always should be followed by health care workers.	

Pet and Animal Related	
Pathogens	<table><tr><td>• *Toxoplasma* • *Cryptosporidium* • *Salmonella* • *Campylobacter* • Shiga toxin-producing *Escherichia coli* • *Bartonella* • *Leptospira*</td><td>• *Brucella* • *Capnocytophaga* • *Cryptococcus* • *Mycobacterium avium* and *marinum* • *H. capsulatum*</td></tr></table>
Transmission	• For the most part, people with HIV infection can and should keep their pets. • HIV-infected persons should be made aware of the potential risks posed by animals and of the avoidance measures for decreasing risks of infection. • Exposure may occur though a lick, a bite or a scratch, or through contact with a pet's stool. Some infections may be spread though contact with an animal's coat or skin. • Fleas may spread some infections to pet owners. • Patients also may be exposed while performing occupational tasks that bring them into contact with animals (e.g., in pet stores, veterinary clinics, farms, and slaughterhouses).

Recommended avoidance measures	• Always wash hands after handling animals, and after cleaning cages or aquariums.
	• When acquiring a new pet, avoid animals <6 months of age (cats younger than 1 year) and those with diarrhea.
	• Stray animals may carry many infections and should be avoided.
	• Avoid contact with animal stool.
	• Avoid animals with diarrhea.
	• Pets with diarrhea should be examined by a veterinarian and should have stool checked for *Cryptosporidium*, *Salmonella*, *Campylobacter*, and Shiga toxin-producing *E. coli*.
	• Wash any bites or scratches with soap and water, and seek medical attention.
	• Animals should not be allowed to lick people in the mouth, or on any open cuts or wounds.
	• Cats may increase risk of *Toxoplasma* and *Bartonella* infection.
	• To minimize risk of *Toxoplasma* exposure:
	  • Litter boxes should be cleaned daily, preferably by someone who is not HIV infected or pregnant.
	  • If an HIV-infected person is cleaning a litter box, gloves should be used, and hands should be washed afterward.
	  • Keep cats indoors and do not allow them to hunt.
	  • Do not feed cats raw or undercooked meat.
	• In areas where histoplasmosis is endemic, avoid contact with bird droppings, including soil under bird roosting sites.
	• Always use gloves when cleaning aquariums to avoid contact with *Mycobacterium marinum*.
	• Avoid contact with reptiles (such as lizards, snakes, and turtles), as well as chicks and ducklings, as these may carry *Salmonella*.
	• Avoid exotic pets such as monkeys, ferrets, and other wild animals.

Contact with Children	
Pathogens	<table><tr><td>• CMV</td><td>• Influenza</td></tr><tr><td>• *Cryptosporidium*</td><td>• VZV</td></tr><tr><td>• *Giardia*</td><td>• Enteric pathogens</td></tr><tr><td>• HAV</td><td></td></tr></table>
Transmission	• HIV-infected persons who work as childcare providers, or who have children in daycare, may be exposed to opportunistic pathogens. • The poor personal hygiene habits of children facilitate spread of infection. • Risks specific to the individual, given his/her immune status and medical history, should be discussed with a health care provider. • CMV infection may occur through contact with many body fluids, including stool, urine, and saliva. • Diapering may bring a person into contact with *Cryptosporidium* and other enteric pathogens. • In addition to opportunistic pathogens, childcare providers are exposed to other illnesses, carried by children, to which they may be more susceptible.
Recommended avoidance measures	• Wash hands thoroughly after contact with stool or urine. • Wash hands after diapering and disinfect changing station often. • Wash hands after contact with saliva or objects covered with saliva, such as cups or pacifiers. • Ensure that the immunization status of HIV-infected persons is up to date, as appropriate for their immune status. • HIV-infected persons who are susceptible to VZV should avoid exposure to people with chickenpox or shingles. • VZV-susceptible household contacts of HIV-infected persons should be vaccinated against VZV if they are HIV negative, so that they will not transmit VZV to their HIV-infected contact.

Travel Related	
Pathogens	<table><tr><td>• Enteric pathogens</td><td>• Dengue virus</td></tr><tr><td>• *Plasmodium* species (malaria)</td><td>• Other geographically specific infections</td></tr><tr><td>• Yellow fever virus</td><td></td></tr></table>
Transmission	• Travelers to developing countries are at risk of foodborne and waterborne infections. • Malaria is transmitted by the bite of an infected female *Anopheles* mosquito. • HIV-infected patients are at higher risk of severe malaria. • Yellow fever and dengue fever are spread by mosquito bites.

Travel Related	

Recommended avoidance measures	• Plan the travel itinerary, vaccinations, and prophylaxis in consultation with a health care provider experienced in travel medicine.
	• Discuss area-specific risks and avoidance measures with the healthcare provider.
	• The U.S. Centers for Disease Control and Prevention (CDC) Traveler's Health website has detailed information on most issues pertaining to infections in travelers (www.cdc.gov/travel).
	• Review and update routine vaccine history prior to travel.
	• Generally, live vaccines for HIV-infected persons should be avoided, with some exceptions:
	  • Measles vaccine is recommended for all nonimmune persons with CD4 counts of ≥200 cells/µL. Measles immune globulin should be considered for those with CD4 counts of <200 cells/µL who are traveling in measles-endemic areas.
	  • Varicella vaccine can be considered for VZV-seronegative persons with CD4 counts of ≥200 cells/µL.
	  • Yellow fever vaccination may be considered, see below.
	• Inactivated (killed) enhanced potency polio and typhoid vaccines should be given instead of the live, attenuated forms.
	• Killed and recombinant vaccines including influenza, diphtheria-tetanus, rabies, HAV, HBV, Japanese encephalitis and meningococcal vaccines should be administered as they would be for HIV-uninfected persons preparing for travel.
	• The oral cholera vaccine (not available in the United States) is not recommended for most travelers by the CDC.
	
	Traveler's diarrhea:
	• See sections on foodborne and waterborne infections (above) for risk reduction strategies.
	• Antimicrobial prophylaxis is not routinely recommended for HIV-infected persons traveling in developing countries.
	• Prophylaxis may be appropriate in select situations (for example, high risk of infection and short length of travel)
	• For those to whom prophylaxis is given, fluoroquinolones (such as ciprofloxacin 500 mg PO once daily) may be considered for nonpregnant patients.
	• HIV-infected patients traveling in developing countries should bring antibiotics to be used empirically in the event of developing diarrhea.
	• Appropriate regimens include:
	  • Ciprofloxacin 500 mg PO BID for 3-7 days
	  • Azithromycin 500 mg PO once daily as an alternative, and for pregnant women
	• Antiperistaltic agents such as loperamide or diphenoxylate can be useful in the treatment of traveler's diarrhea.
	• Do not use antiperistaltic agents if high fever or blood in the stool is present. Stop use if symptoms persist >48 hours.
	• Seek medical care if diarrhea is severe, bloody, accompanied by fever and chills, leads to dehydration, or does not respond to empiric therapy.

Travel Related	
Recommended avoidance measures	**Malaria:** • HIV-infected patients should be advised to avoid travel in malarious areas. • If travel to a malarious area cannot be avoided, effective chemoprophylaxis should be given. Consult the CDC Traveler's Health website for specific information (www.cdc. gov/travel). • Be aware that some malaria prophylaxis medications may have drug-drug interactions with antiretrovirals. • Personal protection measures should be followed, including avoidance of peak biting times and use of insect repellants, protective clothing, and permethrin-soaked bed netting. **Yellow fever:** • HIV-infected patients should be discouraged from visiting areas where yellow fever infection is a risk. • Vaccination may be considered in some HIV-infected persons with high CD4 counts who cannot avoid potential exposure, after discussion of risks and benefits. • Vaccine response may be poor, and serologic testing can be considered. • If vaccination is not administered, patients should be advised about the risk of yellow fever, instructed about avoiding the bites of vector mosquitoes, and provided with a vaccination waiver letter. • Personal protection measures should be followed, including avoidance of peak biting times and use of insect repellants, protective clothing, and permethrin-soaked bed netting. Other geographically specific opportunistic infections include visceral leishmaniasis, *Penicillium marneffei* infection, coccidiomycosis, histoplasmosis, and TB.

References

- Aberg JA, Kaplan JE, Libman H, et al.; HIV Medicine Association of the Infectious Diseases Society of America. *Primary Care Guidelines for the Management of Persons Infected with HIV: 2009 Update by the HIV Medicine Association of the Infectious Diseases Society of America.* Clin Infect Dis. 2009 Sep 1;49(5):651-81.

- Centers for Disease Control and Prevention. *Preventing Infections from Pets.* CDC Brochures for Persons Living with HIV/AIDS. Available at cdc.gov/hiv/resources/brochures/index.htm. Accessed June 30, 2010.

- Centers for Disease Control and Prevention. *Guidelines for Prevention and Treatment of Opportunistic Infections in HIV-Infected Adults and Adolescents: Recommendations from CDC, the National Institutes of Health, and the HIV Medicine Association of the Infectious Diseases Society of America.* April 10, 2009. Available at www.aidsinfo.nih.gov/guidelines/.

- Centers for Disease Control and Prevention. *CDC Health Information for International Travel 2010.* Atlanta: U.S. Department of Health and Human Services, Public Health Service; 2009. Chapter 8. *The Immunocompromised Traveler.*

- Gordon RJ, Lowy FD. *Bacterial infections in drug users.* N Engl J Med. 2005 Nov 3;353(18):1945-54.

Opportunistic Infection Prophylaxis

Background

Prophylaxis against opportunistic infection (OI) is treatment given to HIV-infected individuals to prevent either a first episode of an OI (primary prophylaxis) or the recurrence of infection (secondary prophylaxis). Prophylaxis is recommended to prevent three important OIs: *Pneumocystis jiroveci* pneumonia (PCP), *Mycobacterium avium* complex (MAC), and toxoplasmosis. Prophylaxis also is recommended to prevent tuberculosis (TB) in patients with latent *Mycobacterium tuberculosis* infection (see chapter *Latent Tuberculosis*). In endemic regions, prophylaxis against *Histoplasma capsulatum* and *Coccidioides* species is advised. And in some situations, prophylaxis against other OIs may be reasonable; see the OI prevention recommendations of the U.S. Public Health Service and the Infectious Diseases Society of America (USPHS/IDSA) (reference below) for additional information.

HRSA HAB Core Clinical Performance Measures

Percentage of clients with HIV infection and a CD4 count of <200 cells/μL who were prescribed *Pneumocystis jiroveci* **pneumonia prophylaxis**

(Group 1 measure)

Percentage of clients with HIV infection and a CD4 count of <50 cells/μL who were prescribed *Mycobacterium avium* **complex prophylaxis** within the measurement year

(Group 3 measure)

Pneumocystis jiroveci Pneumonia

Background

PCP remains the most common life-threatening infection among U.S. residents with advanced HIV disease.

Primary Prophylaxis: Indications

- Prophylaxis should be administered to all HIV-infected patients with a CD4 count of <200 cells/μL or a history of oral thrush. PCP prophylaxis may be indicated for patients with CD4 counts of >200 cells/μL in the presence of a CD4 percentage <14%, or a history of an AIDS-defining illness.

- For patients whose CD4 counts are declining toward 200 cells/μL, the CD4 count should be monitored closely. PCP prophylaxis should be considered for patients with a CD4 count of 200-250 cells/μL if laboratory monitoring will not be possible within 3 months.

Prophylaxis Options: Recommended Regimens

- Trimethoprim-sulfamethoxazole (TMP-SMX) (also known as cotrimoxazole, Bactrim, and Septra) one double-strength tablet PO once daily (Note: This regimen also is effective in preventing toxoplasmosis.)

- TMP-SMX one single-strength tablet PO once daily (this lower-dose regimen may be better tolerated) (Note: This also is likely to be effective in preventing toxoplasmosis.)

  - **Warning:** Many patients have adverse reactions to sulfa medications. Severe reactions may include persistent neutropenia, rash (including severe erythroderma), and Stevens-Johnson syndrome (bullae and desquamation of the skin). In patients with milder reactions, chemoprophylaxis with TMP-SMX should be continued if clinically possible. Some patients with a history of serious adverse reaction may undergo desensitization, but this must be done cautiously and it requires diligence from the patient and careful management by the provider (see chapter *Sulfa Desensitization*).

Prophylaxis Options: Alternative Regimens

Other options for prophylaxis include the following:

- TMP-SMX one double-strength tablet TIW (e.g., Monday, Wednesday, and Friday)
  (Note: This regimen also is likely to be effective in preventing toxoplasmosis.)

- Dapsone 100 mg PO once daily or 50 mg PO BID
  (Note: These regimens do not prevent toxoplasmosis.)

- Dapsone 50 mg PO once daily + pyrimethamine 50 mg PO once weekly + leucovorin 25 mg PO once weekly
  (Note: This regimen also is effective in reducing the risk of toxoplasmosis.)

  - **Warning:** Glucose-6-phosphate dehydrogenase (G6PD) deficiency can increase the risk of hemolytic anemia or methemoglobinemia in patients receiving dapsone. Screen for G6PD deficiency before starting dapsone. (G6PD deficiency is found in approximately 10% of African-American males, and in 1-2% of males of Mediterranean, Indian, and Asian descent.)

- Aerosolized pentamidine 300 mg once per month, via Respirgard II nebulizer
  (Note: This regimen does not prevent toxoplasmosis.)

  - **Warning:** Aerosolized pentamidine may increase the risk of extrapulmonary pneumocystosis, pneumothorax, and bronchospasm. It increases the risk of

TB transmission to others if the patient has active pulmonary tubercular disease, unless ventilation (negative-pressurized facility with outside venting) is adequate. Do not use for patients in whom TB is suspected. The availability of treatment facilities offering aerosolized pentamidine may be limited.

- Atovaquone suspension 1,500 mg once daily
  (Note: This also is effective in reducing the risk of toxoplasmosis.)
  Atovaquone is more expensive than dapsone. It should be taken with high-fat meals for optimal absorption.

- Atovaquone suspension 1,500 mg + pyrimethamine 25 mg + folinic acid 10 mg all taken PO once daily
  (Note: This regimen also is effective in reducing the risk of toxoplasmosis.)

Secondary Prophylaxis Indications

Prophylaxis should be given to all patients with a history of PCP.

Discontinuing Prophylaxis

Primary or secondary prophylaxis can be discontinued if the CD4 count has increased to >200 cells/μL for at least 3 months in response to effective antiretroviral therapy (ART), with the following cautions:

- If the patient had PCP in the past and the episode of PCP occurred at a CD4 count of >200 cells/μL, it may be prudent to continue PCP prophylaxis for life, regardless of how high the CD4 count rises as a consequence of ART.

- PCP prophylaxis should be reinitiated if the CD4 count decreases to <200 cells/μL or the patient meets other criteria as indicated above.

Prophylaxis During Pregnancy

TMP-SMX is the recommended agent for use during pregnancy; dapsone may be used as an alternative. Some experts recommend high dose folate supplementation (e.g., 4 mg daily) for pregnant women receiving TMP-SMX, because TMP-SMX may worsen folate deficiency. Prophylaxis that includes pyrimethamine generally should be deferred until after pregnancy. During the first trimester, aerosolized pentamidine (which is not systemically absorbed) can be used if the potential teratogenicity of oral agents is a concern.

Mycobacterium avium Complex

Background

Mycobacterium avium complex (MAC) is common among patients with advanced HIV disease and it occurs in people with CD4 counts of <50 cells/μL.

Primary Prophylaxis: Indications

Prophylaxis should be administered to all HIV-infected patients with CD4 counts of <50 cells/μL. Before starting prophylaxis, rule out active MAC infection by clinical assessment and, if warranted, by acid-fast bacilli (AFB) blood cultures (see chapter *Mycobacterium avium Complex*). Also rule out active TB prior to starting any rifabutin-containing regimen for MAC prophylaxis. Review the current drug regimen for medications that may interact with MAC prophylaxis.

Prophylaxis Options: Recommended Regimens

- Azithromycin 1,200 mg PO weekly
- Clarithromycin 500 mg PO BID (Note: Clarithromycin is not recommended for use during pregnancy, and it can have significant interactions with efavirenz, atazanavir, and other drugs; see chapter *Drug-Drug Interactions with HIV-Related Medications*.)
- Azithromycin 600 mg PO BIW

Prophylaxis Options: Alternative Regimens

Rifabutin 300 mg once daily (Note: Rifabutin has significant interactions with many drugs; certain nonnucleoside reverse transcriptase inhibitors and protease inhibitors should be avoided or dosage adjustment of rifabutin may be required. See chapter *Drug-Drug Interactions with HIV-Related Medications*.)

Secondary Prophylaxis

Patients should receive lifelong chronic maintenance therapy, unless immune reconstitution occurs in response to ART. See chapter *Mycobacterium avium Complex*.

Discontinuing Prophylaxis

Primary prophylaxis for MAC can be discontinued in persons who have responded to effective ART with sustained increases in CD4 counts to >100 cells/μL for at least 3 months. Careful observation and monitoring are required, and prophylaxis should be restarted if the patient's CD4 count decreases to <50 cells/μL.

Secondary prophylaxis can be discontinued in patients who received at least 12 months of treatment for MAC, are asymptomatic, and have sustained (for at least 6 months) CD4 counts of >100 cells/μL on ART. Secondary prophylaxis should be reintroduced if the CD4 count decreases to <100 cells/μL.

Prophylaxis During Pregnancy

Azithromycin is the prophylactic drug of

choice during pregnancy, although evidence for its safety in the first trimester is limited. Clarithromycin is teratogenic in animals.

Toxoplasmosis

Background

Toxoplasmic encephalitis (TE) usually is caused by reactivation of latent *Toxoplasma gondii* infection in patients with advanced immunosuppression (especially those with CD4 counts of <100 cells/μL). The USPHS/IDSA recommendations state that all HIV-infected patients should be tested for *Toxoplasma* immunoglobulin G (IgG) antibody soon after the diagnosis of HIV infection. *Toxoplasma* IgG-negative patients should be counseled to avoid sources of infection (see chapter *Preventing Exposure to Opportunistic and Other Infections*), and should be retested for *Toxoplasma* IgG when CD4 counts fall to <100 cells/μL to determine whether they have seroconverted and are therefore at risk of TE. (See chapter *Toxoplasmosis* for more information on active disease and secondary prophylaxis.)

Primary Prophylaxis: Indications

Prophylaxis should be administered to all HIV-infected patients with CD4 counts of <100 cells/μL who are seropositive for *Toxoplasma*. IgG-negative patients should avoid exposure to *Toxoplasma*; see "Patient Education," below.

Prophylaxis Options: Recommended Regimens

- TMP-SMX one double-strength tablet once daily (Note: This option is also effective in preventing PCP.)

Prophylaxis Options: Alternative Regimens

(Note: The following options also are effective in preventing PCP.)

- TMP-SMX, one double-strength tablet PO TIW
- TMP-SMX, one single-strength tablet PO once daily
- Dapsone 50 mg PO once daily + pyrimethamine 50 mg PO weekly + folinic acid 25 mg PO weekly
- Dapsone 200 mg PO weekly + pyrimethamine 75 mg PO weekly + folinic acid 25 mg PO weekly
  - **Warning:** G6PD deficiency can increase the risk of hemolytic anemia or methemoglobinemia in patients receiving dapsone. Screen for G6PD deficiency before starting dapsone. (G6PD deficiency is found in approximately 10% of African-American males, and in 1-2% of males of Mediterranean, Indian, and Asian descent.)
- Atovaquone 1,500 mg PO once daily, with or without pyrimethamine 25 mg PO once daily + folinic acid 10 mg PO once daily; however, this alternative is quite expensive.
- Neither aerosolized pentamidine nor dapsone alone provides protection against TE.

Secondary Prophylaxis

Patients should receive lifelong chronic maintenance therapy, unless immune reconstitution occurs in response to ART (see chapter *Toxoplasmosis*).

Discontinuing Prophylaxis

Primary prophylaxis for TE can be discontinued in patients who have responded to effective ART with sustained CD4 counts of >200 cells/μL for at least 3 months. CD4 counts should be monitored carefully, and prophylaxis should be restarted in patients whose CD4 counts decrease to <100-200 cells/μL.

Secondary prophylaxis may be discontinued if TE signs and symptoms have resolved with treatment and if patients have sustained (for at least 6 months) CD4 counts of >200 cells/μL on ART. Secondary prophylaxis should be reintroduced if CD4 counts drop to <200 cells/μL.

Prophylaxis During Pregnancy

TMP-SMX may be used as primary prophylaxis during pregnancy. Risks of TMP-SMX in the first trimester must be balanced against the risks of reactivated toxoplasmosis. Some experts recommend high dose folate supplementation (e.g., 4 mg daily) for pregnant women receiving TMP-SMX, because TMP-SMX may worsen folate deficiency. Pyrimethamine has been associated with birth defects in animal studies, but limited data in human studies have not shown an increased risk. Secondary prophylaxis generally should be provided using the same guidelines as for nonpregnant women.

Histoplasmosis

Background

Infection with *Histoplasma capsulatum* is common in several geographic areas including the Ohio and Mississippi River Valleys, as well as parts of Central and South America, Asia, and Africa. Symptomatic disease can occur via primary infection or reactivation of previously silent infection in the setting of waning cellular immunity. CD4 counts of ≤150 cells/μL, along with positive *Histoplasma* serology and environmental exposure, are associated with increased risk of symptomatic disease. Histoplasmosis can cause a range of clinical manifestations including respiratory, gastrointestinal, central nervous system (CNS), and cutaneous disease.

Primary Prophylaxis: Indications

Prophylaxis can be considered for HIV-infected patients with CD4 counts of ≤150 cells/μL who are at high risk because of occupational exposure and for those who live in an area where histoplasmosis is highly endemic. HIV-infected patients with CD4 counts of ≤150 cells/μL should be educated to avoid exposure.

Prophylaxis Options: Recommended Regimens

- Itraconazole 200 mg PO once daily (Note: Itraconazole has significant interactions with many drugs, including nonnucleoside reverse transcriptase inhibitors (NNRTIs), protease inhibitors (PIs), and maraviroc. Dosage adjustments may be required, and some combinations may be contraindicated; consult with a pharmacist or other specialist.)

Secondary Prophylaxis

Patients with a history of severe disseminated disease or CNS infection and those who have relapsed despite receiving appropriate therapy should receive long-term suppressive therapy.

Discontinuing Prophylaxis

Primary prophylaxis can be discontinued once CD4 counts are >150 cells/μL for at least 6 months. CD4 counts should be monitored carefully, and prophylaxis should be restarted for patients whose CD4 counts decrease to ≤150 cells/μL.

Secondary prophylaxis may be discontinued if patients have received at least 1 year of itraconazole, have negative blood cultures, have had CD4 counts ≥150 cells/μL for at least 6 months on ART, and have serum *Histoplasma* antigen <2 units.

Prophylaxis During Pregnancy

Azoles should not be used during the first trimester of pregnancy because of teratogenicity concerns.

Coccidiomycosis

Background

The *Coccidioides* species fungus is endemic to many arid regions. In the United States, it is found primarily in the Sonoran Desert in Arizona and the San Joaquin "Central" Valley in California, but also in areas of New Mexico, western Texas, Nevada, and Utah. It also is endemic to many arid regions in Central and South America. Immune response to *Coccidioides* species declines as CD4 counts decrease, and risk of developing symptomatic disease in endemic areas is increased when the CD4 count is ≤250 cells/µL. In HIV-infected patients, six syndromes have been described: focal pneumonia, diffuse pneumonia, cutaneous involvement, meningitis, liver or lymph node involvement, and positive serology without localized infection.

Primary Prophylaxis: Indications

HIV-infected persons from *Coccidioides*-endemic areas with positive IgM or IgG serologies are at increased risk of developing active infection, especially if their CD4 counts are ≤250 cells/µL. Many experts would recommend primary prophylaxis for such patients. Annual monitoring for seroconversion of HIV-infected patients in endemic areas is prudent. Patients in endemic areas should be educated to avoid exposure.

Prophylaxis Options: Recommended Regimens

- Fluconazole 400 mg PO once daily
- Itraconazole 200 mg PO BID

(Note: Itraconazole has significant interactions with many drugs, including NNRTIs, PIs, and maraviroc. Dosage adjustments may be required, and some combinations may be contraindicated; consult with a pharmacist or other specialist.)

Secondary Prophylaxis

Patients who have completed initial treatment for coccidiomycosis should be considered for lifelong chronic maintenance therapy.

Discontinuing Prophylaxis

Primary prophylaxis can be discontinued once CD4 counts are ≥250 cells/µL for at least 6 months, but should be restarted if the CD4 count drops to <250 cells/µL.

Suppressive therapy should be continued lifelong for patients with a history of diffuse pulmonary, disseminated, or meningeal disease, as these patients are at high risk of relapse. Patients with focal coccidioidal pneumonia who have had good clinical response to antifungals can discontinue secondary prophylaxis once they have received 12 months of therapy, and have CD4 counts >250 cells/µL on ART. These patients should undergo close radiologic and serologic monitoring for recurrence.

Prophylaxis During Pregnancy

Women who acquire coccidiomycosis in the second or third trimester of pregnancy are at increased risk of dissemination. Azoles should not be used during the first trimester of pregnancy because of teratogenicity concerns.

Patient Education

- Discuss adverse effects of the selected medication(s) and how the patient should respond in the event of rashes, diarrhea, and other complications.

- Explain the purpose of each medication, and be sure that patients understand the dosage and frequency of administration.

- Reinforce the need to continue taking the medication indefinitely (potentially for life) to reduce the risk of the OI.

- OIs can occur despite prophylaxis. Instruct patients to contact their health care provider if they become ill.

- Counsel patients who are *Toxoplasma* IgG negative to avoid exposure to *Toxoplasma*. Specifically, they should avoid eating raw or undercooked meat, especially pork, lamb, game, and venison. Patients should wash hands after handling raw meat and after gardening or contact with soil. Encourage patients not to adopt or handle stray cats, and, if they own cats, to wash hands thoroughly after cleaning litter boxes. (See chapter *Preventing Exposure to Opportunistic and Other Infections*.)

- For women of childbearing potential who are taking clarithromycin, emphasize the need for effective contraception to avoid potential teratogenic effects of clarithromycin.

- Educate patients in *Histoplasma-* and *Coccidioides*-endemic areas regarding measures to decrease exposure. (See chapter *Preventing Exposure to Opportunistic and Other Infections*.)

References

- Centers for Disease Control and Prevention. *Guidelines for Prevention and Treatment of Opportunistic Infections in HIV-Infected Adults and Adolescents: Recommendations from CDC, the National Institutes of Health, and the HIV Medicine Association of the Infectious Diseases Society of America.* April 10, 2009. Available at www.aidsinfo.nih.gov/guidelines/.

- Centers for Disease Control and Prevention. *Coccidiomycosis.* In: CDC Health Information for International Travel 2010. Atlanta: U.S. Department of Health and Human Services, Public Health Service, 2009. Available at www.cdc.gov/travel/.

- Centers for Disease Control and Prevention. *Histoplasmosis.* In: CDC Health Information for International Travel 2010. Atlanta: U.S. Department of Health and Human Services, Public Health Service, 2009. Available at www.cdc.gov/travel/.

Latent Tuberculosis Infection

Background

Latent (or inactive) tuberculosis (TB) infection occurs when an individual has dormant *Mycobacterium tuberculosis* organisms and no active disease. It can be diagnosed by a tuberculin skin test (TST) or by a blood test called an interferon-gamma release assay (IGRA); both are described below. HIV-infected persons with latent TB infection (LTBI) have a much higher risk of developing active TB (estimated at 10% per year) than the general population (estimated at 10% in a lifetime). The risk of an individual with LTBI developing active TB can be reduced 90% with treatment of LTBI. Hence, identifying and treating HIV-infected persons with LTBI is a high priority. Treatment of LTBI not only reduces the risk of disease to the individual but also reduces the risk of further TB transmission should the HIV/TB-coinfected person develop active pulmonary TB. Standard treatment with isoniazid (INH) is effective and safe.

Issues of concern regarding treatment of LTBI among HIV-infected persons include the following:

- Excluding active pulmonary or extrapulmonary TB disease before treatment with INH alone
- Assessing the risk of latent infection with drug-resistant TB
- Avoiding or managing drug interactions if regimens containing rifampin or rifabutin are used
- Avoiding (if possible) the use of rifampin or rifabutin with pyrazinamide

HRSA HAB Core Clinical Performance Measures

Percentage of clients with HIV infection who received **testing with results documented for latent tuberculosis infection** since HIV diagnosis

(Group 2 measure)

S: Subjective

Ask about symptoms of active TB, including fever, cough, and weight loss; see chapter *Mycobacterium tuberculosis*. HIV-infected persons who have no symptoms of active TB and have not been treated previously for active or latent TB are eligible for LTBI treatment. When patients do have symptoms that could represent active TB, active TB must be evaluated and ruled out by appropriate diagnostic methods before initiating treatment (see "Assessment," below).

Persons who have had bacillus Calmette-Guérin (BCG) vaccine can be evaluated by an IGRA (preferably) or by a TST with correct interpretation. Immigrants from many countries will have had childhood BCG vaccination.

Health care providers should ask about a history of potential exposure to TB, because that might indicate infection with drug-resistant TB. Such risk may occur when the patient knows a source patient or when the exposure occurs in a setting with known drug resistance or in a location with ongoing TB transmission where others remain at risk of exposure.

O: Objective
Diagnostic Evaluation

Current U.S. Centers for Disease Control and Prevention (CDC) guidelines strongly recommend LTBI testing for all newly diagnosed HIV-infected persons. Repeat testing is recommended for patients whose CD4 lymphocyte count increases from low numbers to counts of >200 cells/μL, and annual testing is suggested for patients whose initial test result is negative.

Provisional recommendations from the CDC state that use of either the TST or any of the three currently available IGRAs is acceptable. The TST evaluates delayed hypersensitivity to antigens from a closely related *Mycobacterium* species whereas the IGRAs are in vitro tests of lymphocyte recognition and response to *M. tuberculosis*. A positive TST or IGRA result indicates previous contact between the patient and *M. tuberculosis* and it implies latent TB infection.

In general, all the licensed IGRA tests are considered interchangeable with the TST. Use of an IGRA is preferred for persons with previous BCG exposure and for patient groups at risk of not returning for TST readings. The TST is preferred for children under 5 years of age. The cost of an IGRA is higher than the cost of a TST, and individual clinics should compare the total costs of both testing approaches, including the costs involved in TST protocols of recalling patients who miss visits, repeating TSTs, and treating persons with prior BCG exposure who may have false-positive TST results.

Tuberculin skin test

The TST is administered as an intradermal injection of 0.1 mL (5 tuberculin units) of purified protein derivative (PPD), which raises a wheal in the skin. This is sometimes referred to as the Mantoux test. Multiple-puncture tests such as tine tests and the use of other strengths of PPD are considered unreliable. Anergy testing is not routinely recommended because a randomized controlled study of HIV-infected patients in the United States did not show an advantage to treating anergic, tuberculin-negative persons.

PPD tests are not designed for reading by the patient; a trained health care worker must measure the area of induration (not erythema) 48-72 hours after the test is administered. Induration of 5 mm or more is considered a positive result for HIV-infected persons, other immunosuppressed persons, anyone with recent TB exposure, and anyone with fibrosis on chest X ray that is consistent with previous TB. For HIV-uninfected health care workers, 10 mm of induration is a positive result; in various other populations, either 10 mm or 15 mm of induration may be considered positive. Care providers at many large HIV clinics find it challenging to ensure that their patients return for the PPD reading. One randomized study found that offering incentives (e.g., a fast-food coupon) plus counseling was more effective than counseling alone in obtaining return visits for PPD readings.

Interferon-gamma release assay

IGRA tests performed on peripheral blood samples are available in the United States from two manufacturers. Although the tests are expensive, results are obtained without the patient having to make a return visit to the clinic, and false-positive readings following BCG vaccination do not occur. Both IGRA tests use specific antigens from *M. tuberculosis* to stimulate the patient's lymphocytes and quantify the production of interferon-gamma in response. QuantiFERON-TB Gold (QFT-G) is performed by incubating a heparinized blood sample for 16-24 hours with the synthetic MTB antigens along with positive and negative controls. The incubation must begin within 12 hours, so the need for proximity to a laboratory that performs the test imposes limits on access. The laboratory calculates the amount of interferon-gamma produced by the patient's cells, providing a quantitative result and an interpretation (positive, negative, or indeterminate). The QuantiFERON-TB Gold In Tube (QFT-GIT) provides the clinician with three prepared tubes (three antigens in one tube and positive and negative controls) into which patient blood samples are placed; these tubes may be held for up to 16 hours at room temperature, incubated at 37°C for 16-24 hours, then centrifuged. After centrifugation, the same tubes can be held again at room temperature for up to 3 days or refrigerated for up to 4 weeks before they are analyzed. This provides much greater flexibility in sending specimens to distant or reference laboratories and it makes the technology useful for a much wider array of clinical sites. Again, quantitative results and an interpretation are provided. The T.SPOT TB (T-SPOT) test requires separation and processing of 4 aliquots of 250,000 peripheral blood mononuclear cells each, a step that requires a sophisticated laboratory setting. The number of cells that produce interferon in response to the two MTB antigens is compared with positive and negative controls; both a quantitative result and its interpretation (positive, negative, borderline, or indeterminate) are provided. Performing the test is very labor intensive, and it must take place within 8 hours of obtaining the sample (within 32 hours if using T-Cell Xtend reagent); thus T-SPOT is the least flexible of the three assays.

Limited data suggest that the QFT-GIT is the most specific test (lowest rate of false-positive results) and the T-SPOT is the most sensitive test (with the lowest rate of false-negative results). However, few studies have compared the IGRA assays, and there is no reliable "gold standard" for sensitivity or specificity for latent TB infection. Although these tests do not detect previous BCG exposure, they will yield positive results in all three TB-causing species of the *Mycobacterium tuberculosis* complex, *M. tuberculosis*, *Mycobacterium bovis*, and *Mycobacterium africanum*, and may yield positive results in persons with exposure to certain rare mycobacteria other than *M. tuberculosis* (*Mycobacterium kansasii*, *Mycobacterium marinum*, and *Mycobacterium szulgai*).

There is limited experience using IGRAs for persons with HIV infection and other immunosuppressed states. The overall frequency of positive and negative results is the same with QFT-GIT and TST. However, there is substantial discordance among HIV-infected patients: many with positive TST results will have negative IGRA results, and vice versa. No data are available to determine which test is more reliable. Indeterminate results with QFT-GIT are more frequent with patients who have lower CD4 lymphocyte counts. Some experts anticipate that the T-SPOT may be more consistent in persons with lower lymphocyte (including CD4 cell) counts because a fixed number of cells are used in the assay; however, lymphocyte function may be altered in any case. It appears that there are higher rates of positive results among HIV patients with the T-SPOT than with the other IGRAs. TSTs are known to yield false-negative results in persons with HIV-associated immunosuppression, yet despite this limitation, TSTs are recommended for use with all newly diagnosed HIV patients and for annual testing in certain patients.

A: Assessment

A chest X ray should be obtained for all HIV-infected persons with positive TST or IGRA tests. Asymptomatic patients with negative chest X-ray results should be offered treatment for LTBI. Persons with symptoms consistent with pulmonary or extrapulmonary TB, and those with abnormal chest radiography, require further assessment. This assessment may include sending three separate sputum specimens collected on three consecutive days, or at least 8 hours apart, including at least one early morning specimen (using saline mist to induce cough for those not coughing spontaneously) for acid-fast bacilli (AFB) stain, nucleic acid amplification test, and culture, or obtaining other specimens depending on the suspected site of extrapulmonary TB. If suspicion of TB is low, patients with negative sputum smears (or other biopsy or tissue samples) can begin LTBI treatment. If suspicion of active disease is high, treatment for active disease should be started while the culture results are pending (see chapter *Mycobacterium tuberculosis*). HIV-infected persons with significant exposure to someone with infectious TB should receive a full course of TB prophylaxis regardless of TST or IGRA results. Health departments can assist clinicians in assessing the degree of exposure for an HIV-infected patient and determining whether there is a need for a full course of treatment.

An HIV-infected person with fibrosis on a chest X ray that is consistent with previous TB and with no history of TB treatment (or a history of inadequate treatment) should be evaluated for active TB regardless of TST or IGRA results. If found not to have active TB, the patient should be treated for LTBI. If the patient is strongly suspected to have active TB, standard treatment for active TB should be given while culture analysis is under way. If cultures are negative, patients may be switched to LTBI treatment. Highly suspect but culture-negative patients may be given a 4-month total course of multidrug TB treatment. (See chapter *Mycobacterium tuberculosis*.)

P: Plan

As with any treatment of TB, adherence to the regimen is required for success. Treatment regimens for LTBI in the United States and other high-income nations are presented in Table 1.

Table 1. Treatment Regimens for Latent Tuberculosis			
Drug	**Dosage (taken orally)**	**Frequency**	**Duration (minimum number of doses for completion)**
Recommended			
INH*	Adults: 300 mg Children: 5 mg/kg	Daily	9 months or 270 doses within 12 months
Alternative			
INH*	Adults: 900 mg Children: 10-20 mg/kg	BIW (DOT)**	9 months or 76 supervised doses within 12 months
Exposure to INH-Resistant TB or INH Intolerance			
Rifampin#	Adults: 600 mg Children: 10-20 mg/kg	Daily	4 months or 120 doses in 6 months If used in children, 6 months is recommended
Exposure to Multidrug-Resistant TB			
Treatment options depend on sensitivity of the organism.	Seek expert advice from public health authorities and those experienced in treatment of multidrug-resistant TB. Treatment may be postponed until sensitivity test results are available or may be based on resistance pattern of index case, if known.		

* 10-25 mg of pyridoxine (vitamin B6) should be given with each INH dose to reduce the risk of INH-induced peripheral neuropathy.

** DOT = directly observed treatment

\# Rifampin has significant interactions with nonnucleoside reverse transcriptase inhibitors and protease inhibitors and with other medications. See text about contraindicated combinations, dosage adjustments, and substitution of rifabutin for rifampin.

For treatment of LTBI in persons exposed to multidrug-resistant TB, there are no data on efficacy of various regimens in preventing progression to disease. Experts agree that it is important to follow those with presumed latent MDR TB infection for a minimum of 2 years following the exposure.

INH may cause liver toxicity and it should be used cautiously in patients with active alcohol use, liver disease, or chronic hepatitis B or C. INH is contraindicated for use in patients with acute hepatitis or decompensated liver disease. Before INH use, baseline liver and renal function should be tested. Routine monthly clinical monitoring for fever, fatigue, anorexia, nausea, vomiting, abdominal pain, jaundice, peripheral neuropathy, and rash should be performed. Alanine aminotransferase (ALT) should be monitored monthly in HIV-infected patients who have a risk of hepatitis. If patients develop abnormalities in liver transaminases while taking INH (ALT or aspartate aminotransferase >3 times the upper limit of normal [ULN] with symptoms, or >5 times above the ULN in the absence of symptoms), the INH should be withheld. Obtain expert consultation before treating patients with abnormal liver function or advanced liver disease.

Rifampin may cause liver and bone marrow toxicity. Before rifampin use, obtain baseline liver and renal function tests and a complete blood count. Follow-up is the same as for INH use.

Potential ARV Interactions

Rifampin and rifabutin have important interactions with certain antiretroviral drugs, and dosage adjustments or treatment modifications may be required. Rifampin reduces the blood levels of nonnucleoside reverse transcriptase inhibitors (NNRTIs), protease inhibitors (PIs), the integrase inhibitor raltegravir, and the CCR5 antagonist maraviroc. Rifampin can be used by persons taking efavirenz although many experts recommend increasing the efavirenz dosage to 800 mg daily. Coadministration of rifampin and maraviroc is not recommended, but may be possible with appropriate dosage adjustment of maraviroc; consult with an expert. Rifampin should not be used with nevirapine, etravirine, or PIs. (In some cases, the adverse pharmacokinetic effect of rifampin on PIs may be overcome with large doses of ritonavir, but consultation with a specialist should be obtained before this approach is undertaken; rifampin should not be used in combination with ritonavir-boosted saquinavir because of high rates of hepatic toxicity.)

No data are available on the use of rifabutin for treatment of LTBI. Nevertheless, rifabutin may be considered in place of rifampin for patients taking antiretroviral combinations that include NNRTIs (other than efavirenz) or PIs (other than ritonavir alone). In these cases, the dosages of both rifabutin and the antiretroviral agent usually require adjustment. (See Table 3 in chapter *Mycobacterium tuberculosis* for details on dosage adjustments).

Other Drug Interactions

Rifampin decreases the blood concentrations of estrogens, anticonvulsants, hypoglycemic agents, and many other drugs. Review all medications a patient is taking before initiating rifampin and make adjustments as necessary. (See Table 12: *Clinically significant drug-drug interactions involving the rifamycins* at www. cdc.gov/mmwr/preview/mmwrhtml/rr5211a1. htm#tab12.)

Pregnancy

HIV-infected pregnant women with positive LTBI test results and no evidence of active TB should receive standard prophylaxis as soon as possible, even during the first trimester.

The preferred prophylaxis during pregnancy is a 9-month isoniazid regimen (with pyridoxine, as above). Alternative agents, such as rifampin or rifabutin, should be used with caution because of limited experience. Neonates born to women who received rifampin during pregnancy should be given vitamin K (10 mg) to reduce the risk of hemorrhagic disease. Pyrazinamide generally is avoided during pregnancy because of lack of information regarding fetal effects.

Patient Education

- Patients should know that TB bacteria in their bodies cannot be passed to others while the TB is latent. However, because they have HIV infection, the TB bacteria is more likely to make them sick at some point in the future.

- Treatment for LTBI will help kill the TB bacteria and reduce patients' chances of becoming sick with active TB.

- Patients must take all of their medicine, every day, to prevent the TB from spreading and making them sick.

- Advise patients to contact their health care provider immediately if they have adverse effects to the medication, such as rash or itching. Occasionally, INH can cause tingling or numbness in the hands or feet. The pyridoxine (vitamin B6) they are taking should help prevent that, but they should let their provider know if it occurs.

- Advise patients to avoid the use of alcohol while taking INH. The medicines for TB are processed by the liver and, when combined with alcohol, they easily can overload the liver. Acetaminophen (Tylenol) also is processed by the liver, so patients should keep their intake to a minimum. (Patients with hepatitis C, liver disease, or chronic alcohol use should not take more than 3 grams per day.)

- Tell patients that blood tests will be done regularly to make sure the liver is working well, so it is important to keep follow-up appointments. They should take all their medications, vitamins, and supplements with them to the clinic so that their health care provider can review them and make sure there are no drug interactions.

- If patients experience nausea, vomiting, poor appetite, or abdominal pain; if they notice their urine darkening or becoming cola colored; or if they notice their eyes or skin yellowing, they should contact the clinic immediately. These problems may indicate that the liver is being overwhelmed, and it is important to find out before permanent damage is done.

- Rifampin will cause sweat, tears, urine, and plastic contact lenses to turn orange.

- Rifampin can make birth control pills ineffective. Patients should use a backup method of contraception until treatment is complete. Condoms can help prevent HIV transmission and reduce the likelihood of pregnancy.

References

- Akolo C, Adetifa I, Sheppard S, et al. *Treatment of latent tuberculosis infection in persons with HIV infection.* Cochrane Database Syst Rev. 2004;(1):CD000171.

- American Thoracic Society. *Targeted tuberculin testing and treatment of latent tuberculosis infection.* MMWR Recomm Rep. 2000 Jun 9;49(RR-6):1-51. Available at www.cdc.gov/mmwr/PDF/rr/rr4906.pdf. Accessed June 30, 2010.

- Blumberg HM, Leonard MK, Jasmer RM. *Update on the treatment of tuberculosis and latent tuberculosis infection.* JAMA. 2005 Jun 8;293(22):2776-84.

- Centers for Disease Control and Prevention. *Guidelines for Prevention and Treatment of Opportunistic Infections in HIV-Infected Adults and Adolescents: Recommendations from CDC, the National Institutes of Health, and the HIV Medicine Association of the Infectious Diseases Society of America.* April 10, 2009. Available at www.aidsinfo.nih.gov/guidelines/.

- Centers for Disease Control and Prevention. *Managing Drug Interactions in the Treatment of HIV-Related Tuberculosis.* 2007. Available at: www.cdc.gov/tb/publications/guidelines/TB_HIV_Drugs/PDF/tbhiv.pdf. Accessed June 30, 2010.

- Centers for Disease Control and Prevention, American Thoracic Society. *Update: adverse event data and revised American Thoracic Society/CDC recommendations against the use of rifampin and pyrazinamide for treatment of latent tuberculosis infection—United States, 2003.* MMWR Morb Mortal Wkly Rep. 2003 Aug 8;52(31):735-9.

- Golub JE, Pronyk P, Mohapi L, et al. *Isoniazid preventive therapy, HAART, and tuberculosis risk in HIV-infected adults in South Africa: a prospective cohort.* AIDS. 2009 Jul 17;23(11):1444-6.

- Golub JE, Saraceni V, Cavalcante SG, et al. *The impact of antiretroviral therapy and isoniazid preventive therapy on tuberculosis incidence in HIV-infected patients in Rio de Janeiro, Brazil.* AIDS. 2007 Jul 11;21(11):1441-8.

- Lobue P. Provisional CDC *Recommendations for the use of interferon-gamma release assays to detect Mycobacterium tuberculosis infection in the United States.* Presented at Infectious Disease Society of America; October 29, 2009; Philadelphia.

- Mazurek GH, Jereb J, Lobue P, et al; Division of Tuberculosis Elimination, National Center for HIV, STD, and TB Prevention, Centers for Disease Control and Prevention. *Guidelines for using the QuantiFERON-TB Gold Test for detecting Mycobacterium tuberculosis infection, United States.* MMWR Recomm Rep. 2005 Dec 16;54(RR-15):49-55.. Available at www.cdc.gov/mmwr/pdf/rr/rr5415.pdf. Accessed June 30, 2010.

- National Tuberculosis Controllers Association; Centers for Disease Control and Prevention. *Guidelines for the investigation of contacts of persons with infectious tuberculosis. Recommendations from the National Tuberculosis Controllers Association and CDC.* MMWR Recomm Rep. 2005 Dec 16;54(RR-15):1-47. Available at www.cdc.gov/mmwr/pdf/rr/rr5415.pdf. Accessed June 30, 2010.

- Pai M, Zwerling A, Menzies D. *Systematic review: T-cell-based assays for the diagnosis of latent tuberculosis infection: an update.* Ann Intern Med. 2008 Aug 5;149(3):177-84.

Smoking Cessation

Jeffery Kwong, MS, MPH, ANP

Background

According to the U.S. Centers for Disease Control and Prevention, smoking prevalence among the general adult population in the United States is approximately 20%. Among HIV-infected persons, the prevalence of cigarette smoking appears to be two to three times greater than in the general population, with estimates ranging from 50% to 70%.

HRSA HAB Core Clinical Performance Measures

Percentage of clients with HIV infection who received **tobacco cessation counseling** within the measurement year.

(Group 3 measure)

The health effects of cigarette smoking are extensive and have been well documented. There are approximately 400,000 smoking-related deaths annually in the United States. HIV-infected smokers appear to be at higher risk of a variety of tobacco-related conditions than HIV-uninfected smokers. These include lung cancer, head and neck cancers, cervical and anal cancers, oral candidiasis, and oral hairy leukoplakia. HIV-infected smokers who smoke are more likely to develop the conditions listed above, as well as bacterial pneumonia, *Pneumocystis jiroveci* pneumonia, other pulmonary conditions, and cardiovascular disease. Additionally, HIV-infected smokers have been shown to have a decreased immunologic and virologic response to antiretroviral therapy.

Thus, for HIV-infected persons, even more so than for HIV-uninfected persons, clinicians should consider smoking cessation a health care priority. Although many care providers may feel that they can do little to affect the smoking behaviors of patients, evidence suggests that brief interventions by physicians are quite effective. Studies indicate that smoking cessation interventions as brief as 3 minutes in duration, when delivered by a physician, have a positive impact on abstinence rates of current smokers. Furthermore, studies have found that more than half of current HIV-infected smokers have expressed interest in, or have thought about, smoking cessation.

Cigarettes are highly addictive; the U.S. Surgeon General has equated the addictive potential of cigarettes to that of heroin and cocaine. This is in part because nicotine stimulates the release of several neurotransmitters in the brain, including dopamine. Over time, chronic exposure to nicotine causes physiologic changes in the brain that contribute to the addictive potential of cigarettes.

Cigarette smoking involves dependence on more than a single chemical compound, however. It is a multidimensional behavior that has both physiologic and psychological components. Therefore, smoking cessation efforts often require a combined approach to be successful.

Behavioral model for smoking cessation

Several behavioral models present a psychological framework for understanding individuals who are attempting to change behaviors. The transtheoretical model of health behavior change is one of the more frequently cited frameworks for understanding the stages of behavior change of smokers. According to this model, there are five phases of behavior change: precontemplation, contemplation, preparation, action, and maintenance. Using this framework, clinicians can devise interventions that are most appropriate for the patient's current stage on the continuum.

- **Precontemplation:** The individual does not expect to make any change in behavior within the next 6 months. At this stage, the individual is resistant to hearing or learning about health behavior change.

- **Contemplation:** The individual plans to make a behavior change within the next 6 months. This stage is characterized by ambivalence about smoking.

- **Preparation:** The individual anticipates making a behavior change within the next month. Individuals in this phase have made plans for taking action and intend to make a change.

- **Action:** The individual has made a significant change; in the case of smoking cessation, this means that the individual has quit completely.

- **Maintenance:** The individual attempts to prevent relapse.

Patients may move back and forth among these stages at various points during the process of smoking cessation.

Cessation interventions in the clinic

As suggested above, brief smoking cessation interventions delivered by clinicians can significantly increase abstinence rates of current smokers. The U.S. Surgeon General has developed guidelines for clinicians to use during clinic visits to help patients who are interested in smoking cessation. These include use of the Five A's model, which provides a brief and structured framework for addressing smoking cessation in clinical settings (see Table 1).

Table 1. The Five A's Model for Treating Tobacco Use and Dependence

Component	Action	Example
ASK every patient about tobacco use	Identify and document tobacco use at **every visit**.	Incorporate questions about tobacco use when obtaining vital signs or when reviewing a patient's history. • "Do you currently use tobacco?" • "Do you currently smoke cigarettes?"
ADVISE to quit	Using **a clear, strong, and personalized message**, urge every tobacco user to quit.	• "It is important for you to quit smoking now." • "Quitting is the most important thing you can do to protect your health." • "I can help you quit." Also link smoking with something specific to the patient, such as secondhand exposure to children or partners, his/her own lung, cardiovascular, or cancer risk, or the expense of cigarettes.
ASSESS readiness to make a quit attempt	Determine whether the tobacco user is **willing and ready** to make a quit attempt within 30 days.	• "Are you willing to give quitting cigarettes a try?"
ASSIST in the quit attempt	For the patient willing to quit, **assist in developing a quit plan.** Provide practical counseling, support, and supplementary materials.	• Have patient set a quit date and enlist the support of his/her family and friends. • Offer pharmacotherapy, as appropriate, including nicotine replacement. • Provide counseling that includes problem solving and skills building.

Component	Action	Example
<u>ARRANGE</u> for follow-up	Arrange for **follow-up contacts** beginning within the first week after the quit date.	• Contact patient via telephone or in person soon after the quit date. This can be done by the primary clinician or other trained staff members. • During the follow-up encounter, assess and identify any problems, review medication use and side effects, provide reminders about additional resources. • Congratulate patients on their successes. • Help those with relapses assess problems with and barriers to quitting, and offer additional or different assistance. • For patients who report a relapse, help them identify the circumstances that led the relapse and assist them with recommitting to smoking abstinence.

Adapted from Fiore MC, Jaén CR, Baker TB, et al. *Treating Tobacco Use and Dependence: 2008 Update.* Clinical Practice Guideline. Rockville, MD: U.S. Department of Health and Human Services, Public Health Service; May 2008. Available at www.ncbi.nlm.nih.gov/bookshelf/br.f cgi?book=hsahcpr&part=A28163. Accessed June 30, 2010.

For patients who are not ready to quit, techniques such motivational interviewing (MI) can be used in conjunction with the stages-of-change model to explore the smokers' beliefs, feelings, and barriers to successful cessation efforts. Components of MI include: a) expressing empathy; b) developing discrepancy; c) rolling with resistance; and d) supporting self-efficacy. Effective use of MI involves specialized training. Partnering with clinic staff or outside agencies that are familiar with MI techniques can help improve behavior change outcomes, such as smoking cessation. (For further information, see "References," below.)

Pharmacologic interventions

In addition to counseling, the use of pharmacologic interventions such as nicotine replacement therapy and other adjuvant therapies should be considered. These therapies were developed for the general population, but current clinical guidelines suggest that they should be efficacious for HIV-infected smokers.

Clinicians should be aware of potential medication adverse effects (see Table 2).

S: Subjective

• Ask all patients about their smoking status at every visit. This can be easily incorporated as part the initial intake when vital signs are obtained.

• Document smoking history, including the number of cigarettes smoked per day.

• If the patient is not ready to quit, use MI techniques to identify beliefs and barriers and to create ambivalence about smoking.

• For the smoker interested in quitting:

  • Help identify triggers to smoking, and develop a quit plan.

  • Assess for contraindications to pharmacologic smoking cessation treatments such as history of seizure disorders, sleep disturbances, mood disorders, and pregnancy.

• For patients who recently quit, congratulate them on their accomplishments and reinforce the benefits of continued cessation.

• For patients who recently relapsed, help them identify what led to the relapse and how to avoid relapses in the future. Assist them in getting back on track with a cessation program.

O: Objective

During the physical examination, assess for evidence of smoking-related illnesses and the comorbid conditions that may be affected by smoking. At a minimum, measure blood pressure and oxygen saturation measurements and examine for oral lesions, abnormal breath sounds, and decreased peripheral perfusion.

A/P: Assessment and Plan

Determine the smoker's readiness to change (see behavioral model for smoking cessation, above). For those smokers in the preparation or action stage, assist with implementing a quit plan. For those who are in the relapse stage, reinforce self-efficacy and encourage them to recommit to cessation. For those in the maintenance stage, congratulate them and reinforce the benefits of smoking cessation.

For patients willing to quit, offer resources and information that will help them to be successful in their quit attempt. Evidence suggests that the combination of counseling and medication is more effective than either intervention alone. Therefore, every effort should be made to combine counseling sessions with pharmacotherapy for patients who are motivated and ready to quit smoking.

Components of effective counseling include problem solving, skills training, and social support. Problem solving and skills training should focus on how to deal with triggers or urges that may lead to relapse. Examples include recognition of situations or events that may prompt a person to smoke (e.g., drinking alcohol, being around other cigarette smokers, situational stress) and means of reducing or coping with these situations. Social support interventions include providing reassurance that the patient has the ability to succeed with smoking cessation, communicating caring and concern, and encouraging the patient to talk about the quit process.

Offer medications, if there are no contraindications to pharmacologic interventions (see Table 2). All currently available over-the-counter and prescription medications have been shown to be effective. However, studies have shown that combination therapy may be more efficacious than monotherapy. The current tobacco cessation guidelines recommend the following combinations, all of which include nicotine preparations: long-term nicotine patch (>14 weeks) with ad lib use of nicotine gum or spray, nicotine patch with nicotine inhaler, and nicotine patch with sustained-release (SR) bupropion.

Both bupropion SR and varenicline may cause sleep disturbance, and varenicline may cause exacerbation of neuropsychiatric symptoms. For HIV-infected patients who take efavirenz as part of their antiretroviral therapy, concomitant use of either bupropion SR or varenicline may increase the possibility of these side effects. Additional research in this area is needed.

Table 2. Pharmacologic Options for Smoking Cessation

Drug	Recommended Dosing	Common Side Effects	Comments
Nicotine Formulations			
			• Use with caution for patients with cardiovascular disease (particularly those within 2 weeks of myocardial infarction), those with serious arrhythmias, and those with unstable angina pectoris (however, note that, for many patients, continued smoking may be more dangerous than nicotine replacement). • The adverse effects of cigarette smoking during pregnancy are well established, and smoking generally is more harmful than the use of nicotine replacements. Smoking cessation aids may help motivated patients quit during pregnancy.
Nicotine Patch (available OTC) *Dosage varies by brand:* **Nicoderm or Habitrol:** • 21 mg/24 hours • 14 mg/24 hours • 7 mg/24 hours **Nicotrol:** • 15 mg/24 hours • 10 mg/24 hours • 5 mg/24 hours	Dosing recommendations vary based on the number of cigarettes smoked. Individualize treatment. Sample treatment recommendation for smokers who smoke ≥10 cigarettes per day: • High-dose patch for 4-6 weeks, then • Medium-dose patch for 2 weeks, then • Low-dose patch for 2 weeks For smokers who smoke <10 cigarettes per day: • Medium-dose patch for 6-8 weeks, then • Low-dose patch for 2 weeks	Local skin reaction, insomnia or vivid dreams	• Apply upon awakening. • Place patch on a relatively hairless location, rotating sites to avoid irritation. • If experiencing sleep disturbance, remove patch prior to bedtime or use the 16-hour patch.

Drug	Recommended Dosing	Common Side Effects	Comments
Nicotine Formulations			
Nicotine Lozenge (available OTC) • 2 mg and 4 mg	• For patients who smoke their first cigarette >30 minutes after waking, start with 2 mg dose. For patients who smoke their first cigarette within the first 30 minutes after waking, start with 4 mg. • Most patients should use 1 lozenge Q1-2H during the first 6 weeks. • Allow lozenges to dissolve, do not chew or swallow. Most individuals use 9 lozenges per day; maximum is 20 per day. • Lozenges should be used for up to 12 weeks, decreasing dosing from 1 lozenge Q1-2H for the first 6 weeks, to 1 lozenge Q2-4H during weeks 7-9, and 1 lozenge Q4-8H during weeks 9-12.	Nausea, hiccups, heartburn, headache, cough	• Do not eat or drink anything except water for 15 minutes before or using a lozenge.
Nicotine Inhaler (prescription only) • 4 mg per inhalation, • 10 mg cartridge	Recommended dosage: 6-16 cartridges per day. Duration of therapy: up to 6 months, taper dosage in last 3 months.	Local irritation in the mouth and throat, cough, rhinitis; may cause bronchospasm (<1%)	• Use caution in persons with severe reactive airway disease.
Nicotine Nasal Spray (prescription only) • 0.5 mg per spray	• Patient should use 1-2 sprays each nostril per hour (total 1-2 mg per hour), increasing as needed for symptom relief. • Minimum recommended treatment is 16 sprays (8 mg) per day, with a maximum limit of 80 sprays per day (10 sprays per hour). • Recommended duration of therapy: 3-6 months. • Do not sniff, swallow, or inhale through the nose while administering doses. Tilt head slightly back when dosing.	Nasal irritation, transient changes in sense of smell and taste; may cause bronchospasm (<1%)	• Use caution in persons with severe reactive airway disease. • Nicotine nasal spray has highest dependence potential of the nicotine replacement therapies.

Drug	Recommended Dosing	Common Side Effects	Comments
Non-Nicotine Medications, First Line			
Bupropion SR • 150 mg	Begin 1-2 weeks before quit date. • Start at 150 mg daily for 3 days, then increase to 150 mg BID for 7-12 weeks. • May consider longer term therapy.	Insomnia, dry mouth	• May lower seizure threshold in certain patients. • Levels increased in patients on P450 3A4 inhibitors. • Use with caution in patients with history of seizures, eating disorders, or who have used a monoamine oxidase (MAO) inhibitor in the past 14 days.
Varenicline • 0.5 mg and 1 mg	Begin 1 week before quit date. • Start with 0.5 mg daily for 3 days, increase to 0.5 mg BID for 4 days, then 1 mg BID for duration of therapy. • Typical duration: 12 weeks. • Varenicline is approved for maintenance therapy for up to 6 months.	Nausea; flatulence; headache; sleep disturbance; abnormal, vivid, or strange dreams; depression; agitation; suicidal ideation; and suicide FDA Black Box warning regarding neuropsychiatric adverse effects	• Use with caution in patients with history of psychiatric illness. Monitor closely for mood and behavior changes. • Dosage reduction recommended for patients who have creatinine clearance (CrCl) of <30 mL/min or are on dialysis. • To reduce nausea, should be taken with food. To reduce insomnia, second pill can be taken at dinner rather than at bedtime. • Dosage may be reduced for patients with adverse effects.
Non-Nicotine Medications, Second Line			
Clonidine • 0.1 mg tablet • 0.1 mg transdermal patch	• 0.1 mg tablet PO BID OR • 0.1 mg transdermal patch per day. Can increase by 0.1 mg/day per week if needed. • Duration of treatment: 3-10 weeks. • Do not discontinue therapy abruptly.	Dry mouth, drowsiness, dizziness, sedation, and constipation Rebound hypertension if discontinued abruptly	• Monitor blood pressure when using this medication. If discontinuing, taper medication to avoid rebound hypertension. • If using patch, place on relatively hairless location between the neck and waist.
Nortriptyline	• Begin 10-28 days before quit date. • Start at 25 mg once daily and increase to target dosage of 75-100 mg once daily if tolerated. • Treatment duration: approximately 12 weeks; some may consider extending treatment up to 6 months.	Sedation, dry mouth, blurred vision, urinary retention, lightheadedness, tremor, cardiac conduction abnormalities	• Use with caution in patients with cardiac conduction abnormalities disease. • Do not coadminister with MAO inhibitors. • Overdose may produce life-threatening cardiovascular toxicity, as well as seizures and coma.

Section 3: Health Maintenance and Disease Prevention

All patients who are actively quitting should have close follow-up, and they should be offered support. Research has shown that ongoing support during the quit phase results in higher abstinence rates.

Follow-up can include telephone calls or in-person evaluation.

For patients who recently quit or relapsed, continue to provide support and encouragement. Assist individuals who relapsed with the opportunity to continue with cessation plans.

Refer patients to smoking cessation groups, classes, and other resources.

Patient Education

- For patients who have decided on pharmacologic interventions and for whom there are no contraindications, provide education regarding medication side effects, anticipated withdrawal symptoms, and strategies for managing withdrawal.

- Review and reinforce strategies in the event of relapse.

- For those who are not ready to quit, inform them of the consequences of continued smoking and remind them about the available resources.

Suggested Resources:

- National Telephone Counseling and Quit Line (800-QUIT-NOW) (800-784-8669)

- American Cancer Society (www.cancer.org)

- American Lung Association (maintains profiles of state tobacco control activities) (www.lungusa.org)

- National Cancer Institute (www.nci.nih.gov)

- Office on Smoking and Health at the Centers for Disease Control and Prevention (www.cdc.gov/tobacco)

References

- Cook PF, Bradley-Springer L, Corwin M. *Motivational Interviewing and HIV: Reducing Risk, Inspiring Change.* Mountain Plains AIDS Education Training Center; August 2009. Available at www.mpaetc.org/scripts/prodView.asp?idproduct=141. Accessed June 30, 2010.

- Crothers K, Goulet JL, Rodriguez-Barradas MC, et al. *Impact of cigarette smoking on mortality in HIV-positive and HIV-negative veterans.* AIDS Educ Prev. 2009 Jun;21(3 Suppl):40-53.

- Fiore MC, Jaen CR, Baker TB, et al. *Treating Tobacco Use and Dependence: 2008 Update. Clinical Practice Guideline.* Rockville, MD: U.S. Department of Health and Human Services, Public Health Service; 2008.

- Prochaska JO. *Decision making in the transtheoretical model of behavior change.* Med Decis Making. 2008 Nov-Dec;28(6):845-9.

- Prochaska JO, Velicer WF. *The transtheoretical model of health behavior change.* Am J Health Promot. 1997 Sep-Oct;12(1):38-48.

- Reynolds NR. *Cigarette smoking and HIV: more evidence for action.* AIDS Educ Prev. 2009 Jun;21(3 Suppl):106-21.

- Vidrine DJ. *Cigarette smoking and HIV/AIDS: health implications, smoker characteristics and cessation strategies.* AIDS Educ Prev. 2009 Jun;21(3 Suppl):3-13.

- Walters ST, Wright JA, Shegog R. *A review of computer and internet-based interventions for smoking behavior.* Addict Behav. 2006 Feb;31(2):264-77.

Nutrition

Background

Maintaining good nutritional status is important to support overall health and immune system function for people with HIV/AIDS. Many HIV-related conditions affect and are affected by the body's nutritional status. These include conditions related to HIV itself (e.g., opportunistic infections and other illnesses), comorbid conditions, and adverse effects of therapies.

Inadequate nutrition in people with HIV infection may result from many factors, including conditions such as nausea, vomiting, and anorexia (see chapter *Nausea and Vomiting*) that may prevent adequate intake of nutrients and medications; diarrheal infections (see chapter *Diarrhea*) that prevent absorption of nutrients and medications; poor oral health conditions that interfere with chewing or tasting food (see chapter *Oral Health*); systemic illnesses (including HIV itself) that create a catabolic state; and psychological conditions (such as depression) that impair patients' ability to nourish themselves. In addition, financial constraints may limit patients' access to nutritious food.

Evaluation and enhancement of patients' nutritional status may help correct or compensate for deficiencies (e.g., in the case of weight loss or nutrient deficits), may be a key treatment modality for certain conditions (e.g., dyslipidemia, hyperglycemia), and may help to maintain good health and immune function. This chapter focuses on the evaluation of patients with nutritional deficiencies, particularly weight loss, and on simple strategies for maintaining good nutrition in individuals with barriers to maintaining adequate weight.

It should be noted that obesity and overweight conditions are increasingly common in HIV-infected individuals; many of the principles described here also may be applied to the evaluation of overweight patients. Recommendations for weight reduction for HIV-infected patients are the same as for the general population and will not be discussed in detail; for overweight patients with lipohypertrophy, diabetes, dyslipidemia, or coronary artery disease, see the respective chapters on these conditions.

Ideally, HIV-infected individuals will receive the services of HIV-experienced nutrition specialists, who may contribute to the patient care team in the following ways:

- Conducting routine screening to identify and treat nutritional problems
- Preparing a tailored nutritional plan to optimize patients' nutritional status, immune status, and overall well-being
- Screening and developing interventions for growth problems in children
- Developing strategies to prevent loss of weight and lean body mass
- Adapting dietary recommendations to help reduce the risk of comorbid conditions such as diabetes and heart disease, or treating these complications
- Educating patients about how to modify their dietary habits to maximize the effectiveness of medical and pharmacologic treatments
- Tailoring nutritional recommendations to fit patients' lifestyles and financial resources
- Counseling patients to promote nutrition self-care using available resources

- Providing nutritional support to patients may help to do the following:

  - Address common problems associated with HIV disease and its treatment (e.g., weight loss, wasting, fatigue, loss of appetite, adverse changes in taste, dental problems, gastrointestinal complaints)

  - Treat chronic comorbid conditions (e.g., cardiovascular disease, hypertension, diabetes, cirrhosis)

  - Improve quality of life

  - Enhance immune responses, slow disease progression, and prolong life

S: Subjective

History

Identify nutrition risk factors at the start of care through interview, questionnaire, or both. Update the history at least annually.

The history should elicit signs and symptoms related to nutrition issues, indications regarding dietary habits, and symptoms that suggest nutritional deficiencies.

Nutrition-Related Questions	
Signs, Symptoms, and Comorbid Conditions:	
• Poor or sporadic appetite • Early satiety • Weight gain or loss • Trouble chewing or swallowing • Dental problems including poor dental hygiene • Gastrointestinal complaints, including nausea, diarrhea, constipation, heartburn, gas	• Changes in body contours with fat gain in abdomen, back of neck, and breasts (lipodystrophy) or fat loss in extremities and face (lipoatrophy) • Depression, stress • Fatigue • Chronic pain • Other diseases affecting diet and nutrition • Medications, including over-the-counter and herbal products
Medication-Related Factors:	**Social and Behavioral Factors:**
• Medication side effects • Difficulty coordinating meals with medicines • Use of nutritional supplements	• Frequent eating out • Smoking • Alcohol or substance abuse • Erratic meal patterns • Unbalanced diet (e.g., high intake of low-nutrient foods; deficiency in key nutrients) • Resources to ensure secure, continued food access • Availability of food storage and preparation facilities • Housing (stable, homeless, marginally housed, or in transition) • Nutrition literacy

To develop a specific dietary history, ask about the following:

Dietary History	
Usual Dietary Intake	**Factors That May Affect or Limit Intake**
• Frequency of intake of foods providing key nutrients (e.g., dairy products, fortified or whole grains, fruits and vegetables, fluids, meat, eggs, beans) as well as those that perhaps should be limited (fast-food items, highly processed or salted products) • Usual meal patterns (number of times per day, snacks) and whether meals are prepared and eaten at home or eaten at restaurants or fast-food establishments • Specific information about nutritional supplements (e.g., vitamins, minerals, herbs, protein), including contents, amounts, formulation (pills, powders, drinks), cost, and overlap among products	• Amount of money available for food, or participation in food assistance programs (e.g., food stamps, food pantries) • Appetite, general well-being (e.g., fatigue, pain, depression) • Food allergies, intolerances • Problems with dentition, swallowing, heartburn, diarrhea, constipation • Coordination of foods and supplements with medications (HIV or other)

Elicit symptoms that may be related to nutritional deficiencies.

Symptoms with Possible Relationship to Nutritional Deficiencies	
• General symptoms (e.g., fatigue, decreased cognitive function, headache) • Behavioral changes (e.g., irritability, apathy, decreased responsiveness, anxiety, attention deficit) • Body habitus changes (e.g., loss or gain of fat) • Gastrointestinal symptoms (e.g., diarrhea, constipation, bloating)	• Changes in skin, nails, hair (e.g., dryness, breaking, thinning) • Muscle loss • Neurologic symptoms (e.g., weakness, sensory changes, gait abnormalities)

O: Objective
Physical Examination

Perform a careful physical examination, if possible with anthropometric and body composition testing as described below (Table 1). Compare current findings with past assessments and review at least every 6 months.

The physical examination should include the following:

- Vital signs, with orthostatic vital signs if dehydration is suspected

- Weight (compare with previous values) and body mass index (BMI)

- General appearance and gross nutritional status (e.g., obesity, cachexia, wasting)

- Body habitus: loss of subcutaneous fat in face, buttocks, arms and legs and/or increased fat in abdomen, breasts, back of neck, and upper back ("buffalo hump")

- Muscle mass

- Mouth: breakdown in oral mucosa, cheilosis, angular stomatitis, glossitis, papillar atrophy

- Abdomen: hepatomegaly (may be caused by fatty infiltration)

- Skin: dryness, peeling, breakdown, pallor, hypopigmentation or hyperpigmentation

- Nails: pale nail beds, fissures or ridges

- Neurologic system, including strength, sensation, coordination, gait, deep tendon reflexes

Anthropometric and body composition tests are usually performed by registered dietitians. They can provide important information about patients' nutritional status.

Table 1. Anthropometric Measurements for Adults and Children

	Height	Weight	Assessment for Changes over Time
Adults	Measure at baseline (self-report is not accurate).	• Measure at least quarterly and consider intervention when small changes are observed. Do not wait until major amounts of weight have been lost or gained. • Record sequentially at the front of the patient's chart and monitor for trends.	Use healthy, premorbid weight to assess change, not the first clinic weight or the ideal weight. (Use the patient's weight at a time when the patient is healthy, feels well, and can easily maintain that weight.) *
Children	Measure at least quarterly using length board (0-2 years) or wall-mounted stadiometer (≥2 years).	• Measure at least quarterly and consider intervention when small changes are observed. Do not wait until the patient has dropped significantly on the growth chart. • Calculate age and plot the measurements on growth charts specific for age, sex, and country.#	Assessment of optimal growth is based on the observed pattern over time. General goals include a weight relatively "matched" for length or height (about the same percentile) and relative stability of percentile tracking over time.* #

* BMI (body mass index) is useful as an evaluative index. See chapter *Initial Physical Examination*, also online calculator at www.cdc.gov/healthyweight/assessing/bmi/.

\# Growth charts for children in the United States are available online from the U.S. Centers for Disease Control and Prevention (CDC) at www.cdc.gov/growthcharts/. A variety of growth charts are available for children from specific ethnic groups (e.g., Chinese, Vietnamese, Thai), children with selected conditions affecting growth (e.g., Down syndrome), or those who are born prematurely. Percentiles for both height and weight should be recorded sequentially.

Body Composition Testing

Body composition commonly is tested by bioelectrical impedance analysis (BIA) (Table 2) or skinfold thickness and circumference (Table 3).

Table 2. Bioelectrical Impedance Analysis

BIA testing is the standard of care for adults but has not been well validated for children:

- BIA is useful for assessing disease progression or health maintenance, documenting response to treatment, and justifying the cost of nutritional supplements and AIDS-wasting medications.
- The test is simple, noninvasive, and quick (<5 minutes). However, staff training and specialized software are required to interpret the results.
- Perform BIA at baseline. Update every 6-12 months or more frequently if the patient is ill, has a decline in immune status, or has a weight change of 5-10%.
- The BIA test reports the following:
  - **Body cell mass (BCM):** the target component, reflecting cells in muscles, organs, and the circulation; losses may indicate AIDS wasting. BCM is recorded in pounds. Monitor for trends.
  - **Fat:** an index of energy stores; recorded in pounds and percentage.
  - **Phase angle:** a measure of cellular integrity, an independent indicator of morbidity and mortality in HIV-infected patients.

Table 3. Skinfold Thickness and Circumference Measures
Skinfold thickness and circumference measures can be used for adults and children in resource-limited settings, and for situations in which bioelectrical impedance analysis is not available. Circumference measures also can be used to monitor changes over time associated with lipodystrophy in adults.   • Skinfold thickness is measured with calipers.   • Circumference measures are taken at specific anatomical landmarks with nonstretchable tape.   • Techniques and protocols for taking anthropometric measurements can be found at www.cdc.gov/nchs/data/nhanes/nhanes_03_04/BM.pdf.

Laboratory Testing

Perform basic laboratory (blood) tests, including the following:

- Hemoglobin and/or hematocrit

- Total protein, albumin

- Fasting blood glucose

- Fasting lipids (triglycerides, total cholesterol, low-density lipoprotein cholesterol [LDL], high-density lipoprotein cholesterol [HDL])

- CD4 cell count and HIV viral load, if no recent values are available

- Specific vitamin and nutrient tests as indicated by symptoms (e.g., iron studies in case of anemia, vitamin B12 in case of peripheral neuropathy)

- Others tests, such as testosterone and thyroid hormone levels as appropriate, to rule out other causes of symptoms

A: Assessment

Assess subjective information and objective findings to evaluate nutritional status.

Identify Nutrition Concerns

Several factors may influence nutrition, including the following:

- Barriers to good nutrition (e.g., lack of knowledge or motivation for self-care, poor appetite, lack of money for food, lack of facilities for food storage and preparation)

- Lifestyle factors (e.g., smoking, substance abuse, frequent eating out, erratic eating patterns, hectic schedule, high stress)

- Physical problems affecting food and nutrient intake (e.g., poor appetite, nausea, fatigue, pain, weakness, mouth or throat pain, acid reflux, missing or decayed teeth, poorly fitting dentures, poor eyesight, constipation)

- Nutrient losses (e.g., owing to diarrhea, vomiting)

- Potential confounding factors (e.g., use of multiple overlapping or questionable supplements, eating disorders)

Evaluate Dietary Intake

Assess the following diet-related issues:

- Expected excesses or deficiencies from dietary history or interview

- Rating of food security, including access to cooking and refrigeration

- Food intolerances, aversions, or allergies likely to affect adequacy of intake

- Special needs related to other conditions (e.g., documented cardiovascular disease, diabetes, hypertension)

Evaluate Weight, Body Composition, and Weight Distribution

Assess physical findings of malnutrition and confirm with nutrition history, laboratory tests, and anthropometric evidence. Normal and abnormal findings of anthropometric tests and recommendations for monitoring changes over time are presented in Table 4.

Table 4. Evaluating the Findings of Anthropometric Tests	
Monitoring Trends and Recommendations	

Adults
• Chart trends over time relative to previous measurements and the following population norms:
   • BMI (healthy range: 19-25)
   • BIA:
     ⊳ BCM (percentage of weight): women 30-35%; men 40-45%
     ⊳ Fat (percentage of weight): women 20-30%; men 15-25%
     ⊳ Phase angle: women >5; men >6
• **Skinfold thicknesses and circumferences:** Chart changes in absolute measures and percentiles
• **Changes in body contours:** Evaluate lipodystrophy (excess accumulation of fat in abdomen, breasts, dorsocervical area) and lipoatrophy (loss of subcutaneous fat in face, extremities, buttocks)
	Children
	• **Plot measurements on growth charts and track percentiles over time** (the consistency of percentiles rather than the absolute percentile is important)
	• **Skinfold thicknesses and circumferences:** Chart changes in absolute measures and percentiles

Abbreviations: BCM = body cell mass; BIA = bioelectrical impedance analysis; BMI = body mass index

Evaluate Laboratory Findings

- Evidence of malnutrition (e.g., low iron or protein stores)

- Evidence of disease or risk of disease for which dietary treatment is indicated (e.g., high fasting glucose, hypertension, hyperlipidemia)

Develop a Problem List

The following suggests a useful format for a nutrition-related problem list.

Problem #	Description of Problem (circle/describe)
	Nutrition barriers: insufficient knowledge, poor appetite, food insecurity, no food preparation or storage facilities, homelessness
	Lifestyle: substance abuse, smoking, erratic eating, frequent fast-food intake, high stress
	Weight or body composition: undesirable weight gain or loss (adult), changes in growth trajectory (children), loss of lean body mass (wasting), gain of excess fat (obesity), lipoatrophy or lipodystrophy
	Physical problems: fatigue, pain, early satiety, poor dentition, clinical signs of malnutrition
	Laboratory findings: low hematocrit or hemoglobin, low protein or albumin, low or high fasting glucose, high total cholesterol, high LDL, high triglycerides, low HDL, low testosterone
	Gastrointestinal: diarrhea, vomiting, reflux, constipation
	Poor diet: poor food choices, bingeing, skipping meals, high sugar intake, high alcohol consumption, high intake of refined foods, low fruit and vegetable intake, insufficient protein, insufficient calcium, food allergies or intolerances that limit intake
	Comorbid conditions: diabetes, hypertension, cardiovascular disease, cancer, gastroesophageal reflux disease (GERD)
	Medications: drug-drug or drug-nutrient interactions or difficulty coordinating medicines with meals
	Supplements: insufficient or excessive intakes, cost of supplements unaffordable, supplements with potential or unknown risks

P: Plan

Develop a nutritional plan and provide practical nutrition education for common problems (see "Resources," below).

Evaluate and treat concurrent medical problems (e.g., diarrhea, nausea, infections, malignancies, depression, pain). For severe or persistent nutritional problems, or for specific needs, refer to a nutrition specialist for evaluation and treatment.

Common nutrition-related problems are presented in Table 5, along with simple management suggestions that may help resolve them and help patients maintain adequate nutrition.

Table 5. Practical Interventions for Common Nutrition-Related Problems

Problem	Suggestions

Weight Loss (decrease in both body cell mass and fat)	• Early identification and ongoing monitoring are key.
	• Identify and treat underlying risk factors.
	• Try to add calories without adding "bulk":
	  • Fat (9 calories/gram): butter, margarine, avocado, cream, mayonnaise, salad dressing
	  • Carbohydrate (4 calories/gram): jam, jelly, sugar, icing, gum drops
	  • Protein (4 calories/gram): protein powders, cheese, nut butters, trail mix, powdered breakfast drinks, nonfat dry milk
	• Eat more frequently.
	• Maximize good days.
	• Use canned supplements (e.g., Ensure, Boost).
	• For wasting or substantial weight loss, consider referral for therapies such as appetite stimulants or human growth hormone.

Diarrhea	• Increase soluble fiber; decrease insoluble fiber. • Replenish beneficial bacteria (e.g., with lactobacilli preparations). • Avoid intestinal irritants and stimulants. • Decrease dietary fat. • Decrease or eliminate lactose. • Increase fluids and provide electrolytes (sodium, potassium). • Treat with pancreatic enzymes.
Early Fullness	• Take small, frequent meals. • Concentrate on solid foods, with liquids between meals. • Eat lower-fat, lower-fiber foods. • Wear loose-fitting clothing. • Sit up while eating. • Eat, walk, and eat again.
Nausea	• Take small, frequent meals. • Try dry snack foods. • Avoid fried foods, very sweet foods, spicy foods, and foods with strong odors. • Try cool, clear beverages, popsicles. • Try ginger-containing foods and drinks. • Keep liquids to a minimum at meals.

Problem	Suggestions
Changes in Taste	• Eat a variety of foods, not only favorite foods. • Try protein sources other than red meat. • Marinate foods, use sauces. • Use more and stronger seasonings. • Try tart foods. • Use sugar or salt to tone down the flavor of foods. • Try a mouth rinse of 1 teaspoon of baking soda in 1 cup of warm water before eating.
Loss of Appetite	• Rely on favorite foods. • Ask family members and friends to prepare meals. • Eat small, frequent meals. • Keep snacks handy for nibbling. • Eat before bedtime. • Eat in a pleasant place, with other people. • Make the most of good days. • Try light exercise to stimulate appetite. • Add extra calories without adding bulk. • Consider appetite stimulants (e.g., megestrol, stimulants).
Difficulty Chewing or Swallowing or Sore Mouth and Throat	• Choose soft, nutritious foods. • Blend or puree foods (e.g., soup or stew, smoothies). • Add cream sauces, butter, or gravy for lubrication. • Sip liquids with foods. • Use a straw or drink foods from a cup. • Choose bland, low-acid foods. • If hot foods cause pain, serve foods cold or at room temperature. • Avoid alcohol and tobacco. • Soothing lozenges or sprays may help.
Food Insecurity	• Refer to social services for assistance with accessing resources such as food stamps, community meals, or a food pantry program. • Refer to a dietitian for assistance with low-cost food ideas. • Use materials at www.cheapcooking.com/index.htm.
Unbalanced Diet and Other Conditions Requiring Dietary Modification	• Refer to a dietitian for counseling and education.

Nutrition Specialists

Whenever possible, nutritional services should be provided by a registered dietitian (RD) who is a qualified HIV care provider. In the United States, holding this status requires a nutrition degree from an accredited college, graduation from an approved internship or master's degree program, and maintenance with 75 continuing-education units every 5 years, including specific and ongoing HIV training. An RD with HIV/AIDS expertise in the United States can be located by going to www. eatright.org, clicking on "Find a Nutrition Professional," entering the patient's zip code or city, and selecting "HIV/AIDS" under areas of specialty. Membership in the HIV/AIDS Dietetic Practice Group (www.hivaidsdpg.org) also may indicate HIV experience.

Resources

The following online resources provide information, guidelines, and tools for providers and patients in managing issues related to nutrition and HIV:

- **2000 CDC Growth Charts: United States** Center for Disease Control and Prevention, National Health and Nutrition Examination Survey. Available at www.cdc.gov/growthcharts/.

- **Center for Disease Control and Prevention National Center for Health Statistics** (www.cdc.gov/nchs/products/pubs/pubd/series/sr11/240-221/240-221.htm)

- **CheapCooking.com.** Website with recipes using low-cost ingredients and tips for frugal meal planning. Available at www.cheapcooking.com.

- **HIV/AIDS Dietetic Practice Group** Affiliate of the American Dietetic Association. Website includes screening tool (Nutrition Screen and Referral Criteria for Adults with HIV/AIDS). Available at www.hivaidsdpg.org/.

- **MyPyramid.gov.** U.S. Department of Agriculture website with dietary guidelines, tips, resources, and consumer-oriented information. Available at www.mypyramid.gov.

- **Health Care and HIV: Nutritional Guide for Providers and Clients** (www.aidsetc.org/aidsetc?page=etres-display&resource=etres-1931)

- **Nutrition and Food Safety** (www.aids.gov/hiv-aids-basics/staying-healthy-with-hiv-aids/taking-care-of-yourself/nutrition-and-food-safety/)

- **Nutrition.gov** (www.nutrition.gov/nal_display/index.php?info_center=11&tax_level=1)

- **Tufts University Nutrition and Infection Unit** (www.tufts.edu/med/nutrition-infection/hiv/health.html)

References

- Association of Nutrition Services Agencies. *ANSA Nutrition Guidelines and Fact Sheets.* Available at www.ansanutrition.org/nutrition/index.cfm. (Select "Nutrition Info.") Accessed June 30, 2010.

- Bartlett JG. *Introduction. Integrating nutrition therapy into medical management of human immunodeficiency virus.* Clin Infect Dis. 2003 Apr 1;36(Suppl 2):S51.

Antiretroviral Therapy

Susa Coffey, MD

Background

Potent combination antiretroviral therapy (ART), typically consisting of three or more antiretroviral (ARV) drugs, has greatly improved the health and survival rates of HIV-infected patients in areas of the world with access to ARVs. More than 20 individual ARVs in six classes are available in the United States,

HRSA HAB Core Clinical Performance Measures

Percentage of clients with AIDS who are prescribed **antiretroviral therapy**

(Group 1 measure)

in addition to several fixed-dose combination preparations. These can be combined to construct a number of effective regimens for initial and subsequent therapy. Although ART has its limitations (see below), it saves lives and improves immune system function, reduces the risk of many HIV-related and "non-AIDS" complications, and reduces the risk of HIV transmission. Increasingly, several lines of evidence point to the benefit of ART even for patients with high CD4 counts.

Mortality and morbidity benefits of ART are particularly obvious in patients with relatively advanced immune suppression or with symptoms related to HIV infection. For asymptomatic patients with higher CD4 counts (e.g., >350 cells/µL), the question of when to initiate ART remains an area of research and debate. It is clear there is a spectrum of risk for adverse outcomes that increases as the CD4 count declines. In persons with CD4 counts of <200 cells/µL, effective ART dramatically decreases morbidity and mortality. For persons with CD4 counts of 200-350 cells/µL, data from randomized controlled studies as well as cohort studies also demonstrate a reduction in both AIDS and non-AIDS events among those who start ART. Although it is not clearly known at what CD4 threshold ≥350 cells/µL therapy should be started, a variety of data from observational cohort studies show a reduction in death as well as in AIDS and non-AIDS related complications among persons who start ART with CD4 counts of >350 cells/µL rather than <350 cells/µL. It should be noted, however, that these findings are not consistent across all studies. For patients with CD4 counts of >500 cells/µL, the limited data that are currently available (from cohort studies) are inconsistent on the question of whether initiation of ART results in better outcomes. A randomized clinical trial of earlier (>500 cells/µL) versus deferred (<350 cells/µL) treatment is under way, and the results of that study along with those from the cohort studies may help define an optimal threshold at which to initiate ART.

Meanwhile, in recent years, a growing body of evidence has demonstrated adverse effects of untreated HIV on many organ systems and aspects of functioning, even in persons with high or relatively high CD4 counts (>350-500 cells/µL). These include the following:

- Cardiovascular disease
- Kidney disease, specifically HIV-associated nephropathy (HIVAN)
- Liver disease, particularly among patients with chronic hepatitis B virus (HBV) or

hepatitis C virus (HCV)

- Neurocognitive deficits, including dementia
- Cancers, both AIDS-malignancies and non-AIDS malignancies

Many of these effects appear to be mediated through persistent immune system activation and ongoing inflammation in various organ systems. ART with virologic suppression appears to reduce immune activation and protect against many of these morbidities, but it may not restore immune system function to normal and may not fully reverse disease processes. The beneficial effects of ART may be attenuated for patients who start ART with lower CD4 cell counts. Additionally, the risk of certain ARV-related adverse events may be greater for those who start ART at lower CD4 levels.

Although ART can confer substantial health benefits, it has significant limitations. ART does not cure HIV infection and it requires that multiple medications be taken for life (i.e., potentially many decades). It may cause a variety of adverse effects (some severe), is expensive, requires close adherence to be effective and to prevent the emergence of resistance, and sometimes fails (because of the patient's imperfect adherence or other factors). The failure of an ARV regimen when accompanied by drug resistance usually means that subsequent regimens are less likely to succeed.

In past years, many of the available ARVs presented challenges in the realms of adverse effects, pill quantity, dosing frequency, and durability. Given these limitations of ART, much attention was devoted to estimating the point at which the potential benefits of ART outweighed the potential risks of ART. Today, the newer ARV regimens, specifically those currently recommended by the U.S. Department of Health and Human Services (DHHS) for initial therapy, are for most patients, simple, tolerable, and effective. As a result of both the availability of ARV regimens that are less toxic and easier to administer, and the increasing appreciation of the adverse impacts of untreated HIV, the tipping point between the potential benefit and the potential risk of ART is shifting. Most HIV experts (as is reflected in the current DHHS *Guidelines for the Use of Antiretroviral Agents in HIV-1-Infected Adults and Adolescents*; see below) recommend earlier initiation of treatment, and many recommend ART for all willing individuals regardless of CD4 count, unless there are compelling reasons not to treat (see "When to Initiate Therapy: DHHS ARV Guidelines," below; also see the DHHS *Guidelines* for a full discussion of these issues). An expected additional benefit of earlier treatment is the likelihood that HIV transmission will be reduced.

Of course, in deciding when to start ART for the individual patient, practitioners must weigh the expected benefits of ART for that person (in terms of morbidity and mortality) against the possible risks of ART (e.g., toxicity, drug resistance, adverse drug interactions).

Although implementing and monitoring ART is complex, a number of guidelines from expert panels are available to help clinicians select effective regimens for particular patients. The DHHS keeps a repository of frequently updated recommendations on the use of ARV medications for adults and adolescents, pregnant women, and children. All clinicians who treat HIV-infected patients should be familiar with the most current versions of these treatment guidelines. They are available on the Internet at the AIDSinfo website (aidsinfo.nih.gov/guidelines/). The DHHS *Guidelines* are referenced frequently in this chapter.

When to Initiate ART: DHHS ARV Guidelines

The following recommendations have been adapted from the DHHS *Guidelines for the Use of Antiretroviral Agents in HIV-1-Infected Adults and Adolescents.*

Indicator	Recommendation
AIDS-defining illness	Strongly recommended
CD4 count <350 cells/μL	Strongly recommended
CD4 count 350-500 cells/μL	Strongly recommended by 55% of the panel, moderately recommended by 45% (more urgent at lower CD4 levels)
CD4 count >500 cells/μL	Moderately recommended by 50% of the panel treatment, considered optional by 50%

Adapted from U.S. Department of Health and Human Services. *Guidelines for the Use of Antiretroviral Agents in HIV-1-Infected Adults and Adolescents;* Table 2. January 10, 2011. Available at www.aidsinfo.nih.gov/guidelines/.

Persons with certain conditions should be treated with ART regardless of CD4 count. These conditions include the following:

- Pregnancy (see chapters *Reducing Maternal-Infant HIV Transmission* and *Care of HIV-Infected Pregnant Women*)
- HIVAN (see chapter *Renal Disease*)
- HBV coinfection, when treatment of HBV is indicated (see chapter *Hepatitis B Infection*)

In some situations, ART may be needed relatively urgently. These include the following:

- AIDS-defining conditions
- Acute opportunistic infections
- Lower CD4 counts (e.g., <200 cells/μL)
- Rapidly declining CD4 counts (e.g., >100 cells/μL/year)
- Higher viral loads (e.g., >100,000 copies/mL)

(Adapted from U.S. Department of Health and Human Services. *Guidelines for the Use of Antiretroviral Agents in HIV-1-Infected Adults and Adolescents;* Table 2a, Conditions Favoring More Rapid Initiation of Therapy. January 10, 2011. Available at www.aidsinfo.nih.gov/guidelines/.)

S: Subjective

Obtain the patient's history and review of systems, including the following (see chapter *Initial History*):

- CD4 cell count history, including nadir
- HIV RNA (viral load) history, including pretreatment values if the patient is currently taking ARVs
- History of HIV-related conditions
- Previous and current ARV regimens, including start and stop dates, regimen efficacy, toxicity, resistance
- Current medications, including herbal preparations, supplements, and over-the-counter medications
- Medication allergies, intolerances, or prominent adverse effects
- Comorbid conditions (e.g., HBV, HCV, depression)
- Current and previous substance use, including alcohol and recreational drugs
- Self-assessment of adherence to previous regimens
- Desire to start or continue an ARV regimen
- Commitment to adherence (see chapter *Adherence*)
- Occupation and daily schedule

- Willingness and indicators of ability to adhere to various types of regimens (e.g., once daily, twice daily, with or without food) given current life situation

- For women of childbearing potential: last menstrual period, current method of birth control (if any), current pregnancy status, thoughts on whether or when to have children

O: Objective

Perform the following objective tests:

- Complete physical examination (see chapter *Initial Physical Examination*).

- Current CD4 count and HIV viral load: preferably two or more separate results approximately 1 month apart.

- Drug resistance test, as appropriate; to look for transmitted ARV resistance mutations, a genotype should be performed for all patients before initiating ART; this should be done as early in the course of infection as possible, because mutations may revert to wild-type. Review the results of previous resistance testing or obtain a baseline resistance test, if this was not done earlier; if a test was done in the past, consider retesting before ART is begun (see chapter *Resistance Testing*). Patients with detectable viral loads on ART also should undergo resistance testing.

- Complete blood count (CBC) and platelet count, liver function tests (LFTs), renal function tests, fasting lipid panel, fasting glucose, rapid plasma reagin (RPR), tuberculin skin test, hepatitis serologies, *Toxoplasma* IgG, urinalysis, (see chapter *Initial and Interim Laboratory and Other Tests*).

A: Assessment

Make the following basic decisions:

- The patient is or is not likely to benefit from ART at this time (i.e., do potential benefits outweigh the risks?). See the DHHS *Guidelines* noted above, which thoroughly address the issue, and note that many experts are increasingly concerned about the potential harm of untreated HIV infection, even in individuals with high CD4 cell counts. See chapters *Risk of HIV Progression/ Indications for ART* and *CD4 Monitoring and Viral Load Testing*.

- The patient is or is not willing to start ARVs at this time (the choice to accept or decline therapy ultimately lies with the patient). If not, work with the patient on readiness issues, with more urgency if the CD4 count is low or the patient has symptoms or comorbidities that suggest treatment is needed.

- The patient is or is not likely to adhere to an ARV regimen (an adherence counselor, with or without a mental health clinician, may be able to assist with this assessment and should be called upon if available). No patient should be automatically excluded from consideration for ART; the likelihood of adherence must be discussed and determined individually (see chapter *Adherence*).

P: Plan

After educating the patient about the purpose and logistics of the proposed regimen and assessing the patient's potential for adherence, ART can be initiated, changed, or postponed accordingly.

The primary goal of therapy is to reduce HIV-related morbidity and mortality through maximal and durable viral suppression; this includes improving immune function and reducing HIV-associated inflammation. Among the secondary goals are improving quality of life and reducing the risk of HIV transmission.

Considerations Before Initiating ART

No "average patient" exists. Some patients will do better during treatment and some will do worse than clinical studies would predict. Health care providers must work with each patient to develop a treatment strategy that is both clinically sound and appropriate for that individual's needs, priorities, and circumstances of daily life. Despite the fact that the regimens currently recommended by the DHHS *Guidelines* are more compact and have fewer adverse effects than earlier regimens, not all patients will be able to take or tolerate all drugs, and the patient's understanding, readiness to commit to the regimen, and history of adherence to previous regimens must be considered when choosing ARV combinations. Major considerations are as follows:

- Degree of immunodeficiency and risk of disease progression as reflected by the CD4 count and HIV RNA level. ART is more urgent for patients with lower or rapidly declining CD4 counts (see "When to Initiate ART: DHHS ARV Guidelines," above, and chapters *Risk of HIV Progression/Indications for ART* and *CD4 Monitoring and Viral Load Testing*)

- Comorbidities

- Potential benefits and risks of ARV drugs

- Resistance, if any, to ARV medications (obtain resistance testing prior to ARV initiation for ARV-naive patients)

Of course, the patient's willingness to begin ART is critical, as mentioned above. Patients have the right to decline or postpone ART. This decision should not affect any other aspect of care, and ART should be offered again at each visit to patients for whom treatment is indicated. If mental health issues, addiction, or the patient's social situation are barriers to adherence, initiate appropriate referrals and reassess adherence barriers at regular intervals.

Preparing the Patient for ART

Before starting ART, it is important to have a detailed discussion with patients about their readiness to commit to a medication regimen, the expected benefits and possible adverse effects, and required monitoring and follow-up visits. Patients must understand that the first treatment regimen offers the best opportunity for effective viral suppression and immune reconstitution, which are the primary goals of ART.

Supporting Adherence

Numerous strategies have been tested for their effectiveness in supporting patients' adherence to the ART regimen. Successful approaches include extensive patient education, telephone contact with office staff members who can answer questions about adverse effects or other difficulties, family meetings, and peer support. Trust and accessibility appear to be important predictors of adherence, and some practitioners see the patient for two or three appointments before starting ART.

Compact regimens consisting of fewer pills and once-daily dosing often encourage adherence. Advise patients about potential adverse effects and at the same time let them know that many adverse effects may be treated or that substitutions often can be made for problematic ARVs. The choice to accept or decline ART ultimately lies with the patient (see chapter *Adherence*).

Anticipating Difficulties

Choosing an initial regimen that fits the patient's lifestyle and that is likely to be tolerable, and easy to take, will improve the likelihood of long-term success with that regimen. If patients develop toxicities to one or more components of an initial regimen, substitutions typically can be made without limiting the success of the regimen. Close monitoring and "check-in" appointments allow these adjustments to be made under clinical supervision. Close monitoring also can help to identify medication toxicities that may limit treatment and to detect early signs of inadequate medication adherence; early intervention to treat adverse effects and to support adherence may increase the likelihood of treatment success.

Considerations in Regimen Selection

Regimens should be selected with consideration of both patient factors and medication factors. The patient's schedule, adherence history, and self-defined goals of ART should be considered in selecting a regimen to which the patient will best adhere. The patient's comorbid conditions and potentially interacting medications should be evaluated for possible contraindications or synergism. The ARV history and all resistance profiles should be reviewed carefully so that a regimen that will be likely to achieve durable viral suppression can be chosen. The CD4 cell count should be reviewed if nevirapine is being considered, and viral tropism and the HLA-B*5701 status should be determined if maraviroc or abacavir, respectively, is being considered. The patient's HBV status will influence selection of NRTIs (tenofovir + emtricitabine or lamivudine should be included in the ART regimen, for co-treatment of HIV and HBV, unless contraindicated). In women who are pregnant or likely to become pregnant, ARV pregnancy categories and ARV teratogenicity should be taken into account. Drug interactions amongst ARVs or between ARVs and other medications should be evaluated, as dosage adjustments may be required or certain combinations may be contraindicated (see Tables (see Tables 14, 15a-e, and 16a-b of the DHHS *Guidelines*).

The advantages and disadvantages of various drug classes and individual drugs recommended for use in initial therapy are reviewed in Table 6 of the DHHS *Guidelines*.

Use of Multiple Classes of Drugs

For initial therapy in patients with wild-type HIV virus, the DHHS *Guidelines* recommend the use of two nucleoside reverse transcriptase inhibitors (NRTIs) in combination with either a nonnucleoside reverse transcriptase inhibitor (NNRTI), a ritonavir-boosted protease inhibitor (PI), or an integrase inhibitor (II). Drug combinations that include only NRTIs generally do not reduce virus levels as effectively as two-class combinations. The question of whether to use an NNRTI, a PI, or an II in initial therapy is a matter of debate. Some clinicians advocate using an NNRTI or II initially to preserve use of the PI class for later and to avoid PI-related toxicities. Others are more concerned about the potential toxicities of NNRTIs or the low genetic barrier to resistance presented by NNRTIs and IIs, and instead recommend starting with a PI-containing regimen. Each of the initial regimens proposed by the DHHS *Guidelines* is highly effective if taken as directed, and each has specific advantages and disadvantages (see Table 6 of the DHHS *Guidelines*). In the end, the regimen should be selected with the individual patient in mind because the only effective combination for that patient is the one that he or she is willing and able to take on a consistent basis. See the information on drug resistance and toxicities below as well as the full text of the DHHS *Guidelines* for more complete discussions.

Salvage therapy for patients with ARV-resistant HIV often comprises agents from three or more ARV classes; consult with an expert.

Boosted Protease Inhibitors

Ritonavir is used at low doses in combination with most other PIs to enhance or "boost" the serum level and prolong the half-life of the PI. This strategy generally decreases the dosing frequency and the number of pills required, and it improves the activity of some PIs. Several currently used PIs require boosting with ritonavir, and some require ritonavir boosting to overcome certain interactions between PIs and other medications (e.g., atazanavir must be boosted with ritonavir if tenofovir also is a component of the ARV regimen); see "Drug Interactions," below, and Tables 13, 14, and 15 in the DHHS *Guidelines*.

Preferred Starting Regimens

More than 20 ARVs in six drug classes have been approved for use in the United States by the U.S. Food and Drug Administration (FDA) (see Appendix B, Tables 1-6 and Tables 11-13 in the DHHS *Guidelines*). In recent years, an increasing number of fixed-dose combinations (FDCs) have become available to simplify dosing and reduce pill burden.

These include four NRTI combinations:

- Abacavir + lamivudine (Epzicom)

- Abacavir + lamivudine + zidovudine (Trizivir)

- Emtricitabine + tenofovir (Truvada)

- Lamivudine + zidovudine (Combivir)

One PI coformulation:

- Lopinavir + ritonavir (Kaletra)

And a one-pill-per-day formulation of two NRTIs and one NNRTI:

- Emtricitabine + tenofovir + efavirenz (Atripla)

Other FDCs are in development and may become available in coming years.

The DHHS *Guidelines* suggest "preferred" and "alternative" components for initial therapy (Table 1). Clinicians should note that these recommendations change over time as new data regarding efficacy or toxicity become available. Among regimens with adequate potency (taking into account possible ARV resistance), regimen selection should be guided by factors such as anticipated tolerability, pill burden, drug interactions, and the patient's comorbid conditions. Other agents or combinations may be appropriate or preferable for individual patients (see Table 5a of the DHHS *Guidelines*).

Table 1. Recommended Regimens for Initial Antiretroviral Treatment

Preferred Regimens	
NNRTI based	Efavirenz[1] + tenofovir/emtricitabine (TDF/FTC)[2]
PI based	Atazanavir/r + TDF/FTC[2]
	Darunavir/r (once daily) + TDF/FTC[2]
II based	Raltegravir + TDF/FTC[2]
Pregnant women	Lopinavir/r (twice daily) + zidovudine (ZDV)/lamivudine (3TC)[2]
Alternative Regimens	
NNRTI based	Efavirenz[1] + (abacavir [ABC]/3TC)[2,3] or (ZDV/3TC)[2]
	Nevirapine[4] + ZDV/3TC[2]
PI based	Atazanavir/r + (ABC/3TC)[2,3] or (ZDV/3TC)[2]
	Fosamprenavir/r (once daily or twice daily) + (ABC/3TC)[2,3] or (ZDV/3TC)[2] or (TDF/FTC)[2]
	Lopinavir/r (once daily or twice daily) + (ABC/3TC)[2,3] or (ZDV/3TC)[2] or (TDF/FTC)[2]

[1] Efavirenz should not be used by women during the first trimester of pregnancy or by those who are trying to conceive or not using effective and consistent contraception.

[2] 3TC can be used in place of FTC and vice versa.

[3] Abacavir should not be used by patients who test positive for HLA-B*5701; use with caution if HIV RNA level is >100,000 copies/mL or if there is a high risk of cardiovascular disease.

[4] Nevirapine should not be started if the pre-ARV CD4 count is >250 cells/μL in women or >400 cells/μL in men.

Abbreviations: /r = low-dose ritonavir; II: integrase inhibitor; NNRTI = nonnucleoside reverse transcriptase inhibitor; NRTI = nucleoside/nucleotide analogue; PI = protease inhibitor

Adapted from U.S. Department of Health and Human Services. Table 5a. Antiretroviral Regimens Recommended for Treatment-Naive Patients. In: *Guidelines for the Use of Antiretroviral Agents in HIV-1-Infected Adults and Adolescents*. January 10, 2011. Available at www.aidsinfo.nih.gov/guidelines/.

Note: The DHHS *Guidelines* also list regimens that "May Be Acceptable" and "Should Be Used with Caution," see Table 5b in the DHHS *Guidelines*.

Once-Daily Regimens

The use of convenient and simplified dosing is an obvious strategy for improving adherence, particularly with the availability of coformulations that reduce pill burden (see "Preferred Starting Regimens," above). The DHHS *Guidelines* currently include three once-daily combinations among "preferred" regimens for initial therapy, and list several other possibilities among "alternative" regimens.

Avoiding Drug Resistance

ARV medications never should be given as single agents, in two-drug regimens, in suboptimal regimens, or in lower dosages than recommended, because of the potential for development of resistance. High-level resistance to NNRTIs, as well as to emtricitabine and lamivudine, may develop quickly (i.e., within days to weeks) in these situations, and the same may be true for the II raltegravir. It may take longer for high-level resistance to develop to other NRTIs and to ritonavir-boosted PIs. Patients must be instructed to take the full dosage of all medications on schedule and to avoid skipping doses or taking "days off" from their regimens. Careful medication dosing is important because resistance to one drug within a particular class may transfer to other drugs in the same class (cross-resistance). Cross-resistance can limit the options for future therapy significantly or necessitate the use of very complicated regimens in the future. Once resistant viral strains have developed, they may be transmitted to other people.

Acquired or "primary" resistance, in which a patient is infected with ARV-resistant virus, is common in parts of the United States. Because both multi- and single-class resistance has been found among ARV-naive persons in many U.S. cities, it is recommended that individuals with newly diagnosed HIV infection and all others entering care should receive a baseline resistance test. This test should be obtained as early as possible, in order to maximize the likelihood of detecting transmitted mutations, and before initiation of ART (see chapter *Resistance Testing*).

Drug Interactions

Many of the ARVs interact with one another as well as with other common medications. When starting or changing an ARV regimen, review all the patient's current medications carefully for possible drug interactions. See chapter *Drug-Drug Interactions with HIV-Related Medications* for a summary of this issue and for references and resources to review medication lists and combinations. For further information on drug interactions involving ARVs, see Tables Tables 15a-e and 16a-b in the DHHS *Guidelines*.

Drugs and Drug Combinations That Should Not Be Used

Most clinicians in the United States avoid using the NRTIs zidovudine (except for pregnant women), stavudine, or didanosine if other options are available, because of the high rates of metabolic and other adverse effects associated with these agents. Stavudine, in particular, is likely to cause peripheral neuropathy and lipoatrophy. Drugs with additive or overlapping toxicities, such as stavudine and didanosine, should not be combined. Zidovudine and stavudine, which compete intracellularly and therefore cause antagonism, should not be used together.

Drugs with similar mechanisms of action and resistance mutations (e.g., lamivudine and emtricitabine, or efavirenz and nevirapine) offer no significant advantage when combined and may increase toxicities. Certain three-drug combinations have suboptimal efficacy and are not recommended (e.g., tenofovir + didanosine + an NNRTI; tenofovir + emtricitabine + nevirapine; and three-NRTI regimens). Some ARVs require specific dosing intervals in particular patients. For example, once-daily dosing of lopinavir/ritonavir is not recommended for patients receiving concomitant efavirenz or nevirapine, and some once-daily PIs or combinations should not be used for treatment-experienced patients. For further information, see Tables 7 and 8 in the DHHS *Guidelines*.

Follow-Up of Patients Starting ART

Patients who start a new ARV regimen ideally should be seen at least twice within the first month to allow for an assessment of their adherence to therapy and the tolerability and adverse effects of the regimen.

When patients have been on a new regimen for 2-8 weeks, clinicians should check the following:

- HIV viral load, to monitor initial virologic response to therapy, then every 4-8 weeks until the viral load is below the level of detection

- CD4 cell count

- CBC with platelets, especially for patients starting a zidovudine-containing regimen, to monitor for anemia

- LFTs, to monitor for hepatotoxicity (patients starting a nevirapine-containing regimen should be monitored closely for the first 18 weeks of treatment)

- Serum electrolytes, blood urea nitrogen, and creatinine (particularly for patients taking tenofovir)

- Fasting glucose and lipids (after 3-6 months)

For further information, and for recommendations about monitoring stable patients, see chapter *Initial and Interim Laboratory and Other Tests.*

Regimen Failure

An ART regimen may fail for several reasons, including the following:

Incomplete virologic response

- Viral load does not decline below the level of detection (i.e., <40-75 copies/mL) within 6 months of initiating therapy. (For some patients with multidrug resistance, it may not be possible to decrease plasma HIV viral load to undetectable levels, and stabilization of viral load below the previous baseline may be an appropriate goal of therapy.)

Virologic rebound

- Virus is repeatedly detected in plasma after suppression to undetectable levels. Confirmatory testing is required to rule out "blips" of virus (isolated elevations in viral load of less than several hundred copies/mL) that are not clinically significant and to ensure that the increase is not caused by infection, vaccination, or problems with test methodology. Note that some patients may have persistently detectable low-level viremia (<200 copies/mL); the clinical significance of this is not clear.

Immunologic failure

- Despite virologic suppression on ART, the CD4 cell count shows an inadequate response or a persistent decline.

Clinical progression

- Recurrent, persistent, or new HIV-related illness occurs after ≥3 months on ART. Note that new or recurrent symptoms of opportunistic illness occurring in the first weeks to months after starting ART, especially in patients with severe immunosuppression, may not reflect a failure of ART. Rather, these symptoms could be attributable to persistence of opportunistic infections that may require longer treatment, or they could be caused by an immune reconstitution inflammatory syndrome (see chapter *Immune Reconstitution Inflammatory Syndrome*).

Responding to Apparent Treatment Failure

- Carefully assess patient adherence, because inadequate adherence to ART is a common reason for regimen failure. In some cases, adherence support, treatment of adverse drug effects, substitution for poorly tolerated ARVs, or other measures to enhance adherence may result in virologic suppression (see chapter *Adherence*). In other cases, ARV resistance may have developed. Poor adherence may affect the decision to change therapy, and adherence issues should be addressed before a new regimen is initiated. If resistance is suspected, obtain an appropriate resistance test (or CCR5 tropism assay, if the patient is taking a CCR5 antagonist) while the patient is on the failing regimen; see below.

- The availability of effective alternative ARVs is a critical consideration in deciding whether or when to change therapies. The development of new ARVs and new ARV classes in recent years has made virologic suppression possible for most patients, even those with extensive resistance. For those few patients in whom treatment possibilities are limited or nonexistent, it may be necessary to weigh the value of partial virologic suppression with the current regimen against the likelihood of further resistance developing. Strongly consider consultation with an experienced HIV provider and the use of HIV resistance testing when considering changes in therapy. When no treatment options remain among currently approved drugs, refer the patient to an appropriate clinical trial, if possible.

Note that the optimal management of immunologic failure is uncertain and is an active area of research. Consult with an HIV expert and consider referral to a research study.

Resistance and Coreceptor Tropism Testing

If resistance is suspected, obtain an appropriate resistance test (see chapter *Resistance Testing*). Resistance testing is recommended, before changing regimens, in cases of virologic rebound during ARV therapy or suboptimal suppression of viral load on ARV therapy. Resistance testing often is crucial in identifying ARVs that are not likely to be effective against the patient's virus. It should be done while the patient is taking the failing regimen (or within 4 weeks of discontinuation) to maximize the likelihood that resistant

viral populations will be present in detectable numbers. In virologic failure of a first regimen, it is fairly common to see resistance to only one or two drugs in a multidrug combination. The test results should be interpreted in the context of the patient's ARV history and the results of previous resistance tests.

Standard genotypes test give information about resistance that may affect NRTI, NNRTI, and PI agents. If integrase inhibitor (or fusion inhibitor) resistance is suspected, a specific genotype test must be ordered. There are no commercially available tests for resistance to CCR5 antagonists. For patients with virologic failure while taking a CCR5 antagonist, a coreceptor tropism assay should be considered (though the result does not rule out the possibility of resistance to CCR5 antagonists).

Cross-resistance exists among ARVs, such that resistance to one drug in a class of agents often extends to other drugs in that class. For example, cross-resistance between efavirenz and nevirapine is almost complete, and resistance mutations to NRTIs and to PIs often decrease viral susceptibility to other drugs in those classes. As a result, selecting a new ARV regimen can be complicated because it requires knowledge of expected resistance patterns. The likelihood of sustained viral suppression is lower when resistant virus is present even if a subsequent regimen contains new ARVs.

If treatment with a CCR5 antagonist is being considered, a tropism test must be obtained to verify that the patient has only CCR5-tropic virus (the currently available agent in this class is not effective in patients with any degree of CXCR4 virus). The standard test requires an HIV viral load of >1,000 copies/mL at the time of testing; a newer proviral DNA assay can identify coreceptor tropism in blood samples with HIV RNA levels below the limit of detection (this has not been clinically validated).

Suggestions for Changing an ARV Regimen for Suspected Drug Failure

The following recommendations are adapted from the DHHS *Guidelines*.

Distinguish between the need to change a regimen because of drug intolerance or inability to adhere to the regimen and the failure to achieve the goal of sustained viral suppression. In the event of intolerability, single agents usually can be changed without resistance testing.

In general, do not change a single drug or add a single active drug to a failing regimen; it is important to use at least two or, preferably, three fully active ARVs (e.g., ARVs selected on the basis of resistance testing or because they are from a drug class to which the patient's virus has not been exposed). If resistance testing (performed while the patient is taking the failing regimen) shows resistance to only one agent in a regimen, it may be possible to replace only that drug; however, consultation with an expert is recommended.

In general, the goal of ART is to suppress HIV RNA to undetectable levels, in order to improve or maintain immune function. This usually is possible even for patients with resistance to multiple drugs as new ARV agents and new classes of ARVs have become available. Nevertheless, some patients have limited options for new regimens that will achieve durable virologic suppression. In some of these cases, it may be reasonable to continue the same regimen if partial virologic suppression and clinical and immunologic stability are maintained. The risk of continuing patients on a partially suppressive regimen, however, is the emergence of additional resistance mutations.

Data on the value of restarting a drug that the patient has previously received are limited. Resistant virus can be archived and will reemerge for patients who are rechallenged with regimens on which they had previously

developed resistance. As a result, resistance tests from previous regimens should be used with current resistance tests to determine what drugs might be active in a new regimen.

Making the decision to change therapy and choosing a new ARV regimen require that the clinician have considerable expertise in the care of people with HIV infection. Those less experienced in the care of persons with HIV are strongly encouraged to obtain assistance by consulting with or referring to an expert.

Follow-Up of Patients Not Started on ART

Patients who are not on ART

These patients should continue their regular visits for monitoring, prophylaxis, and other medical treatment (see section *Testing and Assessment* for chapters on physical examinations and laboratory tests). ART should be discussed again and offered at regular intervals, if it is indicated, to anyone who initially refuses treatment. Routine clinic visits present ongoing chances to educate patients about new medications and research findings and to discuss the benefits of ART and the risks of delayed treatment. Decreases in patients' CD4 count or declines in their condition should be taken as opportunities to reassess their decisions about ARVs. If lack of readiness or probable adherence difficulties are at issue, an adherence counselor (if available) or a mental health provider should be engaged to bolster the patients' support and coping mechanisms (see chapter *CD4 Monitoring and Viral Load Testing* and the DHHS *Guidelines*).

Special Situations for ART

ART during acute or primary HIV infection

It is not yet known whether ART has a long-term benefit when started during primary HIV infection, though there are a number of theoretic reasons why early treatment may reduce the severity of immune system disruption, lessen both the short-term and the long-term impact of HIV infection, and decrease the risk of HIV transmission. The DHHS *Guidelines* state that treatment of acute HIV is optional (except during pregnancy, when ART should be started as quickly as possible to reduce the risk of perinatal HIV transmission). However, for the appropriate patient, it is reasonable to consider starting therapy, with the goal of maximal virologic suppression. Before starting an ARV regimen, patients must be counseled carefully about potential limitations, such as toxicity, pill burden, cost, and the possible development of drug resistance. Patients should be monitored with HIV viral load, CD4 counts, and other parameters, as with patients with established infection who are receiving ART. Because no definitive data showing the clinical benefit of early treatment are available, persons with acute HIV infection ideally should be enrolled in clinical trials, if possible (see chapter *Primary HIV Infection*).

Pregnant women

Combination ARV regimens are recommended for all women during pregnancy, regardless of CD4 count or HIV RNA level. The goal of ART for pregnant women is to reduce the risk of transmission to the infant and to treat HIV infection in the mother, through maximal virologic suppression. Obviously, the decision of whether to start ART during pregnancy is the choice of the woman, and her choice must be respected. There are a number of specific considerations about ART in pregnant women, including the timing of ART initiation (for those not already on treatment), specific ARVs that are recommended or that should be avoided (because of toxicity or teratogenicity concerns), pharmacokinetic variations and dosing requirements in pregnancy, and indications for resistance testing. See chapters *Reducing Maternal-Infant HIV Transmission* and *Care of HIV-Infected Pregnant Women*; also refer to the DHHS *Recommendations for Use of Antiretroviral Drugs in Pregnant*

HIV-1-Infected Women for Maternal Health and Interventions to Reduce Perinatal HIV Transmission in the United States (available at aidsinfo.nih.gov/guidelines).

Acute opportunistic infections

The presence of opportunistic infections is a strong signal of the need for ART and effective immune reconstitution. For some of these infections, ART is the primary therapy, and for others it is adjunctive. Although ART sometimes causes immune reconstitution inflammatory syndromes if initiated in the setting of acute opportunistic infection, limited clinical data for many such infections (including *Pneumocystis jiroveci* pneumonia and tuberculosis in persons with very low CD4 counts) suggest improved outcomes if ART is started early. Exceptions to this recommendation include cryptococcal meningitis, for which most experts recommend a short period of antifungal treatment before ART is started. For further information, see chapter *Immune Reconstitution Inflammatory Syndrome* and the *Guidelines for Prevention and Treatment of Opportunistic Infections in HIV-Infected Adults and Adolescents: Recommendations from CDC, the National Institutes of Health, and the HIV Medicine Association of the Infectious Diseases Society of America* (see "References," below).

Hepatitis B coinfection

If treatment for either HIV or HBV is needed, treatment for both infections generally should be initiated, by including in the ART regimen two NRTIs with activity against both viruses (tenofovir + emtricitabine or tenofovir + lamivudine), if possible. The use of a single NRTI with activity against both viruses (resulting in monotherapy for HBV) is not recommended. If tenofovir is contraindicated, another anti-HBV drug should be used in combination with lamivudine or emtricitabine. Flares of HBV may occur if tenofovir, emtricitabine, or lamivudine is discontinued; monitor closely or consider substitution of another anti-HBV drug. See chapter *Hepatitis B Infection* and the DHHS *Guidelines* for additional information.

HIV-associated nephropathy

ART is a primary treatment for HIVAN and should be started urgently for patients with suspected HIVAN. See chapter *Renal Disease*.

Expert Consultation

The National HIV/AIDS Clinicians' Consultation Center is a valuable resource for any clinician seeking expert advice about ART, HIV clinical manifestations, laboratory evaluations, and other issues. Its National HIV Telephone Consultation Service (Warmline) is staffed by HIV-experienced physicians and pharmacists. The Warmline operates Monday through Friday, 8 AM to 8 PM eastern time and is available free of charge in the United States at 800-933-3413.

Patient Education

- Making the decision to start ART is rarely an emergency situation. Before starting patients on ART, health care providers must work with them to determine how important therapy would be for them, what goals of therapy are likely to be achieved, and which personal issues are pertinent for selecting the best regimen to fit their lifestyles.

- Providers should review the proposed drug regimen with their patients. Be sure patients understand the instructions about dosage, scheduling, food requirements or restrictions, drug storage, adverse effects, toxicities, and type of reactions that must be reported immediately, as well as remedies for common adverse effects.

- Providers should explain to patients that successful ART requires a commitment to taking the medications precisely as prescribed. There is a limited number of ARVs, and if they are taken incorrectly, the virus quickly can become resistant to the medications. This will mean even fewer choices and less effective treatment in the future. It also may mean that they could transmit resistant virus to a partner or, if they are pregnant, to an infant.

- Patients should know that HIV medications do not prevent transmission of infection to others. Safer-sex recommendations must be followed and other high-risk activities (e.g., needle sharing) must be carefully avoided to prevent the transmission of the virus to others (see chapter *Preventing HIV Transmission/Prevention with Positives* for more information).

- Recommend prevention measures such as using latex barriers during sex (safer sex) and not sharing needles or other drug-using equipment, even with other HIV-infected persons.

- Patients should know that, if their virus develops resistance to some ARVs and they pass that virus on to another person, HIV medications may not be effective for that person. If a patient's partner happens to have a drug-resistant strain of HIV, it is possible for the patient to become infected with a resistant virus in addition to the one he or she has already, and that may limit treatment options.

- HCV, HBV, and other sexually transmitted infections such as syphilis and gonorrhea can be transmitted between two HIV-infected partners.

- Patients should be advised to check with their provider before discontinuing ARVs. If ARVs must be discontinued, it is usually best to stop all ARVs at once. The exception to this recommendation may be NNRTI-containing regimens; in this case, the NRTIs should be continued for about 1 week after discontinuation of the NNRTI, if possible. Even carefully managed interruptions can cause drug resistance mutations. Again, this will limit future treatment options, and it should be avoided if possible.

- Patients should be encouraged to advise their providers of all other medications that they take, including over-the-counter medications, herbal remedies and nutritional supplements.

- Discuss contingencies in the event the client is unable to take ARVs for a day or more (e.g., illness, severe adverse effects, hospitalization, or other unexpected circumstances).

References

- Kaplan JE, Benson C, Holmes KH, et al; Centers for Disease Control and Prevention; National Institutes of Health; HIV Medicine Association of the Infectious Diseases Society of America. *Guidelines for prevention and treatment of opportunistic infections in HIV-infected adults and adolescents: recommendations from CDC, the National Institutes of Health, and the HIV Medicine Association of the Infectious Diseases Society of America.* MMWR Recomm Rep. 2009 Apr 10;58(RR-4):1-207. Available at aidsinfo.nih.gov/guidelines.

- McNicholl I. *Database of Antiretroviral Drug Interactions.* HIV InSite. Coffey S, Volberding PA, eds. San Francisco: UCSF Center for HIV Information. Available at hivinsite.ucsf.edu/insite?page=ar-00-02.

- U.S. Department of Health and Human Services. *Antiretroviral Postexposure Prophylaxis After Sexual, Injection-Drug Use, or Other Nonoccupational Exposure to HIV in the United States.* MMWR Recomm Rep. 2005 Jan 21;54(RR02);1-20. Available at aidsinfo.nih.gov/guidelines.

- U.S. Department of Health and Human Services. *Guidelines for the Use of Antiretroviral Agents in HIV-1-Infected Adults and Adolescents.* January 10, 2011. Available at aidsinfo.nih.gov/guidelines.

- U.S. Department of Health and Human Services. *Recommendations for Use of Antiretroviral Drugs in Pregnant HIV-1-Infected Women for Maternal Health and Interventions to Reduce Perinatal HIV Transmission in the United States.* May 24, 2010. Available at www.aidsinfo.nih.gov/guidelines/.

- U.S. Department of Health and Human Services. *Updated U.S. Public Health Service Guidelines for the Management of Occupational Exposures to HIV and Recommendations for Postexposure Prophylaxis.* Available at www.aidsinfo.nih.gov/guidelines/.

- World Health Organization. *Progress on Global Access to Antiretroviral Therapy: An Update on "3 X 5",* June 2005.

Section 4: Health Care Maintenance and Disease Prevention

Reducing Maternal-Infant HIV Transmission

Carolyn K. Burr, EdD, RN

Background

This chapter describes strategies for reducing the risk of perinatal HIV, based on the U.S. Department of Health and Human Services (DHHS) *Recommendations for Use of Antiretroviral Drugs in Pregnant HIV-1-Infected Women for Maternal Health and Interventions to Reduce Perinatal HIV Transmission in the United States*. It is not intended to be a comprehensive discussion of these topics, and all HIV-infected pregnant women should be treated by an HIV-experienced obstetrician and an HIV specialist. For centers that do not have HIV specialists available, experts at the National Perinatal HIV Consultation and Referral Service are available for consultation through the Perinatal HIV Hotline (888-448-8765). For more information on other aspects of caring for HIV-infected pregnant women, see chapter *Care of HIV-Infected Pregnant Women*.

Unless otherwise referenced, the information in this chapter is based on the most recent DHHS perinatal guidelines available at the time this chapter was published. Consult the AIDSinfo website (aidsinfo.nih.gov/guidelines/) for the most current recommendations.

HRSA HAB Core Clinical Performance Measures

Percentage of pregnant women with HIV infection who are prescribed **antiretroviral therapy**

(Group 1 measure)

Overview of Prevention of Perinatal HIV Transmission

In the absence of antiretroviral (ARV) prophylaxis or other interventions, the rate of perinatal HIV transmission in the United States ranges from 16% to 25%. Antiretroviral therapy (ART) is highly effective in reducing the risk of perinatal transmission of HIV, to as low as 1-2%. All pregnant women with HIV infection should be educated about the risks of perinatal HIV transmission and offered ART and other medical management to maintain or improve their own health and to reduce the risk of HIV transmission to their infants.

In 1994, the Pediatric AIDS Clinical Trial Group study 076 (PACTG 076) found that ARV treatment during pregnancy could significantly reduce the risk of HIV transmission to infants. The intervention, consisting of zidovudine (ZDV) given PO to the women during the last weeks of pregnancy and IV during labor and delivery, as well as to the newborns for 6 weeks, reduced the rate of infant infection from 25.5% to 8.3%. The ZDV regimen quickly became the standard of care in the United States and other high-income countries. Subsequent studies showed that combination ARV regimens with suppression of maternal HIV viral load to undetectable levels further reduced the risk of perinatal infection.

Studies in resource-limited countries as well as in resource-abundant areas have examined various ARV strategies for reducing the risk of perinatal HIV transmission. The Petra study, a placebo-controlled trial in a breast-feeding population in Uganda, South Africa, and Tanzania, found a transmission rate of 8.9% among women who received PO ZDV plus lamivudine (3TC) intrapartum and for 1 week postpartum and whose infants also received 1 week of ZDV/3TC, compared with a rate of 15.3% in the placebo group. The HIV NET 012 trial in a breast-feeding population in Uganda compared the efficacy of a single dose of nevirapine given to the mother at the onset of labor plus a single dose given to the newborn 48 hours postpartum with that of PO ZDV given to the mother during labor and to the newborn. The transmission rate was 11.8% in the nevirapine arm compared with 20.0% in the ZDV arm. The results of this study and the low cost of nevirapine prompted a number of resource-limited countries to institute nevirapine prophylaxis as the standard of care for preventing mother-to-child transmission of HIV. Numerous other trials have demonstrated the efficacy of various ARV strategies, combining different ARVs with different treatment durations and given to mothers, newborns, or both, in both breast-feeding and non-breast-feeding populations. Research has shown that ARV interventions even late in the peripartum or newborn periods may decrease the infant's risk of HIV infection. A retrospective study of subjects in New York found that the rate of perinatal HIV transmission was 9.3-10% if ZDV was given either to both the mothers intrapartum and their newborns or to the newborns only, compared with 26.6% if no ARV medication was given. This study underscores the importance of offering ARV interventions to pregnant women with HIV infection whenever they are identified in pregnancy or during labor and delivery, or as an intervention with the newborn.

In the United States, the PACTG 076 regimen remains an important component in the prevention of perinatal HIV transmission, and usually is incorporated into combination ART for pregnant women. For international settings, other guidelines have been developed by global agencies such as the World Health Organization (see "References," below) and by individual governments.

Mother-to-child transmission also can occur through breast-feeding. Recent studies have shown that ART given to the nursing mother and/or to her infant decreases the risk of transmission to the infant. However, because substitute feeding in the United States is safe, affordable, feasible, sustainable, and available, mothers in the United States should not breast-feed.

HIV Testing During Pregnancy

The success of interventions to reduce the risk of perinatal HIV transmission has been achieved through the routine HIV testing and counseling of all pregnant women. Interventions to prevent transmission can be effective only if women know their HIV status and have access to treatment. The DHHS has recommended universal HIV counseling and testing for pregnant women since 1995. Many national professional and governmental organizations, including the American Academy of Pediatrics, the American College of Obstetricians and Gynecologists, and the U.S. Preventive Services Task Force, endorse those recommendations. Current recommendations from the U.S. Centers for Disease Control and Prevention (CDC) feature the following three approaches to HIV testing during pregnancy:

- Routine testing as part of first trimester prenatal screening tests for all pregnant women, using an "opt-out" policy whereby a pregnant woman is tested unless she specifically declines testing

- Routine "opt-out" testing with a rapid HIV test for women who present in labor with unknown or undocumented HIV status, in order to offer ARV prophylaxis during labor for those who test positive for HIV

- Rapid HIV testing for newborns of mothers of unknown HIV status so that they can receive postexposure ARV prophylaxis, if indicated

State laws regarding HIV testing during pregnancy vary widely, and many are currently under review. A number of states have adopted the opt-out approach, whereas some still require written informed consent before an HIV test is done. Others require patient education and a chart note from the providers. Clinicians should be familiar with relevant state laws regarding HIV testing during pregnancy, opt-out or consent provisions, and regulations about rapid HIV testing during the intrapartum or newborn period. (Information on state laws regarding HIV testing during pregnancy can be found at the National HIV/AIDS Clinicians' Consultation Center's Compendium of State HIV Testing Laws at www.nccc.ucsf.edu/.) Whatever the consent process, a woman should know that an HIV test is being done and should receive at least the information outlined below.

HIV Education and Counseling of Pregnant Women

Educating pregnant women about the importance of HIV testing is a critical element in preventing perinatal HIV transmission. However, extensive pretest counseling is not essential. A woman must be told that HIV testing is a standard component of prenatal care, that her clinician recommends the tests, and that all pregnant women should be tested for HIV because knowing about HIV infection is important for their health and the health of their babies. Research has shown that a provider's strong endorsement of HIV testing is a major predictor of whether a woman receives an HIV test. Testing should be voluntary and free of coercion, and a woman should know that she can decline testing without the risk of being denied care. A woman's age, cultural background, educational level, and primary language may influence her knowledge about HIV transmission and her willingness to be tested; the clinician should consider these factors carefully when providing education and information.

The following minimum information should be provided through an educational session with a health care provider or through written or electronic media (e.g., brochures, videos):

- HIV is the virus that causes AIDS. Approximately 25% of women with HIV who are not treated will transmit the virus to their babies during pregnancy, during labor and delivery, or by breast-feeding.

- A woman could be at risk of HIV infection and not know it.

- ART is highly effective in protecting the infant from being infected with HIV and can improve the mother's health.

- HIV testing is recommended for all pregnant women.

- Women who decline testing will not be denied care.

Women should be told that test results are confidential to the extent allowed by law and that medical and other services are available for women with HIV infection. Reporting requirements for the specific state should be explained.

HIV testing should be performed as early in pregnancy as possible to allow for interventions to prevent transmission and for effective management of a woman's HIV infection, if the woman is found to be HIV seropositive. The CDC recommends repeat HIV testing in the third trimester for women who receive health care in jurisdictions with an elevated incidence of HIV or AIDS among women, as well as for women at high risk of acquiring HIV (e.g., a history of injection drug use, exchange of sex for money or drugs, multiple sex partners, or a partner known to be HIV infected). Jurisdictions in which repeat third trimester testing is recommended include Alabama, Connecticut, Delaware, District of Columbia, Florida, Georgia, Illinois, Louisiana, Maryland, Massachusetts, Mississippi, Nevada, New Jersey, New York,

North Carolina, Pennsylvania, Puerto Rico, Rhode Island, South Carolina, Tennessee, Texas, and Virginia. Any pregnant woman with signs or symptoms of acute HIV infection should be evaluated (see chapter *Primary HIV Infection*) and receive an HIV plasma RNA test as well as an antibody test. A number of states mandate a third-trimester HIV test for all pregnant women. If the client declines testing at any point, the clinician should inquire about her reasons and follow up at subsequent visits. If the provider is persistent, the woman may choose to have an HIV test at a later visit.

In the United States, the vast majority of pregnant women who are tested for HIV will be HIV seronegative. When giving test results to an HIV-negative woman, the clinician should take the opportunity to discuss risk-reduction strategies to help ensure that she remains uninfected by HIV. Women at high risk of HIV infection should be referred for more extensive counseling because some research indicates that pregnancy may place them at greater risk of acquiring HIV infection, and acute HIV infection may confer greater risk of transmission to the fetus.

Counseling a pregnant woman with a positive HIV test result requires knowledge and sensitivity. The clinician should explain that, even though the woman may feel well, she is infected with the virus. The woman should be told about the importance of medical management of HIV for her own health and for the prevention of perinatal transmission, and she should be guided to the medical and social services available in her local community. She also should be referred to an HIV obstetric specialist who can work closely with her primary obstetric and HIV providers to manage her care during the pregnancy. The patient may be surprised or shocked upon receiving the HIV diagnosis, or she may have known her status but been reluctant to disclose it. The clinician should emphasize the importance of emotional and social support,

assess the patient's social support resources, and offer her referrals as needed.

Rapid HIV Testing During Labor

As discussed earlier, beginning ART during pregnancy offers the greatest chance for preventing perinatal transmission of HIV, but interventions during the intrapartum and neonatal periods also offer opportunities to decrease the risk of HIV transmission. Rapid HIV testing for women who present in labor with unknown or undocumented HIV status can identify women who are infected with HIV so that interventions can be offered. Available rapid HIV antibody tests are both sensitive and specific and provide results in as little as 20 minutes.

Women who should receive HIV testing during labor include the following:

- Those who have had little or no prenatal care
- Those who were not offered testing earlier in pregnancy
- Those who declined previously
- Those whose HIV test results are not available at the time of labor

Education and counseling for the woman in labor who needs an HIV test should incorporate the information for prenatal education discussed earlier, with consideration given to the special circumstances of labor. Special educational formats such as flip charts have been developed to help with patient education. Confidentiality should be assured for the information and consent process and for treatment. If an opt-out approach is used in the labor setting, a woman of unknown serostatus should be told that no HIV test is found on her chart, that HIV testing is part of routine care, and that she can decline if she wishes, but that experts recommend HIV testing because available interventions can decrease her baby's risk of becoming infected with HIV if she is found to be seropositive.

Factors Influencing Perinatal HIV Transmission

Perinatal transmission is most likely to occur in the intrapartum period. Several factors influence the risk of transmission from mother to infant. One of these is the mother's HIV RNA level (viral load). Clinical trials and observational studies have shown a strong positive correlation between maternal HIV viral load during pregnancy or at delivery and the risk of perinatal HIV transmission, even among women receiving treatment with ARVs. However, HIV transmission may occur at any level of maternal HIV RNA, including (rarely) when the viral load is undetectable. ARV prophylaxis is a critical factor in reducing HIV transmission. For women on effective combination ART with undetectable HIV RNA, the rate of perinatal HIV transmission is approximately 1%. Thus, ARV prophylaxis with full suppression of HIV RNA is recommended for all pregnant women with HIV infection, regardless of HIV viral load. Note that ART may exert protective effects not only by lowering maternal HIV RNA but also (for ARVs with good transplacental passage) by providing preexposure and postexposure prophylaxis.

Other maternal factors associated with increased risk of perinatal transmission include low CD4 cell count, sexually transmitted infections, active genital herpes during labor, illicit drug use, cigarette smoking, and unprotected sex with multiple partners.

Obstetric factors also affect the risk of HIV transmission. Infection risk increases linearly with the increased duration of ruptured membranes, although the effect of ruptured membranes in women with low viral loads is not known. Invasive procedures performed at any time during pregnancy, such as amniocentesis, placement of scalp electrodes, artificial rupture of membranes, episiotomy, or operative (forceps) delivery may increase risk by exposing the fetus to maternal blood; these procedures should be avoided (though the risk of transmission in women on fully suppressive ART is not clear). In addition, the mode of delivery, whether vaginal or cesarean, can influence the risk of HIV transmission. Scheduled cesarean delivery decreases the rate of perinatal infection for women with an HIV RNA level of >1,000 copies/mL, but its efficacy is not clear for women whose labor has begun or for those whose membranes have ruptured; see "Mode of Delivery and Intrapartum Management," below, for further information.

Infant risk factors for HIV infection include premature birth, low birth weight, skin and mucous membrane lesions such as thrush, and breast-feeding. Breast-feeding increases the risk of HIV transmission by 5-20%. In the United States, where safe, affordable replacement feeding and clean water routinely are available, women with HIV should not breast-feed. However, some women with HIV will be under tremendous cultural and familial pressure to breast-feed and will need the clinician's ongoing support to use substitute formula.

Because many factors that affect the risk of perinatal HIV transmission may be modified, clinicians should educate pregnant women carefully about the importance of ARV prophylaxis and other strategies to reduce the risk of maternal-fetal transmission of HIV.

Antiretroviral Therapy During Pregnancy

The goals of ART for the pregnant woman are the same as those for any person living with HIV:

- To suppress the level of HIV as low as possible for as long as possible

- To preserve and restore immune function

- To prolong life and improve quality of life

An additional, and crucial, goal of ART for pregnant women is to reduce the risk of perinatal HIV transmission through maximal HIV suppression. The DHHS recommendations discuss in detail the multiple issues that must be considered when balancing the woman's need for therapy for her own health and the need to decrease the risk of transmission to the infant. Combination ART is recommended for all HIV-infected pregnant women regardless of CD4 count or HIV viral load. Decisions about ART are complex and should be made by the woman and her health care provider after discussing the risks and benefits. Clinicians are urged to consult an HIV specialist and the most current DHHS recommendations when making therapeutic decisions. The Perinatal HIV Hotline (888-448-8765) provides free clinical consultation on all aspects of perinatal HIV care. The following discussion addresses some of the issues in determining ART strategies and is taken from the DHHS *Perinatal ARV Guidelines*.

The DHHS Perinatal HIV Guidelines Working Group recommends fully suppressive combination ART for all pregnant women, unless there are compelling reasons based on pregnancy-specific maternal and fetal safety issues to modify this approach. Key recommendations from the DHHS *Perinatal ARV Guidelines* include the following:

- Assess the woman's HIV disease status and make recommendations about initiating or altering an ARV regimen, as part of the initial evaluation.

- Recommend ARV prophylaxis to all pregnant women regardless of HIV viral load or CD4 count.

- Discuss known benefits and potential risks of ART.

- Include ZDV as part of the antenatal ART regimen, unless there is severe toxicity or the woman is already on a fully suppressive regimen.

- If HIV RNA is >500-1,000 copies/mL, perform drug-resistance testing prior to starting or changing ART.

- Emphasize the importance of adherence to the regimen.

- Ensure that the woman has access to and coordination of services among perinatal, primary care, and HIV providers as well as mental health and drug abuse services and income support as needed.

A fundamental principle of the guidelines is that therapies of known benefit should not be withheld during pregnancy unless they may cause adverse effects to the woman, fetus, or infant, and these adverse effects outweigh the potential benefits. Thus, women should be advised of the potential risks and benefits of ART (to the woman, fetus, and infant) and of the limited long-term data on outcomes for infants with in utero exposure to ARVs, but treatment decisions should be guided by the woman's clinical, virologic, and immunologic status and by the goal of preventing perinatal transmission. Women should be educated and counseled on the importance of close adherence to the ART regimen (see chapter *Adherence*).

Drug-resistance testing should be conducted for all pregnant women before the initiation of therapy, and for women who are already on ART without fully suppressed HIV RNA.

All women receiving ARVs during pregnancy for prophylaxis or for treatment should receive a combination containing at least three agents, with the aim of viral suppression to undetectable levels (i.e., <40-75 copies/mL, depending on the assay). Monotherapy (e.g., with ZDV) and dual therapy are not as effective and generally are not recommended. The regimen should include two nucleoside reverse transcriptase inhibitors (NRTIs) and either a nonnucleoside reverse transcriptase inhibitors (NNRTI) or a protease inhibitor (PI). Regimen selection should be individualized on the basis of factors such as anticipated safety and efficacy, ARV history, results of resistance testing, and comorbidities (e.g., hepatitis B virus [HBV]) (see chapter *Antiretroviral Therapy* for considerations in selecting ARVs). It should be recognized that only limited information is available for many ARVs and ARV combinations regarding potential toxicities for the fetus or infant (see Table 4), and for dosage requirements with pregnant women.

The DHHS *Perinatal ARV Guidelines* offer recommendations on the use of specific ARV agents during pregnancy. The table below shows "recommended" and "alternative" ARVs; others are classified as "Use in special circumstances" or "Insufficient data to recommend use." For more complete information, see Table 5 of the *Guidelines*).

Recommendations for ARV Use During Pregnancy

ARV Class	Recommended Agents	Alternative Agents
NRTI	• Lamivudine • Zidovudine	• Abacavir # • Didanosine • Emtricitabine • Stavudine
NNRTI	• Nevirapine*	
PI	• Lopinavir/ritonavir (Kaletra)	• Atazanavir/ritonavir • Indinavir/ritonavir • Nelfinavir • Ritonavir (full-dose) • Saquinavir/ritonavir

* For women with CD4 counts of >250 cells/µL, nevirapine should be initiated only if benefit clearly outweighs risk, owing to the increased risk of potentially life-threatening hepatotoxicity in women with high CD4 counts. Women who are already taking nevirapine at the start of pregnancy and are tolerating it well may continue nevirapine, regardless of CD4 count.

\# Risk of hypersensitivity reaction; should be given only to patients who test negative for HLA-B*5701. Test for HLA-B*5701 before starting abacavir.

Adapted from U.S. Department of Health and Human Services. *Recommendations for Use of Antiretroviral Drugs in Pregnant HIV-1-Infected Women for Maternal Health and Interventions to Reduce Perinatal HIV Transmission in the United States*; Table 5. May 24, 2010. Available at aidsinfo.nih.gov/guidelines/.

The guidelines' preferred NRTI component is ZDV/3TC, because of data showing safety and efficacy in pregnancy. The specific alternative NRTIs listed above may be used for women with severe intolerance to ZDV (e.g., severe anemia) or documented resistance to ZDV (see "Safety and Toxicity of Antiretroviral Medications During Pregnancy," below).

Of the NNRTIs, nevirapine may be used for women with CD4 counts of <250 cells/µL or continued for women who are already on nevirapine-containing regimens. Nevirapine generally should not be used for treatment-naive women with CD4 counts of >250 cells/µL because of an increased risk of symptomatic and potentially fatal hepatic and rash toxicity. Efavirenz is not recommended for use during the first trimester because of potential teratogenicity, but it can be considered in later stages of pregnancy if other agents are not appropriate (see "Safety and Toxicity of Antiretroviral Medications During Pregnancy," below). There are insufficient pharmacokinetic and safety data to recommend the use of etravirine during pregnancy.

Lopinavir/ritonavir is the recommended PI based on efficacy studies in adults and experience in pregnant women. Alternative PIs include ritonavir-boosted atazanavir, saquinavir, and indinavir, although data during pregnancy are limited and the latter two agents may be less well tolerated. Nelfinavir, another alternative agent, has been used widely for pregnant women but generally is not recommended for nonpregnant adults because of inferior efficacy compared with first-line agents. Darunavir, fosamprenavir, and tipranavir are not recommended because of lack of data in pregnancy, but they may be considered if other agents are not tolerated or are not appropriate.

Pharmacokinetic and safety data in pregnancy are not sufficient to recommend the use of raltegravir, maraviroc, or enfuvirtide, but these may be considered for use by women for

Section 4: Health Care Maintenance and Disease Prevention

whom drugs in other classes have failed; they should be prescribed in consultation with HIV and obstetric specialists.

Some key recommendations of the DHHS guidelines are that ZDV should be included in the ARV regimen if possible, that the ZDV prophylaxis regimen used in PACTG 076 should be administered intrapartum (i.e., IV ZDV during labor), and that PO ZDV should be given to newborns for 6 weeks. The guidelines emphasize that the PACTG 076 regimen is effective not only for women whose clinical status is similar to that of the participants in the original study, but also for women with advanced HIV disease, low CD4 counts, and previous ZDV therapy.

ART Recommendations by Clinical Scenario
Recommendations for ARV Chemoprophylaxis to Reduce Perinatal HIV Transmission

The DHHS *Perinatal ARV Guidelines* offer recommendations on ARV prophylaxis to reduce perinatal HIV transmission based on four clinical scenarios, categorized by whether the mother needs ART for her own health and by her ART status when she presents for care (see Table 6).

HIV-infected pregnant women currently receiving ART

Women already receiving ART should, in general, continue to receive it during pregnancy if it is suppressing viral replication. If the woman has detectable virus (e.g., >500-1,000 copies/mL) on therapy, HIV drug-resistance testing should be performed, and the regimen should be optimized to maximize the likelihood of achieving virologic suppression. Women presenting in the first trimester should be counseled about the risks and benefits of ART during this period. Discontinuation of therapy could lead to increased viral load and potential for transmission to the fetus.

Efavirenz should be avoided or be substituted for in the first trimester. Pregnant women receiving nevirapine-containing regimens should continue them, regardless of CD4 count, if they are virologically suppressed and tolerating the regimen.

HIV-infected pregnant women not on ART who need ART for their own health

Any pregnant woman who meets the standard criteria for ART under the DHHS guidelines for adults and adolescents (aidsinfo.nih. gov/guidelines) should receive standard, potent, combination ART as soon as possible, including during the first trimester. The drug regimen should be based on the recommendations of the *Perinatal ARV Guidelines* (see above and Table 5). As in other scenarios, drug-resistance testing should guide ARV selection. Efavirenz should be avoided during the first trimester.

HIV-infected pregnant women not on ART who need ART solely to prevent perinatal transmission

ART is recommended as perinatal prophylaxis with pregnant women for whom treatment is not required for their own health. This recommendation applies to all pregnant women regardless of viral load. Rates of transmission are very low among women with undetectable or low viral loads (<1,000 copies/mL) but transmission has occurred at all RNA levels. ARV medications decrease the risk of transmission, including in women with low viral loads. Antenatal ART not only lowers maternal viral load but also provides the infant with preexposure prophylaxis during the birth process; the neonate also receives postexposure prophylaxis through neonatal ZDV.

Women should be counseled about the benefits of ART in preventing perinatal transmission. Because the risk of teratogenic effects on the fetus is greatest during the first 10 weeks of gestation, the woman may wish to defer starting a regimen until after 12 weeks' gestation. As discussed above, efavirenz should be avoided during the first trimester.

Consideration can be given to discontinuing ART in women who do not have indications for continued ART; see "Postpartum Follow-Up of HIV-Infected Women," below.

HIV-infected pregnant women who previously have received ART or prophylaxis but are not currently receiving any ARV medications

In some instances, a pregnant woman has been on ART for prophylaxis during a previous pregnancy and subsequently discontinued the medication. ARV drug-resistance testing should be conducted prior to initiating ART. The regimen should be chosen on the basis of previous ART experience and the reasons for stopping and results of past and current resistance testing, with avoidance of drugs and combinations with teratogenic (e.g., efavirenz) or adverse maternal effects. The selection of an ART regimen for women with advanced HIV disease or a history of extensive prior therapy can be challenging, and consultation with an HIV specialist is recommended. As discussed above, efavirenz should be avoided during the first trimester.

Pharmacokinetic Considerations During Pregnancy

Physiologic changes that occur during pregnancy (e.g., prolonged gastrointestinal transit time, increase in body fat and water, and changes in cardiac, circulatory, hepatic, and renal function) may affect the kinetics of drug absorption, distribution, and elimination. Few pharmacokinetic studies have been conducted on levels of ARVs during pregnancy, but available data suggest that altered dosing for some PIs (e.g., lopinavir/ritonavir) may be required (see Table 5 of the *Guidelines*).

Special Circumstances
Hepatitis B coinfection

In selecting ARVs, providers must decide whether to concurrently treat HBV, using NRTIs that have activity against both HIV and HBV (i.e., lamivudine, emtricitabine, and tenofovir). Making these decisions is complicated, and consultation with an expert is recommended. Also see the relevant discussion in the DHHS *Perinatal ARV Guidelines*, and chapter *Hepatitis B Infection* in this manual.

HBV-infected pregnant women who are not immune to hepatitis A should be vaccinated. Infants born to coinfected women should receive HBV immune globulin and start the HBV vaccine series within 12 hours after birth (with subsequent vaccine doses per usual protocol).

Hepatitis C coinfection

Treatment for hepatitis C (HCV) is not recommended during pregnancy. Recommendations for ART during pregnancy are the same for women who are coinfected with HCV as for those without HCV coinfection.

Coninfected pregnant women should be tested for immunity to hepatitis A and HBV; if not immune, they should be vaccinated. Infants born to coinfected women should be evaluated for HCV infection.

See the relevant discussion in the DHHS *Perinatal ARV Guidelines*, and chapter *Hepatitis C Infection* in this manual.

Safety and Toxicity of Antiretroviral Medications During Pregnancy

Limited data are available on the safety of ARVs in pregnancy, particularly when ARVs are used in combination. The existing safety and toxicity information is derived from animal and human studies, clinical trials, registry data, and anecdotal experience.

Several drugs are of special concern when used during pregnancy (see DHHS *Perinatal ARV Guidelines*; Table 4), including the following:

- **Efavirenz:** Efavirenz is classified by the U.S. Food and Drug Administration (FDA) as a Pregnancy Class D drug because malformations have occurred in monkeys receiving efavirenz during the first trimester. Several cases of neural tube defects in humans after first-trimester exposure to efavirenz have been reported. Efavirenz should be avoided during the first trimester, and women taking efavirenz should be counseled about the risks and the importance of avoiding pregnancy. Use of efavirenz can be considered after the second trimester if no alternative is available.

- **Nevirapine:** Women, including pregnant women, who begin nevirapine therapy when their CD4 count is >250 cells/μL have nearly a 10 times higher incidence of hepatotoxicity than women initiated on nevirapine at lower CD4 counts. Symptoms of hepatotoxicity include fatigue, malaise, anorexia, nausea, jaundice, liver tenderness, and hepatomegaly. Nevirapine should be initiated as part of an ARV regimen for pregnant women with CD4 counts of >250 cells/μL only if the benefits clearly outweigh the risks (see Table 5 in the guidelines).

- **Tenofovir:** Tenofovir may cause fetal bone toxicity and should be used only in special circumstances such as intolerance or resistance to ZDV, or coinfection with HBV where treatment of HBV is indicated.

- **Didanosine + stavudine:** The combination of didanosine (ddI) and stavudine (d4T) may cause fatal lactic acidosis and hepatic steatosis and should be avoided unless no alternative is available. Patients may present with symptoms 1-6 weeks in duration that include nausea, vomiting, abdominal pain, dyspnea, and weakness; clinicians should be alert for early signs and symptoms of lactic acidosis and evaluate them promptly.

In addition, PIs have been associated with an increased risk of new-onset diabetes, worsening diabetes, and diabetic ketoacidosis. Of course, pregnancy itself is a risk factor for hyperglycemia. Clinicians should monitor the glucose levels of pregnant women taking PIs and should educate them about the symptoms of hyperglycemia. The DHHS *Perinatal ARV Guidelines* recommend that pregnant women on ART should be screened with a standard 50 g glucose loading test at 24-28 weeks (see chapter *Care of HIV-Infected Pregnant Women*).

Information on ARV toxicity during pregnancy should be consulted carefully before treatment choices are made. The DHHS guidelines provide information on each ARV drug, including preclinical and clinical data, pharmacokinetic and toxicity data, and recommendations regarding use during pregnancy. These guidelines are updated routinely as information is received (see Tables 4 and 5 in the *Guidelines*). Numerous other medications also are contraindicated for use during pregnancy, and potential toxicity should be considered carefully before any medication is given to a pregnant woman.

Adverse Events Related to ARV Drugs During Pregnancy

A European study found an approximately twofold increase in risk of preterm birth among mothers who took combination therapy during pregnancy (whether started before or during pregnancy). A metaanalysis of seven clinical trials in the United States, however, found that ARV use was not associated with preterm labor, low birth-weight, low Apgar scores, or stillbirth. Subsequent data have been conflicting, but clinicians should be aware of a possible small increased risk of preterm birth among women who receive PIs. However, the benefit of PIs for the mother's health and for prevention of perinatal transmission is clear, and PIs should not be withheld. Until more is known, pregnant women who are taking combination regimens should be monitored closely for complications and toxicities and should be educated about the signs of premature labor.

Antiretroviral Pregnancy Registry

The Antiretroviral Pregnancy Registry collects observational data on HIV-infected pregnant women taking ARV medications to determine whether patterns of fetal or neonatal abnormalities occur. This is a project initiated by the pharmaceutical industry and overseen by an advisory committee comprising representatives from the CDC, National Institutes of Health, FDA, pediatric and obstetric providers, and others. Providers who care for pregnant women taking ARVs are encouraged to enroll patients in the registry at the time of initial evaluation. Information is confidential and patients' names are not used. More information can be obtained by visiting the registry website (www.APRegistry.com) or by calling 800-258-4263, 8:30 AM to 5:30 PM eastern time.

Intrapartum Management and Mode of Delivery

All pregnant women with HIV infection should receive the intrapartum and neonatal components of ZDV prophylaxis used in the PACTG 076 protocol, as outlined earlier. IV ZDV should be given to the woman during labor as a 1-hour loading dose of 2 mg/kg followed by a continuous infusion of 1 mg/kg per hour until delivery. Women on ART should continue their regimen on schedule as much as possible during labor, except that women receiving ZDV or a ZDV-containing fixed-dose combination should be given IV ZDV, with other components continued PO. For women on a stavudine-containing regimen, the stavudine component should be discontinued while IV ZDV is being administered.

For women who have detectable viral load at the time of delivery, the addition of the single-dose nevirapine protocol (single dose to the woman during labor, single dose to the neonate) generally is not recommended in the United States, because clinical trials conducted to date, although small, have not shown benefit and there is a risk of nevirapine resistance. However, single-dose nevirapine may be considered in special circumstances for women with high HIV RNA levels, especially when a patient is not on ART and delivery is vaginal rather than via a scheduled cesarean delivery. If single-dose nevirapine is given, most specialists recommend also giving NRTIs (e.g., ZDV/3TC), and continuing the NRTIs for at least 7 days to decrease the risk of nevirapine resistance.

Studies conducted before the availability of viral load testing found that cesarean delivery performed before the onset of labor or rupture of membranes significantly reduced the risk of perinatal transmission. However, now that many HIV-infected pregnant women in the United States and other high-income settings are receiving potent combination ART, rates of HIV transmission rates are very low (about 1.2-1.5%, unadjusted for mode of delivery); it is difficult to determine whether delivery by cesarean section further decreases the risk of peripartum transmission.

For a woman with a viral load of <1,000 copies/mL, the decisions on mode of delivery should be individualized and based on discussions between the woman and her obstetric clinician. The woman and her health care providers should decide about mode of delivery before the onset of labor, based on her current viral load, her health status, and the outcome of discussions about other concerns, which should include counseling about the risks and benefits of cesarean delivery. For women with HIV RNA levels of >1,000 copies/mL at or near the time of delivery (this would apply to many women on ART for whom viral suppression has not been achieved by the time of delivery because of late entry into care, issues of adherence, or viral resistance), the DHHS *Perinatal ARV Guidelines* and the American

College of Obstetricians and Gynecologists recommend delivery by scheduled cesarean section at 38 weeks' gestation. IV ZDV should be started 3 hours before a scheduled cesarean delivery. Prophylactic antibiotics are recommended at the time of cesarean delivery for HIV-infected women to decrease the risk of maternal infection.

It is not clear whether cesarean delivery provides any benefits in preventing perinatal HIV transmission once labor has begun or membranes are ruptured. Management of a woman for whom a scheduled cesarean was planned but who presents in labor or with ruptured membranes should be individualized on the basis of her HIV viral load, current ART regimen, length of time since membrane rupture, duration of labor, and other clinical factors.

The DHHS *Perinatal ARV Guidelines* outline four scenarios in which the clinician must decide whether cesarean delivery is needed (see Table 9 in the *Guidelines*). The data on the benefits of cesarean delivery are complex and must be considered alongside the increased risk to the mother after surgery. The clinician should consult an obstetric/HIV specialist to discuss specific situations.

A woman who presents in labor without a documented HIV status should receive a rapid HIV antibody test and, if the result is positive, should be presumed to be infected until the confirmatory HIV test result is received. She should receive IV ZDV immediately to prevent perinatal transmission. She will need confirmation and staging of her HIV infection (e.g., CD4 cell count, HIV RNA viral load) as well as referral to care for her own health and ongoing psychological support.

Questions remain about the management of labor when a vaginal delivery is planned. Because the duration of ruptured membranes is a risk factor for perinatal transmission, pregnant women with HIV infection should be counseled to go to a hospital for care at the first signs of labor or rupture of membranes. If the membranes rupture spontaneously before labor occurs or early in labor, the clinician should consider interventions to decrease the interval to delivery, such as administration of oxytocin. Procedures that potentially increase the neonate's exposure to maternal blood, such as the use of scalp electrodes or artificial rupture of membranes, should be avoided. Operative interventions with forceps or vacuum extractor and episiotomy should be performed only in select circumstances.

For management of postpartum hemorrhage owing to uterine atony, note that methergine has significant interactions with PIs and with efavirenz and should not be administered to women taking these medications, if possible. If alternative treatments are not available and methergine must be used, it should be given at the lowest possible low dosage and for the shortest duration possible.

Postpartum Follow-Up of HIV-Infected Women

Women with HIV infection who have recently delivered need access to a comprehensive array of services for themselves and their infants. The clinician should refer the postpartum woman not only to her primary obstetric and HIV providers for family planning and HIV management but also to a pediatric HIV specialist for care of her infant. She should be referred as needed for mental health, substance abuse, and social support services. The clinician should be alert for indications of postpartum depression and should offer treatment promptly, if indicated. Adherence to ARV regimens may be particularly difficult for a woman in the immediate postpartum period because of postpartum physical and psychological changes and the demands of caring for a newborn; accordingly, the woman may require new or continued support services.

Women who are diagnosed through preliminary rapid HIV testing in labor will need thorough evaluation and management including confirmatory HIV testing and referral for medical and social services. They should not breast-feed unless the results of the confirmatory tests are received as negative.

Women should be evaluated regarding their ongoing need for ART postpartum. If ART was given only or primarily to reduce the risk of perinatal transmission, and if the woman's CD4 count has always been above the threshold recommended for treatment in the current adult and adolescent guidelines and she does not have other factors that would recommend treatment, the woman and her clinician, in consultation with an HIV specialist, may consider discontinuing therapy after pregnancy, with the option to resume ART in the future. On the other hand, for women with a CD4 nadir below the currently recommended threshold for treatment initiation or a history of symptoms or conditions caused by HIV, long-term ART should be recommended.

If ART is being discontinued, all drugs should be stopped at the same time if they have similar half-lives. NNRTIs have longer half lives than other agents, so a NNRTI should be discontinued at least 7 days before other ARVs, in order to avoid a period of NNRTI monotherapy and the development of NNRTI resistance mutations. Alternatively, a PI may be substituted for the NNRTI several weeks before stopping the ART. Note that, for women with HBV coinfection, discontinuation of NRTIs with anti-HBV activity (e.g., 3TC, emtricitabine, tenofovir) may result in a flare of HBV; consult with an expert before discontinuing ART.

Contraceptive counseling is an important aspect of postpartum care. Women should be offered dual-method contraception if pregnancy is not desired in the short-term future or if the ART regimen contains potentially teratogenic drugs such as efavirenz. (See chapters *Care of HIV-Infected Pregnant*

Women and *Health Care of HIV-Infected Women Through the Life Cycle.*)

Breast-feeding is not recommended in the United States or other parts of the world where replacement feeding is affordable, feasible, acceptable, sustainable, and safe. Women may experience culture-based and family pressure to breast-feed and may need support to use replacement feeding.

Follow-Up of HIV-Exposed Infants

The HIV-exposed neonate born to a mother with HIV infection should receive ZDV syrup at a dosage of 2 mg/kg body weight per dose Q6H beginning as soon as possible after birth, preferably within 6-12 hours, and continuing for 6 weeks. Newborns should be discharged home with a supply of PO ZDV syrup. The use of ZDV for the neonate is recommended regardless of whether the mother has a history of resistance to ZDV. Few data are available to guide decision making regarding the use of additional ARVs (i.e., combination therapy) for neonates; consult with a pediatric HIV expert. Every HIV-exposed infant should be referred to a pediatric HIV specialist for diagnostic testing and monitoring of health status.

For an infant born to a mother whose HIV status is unknown, rapid HIV testing of the mother or the infant should be done as soon as possible. If the result for either is positive, ZDV prophylaxis for the infant should be started immediately. A confirmatory HIV test (e.g., Western blot) should be done at the same time and prophylaxis should be discontinued if the result is negative. If positive, the infant should be tested with an HIV DNA polymerase chain reaction (PCR) assay or an HIV RNA assay. If the newborn's HIV viral load test result is positive, prophylaxis should be discontinued and the infant should be referred urgently to a pediatric HIV specialist for management of HIV infection using combination ART.

Traditional HIV antibody testing cannot be used with infants because maternal antibodies may persist for up to 18 months. Diagnosis of HIV infection in infants requires virologic testing (HIV DNA or HIV RNA). Virologic testing should be performed by age 14-21 days, then at 1-2 months, and at 4-6 months. HIV can be diagnosed in an infant on the basis of two positive results from virologic tests done on separate blood samples at any time. HIV can be excluded presumptively in an infant with two or more negative results from virologic tests, with one done at ≥14 days of age and one done at ≥ 1 month of age, or one negative virologic test done result done at ≥2 months of age, or one negative HIV antibody test result done at ≥ 6 months of age. HIV can be excluded definitively with two or more negative virologic tests, one done at age ≥1 month and one done at ≥4 months, or two negative HIV antibody tests from separate specimens done at age ≥6 months. However these tests may not be accurate in infants who are receiving combination ART. Some experts recommend retesting, using an antibody test, at age 12-18 months as a confirmatory test.

Infants should have a baseline complete blood count and should be monitored for anemia while they are taking ZDV. *Pneumocystis jiroveci* pneumonia (PCP) prophylaxis for HIV-exposed infants is recommended for infants with indeterminate HIV status starting at 6 weeks when the ZDV prophylaxis regimen is completed until they are determined to presumptively or definitively HIV seronegative. Initiation of PCP prophylaxis should be stopped or avoided altogether when HIV has been presumptively excluded.

Parents and family caregivers must be taught how to monitor the infant for signs of illness until an HIV diagnosis is made or ruled out. They also need to know that the infant's exposure to ARV agents in utero is an important part of the infant's medical history and should be shared with future health care providers. Although no enduring consequences of ARV exposure have been

confirmed, the child may be at risk of long-term problems.

Patient Education

- The clinician should provide the pregnant woman with the most current information on the risk of perinatal HIV transmission and the importance of ARV prophylaxis.

- The clinician and the patient should have a detailed discussion about whether she needs ART for her own health as well as about ARV regimens that would help her to decrease the risk of perinatal transmission.

- The clinician should review with the patient the critical importance of her adherence to ART regimens before prescribing a regimen.

- The clinician should review possible adverse effects of the ARVs and give the patient specific instructions about managing them if they are mild or seeking medical advice if they are more serious, such as ongoing fatigue, persistent nausea and vomiting, or signs of hyperglycemia.

- The clinician should explain the signs and symptoms of early labor to the patient and emphasize the importance of seeking medical care if she has signs and symptoms of early labor or premature rupture of membranes.

- Early in the third trimester, the clinician and the patient should discuss the risks and potential benefits of cesarean section based on her viral load and clinical status.

- Intrapartum management, including the use of intrapartum ZDV, should be discussed with the patient so that she knows to tell the delivery team about her HIV status when she presents in labor.

- The clinician should discuss infant feeding plans with the mother and reinforce that she should not breast-feed. The clinician may need to provide ongoing support for formula feeding.

- The clinician should discuss follow-up plans and make referrals for the patient and her infant. If possible, the woman should meet the pediatric HIV team before delivery or in the postpartum period. The importance of ARV prophylaxis and follow-up for the newborn should be emphasized.

References

- American College of Obstetricians and Gynecologists, Committee on Obstetric Practice. *Prenatal and perinatal human immunodeficiency virus testing: expanded recommendations.* ACOG Committee Opinion No. 418. Washington, DC: American College of Obstetricians and Gynecologists; 2008.

- American College of Obstetricians and Gynecologists. *Routine human immunodeficiency virus screening.* ACOG Committee Opinion No. 411. Washington, DC: American College of Obstetricians and Gynecologists; 2008.

- American College of Obstetricians and Gynecologists. *Scheduled cesarean delivery and the prevention of vertical transmission of HIV infection.* ACOG Committee Opinion No. 234. Washington, DC: American College of Obstetricians and Gynecologists; 2000.

- Anderson JR. *HIV and Reproduction.* In: Anderson JR, ed. *A Guide to the Clinical Care of Women with HIV, 2005 Edition.* Rockville, MD: Health Services and Resources Administration; 2005. Available online at hab.hrsa.gov/publications/womencare05.

- Antiretroviral Pregnancy Registry Steering Committee. *Antiretroviral Pregnancy Registry International Interim Report for 1 January 1989 through 31 July 2009.* Wilmington, NC: Registry Coordinating Center; 2009. Available at www.apregistry.com/forms/interim_report.pdf.

- Branson BM, Handsfield HH, Lampe MA, et al.; Centers for Disease Control and Prevention. *Revised recommendations for HIV testing of adults, adolescents, and pregnant women in health-care settings.* MMWR Recomm Rep. 2006 Sep 22;55(RR-14):1-17.

- Bulterys M, Jamieson D, O'Sullivan MJ, et al. *Rapid HIV-1 testing during labor: a multicenter study.* JAMA. 2004 Jul 14;292(2):219-23.

- Centers for Disease Control and Prevention. *U.S. Public Health Service recommendations for human immunodeficiency virus counseling and voluntary testing for pregnant women.* MMWR Recomm Rep. 1995 Jul 7;44(RR-7):1-15.

- Centers for Disease Control and Prevention. *Rapid HIV-1 Antibody Testing during Labor and Delivery for Women of Unknown HIV Status: A Practical Guide and Model Protocol.* January 30, 2004. Available at www.cdc.gov/hiv/topics/testing/resources/guidelines/rt-labor&delivery.htm.

- Centers for Disease Control and Prevention. *Recommendations of the U.S. Public Health Service Task Force on the use of zidovudine to reduce perinatal transmission of human immunodeficiency virus.* MMWR Recomm Rep. 1994 Aug 5; 43(RR-11):1-20.

- Guay LA, Musoke P, Fleming T, et al. *Intrapartum and neonatal single-dose nevirapine compared with zidovudine for prevention of mother-to-child transmission of HIV-1 in Kampala, Uganda: HIVNET 012 randomized trial.* Lancet. 1999 Sep 4; 354(9181):795-802.

- International Perinatal HIV Group. *Duration of ruptured membranes and vertical transmission of HIV-1: a meta-analysis from 15 prospective cohort studies.* AIDS. 2001 Feb 16;15(3):357-68.

- Ioannidis JP, Abrams EJ, Ammann A, et al. *Perinatal transmission of human immunodeficiency virus type 1 by pregnant women with RNA virus loads <1000 copies/ml.* J Infect Dis. 2001 Feb 15; 183(4):539-45.

- Mofenson LM, Lambert JS, Stiehm ER, et al.; *Pediatric AIDS Clinical Trials Group Study 185 Team. Risk factors for perinatal transmission of human immunodeficiency virus type 1 in women treated with zidovudine.* N Engl J Med. 1999 Aug 5;341(6):385-93.

- Petra Study Team. *Efficacy of three short-course regimens of zidovudine and lamivudine in preventing early and late transmission of HIV-1 from mother to child in Tanzania, South Africa, and Uganda (Petra study): a randomised, double-blind, placebo-controlled trial.* Lancet. 2002 Apr 6;359(9313):1178-86.

- Sperling RS, Shapiro DE, Coombs RW, et al.; Pediatric AIDS Clinical Trials Group Protocol 076 Study Group. *Maternal viral load, zidovudine treatment, and the risk of transmission of human immunodeficiency virus type 1 from mother to infant.* N Engl J Med. 1996 Nov 28;335(22):1621-9.

- U.S. Department of Health and Human Services. *Guidelines for the Use of Antiretroviral Agents in HIV-1-Infected Adults and Adolescents.* January 10, 2011. Available at www.aidsinfo.nih.gov/guidelines/.

- U.S. Department of Health and Human Services. *Recommendations for Use of Antiretroviral Drugs in Pregnant HIV-1-Infected Women for Maternal Health and Interventions to Reduce Perinatal HIV Transmission in the United States.* May 24, 2010. Available at aidsinfo.nih.gov/guidelines/.

- U.S. Department of Health and Human Services. *Guidelines for the Use of Antiretroviral Agents in Pediatric HIV Infection.* February 29, 2009. Available at aidsinfo.nih.gov/guidelines/.

- World Health Organization. *Rapid advice: use of antiretroviral drugs for treating pregnant women and preventing HIV infection in infants.* Geneva: World Health Organization; November 30, 2009. Available at www.who.int/hiv/pub/mtct/advice/en/. Accessed June 30, 2010.

Section 4: Health Care Maintenance and Disease Prevention

Care of HIV-Infected Pregnant Women

Background

This chapter describes the elements involved in caring for the pregnant woman with HIV infection, whether the woman was known to be HIV infected before conception or was found to be HIV infected during pregnancy. It is not intended to be a comprehensive discussion of this topic, and an HIV-experienced obstetrician and an HIV specialist should be involved in the management of all HIV-infected pregnant women. For centers that do not have HIV specialists available, experts at the National Perinatal HIV Consultation and Referral Service are available for consultation through the Perinatal HIV Hotline (888-448-8765).

The goals of HIV management during pregnancy are to maintain and support the woman's health, provide optimal antiretroviral treatment (ART) to preserve or restore her immune system and suppress viral replication, and to offer interventions that decrease the risk of perinatal HIV transmission. According to the U.S. Department of Health and Human Services perinatal guidelines, *Recommendations for Use of Antiretroviral Drugs in Pregnant HIV-1-Infected Women for Maternal Health and Interventions to Reduce Perinatal HIV Transmission in the United States,* all HIV-infected pregnant women should be given ART during pregnancy to prevent mother-to-child transmission of HIV, regardless of whether ART is indicated for the woman's own health (see chapter *Reducing Maternal-Infant HIV Transmission*).

The first task in caring for an HIV-infected woman who is pregnant or considering pregnancy is to provide counseling that will allow her to make informed reproductive choices. Taking a careful reproductive history and providing preconception counseling should be part of any woman's routine primary care. To make informed choices about pregnancy, the patient needs education and information about the risk of perinatal transmission of HIV, potential complications of pregnancy, continuation or modification (or possibly, initiation) of ART, and the support she will need to optimize maternal and fetal outcomes. See chapter *Health Care of HIV-Infected Women Through the Life Cycle* for a more detailed discussion of preconception evaluation.

If ART is indicated for the woman's own health, an appropriate regimen should be started before pregnancy, to attain a stable, maximally suppressed maternal viral load prior to conception. Antiretroviral (ARV) resistance testing should be performed before ART is initiated. Particular ARVs should be avoided, including those with increased risk of causing teratogenicity (e.g., efavirenz), hepatotoxicity (e.g., nevirapine), or metabolic complications such as lactic acidosis (e.g., didanosine and stavudine). See chapter *Reducing Maternal-Infant HIV Transmission*. It should be noted that most fetal organogenesis occurs in the early weeks of pregnancy, before most women know that they are pregnant. Thus, any medication with potential teratogenicity or fetal toxicity, whether an ARV or another drug, should not be administered to women who intend to become pregnant or may become pregnant. Certain medications (e.g., ribavirin) also should be avoided by male partners of women who may become pregnant.

Folate supplementation to reduce the risk of neural tube defects in the developing fetus should be started at least 1 month before conception, if possible, because the neural tube forms in the early weeks of pregnancy (see below).

Section 4: Health Care Maintenance and Disease Prevention

Evaluation and Counseling of Pregnant Women

All HIV-infected pregnant women should receive thorough education and counseling about perinatal transmission risks, strategies to reduce those risks, and potential effects of HIV infection or HIV treatment on the course or outcomes of pregnancy.

- The goals of therapy for pregnant women receiving ART, as for all persons being treated for HIV infection, are to suppress the HIV viral load maximally (preferably to undetectable levels) for as long as possible, to improve quality of life, to restore or preserve immune function, and, for pregnant women specifically, to reduce the risk of perinatal transmission as much as possible.

- Therapy-associated adverse effects, including hyperglycemia, anemia, and hepatic toxicity, may have a negative effect on maternal and fetal health outcomes. Pregnant women should be advised about possible ARV-related adverse effects and should be monitored regularly for these events.

- HIV-infected women should receive evaluation and appropriate prophylaxis for opportunistic infections (OIs), as well as the vaccinations indicated for persons with HIV infection (see below).

- Some medications, both ARVs and other drugs, may cause fetal anomalies or toxicity when taken during pregnancy. These should be avoided in pregnant women, unless the anticipated benefit outweighs the risk. Consult with an HIV or obstetric specialist, a pharmacist, or the drug labeling information before prescribing medications for pregnant women.

- Options for mode of delivery should be discussed early. The benefits and risks of vaginal vs. cesarean delivery are outlined in the perinatal guidelines. If the HIV viral load is >1,000 copies/mL at 36 weeks of pregnancy, a scheduled cesarean delivery at 38 weeks' gestation is recommended to further reduce the risk of transmission.

Other evaluation and support measures for pregnant women should include the following:

- Screening for other potential maternal health problems, such as diabetes and hypertension

- Maternal nutritional evaluation and support, including initiation of a prenatal multivitamin containing folate (0.4-0.8 mg PO once daily) to reduce the risk of fetal neural tube defects; for women receiving trimethoprim-sulfamethoxazole, some experts recommend a folate dose of 4 mg daily

- Screening for psychiatric and neurologic disease

- Counseling about the risks of tobacco smoking; smoking cessation support as indicated (see chapter *Smoking Cessation*)

- Counseling about the risks of alcohol or drug use and support for discontinuation of these activities as needed

- Intimate partner violence screening

- Review of medications, including over-the-counter and nutritional agents, and discontinuation of medications with the potential for fetal harm

- Immunizations (e.g., influenza, hepatitis B) as indicated

- Institution of the standard measures for evaluation and management (e.g., assessment of reproductive and familial genetic history, screening for infectious diseases or sexually transmitted infections [STIs])

- Planning for maternal-fetal medicine consultation, if desired or indicated

- Selection of effective and appropriate postpartum contraceptive methods, if desired

Comprehensive Care of Pregnant Women with HIV Infection

Comprehensive care is important for pregnant women with HIV infection to achieve a healthy pregnancy and delivery. A multidisciplinary approach is the most effective way to address the medical, psychological, social, and practical challenges. For example, while her medical care is being managed by her obstetrician and an HIV specialist, the pregnant woman may need help from a social worker to find appropriate social services for food, housing, child care, and parenting issues. The pregnant woman may need counseling and psychological support for herself and her partner, as well as referrals for substance abuse and detoxification programs. Peer counselors may be of particular assistance. Some patients may need legal or domestic violence services during and after pregnancy. Cooperation and communication between the obstetrician or nurse/midwife and the primary HIV provider are imperative throughout the pregnancy and early postpartum period. Referral to a maternal-fetal medicine specialist may be needed in complicated obstetric cases.

Prenatal Care

All of the pregnancy-related complications seen in HIV-uninfected women, such as hypertensive disorders, ectopic pregnancy, psychiatric illness, multiple gestation, preterm delivery, and STIs, also can occur in HIV-infected women. These problems must be recognized quickly and treated appropriately to avoid life-threatening complications. Ideally, HIV-infected pregnant women are managed by both an experienced obstetrician-gynecologist and an HIV specialist. Communication between these specialists about medications, expectations, and complications is vital for the health and well-being of both mother and baby. If complications occur or abnormalities are detected, they should be evaluated and treated as indicated by the condition, and referral should be made to a maternal-fetal medicine specialist, if possible. Antenatal fetal surveillance and testing to identify fetal abnormalities should be carried out using guidelines established by the American College of Obstetricians and Gynecologists.

The suggested testing and monitoring practices for pregnant women with HIV infection, from the first trimester to labor and delivery, are presented in Tables 1 and 2.

Section 4: Health Care Maintenance and Disease Prevention

Table 1. Recommended Evaluation and Routine Monitoring of the Pregnant Woman with HIV Infection

Evaluation		Frequency
History		
HIV History	Date of diagnosis	Initial
	Signs and symptoms	Initial and at every visit
	Nadir CD4 and current CD4 cell count; HIV viral load	Initial
	ARV history, including regimen efficacy, toxicity, and ARV resistance	Initial
	Opportunistic infections and malignancies	Initial and at every visit
	History of STIs	Initial
	Adherence	Initial and at every visit
Obstetric History	Number of pregnancies; complications and outcomes (GPAL [gravida, para, abortion, living children]); mode of deliveries	Initial
	History of genetic disorders	Initial
	Use of ARV prophylaxis during previous pregnancies	Initial
	HIV status of children	Initial
Current Pregnancy	Last menstrual period (LMP)	Initial
	Pregnancy: intended or not	Initial
	Contraceptive methods used, if any	Initial
	Gestational age (can be calculated in a woman with regular menses by counting weeks from LMP)	Initial and at every visit
	Estimated date of delivery	Initial
	Signs or symptoms of maternal complications: elevated blood pressure, headache, significant edema, gastrointestinal or genitourinary symptoms, vaginal discharge or bleeding, decreased fetal movement (fetal movement is usually first detected at 18-24 weeks of pregnancy)	Initial and at every visit
	Screen for depression	Initial
	Screen for intimate-partner violence	Initial and at every visit

	Evaluation	Frequency
Physical Examination		
General	Vital signs and weight	Initial and at every visit
	Fundoscopy, breast examination	Initial and as indicated
Gynecologic/ Obstetric (usually performed by the obstetric provider)	Pelvic examination, STI screening, examination for perineal or vaginal lesions (discoloration, condyloma, ulcerative lesions, vaginal discharge), cervical lesions, discharge or bleeding	Initial and as indicated
	Fundal height, correlating with gestational age (concordant between 18 and 30 weeks)	Every visit starting the second trimester
	Fetal heart beat and rate: may be audible with Doppler devices as early as 12 weeks	Initial and at every visit
	Fetal movements and position in third trimester	Every visit starting at 24 weeks
Laboratory and Other Studies		
HIV	HIV antibody test (if not already documented)	Initial
	HIV viral load and CD4 count (total and percentage); results obtained at 35-36 weeks guide decisions on the mode of delivery	Viral load at initial visit, 2-4 weeks after starting or changing ART, every 4 weeks until undetectable, then at least every 3 months CD4 count at initial visit and at least every 3 months
	Genotype if ARV naive or detectable HIV RNA while on ART	Initial and as indicated
	Cytomegalovirus (CMV) immunoglobulin G (IgG)	Initial
	Toxoplasma IgG	Initial
	G6PD level in appropriate ethnic or racial groups if PCP prophylaxis with dapsone is anticipated	Initial
General	Complete blood count (CBC)	Initial and every 3 months or more frequently, based on ARV regimen or symptoms; check weeks 24-28
	Chemistries, liver enzymes (LFTs)	Initial and every 3 months or more frequently, based on ARV regimen or symptoms If on NRTIs, monitor electrolytes and hepatic enzymes monthly in third trimester
	Fasting lipids and glucose	Initial and as indicated
	Blood group	Initial
	Rh antibody screen	Initial

Section 4: Health Care Maintenance and Disease Prevention

	Evaluation	Frequency
Pregnancy Specific	Ultrasound	First trimester: confirm gestational age and potential timing for cesarean delivery if necessary Second trimester: assess fetal anatomy for women on combination ART during first trimester
	Maternal serum alpha-fetoprotein (AFP) or triple screen (human chorionic gonadotropin [HCG], serum estriol, and alpha-fetoprotein [AFP])	Screen for neural tube and abdominal wall defect, trisomy 21, and trisomy 18; may be done earlier, at 14-15 weeks Abnormal result requires further investigation — consider amniocentesis only if abnormality is detected on expanded triple-screen or level-2 sonogram and the woman is on suppressive ART (to decrease risk of HIV transmission); voluntary and requires counseling
	Diabetes screening	Consider at 20 weeks; check glucose 1 hour after 50 g glucose load; perform 3-hour glucose tolerance test if screen is abnormal If 3-hour test result is abnormal, perform regular glucose monitoring, especially in women taking protease inhibitors (PIs)
	Rubella antibody	Initial
	Varicella IgG for those without history of chickenpox or shingles	Initial
	Screening for syphilis: rapid plasma reagin (RPR) or Venereal Disease Research Laboratory (VDRL)	Initial and during weeks 32-36
	Consider bacterial vaginosis (BV) screening (BV increases risk of preterm labor)	Week 24-28
	Screening for streptococcus B (if result is positive, intrapartum chemoprophylaxis is indicated)	Week 32-36
	Screening with herpes simplex virus-2 serology in high risk patients is recommended by some experts	Initial
	Urinalysis and clean-catch urine culture	Initial and as indicated
	Papanicolaou test	Initial and as indicated (colposcopy is done on pregnant women, but biopsy is avoided; management resumes postpartum, after the 6-week postpartum visit)

Evaluation		Frequency
Hepatitis Serologies	Hepatitis A virus (HAV) antibody (IgG)	Initial
	Hepatitis B virus (HBV): HBsAg, HBcAb , HBsAb	Initial
	Hepatitis C virus (HCV) antibody	Initial
TB Screening	Tuberculin skin test (purified protein derivative [PPD]), more reliable if CD4 count is >200 cells/µL (induration >5 mm is positive); or interferon-gamma release assay (IGRA); note there is little experience with IGRAs in pregnant women	Initial
Disease Specific	Consider hemoglobin electrophoresis, if anemic or at increased risk of hemoglobinopathies	Initial
	Serum screening for Tay-Sachs disease — both partners — if at increased risk	Initial
	Urine toxicology screen	Initial and as indicated

Table 2. Recommended Evaluation and Routine Monitoring of the Pregnant Woman with HIV Infection: Labor and Delivery

Test	Comment
Record Review	• Documentation of HIV serostatus, blood type and Rh, hepatitis serologies, RPR • Review of ART, if any, during pregnancy • Review of HIV viral load results during pregnancy
Physical Evaluation	• Vital signs and fetal heart rate • Frequency and intensity of contractions • Fetal lie, presentation, attitude, and position • Vaginal examination: rule out HSV lesions; detect ruptured membranes; determine cervical effacement, dilatation, and position • Avoid procedures that increase risk of perinatal HIV transmission (e.g., fetal scalp electrodes, scalp sampling, or assisted rupture of membranes)
Admission Laboratory Tests	• Complete blood count • Liver function tests • RPR or VDRL, if not done recently • Repeat hepatitis B and C testing, if at risk of acquisition of hepatitis B or C, to prevent perinatal transmission of these infections • Others, as required by specific state laws

Immunizations and Opportunistic Infection Prophylaxis

Immunizations During Pregnancy

Immunizations should be given before pregnancy, if possible. Immunizations should be considered during pregnancy when the risk of exposure to an infection is high, the risk of infection to the mother or fetus is high, and the vaccine is unlikely to cause harm. Some vaccinations (particularly live-virus vaccines such as measles/mumps/rubella) are contraindicated, and others should be given only if the anticipated benefit of the vaccination outweighs its risk. Special considerations for immunizations in HIV-infected individuals are discussed in chapter *Immunizations for HIV-Infected Adults and Adolescents.*

Some clinicians avoid giving immunizations during the third trimester of pregnancy because vaccinations may cause a transient increase in the HIV viral load and theoretically may increase the risk of perinatal HIV transmission. An increase in viral load may be prevented with effective ART, and some clinicians defer immunizations until ART is under way.

Recommendations related to immunizations during pregnancy are shown in Table 4.

Table 4. Immunizations and Postexposure Prophylaxis in Pregnant Women with HIV Infection

Immunization	Comment
Hepatitis A virus (HAV)	Recommended for susceptible patients at high risk of becoming infected, those with chronic HBV or HCV, those traveling to endemic areas, injection drug users, and those in the setting of a community outbreak.
Hepatitis B virus (HBV)	Generally recommended for susceptible patients.
Influenza (seasonal and H1N1 pandemic)	Generally recommended; give before flu season. As of 2010, H1N1 influenza vaccination also is recommended.
Measles/Mumps/Rubella (MMR)	Contraindicated.
Pneumococcus	Generally recommended; repeat in 5-7 years.
Tetanus-diphtheria (Td); tetanus- diphtheria-pertussis (Tdap)	Recommended; give booster every 10 years. Give a single dose of Tdap for ages >19 to replace a booster dose of Td.
Immune globulins (for postexposure prophylaxis in susceptible individuals)	**Comment**
Measles	Recommended after measles exposure, for symptomatic HIV-infected persons.
Hepatitis A	Recommended after exposure (close contact or sex partner), or in case of travel to endemic areas.
Varicella-zoster virus immune globulin (VariZIG)	Recommended for susceptible individuals after close contact with someone with varicella or herpes zoster (give within 96 hours).
Hepatitis B immune globulin (HBIG)	Recommended for susceptible individuals after needlestick or sexual exposure to a person with hepatitis B infection.

Opportunistic Infection Prophylaxis

Some OIs can have an adverse effect on pregnancy. In turn, pregnancy can affect the natural history, presentation, treatment, and significance of some OIs. Women should be monitored carefully for OIs during pregnancy, with special attention given to nonspecific symptoms such as fatigue, back pain, and weight loss, which may be attributable to HIV-related illness rather than to pregnancy. Respiratory symptoms in particular merit rapid, aggressive investigation. Clinicians should follow the most current recommendations of the U.S. Centers for Disease Control and Prevention (CDC), National Institutes of Health, and Infectious Diseases Society of America, *Guidelines for Prevention and Treatment of Opportunistic Infections in HIV-Infected Adults and Adolescents*, which give special consideration to pregnant women for each OI discussed. The indications and recommendations for OI prophylaxis generally should follow the guidelines for adults (see chapter *Opportunistic Infection Prophylaxis*). However, because of the risks of teratogenicity or harm to the developing fetus, some drugs routinely used for prophylaxis of OIs in nonpregnant adults are contraindicated during the first trimester of pregnancy, whereas others should not be used at any time during pregnancy.

Special Considerations for OI Prophylaxis During Pregnancy

Trimethoprim-sulfamethoxazole

Trimethoprim inhibits the synthesis of metabolically active folic acid. In pregnant women, folate deficiency increases the risk of neural tube defects in the developing fetus. Pregnant women, or women who may become pregnant, who are taking trimethoprim-sulfamethoxazole (Septra, Bactrim, cotrimoxazole) have an increased risk of folate deficiency and should be given folate supplementation to reduce the risk of neural tube defects. Some experts recommend a folate dose of 4 mg daily for women receiving trimethoprim-sulfamethoxazole.

Genital herpes

Women with HIV infection are more likely than HIV-uninfected women to experience outbreaks of genital herpes. If HSV is transmitted to the infant, neonatal infection can be severe, even if it is detected and treated early. In addition, there is increased genital shedding of HIV in those with active genital HSV lesions. Some experts recommend obtaining HSV-2 serologies in a woman whose clinical history is unclear. Treatment for symptomatic HSV infections should be offered during pregnancy, and suppressive therapy should be given to women with frequent recurrences. If a woman has an active outbreak of genital HSV or experiences prodromal symptoms at the time of labor or membrane rupture, delivery by cesarean section is indicated. Prophylaxis with oral acyclovir late in pregnancy to prevent neonatal herpes transmission is controversial and is not recommended routinely.

Tuberculosis

Prophylaxis is recommended for any woman with a positive PPD skin test result (≥5 mm induration), a positive IGRA result, or a history of exposure to someone with active tuberculosis, after active disease has been ruled out. Because of concern about possible teratogenicity from drug exposure, clinicians may choose to delay prophylaxis until after the first trimester. Patients receiving isoniazid also should receive pyridoxine to reduce the risk of neurotoxicity.

Toxoplasmosis

All HIV-infected persons should be tested for IgG antibodies to *Toxoplasma* soon after HIV diagnosis, and this should be a part of antenatal testing for pregnant women with HIV infection. Women with a negative IgG titer should be counseled to avoid exposure to *Toxoplasma* (e.g., by avoiding raw or undercooked meats, unwashed or uncooked vegetables, and cat feces). Women with previous exposure to *Toxoplasma* (positive IgG titer) should be given prophylaxis during pregnancy, if the CD4 count is <100 cells/μL. For women who require prophylaxis, trimethoprim-sulfamethoxazole is the preferred agent; some specialists advise against giving pyrimethamine during pregnancy. If secondary prophylaxis is used to prevent recurrence of toxoplasmosis, sulfadiazine should not be used, as it is contraindicated for use during pregnancy.

Antiretroviral Therapy

Current U.S. Public Health Service guidelines recommend treating HIV infection in all pregnant women, using the same principles and modalities as used for nonpregnant individuals. HIV-infected pregnant women should receive potent combination ART regimens comprising at least three ARVs. The use of zidovudine (ZDV) prophylaxis alone (monotherapy) is not recommended but may be considered for the few women whose HIV RNA levels are <1,000 cells/μL on no ART and who decline combination ART. The choice of ARV regimen should be based on what is likely to be optimal for the woman's health, the potential effect on the fetus and infant, resistance test results, the woman's previous experience, if any, with ART, and her stage of pregnancy. ARV resistance testing should be performed before initiating or changing therapy. ZDV should be included in the regimens of all pregnant women unless there is severe toxicity or documented drug resistance. ARV agents with known teratogenic effects, such as efavirenz, should be avoided, especially in the first trimester. Women who do not need ART for their own health and are taking ART only for the prevention of perinatal transmission may delay initiation of therapy until after the first trimester. This is a period of rapid organogenesis, and there is an increased risk of birth defects if teratogen exposure occurs. For women already taking ART at the time they become pregnant, the regimen should be reevaluated for its appropriateness during pregnancy to avoid potentially toxic medications and to ensure maximal virologic suppression. The ART regimen may be changed if necessary, but should continue without interruption. Discontinuation of ART could lead to an increase in viral load, which could result in a decline in immune status and an acceleration of disease progression, thereby increasing the risk of HIV transmission to the fetus.

For further information about ART during pregnancy, see chapter *Reducing Maternal-Infant HIV Transmission* and the DHHS *Perinatal ARV Guidelines*. The *Guidelines* include recommendations regarding ARV regimens, modes of delivery (vaginal vs. cesarean section), and potential adverse events, as well as a detailed discussion of individual ARV agents. Additionally, the treatment of pregnant women with HIV/HBV coinfection and HIV/HCV coinfection is discussed.

Antiretroviral Pregnancy Registry

To improve tracking of pregnancy-related adverse events and fetal effects, an Antiretroviral Pregnancy Registry has been established as a collaborative project among the pharmaceutical industry, pediatric and obstetric providers, the CDC, and the National Institutes of Health. The registry collects observational data on HIV-infected pregnant women taking ARV medications to determine whether patterns of fetal or neonatal abnormalities occur. Pregnant women taking ARVs can be placed in this confidential follow-up study by calling 800-258-4263, 8:30 AM to 5:30 PM eastern time; the fax number is 800-800-1052. Information is confidential and patients' names are not used. Providers are encouraged to add to the available information on fetal risk by using this registry at first contact with a pregnant woman receiving ART. More information can be obtained at www. APRegistry.com.

Pregnancy-Specific Complications and Management

Nutrition risk and inadequate weight gain

Maternal nutrition and weight must be monitored throughout the pregnancy. A food diary may be a useful tool in assessing intake, and nutritional counseling is recommended.

Nausea and vomiting

Women with signs of dehydration should be assessed and treated appropriately in collaboration with the obstetrician or nurse/midwife. Any medication used for nausea and vomiting must be assessed for drug-drug interactions with all HIV-related medications the patient is taking.

Hyperglycemia

Pregnancy is a risk factor for hyperglycemia, and women treated with PIs may have an even higher risk of glucose intolerance than other pregnant women and must be monitored carefully. New-onset hyperglycemia and diabetes mellitus, and exacerbation of existing diabetes, all have been reported in patients taking PIs. Clinicians should educate women taking PIs about the symptoms of hyperglycemia and closely monitor glucose levels. Some clinicians check glucose tolerance at 20-24 weeks and again at 30-34 weeks if the woman is taking PIs. The newborn should be checked for neonatal hypoglycemia at 1 and 4 hours after birth.

Lactic acidosis

Lactic acidosis is a rare but life-threatening complication that has been reported in pregnant women taking nucleoside reverse transcriptase inhibitors, particularly didanosine and stavudine. The combination of didanosine and stavudine should be avoided during pregnancy. Clinical suspicion of lactic acidosis should be prompted by vague symptoms such as malaise, nausea, or abdominal discomfort or pain. Lactate levels, electrolytes, and liver function should be monitored carefully, including monthly in the third trimester.

Hyperbilirubinemia

Women taking atazanavir or indinavir frequently develop elevated indirect bilirubin, but it is not known whether treatment during pregnancy exacerbates physiologic hyperbilirubinemia in newborns. Women who are taking indinavir may have an increased risk of nephrolithiasis, but evidence of harm to their newborns has not been demonstrated.

Pain management

Pain management during labor and delivery may be complicated by drug interactions with ARV agents and by the higher medication tolerance in women who have addictions. Additional pain medication may be needed for women with histories of drug use.

Invasive perinatal procedures

The risk of HIV transmission to the fetus during invasive procedures (e.g., amniocentesis, chorionic villus sampling, and percutaneous or umbilical cord blood sampling) must be weighed carefully against the possible benefits of these procedures. Current DHHS guidelines suggest that women undergoing such procedures should be on effective ART, preferably with undetectable HIV RNA. The use of fetal scalp electrodes and artificial rupture of membranes should be avoided if possible, and forceps or vacuum extractors and episiotomy should be used only if there are clear obstetric indications.

Postpartum considerations

Because HIV can be transmitted to the infant through breast-feeding, breast-feeding is contraindicated in the United States and other resource-adequate countries where safe replacement feeding is available. Breast-feeding information should be removed from patient educational material pertaining to labor and delivery. Breast binding and ice packs can be used as needed to reduce lactation discomfort. Clinicians should recognize that women in some cultural groups are expected to breast-feed and they may need additional support to use formula rather than breast-feed.

ART should be continued as indicated by the DHHS *Perinatal ARV Guidelines*. Maternal and infant medication adherence must be discussed with the new mother. Adherence barriers for the mother during the postpartum period may be different from those during pregnancy (e.g., because of changes in daily routine, sleep/wake cycles, and meals).

New mothers should be observed carefully for signs of bleeding or infection.

If the mother's glucose tolerance test was abnormal during pregnancy, she should be reevaluated (by 2-hour glucose tolerance test) 6 weeks postpartum and should be screened yearly for diabetes.

At the infant's 2-week follow-up visit, the HIV pediatric clinician should address the mother's concerns, screen for postpartum depression, assess adherence to her own and the infant's ARV medications, and ensure follow-up for the 6-week postpartum visit with the obstetric provider and soon thereafter with the primary HIV care provider. These visits provide an opportunity to address the woman's contraceptive needs and options, if this was not done previously (see chapter *Health Care of HIV-Infected Women Through the Life Cycle*).

Contraception

Many contraceptive choices are available for HIV-infected women; considerations are discussed in chapter *Health Care of HIV-Infected Women Through the Life Cycle*. Depending on the woman's risk factors, consistent condom use should be emphasized, with or without other methods of contraception, to prevent the transmission of HIV and the acquisition or transmission of other STIs.

Patient Education

- Reinforce regularly and clearly the notion that, when the mother cares for herself, she is caring for her infant. Talk with the patient about stress, the importance of adequate mild-to-moderate exercise, and sufficient rest.

- Emphasize that regular prenatal care is extremely important to prevent complications of pregnancy.

- Use of a prenatal vitamin supplement is important, but cannot replace healthy food intake. Develop a plan with the patient for attaining the desired weight gain during pregnancy, while maintaining a healthy nutritional intake.

- Cigarette, alcohol, and drug use contribute to poor maternal nutrition and can harm the developing fetus. Illicit drug use increases the risk of transmitting HIV to the infant. Injection drug use can transmit HBV, HCV, and CMV to the mother and to the baby. Encourage cessation of cigarette, alcohol, and drug use, and offer referrals for treatment, as needed.

- Be sure the woman understands all planned procedures and treatments and understands their potential risks and benefits both to herself and to the fetus.

- Discuss the risks and benefits (to the woman and fetus) of each medication to be taken during pregnancy, including those for which there are limited data on teratogenicity.

- Discuss ART as part of the strategy to reduce the risk of perinatal HIV transmission to the fetus or newborn. For women at risk, diligent use of "safer sex" during pregnancy is important for preventing transmission of STIs and CMV, which can cause more complications when HIV is present. STIs can harm fetal development and may increase the risk of HIV transmission to the baby. New genital herpes infections during pregnancy can cause severe complications and even death in neonates.

- For women with negative *Toxoplasma* titers, explain the need to avoid undercooked meat, soil, and cat feces.

- Teach the pregnant woman how to obtain medical attention quickly at the first signs of OI or other complication. Discuss what to watch for and how to get help when emergencies arise in the evenings or on weekends or holidays.

- Help the patient clarify her child care options and encourage her to begin putting in place long-term child care and guardianship plans in case she becomes too sick to care for her child or children.

References

- American College of Obstetricians and Gynecologists. *Immunization during pregnancy.* ACOG Committee Opinion No. 282; 2003. [Registration required.]

- Anderson JR. *HIV and Reproduction.* In: Anderson JR, ed. *A Guide to the Clinical Care of Women with HIV.* Rockville, MD: Health Services and Resources Administration; 2005. Available online at hab.hrsa.gov/publications/womencare05. Accessed June 30, 2010.

- Antiretroviral Pregnancy Registry Steering Committee. *Antiretroviral Pregnancy Registry International Interim Report for 1 January 1989 — 31 January 2008.* Available at www.apregistry.com/form/exec-summary. pdf. Accessed June 30, 2010.

- Centers for Disease Control and Prevention. *Enhanced Perinatal Surveillance — Participating areas in the United States and dependent areas, 2000-2003.* HIV/ AIDS Surveillance Supplemental Report 2008;13(No. 4).

- Centers for Disease Control and Prevention. *General recommendations on immunization. Recommendations of the Advisory Committee on Immunization Practices (ACIP) and the American Academy of Family Physicians (AAFP).* MMWR Recomm Rep. 2006 Dec 1;55(RR15);1-48.

- Centers for Disease Control and Prevention. *Guidelines for Prevention and Treatment of Opportunistic Infections in HIV-Infected Adults and Adolescents: Recommendations from CDC, the National Institutes of Health, and the HIV Medicine Association of the Infectious Diseases Society of America.* April 10, 2009. Available at www.aidsinfo.nih.gov/ guidelines/.

- Centers for Disease Control and Prevention. *Sexually transmitted diseases treatment guidelines 2006.* MMWR. 2006;55(No. RR-11):1-100.

- Ethics Committee of the American Society for Reproductive Medicine. *Human immunodeficiency virus and infertility treatment.* Fertil Steril. 2004 Sep;82 Suppl 1:S228-31.

- Minkoff H. *Human immunodeficiency virus infection in pregnancy.* Obstet Gynecol. 2003 Apr;101(4):797-810.

- U.S. Department of Health and Human Services. *Guidelines for the Use of Antiretroviral Agents in HIV-1-Infected Adults and Adolescents.* January 10, 2011. Available at www.aidsinfo.nih.gov/ guidelines/.

- U.S. Department of Health and Human Services. *Recommendations for Use of Antiretroviral Drugs in Pregnant HIV-1-Infected Women for Maternal Health and Interventions to Reduce Perinatal HIV Transmission in the United States.* May 24, 2010. Available at aidsinfo.nih.gov/ guidelines/.

Health Care of HIV-Infected Women Through the Life Cycle

Susan Richardson, MN, MPH, FNP-BC

Background

Women with HIV infection have the same reproductive and life cycle health needs and concerns as women without HIV infection. However, for women with HIV infection, certain gynecologic problems may be more common or more frequent. In addition, issues regarding antiretroviral therapy (ART), contraception, and preconception counseling require special attention. This chapter addresses some of the unique health care needs of HIV-infected women across the lifespan, from menarche through postmenopause, and describes the essential elements of care. For further information, see chapters *Reducing Maternal-Infant HIV Transmission, Care of HIV-Infected Pregnant Women*, and *Antiretroviral Medications and Oral Contraceptive Agents.*

Epidemiology and Factors Affecting HIV Transmission

Heterosexual transmission of HIV is more efficient from man to woman than from woman to man. Transmission can occur through intact vaginal tissue; no damage to the vaginal lining is required. Women have specific risks of HIV acquisition at different phases of the lifespan:

- Young adolescents have immature genital tracts and increased cervical ectopy (increased vulnerability to HIV and other sexually transmitted infections [STIs])

- Women of reproductive age may desire pregnancy and childbearing (potentially increasing risky sexual behaviors)

- Married or partnered women may be monogamous with male partners who have risk factors for HIV infection (women may lack awareness of partner's risk behaviors)

- Postmenopausal or posthysterectomy women may have vaginal atrophy (decreasing the anatomic barrier to HIV), or may have no fear of pregnancy or have a perception that they are at low risk of infection (increasing risky sexual behaviors)

- Additionally, woman-to-woman transmission may occur if risk factors are present

Psychosocial/Emotional Factors Unique to Women

Heterosexual women frequently are faced with unequal power and socioeconomic relationships with their male partners. These women may be more likely to exchange sex for money, less likely to successfully negotiate protected sex, and less likely to leave a relationship they perceive as risky. Women may be more vulnerable to domestic violence and sexual coercion, especially those with histories of childhood sexual abuse. Also, women may inherit social roles and responsibilities as caretakers for extended family members and often for friends.

ART Issues Particular to Women

In general, women on ART have virologic and immunologic responses comparable to those of men; however, several studies have shown that women discontinue ART more frequently than men. Women have higher rates of adverse effects from a number of antiretroviral (ARV) medications, in part because serum levels of at least some ARVs are higher in women. Pregnancy may require changes in ART, either because of pharmacokinetic changes or because of toxicity. See below.

Section 4: Health Care Maintenance and Disease Prevention

ARV Issues for Women	Considerations
ARV adverse effects	Some ARV adverse effects may be more severe in women: • Anemia (zidovudine) • Lactic acidosis (particularly with stavudine + didanosine) • Neuropathy (stavudine, didanosine) • Hepatotoxicity (nevirapine) • Severe rash (nonnucleoside reverse transcriptase inhibitors [NNRTIs], darunavir, tipranavir) • Abacavir hypersensitivity • Lipoaccumulation: central fat accumulation in breasts, abdomen; lipoatrophy: face • Bone loss, especially after menopause
Pregnancy	Teratogenicity: • Efavirenz is associated with neural tube defects in women with exposure during the first-trimester; should be avoided in pregnant women during the first trimester, and in women who may become pregnant Pharmacokinetic (PK) changes: • Serum levels of some ARVs may be decreased during pregnancy (e.g., unboosted protease inhibitors [PIs], lopinavir/ritonavir, ritonavir) • Some ARVs should be avoided and certain ARVs may require dosage adjustment in the third trimester • PK studies in pregnancy are not available for some ARVs See chapter *Reducing Maternal-Infant HIV Transmission*
Contraception	There are significant interactions between some hormonal contraceptive agents and certain ARVs; see "Contraception," below

Baseline Reproductive History

Taking a careful reproductive history should be a part of routine primary care for any woman. Important information to gather includes the following:

- Age of menarche

- Menstrual history: last menstrual period (LMP), amenorrhea, menstrual irregularity, uterine fibroids, endometriosis

- Obstetrical history: G-P-A-L

  - G (gravida, or number of pregnancies), P (parity, or number of births), A (abortion; number of miscarriages or terminations), L (number of living children)

  - Pregnancy complications and outcomes: full-term, premature births, mode of deliveries

  - Use of ART during pregnancy

  - HIV status of children

- Sexual activity: vaginal, oral, anal; condom use; number of partners; sex of partners; HIV status of partners

- Contraception, past and current

- Date of last Papanicolau (Pap) test and results; history of abnormal Pap test results

- Gynecologic procedures: colposcopy/biopsy, loop electrosurgical excision procedure (LEEP), cervical surgery, tubal ligation, partial or total hysterectomy; and indication for these

- STIs, bacterial vaginosis, vulvovaginal candidiasis, herpes, warts; especially recurrence

- Current symptoms: vaginal discharge, vulvar/vaginal/anal pain, dysuria, dyspareunia (pain with intercourse), lesions, intermenstrual bleeding, postcoital bleeding

Elements of Gynecological Care

Women with HIV infection should receive routine screening for gynecologic cancers and infections. Cervical dysplasia and cancer continue to be widespread, especially among women with low CD4 counts, and it is not clear that initiation of suppressive ART improves clinical outcomes of women with dysplasia (see chapter *Cervical Dysplasia*). Other common gynecological problems include recurrent yeast vaginitis, pelvic inflammatory disease; vaginal, vulvar, and anal warts, which are potentially oncogenic; and perineal/perianal herpes that may become severe and recurrent.

Women also should be evaluated for risk of breast cancer, for contraceptive needs, and for preconception counseling.

Medical Service	Comments
Cervical and anal cancer screening	Screen all HIV-infected women for cervical cancer, to age 65 (cervical Pap test) • At initial visit, at 6 months, then annually unless abnormal Consider anal cancer screening (anal Pap test) for all HIV-infected women If cervical or anal Pap screen shows atypical squamous cells of undetermined significance (ASCUS) or dysplasia of any grade, seek colposcopy • See chapters *Cervical Dysplasia* and *Anal Dysplasia* Perform pelvic examination • Include vulvar and anal examination at each visit • Assess for potentially dysplastic lesions
STI screening	Gonorrhea, chlamydia, syphilis at least annually, and more frequently depending on risk factors

Medical Service	Comments
Breast cancer screening	Mammography • Mammogram every 1-2 years recommended for women 50-69 years of age • Consider annual mammogram for women 40-50 years of age • Consider starting earlier if risk factors are present • For women ≥70 years of age, decisions about whether to continue screening should take into account the woman's life expectancy and clinical status Clinical breast examination • Annually • Breast self-examination (BSE) monthly (assess technique)
Contraceptive counseling	• Assess life dynamics and need for contraception at every visit • Stop only after hysterectomy or sterilization • See "Contraception," below
Preconception counseling	Annually or more often for all women of reproductive age • Ask about pregnancy desires at every visit • See "Preconception Counseling," below

Contraception

Many contraceptive choices are available for HIV-infected women; some considerations are presented in the table below. For more information about interactions between ARVs and hormonal agents, see chapter *Antiretroviral Medications and Hormonal Contraceptive Agents*. Depending on the woman's (and her partner's) risk factors, consistent condom use should be emphasized, with or without other methods of contraception, to prevent the transmission of HIV and the acquisition or transmission of other STIs.

Advantages and Disadvantages of Various Contraceptives

Contraceptive Type	Advantages	Disadvantages
Barrier Methods		
Male and female condom	• Only method that protects against transmission of HIV and STIs	• Requires partner cooperation and correct technique • High failure rate when used incorrectly
Diaphragm and cervical cap		• Requires correct technique • High failure rate when used incorrectly
Hormonal Methods*		• Do not prevent STI or HIV transmission
Oral	• Very effective • Lighter menstrual flow	• May have significant drug-drug interactions with PIs and NNRTIs that may affect the efficacy and toxicity of estradiol or norethindrone, and of certain PIs* • Consider alternative methods for women taking PIs or NNRTIs
Injectable depot medroxyprogesterone acetate (DMPA, Depo-Provera)	• Effective contraception for 3 months • May cause amenorrhea	• Concern about osteoporosis with long-term use • Irregular bleeding, especially initially • Weight gain
Transdermal (patch)	• Effective • Lighter menstrual flow	• No studies to document pharmacokinetic interactions, but of possible significance
Vaginal ring	• Effective	• Lighter menstrual flow • No studies to document pharmacokinetic interactions, but of possible significance
Intrauterine devices (IUDs)	• Effective for long-term use • No evidence of increased HIV viral shedding • Progestin-releasing IUD may cause lighter menstrual flow	• Possible blood loss with Copper T IUD • Insertion of IUD not recommended for women with advanced immunosuppression
Etonogestrel implant	• Effective • Amenorrhea	• No studies to document pharmacokinetic interactions, but of possible significance
Emergency contraception: • Levonorgestrel	• Effective	• Efavirenz lowers levonorgestrel levels; use alternative method. • Pharmacokinetic interactions with other ARVs have not been studied, but are of possible significance
• Copper T IUD	• Appropriate for women who present 4-5 days after intercourse	• Heavy blood loss
Surgical Methods		
Bilateral tubal ligation (female)	• Effective; permanent	• Does not prevent transmission of HIV or other STIs • No future fertility (usually not reversible)
Vasectomy (male)	• Effective; permanent	• Does not prevent transmission of HIV or other STIs • No future fertility (usually not reversible)

Contraceptive Type	Advantages	Disadvantages
Spermicides		
Spermicides		• Not currently recommended • Nonoxynol-9 causes mucosal damage to vagina • Do not prevent transmission of HIV or other STIs

* See chapter *Antiretroviral Medications and Hormonal Contraceptive Agents* and *U.S. Department of Health and Human Services Guidelines for the Use of Antiretroviral Agents in HIV-1-Infected Adults and Adolescents.* January 10, 2011. Available at www.aidsinfo. nih.gov/guidelines/.

Preconception Counseling

As discussed above, every visit with an HIV-infected woman in her reproductive years presents an opportunity to discuss pregnancy desires and options, including gathering information about her partner. It is important to assess the couple's sexual history, sexual decision making, and control of reproductive options. When a woman desires pregnancy, it is important to discuss the following, with the goals of educating her and decreasing risk of HIV transmission to an HIV-uninfected partner and to the fetus. Ideally, the partner will take part in the discussion.

- Options for conception that decrease risk of HIV transmission to an HIV-uninfected partner

- Recommendations for ART before and during pregnancy and delivery

- Mode of delivery

- Treatment of an infant, both HIV exposed and HIV infected

- Risk of the infant being infected with HIV

- Care of an HIV-infected child

- Discouragement of breast-feeding

- Disclosure of the child's HIV status

- Guardianship of a child if one or both parents were to become ill or die

Any history of infertility or low fertility in either the patient or her partner should be evaluated and options for having children should be discussed, including current information on gamete donation, other assisted reproductive techniques, and adoption.

If the heterosexual couple is serodiscordant, techniques to minimize the risk of transmission to the uninfected partner should be discussed. These same techniques should be explained to couples when both partners are HIV infected, if there is a risk of transmitting different HIV "strains." Some of these techniques include the following:

- Treatment of STIs

- Maximal suppression of the HIV viral load with ART

- Self-insemination of ejaculate using a syringe

- Estimating the time of ovulation; limiting intercourse to this time

- Pre- and/or post-exposure prophylaxis with ART by an uninfected partner

- Sperm washing

- In vitro fertilization

If the HIV-infected woman elects to initiate ART, an appropriate regimen should be started before pregnancy, avoiding agents with increased risk of teratogenicity (e.g., efavirenz), hepatotoxicity (e.g., nevirapine, in women with CD4 counts of >400 cells/µL), or metabolic complications such as lactic acidosis (e.g., didanosine and stavudine). See chapter *Reducing Maternal-Infant HIV Transmission* and the U.S. Department of Health and Human Services *Perinatal HIV Guidelines* (see "References," below). It should be noted that most fetal organogenesis occurs in the early weeks of pregnancy, before most women know that they are pregnant. Thus, any medication with potential teratogenicity or fetal toxicity, whether an ARV or another drug, should be avoided for use by women who are intending to become pregnant or have the potential for pregnancy. Certain medications (e.g., ribavirin) should be avoided by male partners of women who may become pregnant.

Folate supplementation to reduce the risk of neural tube defects in the developing fetus should be started at least 1 month before conception, if possible, because the neural tube forms in the early weeks of pregnancy (see chapter *Care of HIV-Infected Prenatal Women*).

Menopause

There is evidence that HIV-infected women may be more likely to undergo premature physiologic menopause. Menopausal women are more at risk of premature bone loss, osteopenia, and osteoporosis; this risk may be increased by HIV infection. If indicated, bone density screening (DEXA) should be considered.

Hormone replacement therapy (HRT), especially of long duration, has been associated with an increased risk of breast cancer and cardiovascular and thromboembolic events, and its routine use is not currently recommended. HRT may be considered for women who experience severe vasomotor symptoms and vaginal dryness, but should be used only for a limited period of time and at the lowest effective dosage.

References

- Aaron EZ, Criniti SM. *Preconception health care for HIV-infected women.* Top HIV Med. 2007 Aug-Sep;15(4):137-41.

- Aberg JA, Kaplan JE, Libman H, et al.; HIV Medicine Association of the Infectious Diseases Society of America. *Primary care guidelines for the management of persons infected with human immunodeficiency virus: 2009 update by the HIV medicine Association of the Infectious Diseases Society of America.* Clin Infect Dis. 2009 Sep 1;49(5):651-81.

- Cejtin HE. *Gynecologic issues in the HIV-infected woman.* Infect Dis Clin North Am. 2008 Dec;22(4):709-39, vii.

- Collazos J, Asensi V, Cartón JA. *Sex differences in the clinical, immunological and virological parameters of HIV-infected patients treated with HAART.* AIDS. 2007 Apr 23;21(7):835-43.

- Holstad MM, DiIorio C, Magowe MK. *Motivating HIV positive women to adhere to antiretroviral therapy and risk reduction behavior: the KHARMA Project.* Online J Issues Nurs. 2006 Jan 31;11(1):5.

- Kojic EM, Wang CC, Cu-Uvin S. *HIV and menopause: a review.* J Womens Health (Larchmt). 2007 Dec;16(10):1402-11.

- McNicholl I. *Database of Antiretroviral Drug Interactions.* HIV InSite. San Francisco: UCSF Center for HIV Information. Available at hivinsite.ucsf.edu/insite?page=ar-00-02. Accessed June 30, 2010.

- North American Menopause Society. *Estrogen and progestogen use in peri- and postmenopausal women: March 2007 position statement of The North American Menopause Society.* Menopause. 2007 Mar-Apr;14(2):168-82.

- U.S. Department of Health and Human Services. *Guidelines for the Use of Antiretroviral Agents in HIV-1-Infected Adults and Adolescents.* January 10, 2011. Available at www.aidsinfo.nih.gov/ guidelines/.

- U.S. Department of Health and Human Services. *Recommendations for Use of Antiretroviral Drugs in Pregnant HIV-1-Infected Women for Maternal Health and Interventions to Reduce Perinatal HIV Transmission in the United States.* May 24, 2010. Available at aidsinfo.nih.gov/ guidelines/.

- Whetten-Goldstein K, Nguyen TQ. *You're the First One I've Told: New Faces of HIV in the South.* New Brunswick, NJ: Rutgers University Press; August 2002.

- World Health Organization. *Medical Eligibility Criteria for Contraceptive Use: Update 2008.* Geneva: World Health Organization; 2008.

Section 4: Health Care Maintenance and Disease Prevention

Palliative Care and HIV

Background

Palliative care is not curative care, but is supportive, symptom-oriented care. It may be needed at any point in the course of disease progression to relieve patients' suffering and promote quality of life. Palliative care is important for patients with any medical condition, even if they are not actively in hospice. It may be used in conjunction with disease-specific care or as the sole approach to care. Palliative care includes the following:

- Management of symptoms (e.g., fatigue, pain)

- Treatment of adverse effects (e.g., nausea, vomiting)

- Psychosocial support (e.g., depression, advance care planning)

- End-of-life care

The U.S. Health Resources and Services Administration (HRSA) HIV/AIDS Bureau Working Group on Palliative Care in HIV has provided the following working definition of palliative care:

> Palliative care is patient- and family-centered care. It optimizes quality of life by active anticipation, prevention, and treatment of suffering. It emphasizes use of an interdisciplinary team approach throughout the continuum of illness, placing critical importance on the building of respectful and trusting relationships. Palliative care addresses physical, intellectual, emotional, social, and spiritual needs. It facilitates patient autonomy, access to information, and choice.

> (Excerpted from: *HRSA Working Group on HIV and Palliative Care. Palliative and Supportive Care.* HRSA Care ACTION, July 2000)

Palliative care for patients with HIV infection comprises a continuum of treatment consisting of therapy directed at AIDS-related illnesses (e.g., infection or malignancy) and treatments focused on providing comfort and symptom control throughout the lifespan. This care may involve multidimensional and multidisciplinary services, including HIV medicine, nursing, pharmacy, social work, complementary or alternative medicine, and physical therapy.

Palliative Care in the Era of Antiretroviral Therapy

With advances in HIV-specific therapy and care, HIV infection is no longer a rapidly fatal illness. Instead, patients who are able to tolerate antiretroviral therapy (ART) often experience a manageable, chronic illness.

The death rate from AIDS, however, continues to be significant: approximately 14,000 per year in the United States. In many parts of the world, patients still are not able to obtain specific treatments for HIV or for opportunistic illnesses, and supportive or palliative care may be the primary mode of care available to patients with advanced AIDS. Regardless of access to disease-specific treatment, people living with HIV continue to experience symptoms from HIV disease and its comorbid conditions, and those taking ART may experience adverse effects. Integrating palliative care and disease-specific care is important for treating patients with HIV in order to promote quality of life and relieve suffering.

S: Subjective

The patient with advanced HIV disease complains of one or more of the following:

- Agitation
- Anorexia
- Chronic pain
- Constipation
- Cough
- Decubitus ulcers or pressure sores
- Delirium
- Dementia
- Depression
- Diarrhea
- Dry mouth
- Dry skin
- Dyspnea
- Fatigue
- Fever
- Hiccups
- Increased secretions ("death rattle")
- Nausea
- Pruritus
- Sleep disturbance
- Sweats
- Vomiting
- Weakness
- Weight loss

O: Objective

Conduct a complete symptom-directed physical examination.

To evaluate pain, please refer to chapter *Pain Syndrome and Peripheral Neuropathy.*

A/P: Assessment and Plan
Treatment

Common symptoms of persons with late-stage HIV infection and their possible causes are listed in Table 1. Also included are disease-specific treatments and palliative interventions. Depending on the situation, either or both of these types of treatments may be appropriate. Consider the patient's disease stage and symptom burden, the risks and benefits of therapies, and the patient's wishes.

When assessing each of the patient's symptoms, include the psychiatric review of symptoms (depression, anxiety, psychosis), and consider the following aspects of each symptom:

- Onset, progression, frequency, severity
- Degree of distress and impact on function
- Aggravating and alleviating factors
- Previous treatments and their efficacy
- What the patient believes is causing the symptom
- Coping strategies and supports
- The patient's personal goals of care with this particular symptom

Practitioners should note that some of the palliative treatments may have substantial long-term adverse effects and should be used to alleviate symptoms only in late-stage or dying patients.

Table 1. Common Symptoms in Patients with AIDS and Possible Disease-Specific and Palliative Interventions

Symptom	Possible Causes	Disease-Specific or Curative Treatment	Palliative Treatment
CONSTITUTIONAL			
Fatigue, weakness	• AIDS • Opportunistic infection • Anemia • Hypoandrogen-ism	• ART • Treat specific infections • Erythropoietin, transfusion • Testosterone/androgens in men with concomitant hypogonadism; for women, androgens are investigational and not approved by the U.S. Food and Drug Administration for this use	• Psychostimulants: give in the morning; also useful as treatment for depression and sedation owing to opioids; avoid in patients with anxiety and agitation (methylphenidate, dextroamphetamine, modafinil; pemoline is not first-line because of hepatotoxicity risk) • Corticosteroids (prednisone, dexamethasone)
Weight loss/anorexia	• HIV • Malignancy	• ART • Specific treatment of malignancy • Nutritional support	• Testosterone/androgens in men with hypogonadism (see above) • Oxandrolone for 2-4 weeks courses; an anabolic steroid that may be a useful adjunct, can help increase lean body mass but also has virilizing effects • Megestrol acetate can improve appetite and fatigue but has not been shown to improve nutritional status; possible adverse effects include deep vein thrombosis, glucose intolerance, and hypoandrogenism in men • Dronabinol is a cannabinol derivative that helps increase appetite but over the long term (≥12 months) does not significantly increase weight • Recombinant human growth hormone can improve lean body mass, but is associated with significant side effects (headache, edema, myalgias) and is expensive; consider for patients with severe wasting if no other therapies are effective • Corticosteroids can help increase appetite in the short term but not increase weight, and the duration of effect is short-lived

Symptom	Possible Causes	Disease-Specific or Curative Treatment	Palliative Treatment
Fevers, sweats	• Disseminated Mycobacterium avium complex and other infections • HIV lymphoma, and other malignancies	• Specific treatment of opportunistic infection or malignancy • ART	• Acetaminophen • NSAIDs (ibuprofen, naproxen, indomethacin) • Anticholinergics can be useful for sweats (hyoscyamine, glycopyrrolate) • H2-antagonists can be useful for sweats (ranitidine, famotidine; dose at least 12 hours apart from atazanavir; note that cimetidine should be avoided in patients taking fosamprenavir or delavirdine because of drug interactions)
PAIN			
Nociceptive, somatic, visceral	• Opportunistic infections • HIV-related malignancies, nonspecific	• Specific treatment of disease entities	• See chapter *Pain Syndrome and Peripheral Neuropathy* for detailed treatment options • Refer to the World Health Organization (WHO) analgesic ladder: NSAIDs and opioids • Corticosteroids can be useful for treating inflammatory-mediated pain, often as an adjunct to opioids (may worsen some conditions) • Benzodiazepines or muscle relaxants for muscle spasms (clonazepam, diazepam, baclofen) • Nonpharmacologic therapies (e.g., massage, physical therapy)
Neuropathic	• HIV-related peripheral neuropathy • Cytomegalovirus • Varicella zoster virus • Medications (e.g., stavudine, isoniazid, vincristine)	• ART • Discontinue offending medication • Change antiretroviral or other regimen	• See chapter *Pain Syndrome and Peripheral Neuropathy* for detailed treatment options • Refer to the WHO analgesic ladder: NSAIDs and opioids • Neuropathic pain medications: • Tricyclics (nortriptyline, imipramine) • Anticonvulsants (gabapentin, pregabalin, lamotrigine) • Benzodiazepines can be useful adjuncts (clonazepam) • Corticosteroids can be useful for treating inflammatory-mediated pain, often as an adjunct to opioids (may worsen some conditions) • Acupuncture

Symptom	Possible Causes	Disease-Specific or Curative Treatment	Palliative Treatment
GASTROINTESTINAL			
Nausea, vomiting	• Antiretroviral medications • Esophageal candidiasis • Cytomegalovirus	• Specific treatment of disease entities • Change antiretroviral regimen	• Dopamine antagonists (prochlorperazine, haloperidol) • Prokinetic agents (metoclopramide) • Antihistamines (diphenhydramine, promethazine, meclizine) • Anticholinergics (hyoscyamine, scopolamine) • Serotonin antagonists (granisetron, ondansetron, dolasetron) • Somatostatin analogues in patients with bowel obstruction, to reduce gut motility; can be used with anticholinergics (octreotide) • Benzodiazepines (lorazepam) • Marijuana, dronabinol can help increase appetite
Diarrhea	• *Mycobacterium avium* complex • Cryptosporidiosis • Cytomegalovirus • Microsporidiosis • Other intestinal infections • Malabsorption • Medications (e.g., protease inhibitors)	• Specific treatment of disease entities • Discontinue offending medication	• Bismuth, methylcellulose • Psyllium • Kaolin • Diphenoxylate + atropine • Loperamide • Calcium carbonate • Ferrous sulfate • Tincture of opium for severe chronic diarrhea unresponsive to other therapies • Octreotide for profuse, refractory watery diarrhea; expensive and needs subcutaneous administration
Constipation	• Dehydration • Malignancy • Anticholinergic medications • Opioids • Reduced activity	• Hydration • Radiation and chemotherapy • Medication adjustment	• Activity/diet modification • Prophylaxis for patients taking opioids with docusate + senna • Peristalsis-stimulating agents: • Anthracenes (senna) • Polyphenolics (bisacodyl) • Softening agents: • Surfactant laxatives (docusate) • Bulk-forming agents (bran, methylcellulose) • Osmotic laxatives (lactulose, sorbitol) • Saline laxatives (magnesium hydroxide)

Section 4: Health Care Maintenance and Disease Prevention

Section 4: Health Care Maintenance and Disease Prevention

Symptom	Possible Causes	Disease-Specific or Curative Treatment	Palliative Treatment
RESPIRATORY			
Dyspnea	• *Pneumocystis jiroveci* pneumonia • Bacterial pneumonia • Anemia • Pleural effusion, mass, or obstruction • Decreased respiratory muscle function	• Specific treatment of disease entities • Erythropoietin, transfusion • Drainage, radiation, or surgery	• Use of fan, open windows • Relaxation techniques, massage, guided imagery • Oxygen supplement titrated to comfort, if the patient is hypoxic • Bronchodilators (albuterol, ipratropium, inhaled steroids) if there is bronchospasm • Opioids, particularly morphine, to decrease sense of air hunger and respiratory rate • Benzodiazepines (e.g., lorazepam) to reduce the anxiety that often accompanies dyspnea
Cough	• *Pneumocystis jiroveci* pneumonia • Bacterial pneumonia • Tuberculosis • Acid reflux • Postnasal drip	• Specific treatment of disease entities	• Cough suppressants (dextromethorphan, codeine, hydrocodone, morphine, aerosolized lidocaine) • Bronchodilators (albuterol, ipratropium, inhaled steroids) if there is bronchospasm • H2-blockers or proton-pump inhibitors (ranitidine, omeprazole) if there is acid reflux (caution: possible interactions with atazanavir) • Decongestants (pseudoephedrine, phenylephrine, steroid nasal sprays) for postnasal drip
Increased secretions ("death rattle")	• Fluid shifts • Ineffective cough • Sepsis • Pneumonia	• Antibiotics as indicated	• Atropine, hyoscyamine, transdermal scopolamine, glycopyrrolate • Fluid restriction, discontinue intravenous fluids
Hiccups	• Aerophagia (swallowing air) • *Candida* and other causes of esophagitis including GERD • Vagus and phrenic nerve irritation • CNS mass lesions • Uremia • Alcohol intoxication • Anesthesia	• Treatment of underlying etiology (e.g., antifungals for *Candida* esophagitis, acid reducers for GERD)	• Metoclopramide can promote gastric emptying • Chlorpromazine (antipsychotic) can reduce the CNS response, start at low dosage to reduce the risk of dystonia and drowsiness • Baclofen can reduce the CNS response

Symptom	Possible Causes	Disease-Specific or Curative Treatment	Palliative Treatment
DERMATOLOGIC			
Dry skin	• Dehydration • End-stage renal disease • End-stage liver disease • Malnutrition medications (e.g., indinavir)	• Hydration • Dialysis • Nutritional support • Discontinue offending medication	• Avoid soaps, most of which dry the skin further • Emollients with or without salicylates • Emollients with urea (e.g., Ultra Mide 25) • Emollients with lactate (e.g., Lac-Hydrin) • Lubricating ointments or creams (e.g., petrolatum, Eucerin)
Pruritus	• Fungal infection • End-stage renal disease • End-stage liver disease • Dehydration; dry skin • Eosinophilic folliculitis • Opioid side effect	• Antifungal agents (e.g., itraconazole for eosinophilic folliculitis) • Dialysis • Hydration • Topical corticosteroids	• Avoid soaps and hot baths/showers • Warm compresses • Treatments for dry skin, as above • Topical agents (menthol, phenol [e.g., Sarna lotion], calamine, doxepin, capsaicin) • Antihistamines (hydroxyzine, doxepin, diphenhydramine) • Corticosteroids (topical or systemic) • Opioid antagonists (naloxone, naltrexone) can be useful for treating uremic and biliary-associated pruritus • Antidepressants • Anxiolytics • Thalidomide in intractable pruritus, but beware of side effects, including neuropathy
Decubitus ulcers, Pressure sores	• Poor nutrition • Decreased mobility, prolonged bed rest	• Increase mobility • Enhance nutrition	• Prevention (nutrition, mobility, skin integrity) • Wound protection (semipermeable film, hydrocolloid dressing) • Debridement (normal saline, enzymatic agents, alginates)

Section 4: Health Care Maintenance and Disease Prevention

Section 4: Health Care Maintenance and Disease Prevention

Symptom	Possible Causes	Disease-Specific or Curative Treatment	Palliative Treatment
NEUROPSYCHIATRIC			
Delirium/ agitation	• Electrolyte imbalances, glucose abnormalities • Dehydration • Hypoxia • Toxoplasmosis • Cryptococcal meningitis • CNS masses and metastases • Sepsis • Medication adverse effects (e.g., benzodiazepines, opioids, efavirenz, corticosteroids) • Intoxication or withdrawal	• Correct imbalances • Hydration • Oxygen supplementation • Specific treatment of disease entities • Discontinue offending medications	• Neuroleptics (haloperidol, risperidone, chlorpromazine) to induce sedation in severe agitation • Benzodiazepines (e.g., lorazepam, diazepam, midazolam) in the "terminal restlessness" of the last few days of life to relieve myoclonus, seizures, restlessness (Note: in some patients, these may have adverse effects)
Dementia	• HIV-associated dementia • Other dementia (e.g., Alzheimer dementia, Parkinson dementia, multi-infarct dementia)	• ART	• Psychostimulants (methylphenidate) • Memantine (NMDA antagonist) has been used in patients with Alzheimer dementia but has unclear benefit for patients with HIV-associated dementia • Low-dose neuroleptics (haloperidol, chlorpromazine) can be useful in psychotic delirium

Symptom	Possible Causes	Disease-Specific or Curative Treatment	Palliative Treatment
Depression	• Chronic illness • Reactive depression, major depression	• Antidepressants	• Antidepressants are useful when the patient has a life expectancy of several months or more: SSRIs, SNRIs, mirtazapine (useful in lowest dosages for insomnia), bupropion, (though beware of lowering the seizure threshold); note that tricyclic antidepressants are not considered first- or second-line therapy owing to side effects though they may be useful for treating refractory melancholic or delusional depression (see chapter *Depression* for further information, including dosages) • Psychostimulants are useful for patients who have urgent, severe depression or are weeks from death (methylphenidate, pemoline, dextroamphetamine, modafinil)

Abbreviations: ART = antiretroviral therapy; CNS = central nervous system; GERD = gastroesophageal reflux disease; NMDA = N-methyl-D-aspartate; NSAID = nonsteroidal antiinflammatory drug; SNRI = serotonin norepinephrine reuptake inhibitor; SSRI = selective serotonin reuptake inhibitor

Adapted from Selwyn PA, Rivard M. *Palliative care for AIDS: Challenges and opportunities in the era of highly active anti-retroviral therapy.* Innovations in End-of-Life Care. 2002;4(3). Available at www.edc.org/lastacts.

Advance Care Planning

Advance care planning involves planning for future medical care. Two main documents are produced:

• Advance directive (living will)

• Health care proxy (a person to speak for the patient or make decisions if the patient is too sick to do so)

The clinician should initiate these conversations and make referrals to helpful resources.

Patient Education

• Discuss advance care planning with patients, and the option of hospice care, if appropriate.

• Provide patients and their family members with detailed information so that they understand the illness and associated treatments.

• Instruct patients to discuss their pain or other bothersome symptoms with their health care providers.

• Encourage patients to talk with their health care providers if they are feeling anxious, depressed, or fearful.

• Discuss with patients what their death might be like. Some patients may feel relieved to be able to talk openly about their last days. Assure them that their pain will be controlled and that their health care providers will be there to help them.

Section 4: Health Care Maintenance and Disease Prevention

References

- American Academy of HIV Medicine. *Palliative Care*. In: *The HIV Medicine Self-Directed Study Guide* (2003 ed.). Los Angeles: American Academy of HIV Medicine; 2003.

- American Academy of HIV Medicine. *Palliative Care and End-of-Life Support*. In: *AAHIVM Fundamentals of HIV Medicine (2007 ed.)*. Washington: American Academy of HIV Medicine; 2007.

- National Hospice Organization. *Guidelines for Determining Prognosis for Selected Non-Cancer Diagnoses*. Alexandria, VA: National Hospice Organization; 1996.

- O'Neill JF, McKinney M. *Caring for the Caregiver*. In: O'Neill JF, Selwyn PA, Schietinger H, eds. *The Clinical Guide to Supportive and Palliative Care for HIV/ AIDS*. Rockville, MD: Health Resources and Services Administration; 2003. Available at ftp://ftp.hrsa.gov/hab/PGuide_2003.pdf. Accessed June 30, 2010.

- Selwyn PA, Rivard M. *Palliative care for AIDS: challenges and opportunities in the era of highly active anti-retroviral therapy.* J Palliat Med. 2003 Jun;6(3):475-87.

- University of Washington Center for Palliative Care Education. *Module 1: Overview of HIV/AIDS Palliative Care.* Available at depts.washington.edu/pallcare/. Accessed June 30, 2010.

- U.S. Health Resources and Services Administration. *A Guide to Primary Care of People with HIV/AIDS, 2004 Edition.* Rockville, MD: Health Resources and Services Administration; 2004;123-131. Available online at hab.hrsa.gov/tools/ primarycareguide/. Accessed June 30, 2010.

- Weinreb NJ, Kinzbrunner BM, Clark M. *Pain Management.* In: Kinzbrunner BM, Weinreb NJ, Policzer JS, eds. *20 Common Problems: End-of-life Care.* New York: McGraw Hill Medical Publishing Division; 2002;91-145.

- World Health Organization. *Cancer Pain Relief and Palliative Care, Report of a WHO Expert Committee.* Geneva: World Health Organization; 1990.

Adherence

Background

For HIV-infected patients with wild-type virus who are taking antiretroviral therapy (ART), adherence to ART is the major factor in ensuring the virologic success of an initial regimen and is a significant determinant of survival. Adherence is second only to the CD4 cell count as a predictor of progression to AIDS and death. Adherence rates approaching 100% are needed for optimal viral suppression, yet the average ART adherence in the United States is approximately 70%. Individualized assessment of and support for adherence are essential for patients to be successful with ART.

Patients with suboptimal adherence are at risk not only of HIV progression, but also of the development of drug resistance (see chapter *Resistance Testing*) and consequent narrowing of options for future treatment. In one cohort study it was estimated that drug-resistant mutations will occur in 25% of patients who report very high but not perfect (92-100%) adherence to ART. It is important to note, though, that the relationship between suboptimal adherence and resistance to antiretroviral (ARV) medications is very complex and is not thoroughly understood.

Characteristics of the ARV regimen and individual patient pharmacokinetic variables also influence the likelihood of both virologic suppression and the development of resistance mutations. For example, in patients with wild-type virus on initial ART regimens, it appears that more drug resistance occurs in regimens that are based on an unboosted protease inhibitor or a nonnucleoside reverse transcriptase inhibitor, where the genetic barrier to resistance is relatively low, than in regimens that include a ritonavir-boosted protease inhibitor. In patients with suboptimal adherence, these factors can influence outcomes of therapy more strongly.

HRSA HAB Core Clinical Performance Measures

Percentage of clients with HIV infection on ARVs who were **assessed and counseled for adherence** two or more times in the measurement year

(Group 2 measure)

Section 4: Health Care Maintenance and Disease Prevention

S: Subjective

Studies indicate that health care providers' assessments of their patients' adherence often are inaccurate, so a calm and open approach to this topic is very important.

Adherence assessment is most successful when conducted in a positive, nonjudgmental atmosphere. Patients need to know that their provider understands the difficulties associated with taking an ARV regimen. Within a trusting relationship, a provider may learn what is actually happening with the patient's adherence rather than what the patient thinks the provider wants to hear. See Table 1 for examples of questions to assess adherence in patients who are on ART. For patients who are considering initiation of ART, it is important to lay the groundwork for optimal adherence in advance, and to anticipate barriers to adherence; see Table 2 for exploratory questions.

Common reasons for nonadherence include the following: experiencing adverse drug effects, finding the regimen too complex, having difficulty with the dosing schedule (not fitting into the daily routine), forgetting to take the medications, being too busy with other things, oversleeping and missing a dose, being away from home, not understanding the importance of adherence, and being embarrassed to take medications in front of family, friends, or coworkers. Other contributors to incomplete adherence include psychosocial issues (e.g., lack of social support, homelessness), psychiatric illness, and active substance abuse. It is important to look for these and other potential barriers to adherence. (See chapter *Initial History*.)

O: Objective

Evaluate the following:

- CD4 cell count

- HIV viral load (indicating the effectiveness of ART in suppressing viremia; an indirect indicator of adherence)

- Current drug list (including over-the-counter medications, vitamins, and herbal remedies); check for potential adverse drug-drug interactions with ARV medications

- Pharmacy refill records or missed doses remaining in medi-set pill boxes

A: Assessment

Assess adherence at each visit using questions such as those in Tables 1 and 2, and assessment scales such as those found in Tables 4, 5, and 6 (Appendix). Ask these questions in a simple, nonjudgmental, structured format and listen carefully to the patient to invite honesty about issues that may affect adherence. Asking about adherence over the last 3 to 7 days gives an accurate reflection of longer-term adherence.

Ideally, a multidisciplinary team that includes primary providers as well as nurses, pharmacists, medication managers, and social workers works together to evaluate and support patient adherence.

Table 1. Important Questions to Ask Patients Taking ART

- Do you manage your own medications? If not, who manages them for you?
- What HIV medications do you take and what is their dosage? When do you take these?
- What is your average daily schedule like? How well does taking your HIV medications at this time fit into your daily schedule?
- How do you remember to take your medications?
- How many doses of your HIV medication have you missed in the past 72 hours, past week, past 2 weeks, and past month?
- On a scale of 1 to 10, where would you say you are? A score of 1 indicates that you do not take your medicines as directed at all; for example, not every day or not at the same time every day; 10 indicates that you take your medications perfectly every day, at the same time every day. (Visual analog scales are also used to assess adherence; see Appendix 1.)
- If not a 10, what causes you not to be a 10?
- When are you most likely to miss doses?
- Do you have any adverse effects from your HIV medications? If so, what are they?
- Are you comfortable taking medications in front of others?
- What is most difficult about taking your medications?
- How do you like working with your pharmacy?

Table 2. Important Questions to Ask Patients Considering Initiation of ART

- What is your attitude toward ART?
- Do you believe that ART is effective?
- What are your biggest concerns about starting ART?
- What do you hope these medications will do for you?
- Are you ready to take the medication every day, around the same time each day?
- Are you committed and motivated to take the medication every day for the rest of your life?
- Who knows about your HIV status?
- What other medications are you taking: prescription, over-the-counter, herbals?
- Are you a morning or afternoon person?
- What is your daily routine, including waking and bed times?
- How many meals and snacks do you eat per day, and at what times?
- Do you use alcohol, marijuana, cocaine, or injectable drugs? If so, how much do you use and how long have you used them?
- What are your ARV regimen preferences? What are some of the most important things you want to avoid in an ARV regimen (e.g., specific side effects, number of pills, frequency of dosing)?

The patient's self-report has been shown to be the most effective measure of adherence. Although, according to some studies, self-report of good adherence has limited value as a predictor of good adherence; self-report of suboptimal adherence should be taken seriously and considered a strong indicator of nonadherence.

Before initiating (or changing) ART, it is important to assess the patient's readiness for ART. Patient factors that have been associated with poor adherence in the United States and western Europe include:

- Depression
- Active alcohol or drug use
- Low literacy
- Lack of social support
- Lack of support from a partner
- More advanced HIV infection
- Young age
- Lack of belief in treatment efficacy
- Unstable housing
- Competing priorities (e.g., housing, childcare, food, work)

Most of these factors are modifiable. Before starting ART, appropriate interventions should be made, and sources of adherence support should be identified to help patients overcome potential barriers to adherence.

It is important to note that sociodemographic variables such as sex, HIV risk factors, and education level generally are not associated with adherence. In addition, a history of substance or alcohol abuse is not a barrier to adherence.

Assess the patient's support system, and ask who knows about his or her HIV status. Supportive family members or friends can help remind patients to take their medications and assist with management of adverse effects. For patients who have accepted their HIV infection

as an important priority in their lives, taking medications can become routine despite other potential adherence barriers such as alcohol or drug use.

Assess patients' willingness to accept and tolerate common adverse effects of ART. Patients may identify some adverse effects that they wish to avoid completely and others that they are willing to accept and manage; this may help in tailoring the selection of ARV medications to the individual patient. Describe strategies for the management of adverse effects before starting a regimen (see chapters *Patient Education* and *Adverse Reactions to HIV Medications*), and emphasize that adverse effects often can be treated quite effectively, and that they should notify their providers if they experience them.

For patients taking ART, it is important to assess adherence at every clinic visit. Tools such as those in the Appendix to this chapter may be useful in predicting adherence. Adverse effects are a common cause of suboptimal adherence to ART. Continue to ask whether the patient has adverse effects from the ARV medications and assess his or her ability to accept and tolerate these. Work closely with the patient to treat adverse effects, and consider changes in ART if adverse effects are not tolerated. Continue to offer support to improve or maintain optimal adherence.

Before prescribing ARVs, some clinicians have their patients conduct adherence trials using placebo tablets or jelly beans to measure the patients' readiness to start therapy and their ability to adhere to a regimen. Such a trial allows patients to experience what a regimen will entail in real life, how therapy will affect their daily lifestyles, and what changes will be needed to accommodate the regimen. The shortcoming of placebo trials is that patients are not challenged with adverse effects as they might be with an actual regimen.

P: Plan

Start the ARV regimen only when the patient is ready. Starting it too early may result in poor adherence, failure of the regimen, and increased risk of ARV resistance. Comorbid conditions that interfere with adherence, such as mental health issues or depression, must be treated initially. It is important to consider the patient's preferences and to involve her or him in selecting the drug regimen. The regimen must fit into the patient's daily routine, and the patient must believe in the potential success of ART. Simplifying the ARV regimen to the extent possible with once-daily regimens and the lowest number of pills (and lowest total expense to the patient), while maintaining efficacy and minimizing adverse effects, is important for maximizing adherence and avoiding pill fatigue. Starting ART is rarely an emergency situation, so taking time to identify the patient's wishes for care, making a thorough readiness assessment, selecting the ARV regimen, and planning for adherence support are important measures for maximizing the likelihood of treatment success. (See Table 3 for additional suggestions.)

Table 3. Strategies for Improving Adherence to ART
• Use a multidisciplinary team approach
• Establish a trusting relationship with the patient
• Establish readiness to start ART
• Involve the patient in ARV regimen selection
• Identify potential barriers to adherence prior to starting ART
• Provide mental health and substance abuse resources for the patient if needed
• Anticipate and treat adverse effects
• Assess adherence at every clinic visit
• Use educational aids including pictures, pillboxes, and calendars
• Identify the type of nonadherence and the reasons for nonadherence
• Simplify regimens if possible

Adapted from U.S. Department of Health and Human Services. *Guidelines for the Use of Antiretroviral Agents in HIV-1-Infected Adults and Adolescents*; Table 11. January 10, 2011. Available at www.aidsinfo.nih.gov/guidelines/.

Patients who can identify their medications (in their own words) and describe the proper dosing and administration have higher adherence rates. Providing patient education before writing a prescription helps ensure adherence to ARV regimens. Education can be provided in oral, written, or graphic form to assist the patient's understanding of the medications and their dosing. Basic information, including number of pills, dosages, frequency of administration, dietary restrictions, possible adverse effects, tips for managing adverse effects, and duration of therapy, will help patients to understand their ARV regimens. Patients should understand that the success of ART depends upon taking the medications every day and that adherence levels of >95% may be important in preventing virologic failure.

Close follow-up by telephone, clinic visits, or other contact with the patient during the first few days of therapy is useful in identifying adverse effects, assessing the patient's understanding of the regimen, and addressing any concerns before they become significant adherence barriers. Individualized interventions should be designed to optimize outcomes for each patient. Pharmacists, peer counselors, support groups, adherence counselors, behavioral intervention counselors, and community-based case managers are useful in supporting adherence for the HIV-infected patient. Multidisciplinary teams that include nurses, case managers, nutritionists, and pharmacists, in which each care provider focuses on adherence at each contact with the patient, are extremely effective, and peer support groups, in which patients share with one another their strategies for improving adherence, may be beneficial.

Many physical devices can be used to support adherence. The following are simple, inexpensive, and easy to incorporate into the routine of the HIV patient:

- Medication organizers include pillboxes and medi-sets. These are available in several shapes and sizes to fit the needs of the individual patient. They can be filled weekly so that the patient can easily determine whether a dose of medication was missed.

- Reminder devices include alarm watches, beepers, and cell phone alarms. They are effective in reminding the patient when to take medications. Medication diaries may be used for the patient to record doses that were taken.

- Visual medication schedules are calendars featuring photos or images of the patient's medications to remind the patient which drugs to take and at what dosages.

Interventions for successful adherence are an ongoing effort, not one-time events. Studies have suggested that adherence rates decline when patient-focused interventions are discontinued. Therefore, positive reinforcement at each clinic visit or contact is extremely important. Reinforce what the patient has done well and assist the patient in identifying and problem-solving areas for improvement. Whenever possible, share positive information about the patient's health, such as improvements in quality of life, CD4 cell count, and viral load, to encourage a high level of adherence.

Special Populations and Issues

Mental Illness

Patients with mental health issues may have difficulty with adherence. In this population, it is particularly important to incorporate ARV medications into structured daily routines. Medication cassettes, reminder signs, and calendars have been very effective for these patients. Nursing care providers and family members may be instrumental in filling medication boxes or ordering prescription refills.

Pediatrics

Adherence can be a challenge for young children who rely on parents and caregivers to provide their medications, but adolescents are more likely than younger children to have poor adherence. To improve adherence in this population, it is important to support the family. The U.S. Department of Health and Human Services *Guidelines for the Use of Antiretroviral Agents in Pediatric HIV Infection* address some of the adherence issues and considerations for this patient population.

Low Literacy

Health literacy is an important predictor of treatment adherence, particularly in low-income populations. Adherence interventions are necessary in this population to accommodate individuals who have difficulty reading and understanding medical instructions. Providers often fail to recognize this disability. In addition, adherence support is needed for patients who have difficulty navigating the health care system.

Resource-Limited Settings

Research has shown that the level of adherence in resource-limited countries is at least as good as in resource-rich settings and that rates of virologic suppression are equivalent or better. Lack of access to a consistent supply of ARV medications, including financial barriers that may cause interruptions in treatment, appears to be the primary obstacle to adherence in resource-limited settings.

Patient Education

- Educate patients about the importance of adherence and the need to take their ARV medications exactly as prescribed and to take every dose, every day.

- Advise patients that, if they miss an ARV dose on a rare occasion, that usually will not result in failure of the regimen. On the other hand, if they frequently miss or skip doses of their ARV medications, the regimen may become ineffective, and the HIV may develop resistance to ARVs.

- Tell patients to notify the clinic if they miss doses of the ARV medications.

- Work with patients to devise ways to improve their adherence, and reinforce good adherence behavior.

- Advise patients in advance that some people have adverse effects from the medications, and tell them to notify the clinic if they develop adverse effects. Discuss ways to reduce these effects.

Appendix. Scales to Assess Adherence to HIV Medication Regimens

Table 4. Visual Analog Scale Used in a Research Study to Assess Adherence to HIV Medication Regimens

Script for Interviewing Patients About Adherence	
Interviewer	Now I'm going to ask some questions about your HIV medications.
	Most people with HIV have many pills or other medications to take at different times during the day. Many people find it hard to always remember to take their pills or medicines. For example:
	• Some people get busy and forget to carry their pills with them.
	• Some people find it hard to take their pills according to all the instructions, such as "with food" or "on an empty stomach," "every 8 hours," or "with plenty of fluids."
	• Some people decide to skip taking pills to avoid adverse effects or to just not take pills that day.
	We need to understand what people with HIV are really doing with their pills or medicines. Please tell us what you are actually doing. Don't worry about telling us you don't take all your pills or medicines. We need to know what is really happening, not what you think we "want to hear."
	Which antiretroviral medications have you been prescribed to take within the last 30 days?
INTERVIEWER: LIST CODES FOR ALL ANTIRETROVIRALS THAT SUBJECT WAS PRESCRIBED TO TAKE IN LAST 30 DAYS. IDENTIFY UP TO 4 DRUGS.	
	DRUG A: DRUG C:
	DRUG B: DRUG D:
Interviewer	Now, I am going to ask you some questions about these drugs. Please put an "X" on the line below at the point showing your best guess about how much (DRUGS A-D) you have taken in the last 3-4 weeks. We would be surprised if this were 100% for most people.
HAND INSTRUMENT AND PEN TO RESPONDENT	
Interviewer	• 0% means you have taken no (DRUG A)
	• 50% means you have taken half your (DRUG A)
	• 100% means you have taken every single dose of (DRUG A)
Adherence Self-Assessment Instrument	
Instructions for Patient:	Put an "X" on the line below at the point showing your best guess about how much of each drug you have taken in the last 3 to 4 weeks.
	• 0% means you have taken none of the drug
	• 50% means you have taken half of the drug
	• 100% means you have taken every single dose of the drug
DRUG A:	0% 10% 20% 30% 40% 50% 60% 70% 80% 90% 100%
DRUG B:	0% 10% 20% 30% 40% 50% 60% 70% 80% 90% 100%
DRUG C:	0% 10% 20% 30% 40% 50% 60% 70% 80% 90% 100%
DRUG D:	0% 10% 20% 30% 40% 50% 60% 70% 80% 90% 100%

Adapted from Machtinger EL, Bangsberg DR. *Adherence to HIV Antiretroviral Therapy.* In: Coffey S, Volberding PA, eds. *HIV InSite Knowledge Base* [textbook online]; San Francisco: UCSF Center for HIV Information; May 2005. Available at hivinsite.ucsf.edu/InSite?page=kb-00&doc=kb-03-02-09. Accessed June 30, 2010.

Table 5. Morisky Scale to Assess Adherence to HIV Medications: Dichotomous Response Options

Subjects were asked: "Thinking about the medications PRESCRIBED to you by your doctor(s), please answer the following questions."	**NO**	**YES**
Do you ever forget to take your medications?		
Are you careless at times about taking your medications?		
When you feel better, do you sometimes stop taking your medications?		
Sometimes if you feel worse when you take your medications, do you stop taking them?		

Adapted from Morisky DE, Green LW, Levine DM. *Concurrent and predictive validity of a self-reported measure of medication adherence.* Med Care 1986;24:67-74.

Table 6. Morisky Scale to Assess Adherence to HIV Medications: 5-Point Response Options

Subjects were asked: "Thinking of the medications PRESCRIBED to you by your doctor(s), please answer the following questions."					
Response options: never = 0; rarely = 1; sometimes = 2; often = 3; always = 4	**0**	**1**	**2**	**3**	**4**
Do you ever forget to take your medications?					
Are you careless at times about taking your medications?					
When you feel better, do you sometimes stop taking your medications?					
Sometimes, if you feel worse when you take your medications, do you stop taking them?					

Adapted from Morisky DE, Green LW, Levine DM. *Concurrent and predictive validity of a self-reported measure of medication adherence.* Med Care 1986;24: 67-74.

References

- Bangsberg DR, Moss AR, Deeks SG. *Paradoxes of adherence and drug resistance to HIV antiretroviral therapy.* J Antimicro Chemother 2004: 53: 696-99.

- Brummet L. *AIDS care: adhering to antiretroviral therapy.* Nurs BC. 2002 Oct;34(4):24-5.

- Gaithe J Jr. *Adherence and potency with antiretroviral therapy: a combination for success.* J Acquir Immune Defic Syndr. 2003 Oct 1;34 Suppl 2:S118-22.

- Golin CE, Smith SR, Reif S. *Adherence counseling practices of generalist and specialist physicians caring for people living with HIV/AIDS in North Carolina.* J Gen Intern Med. 2004 Jan;19(1):16-27.

- Machtinger EL, Bangsberg DR. *Adherence to HIV Antiretroviral Therapy.* In: Coffey S, Volberding PA, eds. *HIV InSite Knowledge Base* [textbook online]; San Francisco: UCSF Center for HIV Information; May 2005. Available at hivinsite.ucsf.edu/InSite?page=kb-00&doc=kb-03-02-09. Accessed June 30, 2010.

- Malcolm SE, Ng JJ, Rosen RK, et al. *An examination of HIV/AIDS patients who have excellent adherence to HAART.* AIDS Care. 2003 Apr;15(2):251-61.

- Protopopescu C, Raffi F, Roux P, et al.; ANRS CO8 APROCO-COPILOTE Study Group. *Factors associated with non-adherence to long-term highly active antiretroviral therapy: a 10 year follow-up analysis with correction for the bias induced by missing data.* J Antimicrob Chemother. 2009 Sep;64(3):599-606.

- Stone VE, Smith KY. *Improving adherence to HAART.* J Natl Med Assoc. 2004 Feb;96(2 Suppl):27S-29S.

- U.S. Department of Health and Human Services. *Guidelines for the Use of Antiretroviral Agents in HIV-1-Infected Adults and Adolescents.* January 10, 2011. Available at www.aidsinfo.nih.gov/guidelines/.

Section 4: Health Care Maintenance and Disease Prevention

Diarrhea

Background

Diarrhea is a common complaint among HIV-infected individuals, and it has a variety of causes. Episodes may be acute and brief, intermittent or recurrent, or, in some cases, chronic and severe. If diarrhea persists, it may cause dehydration, poor nutrition, and weight loss. Diarrhea may diminish patients' quality of life significantly, and may interfere with adherence to and efficacy of antiretroviral (ARV) medications.

Diarrhea is defined in various ways, but commonly as more than four loose or watery stools per day for more than 3 days. Duration is classified as follows:

- Acute: <2 weeks

- Persistent: 2-4 weeks

- Chronic: >4 weeks

The causes of diarrhea, both infectious and noninfectious, found in HIV-infected individuals with normal or mildly depressed CD4 cell counts are likely to be similar to those in HIV-uninfected persons. Among the noninfectious causes of diarrhea, adverse effects of ARVs and other medications are particularly common. Persons with advanced immunodeficiency are more likely to have infections, including opportunistic infections, as the cause of diarrhea.

Infectious diarrhea typically involves either the small or the large intestine, and the patient's history often suggests the site of the problem. Infections of the small intestine (enteritis) commonly produce generalized or periumbilical abdominal cramps, large-volume diarrhea without blood, and frequently dehydration. Large-intestine infections (colitis) often produce lower abdominal pain, an unproductive urge to defecate, and frequent small-volume stools with blood and pus.

S: Subjective

The patient complains of diarrhea. Take a thorough history, including the following:

- Onset of diarrhea: sudden or gradual

- Frequency (times per day, last episode)

- Stool consistency (soft vs. liquid)

- Stool color (gray, white, or greasy stools: possible cholelithiasis or pancreatitis; dark stools: possible gastrointestinal bleeding)

- Bloody stools (may indicate invasive organisms, inflammation, ischemia, or neoplasm)

- Rectal bleeding

- Straining at stool

- Pain with defecation, rectal discharge (consider sexually transmitted infections, herpes simplex virus)

- Nausea or vomiting (within 6 hours of ingesting food, consider foodborne illness, gastroenteritis)

- Weight loss: quantify amount and time frame

- Abdominal pain or cramping; location if present

- Fever (consider invasive pathogens: *Shigella, Campylobacter, Salmonella, Clostridium difficile*)

- Other associated symptoms (e.g., bloating, flatus)

- Allergies (to foods or medications)

- Aggravating factors (e.g., dairy products, fatty or spicy foods)

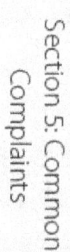

- Alleviating factors (e.g., fasting)
- Treatments tried (e.g., over-the-counter antidiarrheals)
- Contact with others with similar symptoms
- Previous episodes of diarrhea
- History of cytomegalovirus (CMV), *Mycobacterium avium* complex (MAC), or other infections involving the gastrointestinal tract
- Family history of inflammatory bowel disease, celiac disease
- Oral-anal sexual contact (males and females)
- Receptive anal intercourse
- Exposure to unsafely prepared food (e.g., raw, undercooked, spoiled), unpasteurized milk or juices
- Exposure to possibly contaminated water (swimming in or drinking from well, lake, or stream) (consider parasites, including *Giardia*)
- Exposure to non-toilet-trained infants and children (e.g., at a daycare facility), pets, farm animals, reptiles (consider *Giardia, Salmonella*)
- Recent travel (enterotoxigenic *Escherichia coli, Shigella, Rotavirus, Salmonella, Campylobacter, Giardia, Entamoeba histolytica*)
- Antibiotic use or exposure in recent weeks or months or recent hospitalization (consider *C. difficile*)
- ARV medications, especially ritonavir-boosted protease inhibitors; check relationship of diarrhea onset to initiation of ARVs
- Other current and recent medications (prescribed or over-the-counter), including supplements and herbal preparations

- Dietary factors, especially "sugar-free" foods (containing nonabsorbable carbohydrates), fat substitutes, milk products, and shellfish, or heavy intake of fruits, fruit juices, or caffeine
- Alcohol and recreational drug use; withdrawal

O: Objective

Record vital signs, including temperature, orthostatic heart rate, blood pressure measurements, and weight. Compare these with recent or baseline values. Perform a thorough physical examination, including evaluation of the following:

- Hydration status (skin turgor, mucous membrane moistness)
- Nutritional status (body habitus, muscle mass, skin and hair integrity)
- Oropharynx (lesions, candidiasis, ulcerations, Kaposi sarcoma)
- Optic fundi (signs of CMV infection)
- Abdomen (distention, bowel sounds, tenderness, organomegaly, masses, adenopathy)
- Rectum (masses, tenderness, bloody stool)
- Review recent CD4 cell counts. Low CD4 counts increase the risk of chronic or systemic illnesses and opportunistic infections.

A: Assessment

The differential diagnosis of diarrhea is broad and includes the following infectious and noninfectious causes. The CD4 cell count is important in stratifying risk of infection with opportunistic pathogens; some organisms cause disease only with severe immunosuppression.

Infectious Causes

Acute diarrhea, any CD4 count

- Viruses (especially Norwalk virus)
- Viral hepatitis
- Herpes enteritis
- *C. difficile* (suspect in patients who have recently undergone treatment with antibiotics, or hospitalization)
- *Salmonella*
- *Shigella*
- *Campylobacter*
- *E. coli* O157:H7

Chronic diarrhea, any CD4 count

- *C. difficile* (suspect in patients who have recently been treated with antibiotics)
- *Giardia lamblia*
- *E. histolytica*

Chronic diarrhea, CD4 count <300 cells/µL

- Microsporidia
- *Cryptosporidium parvum*
- MAC (CD4 count <50 cells/µL)
- *Isospora belli*
- CMV (CD4 count <50 cells/µL)

Adapted from: Infectious Causes of Diarrhea in Patients with HIV, Table 8-8. In: Bartlett JG, Cheever LW, Johnson MP, et al., eds. *A Guide to Primary Care of People with HIV/AIDS*. Rockville, MD: U.S. Department of Health and Human Services, Health Resources and Services Administration; 2004.

Noninfectious Causes

- Medication adverse effects, common with many medications including some ARVs:
  - Protease inhibitors (especially ritonavir and nelfinavir)
  - Didanosine buffered tablets (no longer available in the United States)
- Irritable bowel syndrome
- Inflammatory bowel disease (ulcerative colitis, Crohn disease)
- Lymphoma
- Lactose intolerance
- Celiac disease
- Small-bowel overgrowth
- Pancreatic insufficiency
- Diverticulitis
- Fecal incontinence
- Laxative abuse

P: Plan

Diagnostic Evaluation

For suspected infections, perform laboratory studies including complete blood count with differential, serum electrolyte panel, and liver function tests. Check stool for white blood cells and blood. Perform stool studies as indicated by the patient's presentation (bacterial culture, ova and parasites, microsporidia, cryptosporidia, *Giardia* antigen, *C. difficile* toxin assay). Order additional studies as suggested by the history (e.g., blood cultures, MAC cultures, hepatitis serologies, retinal examination for CMV). If noninfectious causes are suspected, perform evaluation for these etiologies as indicated (e.g., fecal fat concentration [for steatorrhea], stool osmolar gap [for osmotic diarrhea], anti-tissue transglutaminase [TTG] antibody [for celiac disease], or D-xylose [for pancreatic insufficiency]).

If the patient is febrile, perform a complete fever workup as appropriate (see chapter *Fever*).

Check the CD4 cell count and HIV viral load, if not checked recently.

If stool study results are negative (ova and parasite negative in three successive samples) and the patient has severe symptoms, particularly in the case of advanced immunodeficiency, refer to a gastroenterologist for colonoscopy or flexible sigmoidoscopy with biopsy. Endoscopy with biopsy is the best procedure for identifying certain conditions, including CMV colitis and inflammatory bowel disease. If all study results are negative but the diarrhea persists, repeat endoscopy in 6-8 weeks regardless of the level of immunodeficiency. Pathogens may be difficult to identify.

Treatment

Once a diagnosis is made, initiate appropriate treatment. For seriously ill patients, presumptive treatment may be started while diagnostic tests are pending. If the cause of the diarrhea cannot be identified, consult with an HIV expert or a gastroenterologist.

- For moderate to severe acute diarrhea, including dysentery (bloody diarrhea), empiric treatment can be given pending stool study results or in settings with limited resources for workup. If bacterial pathogens are suspected, use oral fluoroquinolones (e.g., ciprofloxacin 500 mg BID, norfloxacin 400 mg BID, or levofloxacin 500 mg once daily) for 5 days. Monitor effectiveness and adjust therapy according to the results of diagnostic studies and clinical response. Specific treatment with antimicrobials is guided by the pathogens identified in stool studies or on biopsy.

- For mild persistent diarrhea with no identified pathogen, treat with an antidiarrheal agent (see below). For patients whose diarrhea is suspected to be caused by ARV agents or other medications, symptomatic treatment also may be tried. Diarrhea owing to protease inhibitors often decreases after a few weeks without treatment. For persistent daily ARV-associated diarrhea, antidiarrheal agents may be given on a scheduled basis (rather than as needed). If the diarrhea cannot be controlled, a change in ARV regimen should be considered.

Symptomatic treatments

- Antimotility agents such as loperamide (Imodium) in over-the-counter or prescription strengths and atropine/diphenoxylate (Lomotil) are useful for many patients. The suggested dosage is 2 tablets after each loose bowel movement, not to exceed 8 tablets per day. These agents should not be used if patients have bloody diarrhea or if the presence of *C. difficile* is suspected.

- Pharmaconutritional approaches include the use of calcium supplementation (500 mg BID or TID). Patients with diarrhea related to protease inhibitors may find that taking calcium with each dose of protease inhibitors can decrease or prevent diarrhea. Note that magnesium supplements may worsen diarrhea.

- Pancrelipase can be useful in managing chronic diarrhea caused by malabsorption. These come in different formulations with differing amounts of pancreatic enzymes; usual dosage is 2-3 capsules TID with meals, titrated downward according to response.

- Cholestyramine or psyllium (e.g., Metamucil) may reduce diarrhea by slowing peristalsis and adding bulk to stools. Avoid administering cholestyramine with other medications because it may impair their absorption.

- A combination of these treatments may be needed to control chronic diarrhea, and they can be continued for patients after an infectious process has been ruled out.

Nutrition and hydration

Encourage frequent intake of soft, easily digested foods such as bananas, rice, wheat, potatoes, noodles, boiled vegetables, crackers, and soups. Encourage hydration with fruit drinks, tea, "flat" carbonated beverages, and water. Patients should avoid high-sugar drinks, caffeinated beverages, alcohol, high-fiber foods, greasy or spicy foods, and dairy products. Many patients may benefit from a trial of a lactose-free, low-fiber, or low-fat diet. Patients should use nutritional supplements as needed or as recommended by a dietitian. In case of chronic or severe diarrhea, or significant weight loss, refer to a dietitian for further recommendations.

Patients with severe diarrhea must maintain adequate hydration, by mouth if possible. In severe cases, IV administration of fluids may be necessary. Oral rehydration solutions include the World Health Organization formula, Pedialyte, Rehydralyte, Rice-Lyte, and Resol. Homemade alternatives include the following:

- Combine 1/2 teaspoon of salt, 1 teaspoon of baking soda, 8 teaspoons of sugar, and 8 ounces of orange juice; add water to make 1 liter and drink.

- Drink 1 glass containing 8 ounces of apple, orange, or other juice; 1/2 teaspoon of corn syrup or honey; and a pinch of salt; then drink 1 glass containing 8 ounces of water and 1/4 teaspoon of baking soda.

- Mix 1/2 cup of dry, precooked baby rice cereal with 2 cups of water (boil first in areas with poor water quality); add 1/4 teaspoon of salt and drink.

Patient Education

- Diarrhea can have many causes. Instruct patients to notify their health care provider if they develop new or worsening symptoms.

- Instruct patients to take their medications exactly as directed and to call their health care provider if they experience worsening diarrhea, or other symptoms such as fever, nausea, vomiting, or pain.

- Patients must stay nourished and well hydrated even if they are having diarrhea. Instruct patients to eat small, frequent meals and to avoid dairy products, greasy food, and high-fat meals.

- Instruct patients to maintain good handwashing practices during diarrheal

illnesses to prevent infection in close contacts or household members.

- Some diarrheal illnesses are reportable; advise patients that they may be contacted by the local health department.

References

- American Medical Association, American Nurses Association—American Nurses Foundation, Centers for Disease Control and Prevention, Center for Food Safety and Applied Nutrition, Food and Drug Administration, Food Safety and Inspection Service, US Department of Agriculture. *Diagnosis and Management of Foodborne Illnesses.* MMWR 2004; 53(RR04);1-33. Available at www.cdc.gov/mmwr/preview/mmwrhtml/rr5304a1.htm.

- Beatty GW. *Diarrhea in patients infected with HIV presenting to the emergency department.* Emerg Med Clin North Am. 2010 May;28(2):299-310.

- Centers for Disease Control and Prevention. *Guidelines for Prevention and Treatment of Opportunistic Infections in HIV-Infected Adults and Adolescents: Recommendations from CDC, the National Institutes of Health, and the HIV Medicine Association of the Infectious Diseases Society of America.* April 10, 2009. Available at www.aidsinfo.nih.gov/guidelines/.

- Nysoe TE, Paauw DS. *Symptom Management.* In: Bartlett JG, Cheever LW, Johnson MP, et al., eds. *A Guide to Primary Care of People with HIV/AIDS.* Rockville, MD: U.S. Department of Health and Human Services, Health Resources and Services Administration; 2004;55-65. Available at hab.hrsa.gov/tools/primarycareguide.

- Wilcox CM. *Diseases of the Esophagus and Stomach and Bowel.* In: Dolin R, Masur H, Saag M, eds. *AIDS Therapy, 3rd Edition.* New York: Churchill Livingstone Elsevier; 2008.

Ear, Nose, Sinus, Mouth

Background

HIV-infected individuals frequently experience infections and neoplasms that affect the ears, nose, sinuses, and mouth. The degree of immunosuppression, as reflected by a patient's CD4 cell count, can affect the severity, likelihood of recurrence, and response to therapy for various infections and neoplasms.

Patients may present with ear, nose, sinus, or mouth complaints early in the course of HIV infection, perhaps even before they are aware of their infection. Some conditions arise more commonly in patients with advanced HIV infection. Certain complaints (e.g., oral candidiasis) should prompt consideration of HIV testing in patients without known infection.

Ears

HIV-infected patients may experience recurrent acute otitis media and serous otitis media. Nasopharyngeal lymphoid hyperplasia, sinusitis, or allergies may contribute to dysfunction of the eustachian tubes. Unilateral and bilateral sensorineural hearing loss has been reported and may be caused by HIV infection involving the central nervous system (CNS) or the auditory nerve. Hearing loss also may be caused by syphilis, other CNS infections, chronic otitis media, neoplasms, and certain medications (including some nucleoside analogues in rare cases). The pathophysiology, causative organisms, and incidence of external-ear infections appear to be the same in HIV-infected patients as in HIV-uninfected individuals.

S: Subjective

The patient may complain of ear pain, decreased hearing or hearing loss, a feeling of fullness in the ear, vertigo, or a popping or snapping sensation in the ear.

Obtain information regarding the following during the history:

- Medications (prescription and over-the-counter) and herbal supplements, current and past

- Current or recent sinus infection

- Associated symptoms

- Drainage or blood from the ear

- Head or ear trauma

O: Objective

Recent CD4 count is an important measure of immunosuppression and is important in determining whether the patient is at risk of opportunistic infections as causes of ear complaints.

Perform visual and otoscopic inspection, including evaluation for skin abnormalities, lesions, cerumen impaction or foreign body, lymphadenopathy, and adenotonsillar hypertrophy.

If hearing loss is reported or suspected, evaluate hearing and refer the patient for an audiogram. Perform a neurologic examination and draw rapid plasma regain (RPR) or Venereal Disease Research Laboratory (VDRL) test.

A/P: Assessment and Plan
Otitis Externa/Interna

Proceed as with an immunocompetent patient. A chronic or atypical presentation in an HIV-infected patient warrants a thorough evaluation, including cultures, biopsy, radiographic scans, and referral to an ear, nose, and throat (ENT) specialist.

Hearing Loss

A patient with hearing loss should be referred for evaluation or treated, depending on the cause. Avoid ototoxic medications (e.g., furosemide, aminoglycosides).

Nose and Sinuses

Nasal and paranasal sinus conditions occur frequently in HIV-infected patients. Sinusitis, nasal obstruction, allergic rhinitis, and nasal lesions are common. Epistaxis can occur in patients with platelet disorders (e.g., idiopathic thrombocytopenic purpura [ITP]).

S: Subjective

The patient may complain of "stuffy nose," rhinorrhea, epistaxis, frontal or maxillary headaches (worse at night or early morning), pain in the nostrils, persistent postnasal drip, mucopurulent nasal discharge, general malaise, aching or pressure behind the eyes, or toothache-like pain.

Obtain information regarding the following during the history:

- Medications (prescription and over-the-counter) and herbal supplements, current and past
- Current or recent sinus infection
- Previous sinus surgery
- Recent or current upper respiratory infection (URI)
- Nasal bleeding or discharge
- Facial trauma
- Allergic rhinitis
- Positional pain; worse when patient bends forward?
- Tobacco use

- Fever
- Headache
- Mucopurulent nasal drainage

O: Objective

Recent CD4 count is an important measure of immunosuppression and is a key element in determining whether the patient is at risk of opportunistic infections as causes of nasal and sinus complaints.

Examine the nose and sinuses. Check the nasal mucosa with a light and a speculum, looking for areas of bleeding, purulent drainage, ulcerated lesions, or discolored areas. Palpate or percuss the sinuses for areas of tenderness, look for areas of swelling over the sinuses, and visualize the posterior pharynx for mucopurulent drainage. Transillumination may be helpful. Examine the teeth and gums for caries and inflammation of the gingivae. Check maxillary teeth with the use of a tongue blade (5-10% of maxillary sinusitis is attributable to dental root infection). Refer to a dentist for tooth sensitivity or caries.

A: Assessment

- Possible causes of epistaxis include coagulopathy, ITP, tumor, lesions of herpes simplex virus (HSV), and Kaposi sarcoma (KS). Suspect ITP if the platelet count is low and bleeding is difficult to control.

- Acute infection of one or more of the paranasal sinuses is common. *Streptococcus pneumoniae, Haemophilus influenzae,* and *Moraxella catarrhalis* are seen in both HIV-uninfected and HIV-infected patients, whereas *Staphylococcus aureus* and *Pseudomonas aeruginosa* are found more often in HIV-infected patients. Fungi may be the causative agents, especially in patients with severe immunosuppression.

- Chronic sinusitis occurs frequently in patients with HIV infection and may be polymicrobial or anaerobic. In patients with low CD4 cell counts, fungal sinusitis may occur.

- Nasal obstruction may be caused by adenoidal hypertrophy, chronic sinusitis, allergic rhinitis, or neoplasm.

- Tumors may be caused by KS, squamous papilloma, or lymphoma; biopsy is necessary for determining the cause.

- Painful, ulcerated vesicles in the nasal mucosa may be caused by HSV or other infections.

P: Plan
Acute Sinusitis

Combination therapy with antibiotics, decongestants, mucolytics, saline nasal spray, and topical nasal steroids may be effective. See chapter *Sinusitis* for details. Note: For patients taking ritonavir or ritonavir-boosted protease inhibitors, fluticasone (Flonase) nasal spray should not be used, and budesonide (Rhinocort Aqua) should be avoided if possible; see "Potential ARV Interactions," below.

Chronic Sinusitis

Treat with a systemic decongestant (guaifenesin), saline nasal spray BID, and topical nasal saline spray. Patients with exacerbations of sinusitis should be treated as for acute sinusitis. For more detailed information, see chapter *Sinusitis*. With patients taking ritonavir-boosted PIs, avoid fluticasone and budesonide nasal sprays; see "Potential ARV Interactions," below.

Allergic Rhinitis

Patients should avoid exposure to known or suspected allergens. Nasal steroids may be very effective, but avoid fluticasone and budesonide nasal sprays with patients taking ritonavir (see "Potential ARV Interactions," below). Second-generation nonsedating antihistamines such as cetirizine, fexofenadine, and loratadine are not as effective as nasal steroids, but may give additional symptom relief. Note that ritonavir may increase the serum levels and half-life of cetirizine. Daily nasal lavage with normal saline often is beneficial.

Nasal Obstruction

Perform magnetic resonance imaging (MRI) or computed tomography (CT) scan with biopsy for mass lesions or asymmetric nasal lymphoid tissue. Refer to an ENT specialist.

Epistaxis

Epistaxis caused by coagulopathy or tumor is managed the same as for immunocompetent patients with these conditions. Cauterization of an identified bleeding point or packing may be necessary. ITP should be managed in collaboration with a hematologist; antiretroviral therapy (ART) typically is used for chronic management, and corticosteroids or other therapies may be used for acute management.

Potential ARV Interactions

Caution: Protease inhibitors (PIs), particularly ritonavir-boosted PIs, may increase serum glucocorticoid levels if used concurrently with nasal steroids. Fluticasone (Flonase) nasal spray should not be used with ritonavir-boosted PIs unless expected benefits out weigh possible risks, and should be avoided, if possible, in patients taking unboosted PIs. Budesonide (Rhinocort Aqua) nasal spray should be avoided with ritonavir-boosted PIs. Interactions between PIs and other nasal steroids have not been well studied.

Ritonavir may increase serum levels of cetirizine and may prolong its half-life; start with low dosage and monitor for adverse effects.

Mouth and Throat

The oral cavity is one of the most common areas of symptoms in patients with HIV infection. Conditions that arise in the oral cavity may be infectious, benign inflammatory, neoplastic, or degenerative processes.

S: Subjective

The patient may complain of white patches and red areas on the dorsal surface of the tongue and the palate, decreased taste sensation, white lesions along the lateral margins of the tongue, ulcers, nonhealing lesions at the corners of the mouth, sore gums, loose teeth, dysphagia, or odynophagia.

Obtain information regarding the following during the history:

- Medications (prescription and over-the-counter) and herbal supplements (note that some medications may cause aphthous ulcers)

- Usual oral hygiene (toothbrushing, tongue brushing or scraping, flossing, use of mouthwash)

- Date of last dental examination

- Use of tobacco (cigarettes, chewing tobacco)

- Involuntary weight loss

O: Objective

Recent CD4 count reflects degree of immunosuppression and is helpful in determining whether the patient is at risk of opportunistic infections as causes of oral complaints.

Thorough examination of the mouth and throat with a tongue depressor and a good light is mandatory. Observe for white patches or plaques on the mucous membranes that can be partially removed by scraping with a tongue blade (candidiasis). Examine the dorsal surface of the tongue and hard and soft palates for red, flat, subtle lesions (erythematous candidiasis). Look for ribbed, whitish lesions on the lateral aspects of the tongue that cannot be scraped off (oral hairy leukoplakia). Check for ulcerations, inflamed gums, and loose teeth (see section *Oral Health*). Look for discoloration or nodular lesions on the hard palate (Kaposi sarcoma). Check the pharynx for adenotonsillar hypertrophy. Rule out HIV-unrelated causes of pharyngitis, including streptococci or respiratory viruses.

A/P: Assessment and Plan

Perform biopsy, culture, and potassium hydroxide (KOH) preparation of lesions as indicated.

Oral Candidiasis (Thrush)

Oral candidiasis is most likely to occur when the CD4 count is <200 cells/µL, but it can occur at any CD4 level and in HIV-uninfected individuals. It may appear as creamy white plaques on the tongue or buccal mucosa or as erythematous lesions on the dorsal surface of the tongue or the palate. The most common treatment strategy is empiric therapy with topical or systemic antifungal agents. For more details, see chapter *Candidiasis, Oral and Esophageal*.

Angular Cheilitis

Angular cheilitis is also caused by *Candida* species, and it is characterized by fissuring at the corners of the mouth. For information on treatment, see chapter *Candidiasis, Oral and Esophageal*.

Oral Hairy Leukoplakia

Oral hairy leukoplakia (OHL) is caused by Epstein-Barr virus and appears as raised, ribbed, "hairy" white lesions along the lateral margins of the tongue. Lesions are primarily asymptomatic, and treatment generally is not needed. Lesions often resolve with effective ART. For more details, see chapter *Oral Hairy Leukoplakia*.

Kaposi Sarcoma

KS appears as red, blue, or purplish lesions that are flat or nodular, and solitary or multiple. Lesions appear most commonly on the hard palate but also occur on the gingival surfaces and elsewhere in the mouth. A definitive diagnosis requires biopsy and histologic examination. KS often resolves with ART and successful immune reconstitution. If lesions do not respond to ART or if they are severe or numerous, refer to an oncology specialist for chemotherapy. For more details, see chapter *Kaposi Sarcoma.*

Gingivitis

See chapter *Necrotizing Ulcerative Periodontitis and Gingivitis* for details.

Herpes Simplex Virus

HSV lesions occur on the palate, gingivae, or other mucosal surfaces. They appear as single or clustered vesicles and may extend onto adjacent skin of the lips and face to form a large herpetic lesion. Lesions tend to be more common, persist longer, recur more often, and be larger and more numerous in HIV-infected patients, especially those with significant immunosuppression, than in healthy individuals. Empiric treatment with valacyclovir, famciclovir, or acyclovir is appropriate. For more details, see chapter *Herpes Simplex, Mucocutaneous.*

Aphthous Ulcers

Aphthous ulcers are eroded, well-defined lesions surrounded by erythema, ranging in size from <6 mm to several centimeters in diameter. The ulcers can appear anywhere in the oral cavity or pharynx and may be recurrent; they are extremely painful. Treatment may involve topical steroids or other methods. For more details, see chapter *Oral Ulceration.*

Oral Warts (Human Papillomavirus)

Oral warts may appear as solitary or multiple nodules. The lesions may be smooth, raised masses resembling focal epithelial hyperplasia, or small papuliferous or cauliflower-like projections. See chapter *Oral Warts.*

Neisseria gonorrhoeae Pharyngitis

Neisseria gonorrhoeae may be transmitted by orogenital exposure; the patient may have mild symptoms (e.g., sore throat) or be asymptomatic. Physical examination may reveal an erythematous pharynx or exudates. Anterior cervical lymphadenopathy also may be present. Most cases of *N. gonorrhoeae* pharyngeal infection will resolve spontaneously without treatment and usually do not cause adverse sequelae. However, treatment should be initiated to reduce the spread of the infection (see chapter *Gonorrhea and Chlamydia*). Regular screening is recommended for patients at risk of *N. gonorrhoeae* infection.

Medication-Related Mouth or Throat Lesions

- Candidiasis: antibiotics
- Xerostomia: antihistamines, anticholinergics, tricyclics, antipsychotic
- Gingival hyperplasia: phenytoin, calcium channel blockers

Other Conditions

Most of these complications also can occur in the esophagus. See chapters *Esophageal Problems, Candidiasis, Oral and Esophageal,* and *Cytomegalovirus Disease.*

If patient is having mouth pain, anorexia, or problems with taste, treat the condition appropriately and refer to an HIV-experienced dentist for evaluation and further treatment as needed. Refer to a dietitian for assistance with dietary needs (e.g., nutritional supplements).

References

- Greenspan JS, Greenspan D. *Oral Complications of HIV Infection.* In: Sande MA, Volberding PA, eds. *Medical Management of AIDS,* 6th ed. Philadelphia: WB Saunders; 1999:157-169.

- Gurney TA, Murr AH. *Otolaryngologic manifestations of human immunodeficiency virus infection.* Otolaryngol Clin North Am. 2003 Aug;36(4):607-24.

- Lee K, Tami T. *Otolaryngologic Manifestations of HIV.* In: Coffey S, Volberding PA, eds. *HIV InSite Knowledge Base* [textbook online]; San Francisco: UCSF Center for HIV Information; August 1998. Available at hivinsite.ucsf.edu/. Accessed June 30, 2010.

- Miller KE. *Diagnosis and Treatment of Neisseria gonorrhoeae Infections.* American Family Physician; 2006. Available at www.aafp.org/afp/. Accessed June 30, 2010.

- Sande MA, Eliopoulos GM, Moellering RC, et al. *The Sanford Guide to HIV/AIDS Therapy.* Hyde Park, VT: Antimicrobial Therapy, Inc.; 2008.

- Workowski KA, Berman SM. *Sexually Transmitted Diseases Treatment Guidelines, 2006.* Atlanta: Division of STD Prevention, National Center for HIV/AIDS, Viral Hepatitis, STD, and TB Prevention; August 2006. Available at www.cdc.gov/mmwr/preview/mmwrhtml/rr5511a1.htm.

Esophageal Problems

Background

Esophageal problems in HIV-infected patients include difficulty swallowing (dysphagia) or midline retrosternal pain when swallowing (odynophagia). Pain may be diffuse throughout the esophagus or localized in specific areas.

Several conditions may cause esophageal problems. Of the infectious causes of dysphagia in HIV-infected patients, *Candida* is the most common (50-70%). Drug-induced dysphagia, gastroesophageal reflux disease (GERD), vomiting, and hiatal hernia also can cause esophagitis. Less commonly, esophageal cancer or another cause of stricture may produce symptoms. Neuromuscular or neurological causes may be seen in patients with advanced AIDS.

If untreated, esophageal problems may result in esophageal ulcers, scarring of the esophagus, dehydration, and weight loss.

S: Subjective

The patient may complain of difficulty swallowing, a feeling of something being "stuck in the throat," retrosternal pain when eating, "hiccups," indigestion ("heartburn"), retrosternal burning, acid reflux, nausea, vomiting, or abdominal pain.

The history should include the following:

- Medications (prescription and over-the-counter) and herbal supplements, current and past
- Concurrent gastrointestinal (GI) symptoms, such as abdominal pain or diarrhea
- Recent dietary history
- Location and characteristics of pain (diffuse or focal)
- Oral thrush
- Aphthous ulcers
- Cytomegalovirus (CMV)
- *Candida* esophagitis
- Gastroesophageal reflux disease (GERD)
- Hiatal hernia
- Presence of dysphagia to solids, liquids, or both
- Hematemesis or melena

O: Objective

Include the following in the physical examination:

- Measure vital signs (temperature may be elevated with certain infections, such as CMV, but not with herpes simplex virus [HSV], candidiasis, or idiopathic ulcers).
- Record weight (and compare with previous weights).
- Assess for oral candidiasis, lesions, and masses.
- Examine optic fundi to evaluate for CMV retinitis (in patients with CD4 counts of <50-100 cells/μL).
- Palpate for thyroid enlargement.
- Palpate the neck and supraclavicular and infraclavicular areas for lymphadenopathy.
- Assess the abdomen for masses, tenderness, and organomegaly.
- Perform a rectal examination to obtain stool for occult blood.
- Perform a neurologic examination.
- Check the CD4 cell count and HIV viral load to determine the level of immunosuppression and assess the risk

Section 5: Common Complaints

of opportunistic infections as causes of esophageal complaints.

A: Assessment

Common causes of esophageal problems are as follows:

- Candidiasis (common with a CD4 count of <200 cells/μL or recent exposure to steroids or antibiotics)

- Most medications, including antiretroviral agents, can cause nausea and GI-related symptoms; the following medications are commonly associated with difficulty swallowing or heartburn: aspirin, nonsteroidal antiinflammatory drugs, potassium chloride, iron, tetracycline, theophylline, anticholinergic agents, calcium channel blockers, meperidine, and progesterone tablets

- Foods can irritate the esophagus, including citrus fruits, mints, coffee, chocolate, and spicy foods

- GERD

Less common causes of esophageal problems include:

- CMV, HSV, idiopathic or aphthous ulcers

- Kaposi sarcoma, lymphoma, tuberculosis, *Mycobacterium avium* complex (MAC), histoplasmosis

- Cardiac chest pain

P: Plan

Diagnostic Evaluation

Diagnosis often can be made on clinical grounds; in this case, empiric treatment may be initiated (see below). If the diagnosis is unclear, consider endoscopy or radiographic imaging (e.g., computed tomography or barium swallow).

If the patient has dysphagia, odynophagia,

unexplained weight loss, GI bleeding, anemia, or atypical symptoms, refer promptly for GI evaluation and endoscopy, or other evaluation as suggested by symptoms.

Treatment

Determine whether the patient is able to swallow pills before giving oral medications. If pills are not tolerated, the patient may need liquids or troches.

For patients with severe oral or esophageal pain, viscous lidocaine 1% 5-10 mL 2-4 times daily (with swallowing precautions) or Magic Mouthwash (viscous lidocaine 1%, tetracycline, diphenhydramine, and nystatin compounded 1:1:1:1) may be tried.

Other treatments may depend on the underlying cause:

- **Esophageal candidiasis:** Fluconazole is the drug of choice. If symptoms resolve within 7-10 days, no further testing is required. See chapter *Candidiasis, Oral and Esophageal* for more treatment options and for dosing information.

- **Medication related:** Remove the offending drug(s), and institute a trial of H2 blockers or proton pump inhibitors (PPIs) as appropriate (caution: see "Potential ARV Interactions," below).

- **Food related:** Modify the diet and institute a trial of H2 blockers or PPIs as appropriate (caution: see "Potential ARV Interactions," below).

- **"Heartburn" or GERD:** Patients whose primary symptoms are more typical of "heartburn" or reflux, especially those with a history of GERD, should receive a trial of H2 blockers or a PPI as appropriate (these may decrease absorption of atazanavir; see "Potential ARV Interactions," below). Reevaluate after 2-4 weeks; if symptoms are controlled, treat for 4-8 weeks, then reduce the dosage to the lowest effective amount.

Patients may require maintenance therapy for an indefinite period because of the high likelihood of recurrence. If symptoms do not respond to full-dose acid-blocking therapy, refer for GI evaluation.

- **GERD:** For nonpharmacologic treatment, in cases of obesity, counsel patients to lose weight, stop smoking, elevate the head of the bed, eat smaller meals, avoid eating food 2-3 hours before bedtime, and reduce fat in the diet to ≤30% of calorie consumption.

- **CMV:** Treat with anti-CMV medications (e.g., oral valganciclovir). See chapter *Cytomegalovirus Disease* for details.

- **HSV:** Treat with antiviral medications, including acyclovir, famciclovir, and valacyclovir. See chapter *Herpes Simplex, Mucocutaneous.*

- **Aphthous ulcers:** These may respond to oral corticosteroids (consult with a specialist before this is undertaken. Alternatively, a combination of H2 blockers and sucralfate may be effective. In some circumstances, thalidomide 200 mg Q24H may be used. (**Note:** Thalidomide is teratogenic, and women of childbearing potential are not candidates for this therapy unless the potential benefits clearly outweigh the risks and appropriate prevention of pregnancy is undertaken.) Up to 40-50% of patients with aphthous ulcers experience relapse and require repeat treatment.

- **Neoplastic disease:** Treating this condition requires referral to an oncologist.

Esophageal conditions that do not resolve with treatment require referral to a GI specialist for diagnostic endoscopy, with biopsy and brushing for histopathology and cultures as appropriate.

Diet

It is important that patients maintain adequate caloric intake, preferably with foods and liquids that can be swallowed easily. Nutritional supplements along with soft, bland, high-protein foods are recommended. Refer to a nutritionist as needed.

Potential ARV Interactions

Caution: H2 blockers and PPIs interfere with the absorption of atazanavir and several other PIs. For atazanavir, specific dosing strategies are required, and some combinations are contraindicated. See atazanavir package insert for dosage recommendations.

References

- DeVault KR, Castel DO; American College of Gastroenterology. *Updated guidelines for the diagnosis and treatment of gastroesophageal reflux disease.* Am J Gastroenterol. 2005 Jan;100(1):190-200.

- Dieterich DT, Poles MA, Cappell MS, et al. *Gastrointestinal Manifestations of HIV Disease, Including the Peritoneum and Mesentery.* In: Merigan TC, Bartlett JG, Bolognesi D, eds. *Textbook of AIDS Medicine,* 2nd ed. Baltimore: Williams & Wilkins, 1999;542-6.

- Wilcox CM, Monkemuller KE. *Gastrointestinal Disease.* In: Dolin R, Masur H, Saag MS, eds. *AIDS Therapy.* New York: Churchill Livingstone, 1999;752-56.

Eye Problems

Background

The immunosuppression caused by HIV infection increases the incidence of eye infections. However, the risk of serious eye problems associated with advanced immunosuppression, such as blindness caused by cytomegalovirus (CMV) retinitis, is much lower in patients treated with effective antiretroviral therapy (ART). Common problems not unique to HIV-infected patients include dry eye, blepharitis, keratitis, and presbyopia. Infections that may affect the eye include herpes simplex virus (HSV), herpes zoster virus (HZV), and syphilis. More severely immunocompromised patients (CD4 count <100 cells/μL) may experience CMV retinitis, *Toxoplasma* retinochoroiditis, cryptococcal chorioretinitis, and other conditions. Retinal detachment can result. Kaposi sarcoma (KS) also can affect the eye.

Immune reconstitution inflammatory syndrome (IRIS) may affect the eye in patients with advanced HIV disease soon after the initiation of effective ART. IRIS may lead to exacerbation of a previously treated opportunistic infection or a new presentation (often with unusual manifestations) of a previously subclinical infection. In the case of CMV, IRIS may present as retinitis, or less commonly as uveitis or vitreitis. IRIS retinitis typically occurs in patients whose CD4 counts have increased from <50 cells/μL to 50-100 cells/μL while receiving ART.

Drug-induced ocular toxicity can be caused by rifabutin, ethambutol, and cidofovir, and less often by high-dose didanosine (ddI, Videx), IV ganciclovir, IV acyclovir, and atovaquone.

S: Subjective

The patient complains of dry eyes, blurred vision, floaters, sharp pains, flashing lights, central vision loss ("black holes"), vision field defects ("can only see half the page"), or peripheral vision loss ("looks like I'm in a tunnel").

Ascertain the following during the history:

- Pain: clarify type and characteristics
- Unilateral or bilateral problem
- Visual defects (central or peripheral vision loss or distortion), scotomata (an area of lost or depressed vision surrounded by an area of less depressed or normal vision); occurs with reading, distance, or both?
- Time course of symptoms
- Fever
- Headache
- Previous eye or vision problems
- Medications (prescription and over-the-counter) and herbal supplements, current and past
- Use of corrective lenses
- Date of last eye examination
- Recent or current varicella-zoster virus (VZV) or HSV infection

O: Objective

Evaluate recent CD4 cell count and HIV viral load to determine whether the patient is at risk of opportunistic infections as causes of eye complaints. Also, do the following:

- Consider the patient's age.
- Check vital signs, including blood pressure and temperature.
- Administer a visual acuity examination using the Snellen chart. Test the patient's ability to read small print, such as classified ads.

- Consider using an Amsler grid to locate areas of retinal pathology.

- Examine the eyelids for lesions, inflammation, and swelling.

- Examine the external eye for edema, ptosis, conjunctival injection, and corneal clarity.

- Test cranial nerves II, III, IV, and VI.

- Perform funduscopic examination with pupillary dilatation, if available. Note retinal appearance, lesions, and condition of the disc, vessels, and macula.

- Examine the temples and scalp for tenderness

A/P: Assessment and Plan

Refer to an HIV-experienced ophthalmologist for dilated retinal or slit-lamp examination and definitive diagnosis. If symptoms raise suspicion of serious or vision-threatening conditions such as herpes ophthalmicus, CMV retinitis, or retinal necrosis, ophthalmologic evaluation should occur within 24-72 hours. Note that patients with HSV or VZV lesions in the V1 distribution (including the forehead, eyelids, or nose) should receive urgent ophthalmologic evaluation.

The differential diagnosis includes the following conditions:

Dry Eye (Keratoconjunctivitis Sicca)

The patient may complain of intermittent eye pain, intermittent blurred vision that clears with blinking, and mild eye irritation. The condition worsens with extended reading or computer use. Keratoconjunctivitis sicca is related to HIV-mediated inflammation with damage to the lacrimal glands. It occurs in 10-20% of HIV-infected patients, most often in those with advanced HIV disease. In patients with a CD4 count of >400 cells/μL and no other signs or symptoms, confirm that results of a recent eye examination were normal or refer for same, prescribe artificial tears, and monitor.

Blepharitis

Blepharitis is inflammation of the eyelids, a common condition with dry eyes. The patient may complain of discharge and erythema of the eyes or eyelids. Of the bacterial causes, *Staphylococcus aureus* is the most common. Treatment includes cleaning of the eyelashes with warm water and mild shampoo, and applying antibiotic ointment if indicated.

Infectious Keratitis

The patient may complain of photophobia, eye pain, decreased vision, and irritation. Infectious keratitis may be caused by VZV, HSV, CMV, bacteria, fungi, or *Microsporidia*. VZV and HSV are the most common infectious causes of keratitis in HIV-infected patients. Bacterial and fungal keratitis occur equally in HIV-infected and HIV-uninfected persons. Fungal infections are caused most frequently by *Candida* species, especially in intravenous drug users. Keratitis may be more severe and may recur more frequently in HIV-infected patients than in HIV-uninfected persons. Evaluation should include slit-lamp examination by an ophthalmologist.

Refraction Problems

The patient may complain of blurring vision with near or distance vision. Other findings include an abnormal Snellen test or inability to read fine print. The condition may be attributable to presbyopia or other causes. Refer for ophthalmologic examination.

Iridocyclitis/Anterior Uveitis

The patient may complain of redness or watering of the eyes, constriction of the pupil, and blurred vision. Anterior-chamber inflammation is fairly common among patients with HIV infection and is often associated with CMV or HSV retinitis. Ocular bacterial infections, syphilis, toxoplasmosis, and tuberculosis can cause severe symptoms. Fungal retinitis rarely causes iridocyclitis. Other causes include other systemic conditions (e.g., reactive arthritis, sarcoidosis) and drug toxicity (e.g., rifabutin, cidofovir, ethambutol). Evaluation should include slit-lamp examination by an ophthalmologist.

Treatment should be directed at the causative pathogen or illness. If drug toxicity is suspected, the offending drug should be discontinued or reduced in dosage, if possible. Topical steroids may be indicated as an adjunctive measure. CMV IRIS may present as posterior uveitis; for suspected IRIS, consult an HIV-experienced ophthalmologist.

HIV Retinopathy

The patient typically has no symptoms, but may complain of blurred vision, visual field defects, floaters, or flashing lights. Cotton wool spots on the retina appear as small fluffy white lesions with indistinct borders and without exudates or hemorrhages. Usually, these findings are benign and do not progress. Refer for ophthalmologic examination to rule out other causes.

CMV Retinitis

Patients with retinitis caused by CMV infection may be asymptomatic or may experience blurred vision, floaters, scotomata, or central or peripheral vision loss or distortion. Retinal examination shows creamy to yellowish lesions, white granular areas with perivascular exudates, and hemorrhages ("cottage cheese and ketchup"). The abnormalities initially appear in the periphery, but progress if untreated to involve the macula and optic disc. CMV is a common complication of advanced HIV infection in patients with CD4 counts of <50 cells/μL. Vision loss usually is permanent. Urgent ophthalmology consultation and initiation of anti-CMV therapy are required. See chapter *Cytomegalovirus Disease*.

Acute Retinal Necrosis

The patient may complain of eye pain, decreased visual acuity, and floaters. Rapidly progressing peripheral necrosis frequently causes blindness. Retinal necrosis usually is caused by VZV, although HSV and CMV also have been implicated. Treatment should be initiated urgently.

Toxoplasma Retinochoroiditis

Toxoplasma retinochoroiditis may occur in patients with CD4 counts of <100 cells/μL and cause blurred vision, visual field defects, floaters, or flashing lights. In HIV-infected patients, ocular manifestations often appear after the infection of the central nervous system with *Toxoplasma* (see chapter *Toxoplasmosis*). Retinal examination may reveal yellow-white infiltrates without hemorrhage and active vitreous inflammation. Evaluation requires consultation with an HIV-experienced ophthalmologist. If toxoplasmosis is confirmed or strongly suspected, treatment should be initiated as quickly as possible.

Neuro-Ophthalmologic Manifestations

Symptoms or signs of papilledema, optic neuritis, cranial nerve palsies, and visual field defects may indicate encephalopathy, increased intracranial pressure, neurosyphilis, toxoplasmosis, progressive multifocal leukoencephalopathy, meningitis, or central nervous system lymphomas. A thorough neurologic examination is required to determine whether additional diagnostic testing, such as imaging studies or cerebrospinal fluid testing, is needed in addition to ophthalmologic evaluation.

Retinal Detachment

The patient may complain of flashes of light, sudden loss of vision, or both. This condition requires immediate referral to an emergency department.

Patient Education

- Patients should report any changes in vision to their health care provider as soon as possible.

- Routine eye examinations should be part of the patient's primary care.

- Patients with CD4 counts of <50 cells/µL should be examined by an ophthalmologist at baseline and every 6 months thereafter.

References

- Ahmed I, Ai E, Chang E, et al. *Ophthalmic Manifestations of HIV.* In: Coffey S, Volberding PA, eds. *HIV InSite Knowledge Base* [textbook online]; San Francisco: UCSF Center for HIV Information; August 2005. Accessed June 30, 2010.

- Centers for Disease Control and Prevention. *Guidelines for Prevention and Treatment of Opportunistic Infections in HIV-Infected Adults and Adolescents: Recommendations from CDC, the National Institutes of Health, and the HIV Medicine Association of the Infectious Diseases Society of America.* April 10, 2009. Available at www.aidsinfo.nih.gov/guidelines/.

- Copeland R. Ocular *Manifestations of HIV.* eMedicine.com [online medical reference]; January 20, 2005. Accessed June 30, 2010.

- Cunningham Jr ET. *Ocular Complications of HIV Infection.* In: Sande MA, Volberding PA, eds. *Medical Management of AIDS*, 6th ed. Philadelphia: WB Saunders, 1999;171-184.

- Gnann JW Jr. *Varicella-Zoster Virus Infections.* In Dolin R, Masur H, Saag MS, eds. *AIDS Therapy.* New York: Churchill Livingstone; 1999.

- Jacobson M. *Clinical Implications of Immune Reconstitution in AIDS.* In: Coffey S, Volberding PA, eds. *HIV InSite Knowledge Base* [textbook online]; San Francisco: UCSF Center for HIV Information; January 2005. Accessed June 30, 2010.

Fatigue

Background

Fatigue is one of the most common and debilitating complaints of HIV-infected people, with an estimated prevalence of 20-69%. It is defined by Aaronson et al. as "a decreased capacity for physical and/or mental activity due to an imbalance in the availability, utilization, and/or restoration of resources needed to perform activity." The consequences of severe fatigue may include curtailment of work and other activities, need for frequent breaks, limitations in involvement with family and friends, and difficulty completing even the simplest household chores.

In HIV-infected individuals, fatigue may be caused by several comorbid conditions or by HIV itself. HIV-related fatigue is a broad term referring to fatigue that begins or significantly worsens after the patient is infected with HIV and that has no other identifiable causes. HIV-infected people with fatigue should be evaluated carefully for reversible causes, such as depression, anemia, hypogonadism, insomnia, and medication adverse effects, and should be treated aggressively if these are found. In some patients, fatigue may be related to advanced immunosuppression (with low CD4 cell counts) or to high levels of circulating HIV virus. Unfortunately, for many patients, a specific cause of fatigue is not identified. Research to date suggests that fatigue in many HIV-infected individuals may result from a complex interplay between physiologic and psychosocial variables, and studies are being conducted to define factors related to the onset or worsening of fatigue.

S: Subjective

The patient complains of tiredness, easy fatigability, a lack of energy, a need for frequent rest or naps, or waking in the morning feeling unrefreshed. The patient may report difficulty working, difficulty concentrating, inability to exercise without experiencing profound fatigue, or impairment in social relations because of fatigue.

Consider the following during the history:

- No objective clinical indicators exist for fatigue; thus, making a diagnosis of fatigue rests on subjective data.

- Fatigue assessment tools may help in diagnosing fatigue and estimating its severity. One such tool, the HIV-Related Fatigue Scale, was developed specifically for use with HIV-infected individuals (see Barroso and Lynn in "References," below); this assesses the intensity of fatigue (on the day of the assessment and during the previous week), the circumstances surrounding fatigue (including patterns), and the consequences of fatigue.

- Take a thorough history of the fatigue symptoms, including onset, duration, exacerbating and alleviating factors, and associated symptoms. Evaluate for symptoms of other conditions that cause fatigue (e.g., hypothyroidism, hypogonadism, anemia, heart failure, poor nutrition).

- Depression can cause significant fatigue and is common among HIV-infected patients with fatigue. Screen the patient for depression. A single question — "Are you depressed?" — has been shown to be as valid and reliable as most depression instruments. See chapter *Depression* for further information.

- Inquire about social history, specifically any life stressors including those related to housing status, work stress, personal relationships, etc.

- Evaluate the patient's sleep patterns. HIV infection can interfere with sleep architecture early in the illness.

- Inquire about substance use or abuse.

- Obtain a list of all current medications, including herbal and over-the-counter preparations.

- Conduct a nutritional assessment.

O: Objective

Check vital signs and orthostatic blood pressure and heart rate measurements, if indicated. Perform a physical examination including evaluation of nutritional status, affect, conjunctivae and skin (for pallor), thyroid, lungs and heart, and deep tendon reflexes.

A: Assessment

The differential diagnosis includes the following:

- Anemia

- Hypothyroidism

- Hypogonadism

- Depression

- Insomnia or poor-quality sleep

- Substance use or abuse

- Malnutrition

- Medication adverse effects (e.g., zidovudine, interferon)

- Opportunistic infections, malignancy, chronic hepatitis B or C, mononucleosis, other illnesses

- Pregnancy

P: Plan

Diagnostic Evaluation

To rule out reversible causes of fatigue, perform laboratory tests, including:

- Hemoglobin and hematocrit

- Thyroid function tests

- Testosterone (in both men and women)

- Pregnancy test, if applicable

Fatigue assessment tools, as mentioned above, may be used to assess the intensity of fatigue, the circumstances surrounding fatigue, and the consequences of fatigue.

Treatment

If testing reveals a specific cause of fatigue, treat appropriately. For example:

- Treat anemia, hypothyroidism, or hypogonadism, as indicated.

- Treat depression with antidepressant medication, psychotherapy, or both; see chapter *Depression*.

- Treat insomnia and review good sleep-hygiene practices with the patient; see chapter *Insomnia*.

- Refer for treatment of substance use or abuse, if possible.

- Provide counseling regarding any current life stressors that may be contributing to fatigue. Involve social work and case management services regarding housing issues or other social needs that may be contributing to fatigue.

- Treat malnutrition, ideally in conjunction with a nutritionist.

- Treat opportunistic infections and other illnesses. (See section *Comorbidities, Coinfections, and Complications*.)

- Control other symptoms that could be causing fatigue (e.g., diarrhea).

- If fatigue seems to be related to antiretroviral medication(s), weigh the benefits of the medication(s) against the possible adverse effects, and discuss these with the patient.

After appropriate evaluation, if the fatigue is thought to be related to HIV infection or if no specific cause is identified, consider the following:

- If HIV infection is inadequately controlled, particularly if the CD4 count is low or the HIV viral load is high, initiate or optimize antiretroviral therapy (ART), if otherwise appropriate.

- Patients taking effective ART may still experience HIV-related fatigue. Prepare patients for the possibility that fatigue may persist despite ART initiation.

- Encourage patients to track their patterns of fatigue with a fatigue diary if necessary. Once patients recognize their individual patterns, they can better cope with fatigue by planning their daily activities accordingly (e.g., performing the most strenuous tasks during times of peak energy or staggering activities to avoid excessive fatigue).

- Ask patients what seems to aggravate their fatigue. This information, too, will help patients determine their patterns of fatigue and identify self-care actions they might take to avoid triggers that will worsen the fatigue.

- Recommend moderate exercise and frequent rest.

- Refer the patient to community-based agencies for assistance with housekeeping.

- Evaluate the need for occupational therapy (e.g., energy conservation techniques) or physical therapy (e.g., reconditioning and strengthening exercises).

- Medications such as stimulants (e.g., methylphenidate, modafinil) may be helpful for some patients with severe or debilitating fatigue.

Patient Education

- Fatigue is often unrelated to the CD4 cell count or HIV viral load. Teach patients not to dismiss feelings of fatigue if they have higher CD4 counts and lower viral loads. Encourage them to discuss their symptoms with a provider.

- For patients with depression, advise them that appropriate treatment may reduce fatigue.

- Help patients identify how current life circumstances and stressors may contribute to fatigue and encourage them to seek the appropriate social services to help manage appropriately.

- Talk to patients about their sleep habits and recommend changes, as appropriate, to improve their sleep hygiene.

- Prepare patients to accept the fact that their fatigue (in some cases) may be a chronic condition, in which case it can be best managed by maintaining open communication with their provider and remaining engaged in care.

References

- Aaronson LS, Teel CS, Cassmeyer V, et al. *Defining and measuring fatigue.* Image J Nurs Sch. 1999;31(1):45-50.

- Barroso J. *Just Worn Out: A Qualitative Study of HIV-Related Fatigue.* In: Funk SG, Tornquist EM, Leeman J, et al., eds. *Key Aspects of Preventing and Managing Chronic Illness.* New York: Springer, 2001;183-194.

- Barroso J, Carlson JR, Meynell J. *Physiological and psychological markers associated with HIV-related fatigue.* Clin Nurs Res. 2003 Feb;12(1):49-68.

- Barroso J, Lynn MR. *Psychometric properties of the HIV-Related Fatigue Scale.* J Assoc Nurses AIDS Care. 2002 Jan-Feb;13(1):66-75.

- Barroso J, Preisser JS, Leserman J, et al. *Predicting fatigue and depression in HIV-positive gay men.* Psychosomatics. 2002 Jul-Aug;43(4):317-25.

- Breitbart W, McDonald MV, Rosenfeld B, et al. *Fatigue in ambulatory AIDS patients.* J Pain Symptom Manage. 1998 Mar;15(3):159-67.

- Chochinov HM, Wilson KG, Enns M, et al. *"Are you depressed?" Screening for depression in the terminally ill.* Am J Psychiatry. 1997 May;154(5):674-6.

- Darko DF, Miller JC, Gallen C, et al. *Sleep electroencephalogram delta-frequency amplitude, night plasma levels of tumor necrosis factor alpha, and human immunodeficiency virus infection.* Proc Natl Acad Sci USA. 1995 Dec 19;92(26):12080-4.

- Duran S, Spire B, Raffi F, et al. *Self-reported symptoms after initiation of a protease inhibitor in HIV-infected patients and their impact on adherence to HAART.* HIV Clin Trials. 2001 Jan-Feb;2(1):38-45.

- Fontaine A, Larue F, Lassauniere JM. *Physicians' recognition of the symptoms experienced by HIV patients: how reliable?* J Pain Symptom Manage. 1999 Oct;18(4):263-70.

- Molassiotis A, Callaghan P, Twinn SF, et al. *Correlates of quality of life in symptomatic HIV patients living in Hong Kong.* AIDS Care. 2001 Jun;13(3):319-34.

- Phillips KD, Sowell RL, Rojas M, et al. *Physiological and psychological correlates of fatigue in HIV disease.* Biol Res Nurs. 2004 Jul;6(1):59-74.

- Sullivan PS, Dworkin MS, Adult and Adolescent Spectrum of HIV Disease Investigators. *Prevalence and correlates of fatigue among persons with HIV infection.* J Pain Symptom Manage. 2003 Apr;25(4):329-33.

- Vogl D, Rosenfeld B, Breitbart W, et al. *Symptom prevalence, characteristics, and distress in AIDS outpatients.* J Pain Symptom Manage. 1999 Oct;18(4):253-62.

- Voss JG. *Predictors and correlates of fatigue in African-Americans with HIV/AIDS.* Paper presented at the Association of Nurses in AIDS Care 15th Annual Conference; November 7-10, 2002; San Francisco.

Fever

Background

Although fever may accompany HIV infection at various stages of disease, fever in a patient with a low CD4 count (<200 cells/μL) should prompt the clinician to rule out opportunistic infections.

S: Subjective

The patient complains of persistent fever, or new-onset fever of >101°F (38.3°C).

Assess the following during the history:

- Duration of fever
- Associated symptoms, including chills, sweats, weight loss
- Visual disturbances (see chapter *Eye Problems*)
- Nasal or sinus symptoms
- Asymmetric, tender, or new lymphadenopathy
- Cough or shortness or breath (see chapter *Pulmonary Symptoms*)
- Diarrhea, tenesmus (see chapter *Diarrhea*)
- Rash, lesions, soft-tissue inflammation
- Pain (for headache, see chapter *Headache*)
- Neurologic symptoms (see chapter *Neurologic Symptoms*)
- Vaginal or urethral discharge
- Other localizing symptoms
- Unprotected sexual contacts
- Recent injection drug use
- Intravenous line or venous access device
- Travel within the past 6-12 months
- Medications (as a cause of fever)
- Use of antipyretic agents including aspirin, nonsteroidal antiinflammatory drugs (NSAIDs), and acetaminophen; when was most recent dose taken?

O: Objective

Document fever. Check other vital signs, including orthostatic measurements. Check weight and compare with previous values.

Search for evidence of an infectious focus. Perform a complete physical examination, including evaluation of the eyes (including fundus), sinuses, oropharynx, lymph nodes, lungs and heart, abdomen, joints, genitals, uterus, rectum, skin, and neurologic system.

Review recent CD4 measurements, if available, to determine the patient's risk of opportunistic illnesses as a cause of fever.

A: Assessment

The differential diagnosis varies depending on the CD4 count. Possibilities include the following:

Conditions More Likely with Low CD4 Count

- Aspergillosis
- Cryptococcosis
- Cytomegalovirus infection (CMV)
- Disseminated *Mycobacterium avium* complex (MAC)
- Disseminated histoplasmosis
- HIV infection itself
- Lymphoma, other neoplasms
- *Pneumocystis jiroveci* pneumonia (PCP)
- Sinusitis
- Toxoplasmosis
- Tuberculosis (atypical or extrapulmonary)

Conditions That May Occur with Any CD4 Count

- Abscess, cellulitis
- Acute hepatitis
- Autoimmune process
- Bacteremia or sepsis
- Bacterial pneumonia or bronchitis
- Disseminated herpes simplex virus; chicken pox
- Drug-induced fever (common culprits include abacavir, nevirapine, sulfonamides, dapsone, amphotericin, pentamidine, thalidomide, penicillin, clindamycin, carbamazepine, phenytoin, barbiturates, and bleomycin)
- Endocarditis
- Immune reconstitution syndromes, related to opportunistic infections, are often associated with fever (see chapter *Immune Reconstitution Inflammatory Syndrome*)
- Influenza
- Otitis
- Malaria
- Pelvic inflammatory disease (PID)
- Sexually transmitted infections
- Tuberculosis (pulmonary)
- Urinary tract infection (UTI)

P: Plan

Diagnostic Evaluation

Perform laboratory work and other diagnostic studies as suggested by the history, physical examination, and differential diagnosis. These may include the following:

- CD4 count (if not done recently) to help with risk stratification for opportunistic illnesses
- Complete blood count (CBC) with differential

- Blood cultures (bacterial, mycobacterial, fungal)
- Urinalysis, urine culture if UTI symptoms are present
- Liver transaminases, renal panel
- Chest X ray
- Sinus films if indicated by symptoms and physical examination findings
- If respiratory symptoms and signs are present: sputum evaluation (Gram stain and acid-fast bacilli smear, evaluation for PCP), with culture of sputum for bacterial pathogens, acid-fast bacilli, viruses, and fungi as indicated; consider sputum induction or bronchoscopy if indicated
- Serum cryptococcal antigen, if CD4 count is <100 cells/μL and symptoms are consistent with cryptococcosis
- If neurological symptoms and signs are present: computed tomography (CT) or magnetic resonance imaging (MRI) of head, lumbar puncture
- For new lymphadenopathy: aspirate with culture, including acid-fast bacilli and fungal cytology
- For cytopenias: bone marrow aspirate and biopsy may be needed; see applicable treatment guidelines
- For fever of unknown origin (FUO), defined as persistent fever >101°F for >3 weeks without findings on initial workup, more intensive workup may be needed, such as lumbar puncture, other scans or biopsies; consult with a specialist in infectious diseases or an HIV expert to determine whether hospitalization or other laboratory tests are needed
- For patients who recently started abacavir or nevirapine, or other medications, rule out hypersensitivity reactions (see chapter *Adverse Reactions to HIV Medications*)

Treatment

Once a diagnosis is made, appropriate treatment should be initiated. In seriously ill patients, presumptive treatment may be started while diagnostic tests are pending. In some cases, the source of fever cannot be identified. Consult with an HIV expert.

Symptomatic treatment may include NSAIDs (e.g., ibuprofen, naproxen), acetaminophen, and analgesics. Monitor for gastrointestinal adverse effects with NSAIDs. Cold compresses also can be used to relieve fever symptoms. Refer to a dietitian to avoid weight loss during the hypermetabolic state. See section *Disease-Specific Treatment* in this manual if an HIV-related cause is identified.

Patient Education

- Patients should report any new fever to their health care provider. They should measure their temperature using a thermometer at home in order to report actual temperatures.

- Patients should know that fever usually is a sign that their bodies are battling an infection. Their health care providers may need to do special tests to find out what could be causing the fever.

- Many over-the-counter remedies are available to treat fevers. Patients should check with their care provider before taking these. Acetaminophen-containing products (e.g., Tylenol) generally are well tolerated. Persons with liver disease should use acetaminophen only as prescribed. NSAIDs (ibuprofen, naproxen, etc.) may be used, but they can cause gastrointestinal adverse effects, especially if taken without food. Patients should let their care provider know if they need to take these medicines for more than 2 or 3 days.

References

- Bartlett JG, Gallant JE, Pham PA. 2009-2010 *Medical Management of HIV Infection.* Baltimore: Johns Hopkins University School of Medicine; 2009. Available online at hopkins-aids.edu.

- Cross KJ, Hines, JM, Gluckman SJ. *Fever of Unknown Origin.* In: Buckley RM, Gluckman SJ, eds. *HIV Infection in Primary Care 2002.* Philadelphia: WB Saunders; 2002.

Headache

Background

Headache in HIV-infected persons may result from many causes, particularly if the CD4 cell count is low. Possible causes include infections (opportunistic and other) and central nervous system malignancies, HIV-related systemic illnesses, and medication toxicity. In addition, of course, headache may be caused by any of the processes that cause headache in HIV-uninfected individuals. New or severe headache should be evaluated carefully.

S: Subjective

The patient complains of a new type of headache.

Determine the following during the history:

- History of headaches or migraines
- Characteristics of the headache (location, quality of pain, timing, duration, etc.)
- Recent head trauma
- Fever
- History of sinusitis
- Allergies
- Visual changes
- Dizziness, vertigo, nausea
- Mental status changes
- Seizures
- Focal or other neurologic symptoms (see chapter *Neurologic Symptoms*)
- New rashes or ulcerations
- Other symptoms
- Caffeine intake; recent changes in intake
- New medications (e.g., zidovudine)
- Relief of headache by any medication
- Unprotected sex, new sex partner

O: Objective

Perform a physical examination as follows:

- Check vital signs. Look for fever, orthostasis, and hypertension.
- Examine the head and neck for trauma, sinus tenderness, scalp or temple tenderness, and neck mobility; check lymph nodes.
- Check the eyes, including funduscopic examination, for lesions or papilledema.
- Look for oral lesions, dental abscess, thrush, and pharyngeal drainage.
- Examine the lungs for abnormal sounds.
- Check the skin, including palms and soles, for rashes or lesions.
- Perform a complete neurologic examination, including mental status examination.
- Review recent CD4 measurements, if available, to determine the patient's risk of opportunistic illnesses as a cause of headache.

A: Assessment

A partial differential diagnosis includes the following:

- Cryptococcal meningitis
- Neurosyphilis
- Tuberculous meningitis; other meningitis
- Progressive multifocal leukoencephalopathy (PML)
- Toxoplasmic encephalitis
- Cytomegalovirus (CMV) meningoencephalitis or retinitis
- Other encephalitis
- Central nervous system lymphoma
- Systemic infection
- Sinusitis
- Anemia
- Fever
- Medication adverse effect
- Stress or tension headache
- Migraine or cluster headache
- Temporal arteritis
- Depression, anxiety disorder
- Caffeine withdrawal
- Hypertension
- Dehydration

Other causes of headache unrelated to HIV should be considered.

P: Plan

Diagnostic Evaluation

Evaluation should include the following:

- CD4 cell count (if not done recently), to help with risk stratification for opportunistic illnesses
- Complete blood count with differential (if fever or suspected anemia); see chapter *Fever*
- Blood chemistries, including liver function tests, electrolytes, creatinine, glucose
- Serum cryptococcal antigen (if fever is present and CD4 count is <100 cells/µL); see chapter *Cryptococcal Disease*
- *Toxoplasma* immunoglobulin G (if previously negative and CD4 count is <200 cells/µL); see chapter *Toxoplasmosis*
- Syphilis testing: rapid plasma reagin (RPR) or Venereal Disease Research Laboratory (VDRL) test; see chapter *Syphilis*

When indicated, also consider:

- Computed tomography (CT) scan with contrast or magnetic resonance imaging of the head; see chapter *Neurologic Symptoms*
- Lumbar puncture with cerebrospinal fluid (CSF) studies to include opening pressure, cell count, chemistries, bacterial cultures; fungal and acid-fast bacilli evaluations and cultures; India ink stain; cryptococcal antigen, VDRL, as indicated
- Sinus imaging
- Erythrocyte sedimentation rate, if temporal arteritis is suspected

Treatment

- Once a diagnosis is made, appropriate treatment should be initiated. In seriously ill patients, presumptive treatment may be initiated while diagnostic test results are pending. In some cases, the source of headache cannot be identified. Consult with an HIV expert or a neurologist.

- Refer to disease-specific treatment guidelines or primary care management guidelines as appropriate.

- Treat symptomatically with nonsteroidal antiinflammatory drugs (NSAIDs), acetaminophen, or narcotics, if indicated, to control pain.

Patient Education

- Headache can be a sign of an opportunistic infection, especially in patients with low CD4 cell counts. Patients should notify their health care provider if they develop a new headache.

- Providers should inform patients that they may have to do additional tests to determine the cause of the headache.

- Many over-the-counter remedies are available for headache. Patients should check with their health care providers before taking these. Acetaminophen-containing products (e.g., Tylenol) generally are well tolerated. Persons with liver disease should use acetaminophen only as prescribed. NSAIDs (e.g., ibuprofen, naproxen) may be used, but these agents can cause gastrointestinal adverse effects, especially if taken without food. Patients should inform their care provider if they need to take these medicines for more than 2 or 3 days.

References

- McGuire D. *Neurologic Manifestations of HIV.* In: Coffey S, Volberding PA, eds. *HIV InSite Knowledge Base* [textbook online]; San Francisco: UCSF Center for HIV Information; June 2003.

Lymphadenopathy

Background

Lymphadenopathy is very common among HIV-infected individuals and may occur at any stage of HIV infection. It may be the first indication of a serious local or systemic condition, and it should be evaluated carefully. Rapid enlargement of a previously stable lymph node or a group of nodes requires evaluation to identify the cause and to determine whether treatment is needed. Similarly, nodes that are abnormal in consistency, tender to palpation, fluctuant, asymmetrical, adherent to surrounding tissues, or accompanied by other symptoms should be evaluated promptly.

Lymphadenopathy may be generalized or localized and usually is characterized by lymph nodes that are >1 cm in diameter. A multitude of conditions can cause lymphadenopathy, including HIV itself, opportunistic or other infections, and malignancies. The likely causes of lymphadenopathy, and thus the diagnostic workup, will depend in part on the patient's degree of immunosuppression. The risk of opportunistic and certain malignant conditions increases at lower CD4 cell counts (see chapter *Risk of HIV Progression/Indications for ART*).

Many individuals with primary HIV infection (see chapter *Primary HIV Infection*) have generalized lymphadenopathy that may resolve or may persist for months to years. If lymphadenopathy of >2 cm in size occurs in two or more noncontiguous sites and persists for more than 3 months, and if appropriate evaluation reveals no other cause, the patient is diagnosed with persistent generalized lymphadenopathy (PGL). PGL usually is caused by follicular hyperplasia from chronic HIV infection. As long as enlarged nodes are stable in number, location, and size, persons with PGL require no specific management other than monitoring of nodes at each physical examination (though consideration should be given to initiation of antiretroviral therapy [ART]). Changes in the character of the lymph nodes should prompt further evaluation. Rapid involution of PGL may occur with advanced HIV disease and is a poor prognostic sign.

S: Subjective

The patient complains of new, worsening, or persistent glandular swellings in the neck, axilla, groin, or elsewhere.

Ascertain the following during the history:

- Symptoms that accompany the lymphadenopathy, particularly constitutional symptoms such as fever, sweats, fatigue, and unintentional weight loss
- Localized symptoms or conditions that involve areas of the body with lymphatic drainage into the area of abnormal lymph nodes (e.g., in the case of axillary lymphadenopathy, ask about breast masses and skin conditions or trauma involving the arm)
- A full review of systems
- HIV-related or other malignancies, opportunistic illnesses
- Recent travel, country or region of origin, disease exposures (e.g., tuberculosis [TB], sexually transmitted infections), and risk behaviors (e.g., injection drug use)
- Recent initiation of ART (may indicate immune reconstitution inflammatory syndrome [IRIS])
- Trauma or injury (including cat scratches)
- Exposure to household pets
- Current medications

O: Objective

Review recent CD4 cell counts and HIV viral load measurements.

- Check vital signs.

- Perform a complete examination of lymph nodes, including the cervical, submandibular, supraclavicular, axillary, epitrochlear, and inguinal sites. Document the location, size, consistency, mobility, and presence or absence of tenderness of all abnormal nodes. In cases of localized lymphadenopathy, examine the area drained by the node.

- Check for hepatosplenomegaly.

- Perform a focused examination (e.g., lung, breast, skin, genitals) to identify signs of local or systemic illness.

A: Assessment

The differential diagnosis of lymphadenopathy in HIV-infected patients depends in part on the degree of immunosuppression. For further information, see chapter *Risk of HIV Progression/Indications for ART.*

Infectious Causes
Generalized lymphadenopathy

- HIV infection, including PGL

- Mononucleosis; Epstein-Barr virus

- *Mycobacterium avium* complex

- TB

- Cytomegalovirus

- Secondary syphilis

- Toxoplasmosis

- Histoplasmosis, other fungal diseases

- *Bartonella* infection

- Hepatitis B

- Lyme disease

- Widespread skin infections

- IRIS involving various infections

- Follicular hyperplasia

- Castleman disease

Localized lymphadenopathy

- Any of the above

- Oropharyngeal and dental infections

- Cellulitis or abscesses

- TB (scrofula)

- Chancroid

- Chlamydia (lymphogranuloma venereum [LGV])

- Other STIs

Neoplastic Causes

- Lymphoma

- Acute and chronic lymphocytic leukemias

- Other malignancy; metastatic cancer

- Kaposi sarcoma

Other Causes

- Reactive process (benign)

- Sarcoidosis

- Hypersensitivity reaction to medications

- Serum sickness

- Rheumatoid arthritis

P: Plan

Diagnostic Evaluation

After the history and physical examination, the cause of lymphadenopathy may be clear and further diagnostic testing may not be necessary. If the cause of the lymphadenopathy is still uncertain, perform diagnostic testing as indicated by the patient's presentation. This may include the following tests:

- CD4 count (with or without HIV viral load), to determine the risk of opportunistic illnesses

- Complete blood count with differential; liver function tests; urinalysis

- Chest X ray

- TB screening (tuberculin skin test [TST] or interferon-gamma release assay [IGRA])

- Syphilis screening (rapid plasma reagin [RPR] or Venereal Disease Research Laboratory [VDRL] test)

- Blood cultures, if patient is febrile (bacterial, mycobacterial, and fungal, as indicated)

- Testing for specific infections if suspected (e.g., *Bartonella*, LGV)

If a node is large, fixed, nontender, or otherwise worrisome, or if the diagnosis is unclear after initial evaluation, fine-needle aspiration (FNA) biopsy may provide a diagnosis. If FNA is nondiagnostic (false-negative results are relatively common), obtain an excisional biopsy for definitive evaluation. Biopsy specimens should be sent for bacterial, mycobacterial, and fungal cultures; acid-fast staining for mycobacteria; and cytologic examination.

If a node is large, inflamed, tender, or fluctuant, and a bacterial infection is suspected, consider initiating empiric antibiotic treatment and monitoring the patient over the course of 1-2 weeks. If the node does not respond to antibiotic treatment or the patient becomes more symptomatic, arrange for FNA or open biopsy to establish the diagnosis.

Treatment

Treatment will depend on the cause of lymphadenopathy. Refer to section *Comorbidities, Coinfections, and Complications* or to OI management guidelines as appropriate. In the case of HIV-related lymphadenopathy, ART may be effective.

Patient Education

- Lymphadenopathy may come and go throughout the course of HIV infection, but it may be a sign of a serious condition.

- Advise patients to notify their care provider if lymph nodes increase in size or change in character.

References

- Boswell SL. *Approach to the Patient with HIV Infection*. In: Goroll AH, Mulley AG, eds. *Principles of Primary Care*, 5th ed. Philadelphia: JB Lippincott, 2005;78-91.

- *Evaluation of Lymphadenopathy*. In: Goroll AH, Mulley AG, eds. *Principles of Primary Care*, 5th ed. Philadelphia: JB Lippincott, 2005;73-77.

- Kocurek K, Hollander H. *Primary and Preventive Care of the HIV-Infected Adult*. In: Sande MA, Volberding PA, eds. *Medical Management of AIDS*, 6th ed. Philadelphia: WB Saunders, 1999;125-126.

Nausea and Vomiting

Background

Nausea with or without vomiting, and occasionally vomiting without nausea, can occur at any stage of HIV infection. Nausea is a common adverse effect of many antiretroviral (ARV) and other medications, and it often occurs within weeks of starting new medications. In some cases, nausea causes significant discomfort and may interfere with medication adherence. Nausea and vomiting also may be symptoms of a serious complication of ARV therapy, or signs of an opportunistic infection or neoplasm in patients with late-stage AIDS. Clinicians must identify the cause of nausea and vomiting and initiate appropriate treatment.

S: Subjective

The patient experiences nausea with or without vomiting, or vomiting without nausea.

Ascertain the following during the history:

- Duration of symptoms
- Characteristics, timing, and precipitating factors
- Vomiting, including hematemesis
- Diarrhea
- Abdominal pain
- Fever
- Jaundice
- Lightheadedness, dizziness, vertigo, or orthostatic symptoms
- Polyuria
- Polydipsia
- Headache
- Changes in vision
- Neck stiffness
- Pruritus
- Medications, new and ongoing
- Nutritional supplements and nonprescription medications
- Possibility of pregnancy (for women) (e.g., missed menses)
- Alcohol intake, substance use or abuse

- History of:
  - Hepatitis
  - Kidney disease
  - Pancreatitis
  - Cytomegalovirus
  - Central nervous system (CNS) infections, including toxoplasmosis, cryptococcosis, chronic meningitis
  - CNS lymphoma

O: Objective

Check vital signs, including orthostatic blood pressure and heart rate measurements.

Conduct a thorough physical examination, including evaluation of the following:

- Skin turgor
- Eyes and fundi (retinal abnormalities such as papilledema)
- Oropharynx (dryness of oral mucosa, thrush, ulcerations)
- Neck (stiffness or other signs of meningeal irritation)
- Abdomen (tenderness, distention, masses, organomegaly)
- Pelvis (tenderness, masses)
- Neurologic system (mental status, focal neurologic abnormalities)

Section 5: Common Complaints

Review recent CD4 measurements, if available, to determine the patient's risk of opportunistic illnesses.

A: Assessment

A partial differential diagnosis includes the following conditions:

- Medication effect or reaction
- Foodborne illness
- Pancreatitis
- Hepatitis, infectious or drug related (see chapters *Hepatitis B Infection* and *Hepatitis C Infection*)
- Appendicitis
- Esophagitis (see chapter *Esophageal Problems*)
- Lactic acidosis attributable to nucleoside analogues
- Pregnancy
- Adrenal insufficiency
- CNS lymphoma
- Meningitis
- Uremia
- Diabetic ketoacidosis
- Influenza
- Pelvic inflammatory disease (see chapter *Pelvic Inflammatory Disease*)
- Myocardial infarction

P: Plan

Diagnostic Evaluation

Perform laboratory work and other diagnostic studies as suggested by the history, physical examination, and differential diagnosis. Tests may include the following:

- Complete blood count with differential
- Electrolytes, creatinine, blood urea nitrogen

- Glucose
- Amylase and lipase if symptoms of pancreatitis are present
- Liver function tests and hepatitis serologies for possible acute or chronic hepatitis
- Blood cultures and other fever workup as needed (see chapter *Fever*)
- Computed tomography scan of the brain if neurologic symptoms are present (see chapter *Neurologic Symptoms*)
- Cortisol and cosyntropin stimulation test if indicated (e.g., fatigue, weakness, unexplained abdominal pain, weight loss, orthostasis; usually in late-stage AIDS)
- If odynophagia or dysphagia is present, see chapter *Esophageal Problems*
- Lactic acid levels if lactic acidosis is suspected
- Pregnancy test if indicated
- Electrocardiogram if patient has chest pain or suspicious symptoms
- Consult with an HIV expert to determine whether hospitalization or other laboratory tests are needed

Treatment

Once the diagnosis is made, appropriate treatment should be initiated. In seriously ill patients, presumptive treatment may be started while diagnostic test results are pending. See appropriate chapters in section *Comorbidities, Coinfections, and Complications* and relevant guidelines.

In the case of significant adverse effects from ARVs or other medications, substitute a less emetogenic ARV for the problematic medication, if possible (without compromising the efficacy of the treatment regimen). In the case of serious or life-threatening medication toxicities (e.g., lactic acidosis or abacavir hypersensitivity reaction), discontinue the problematic medication (see chapter *Adverse Reactions to HIV Medications*).

After the workup and exclusion of life-threatening illness, symptomatic treatment can be considered. If nausea and vomiting are attributable to medications that are vital to the patient, and these complications are not life-threatening, antiemetic therapy may be the best treatment. Chronic therapy is not always necessary. Some patients obtain adequate relief by breaking the "nausea cycle" with effective antiemetics for 1-2 days and then establishing meals or snacks with medications. Patients with dehydration may require administration of fluids (PO or IV) to relieve nausea. For patients with chronic nausea resulting in weight loss, refer to a nutritionist for assessment and nutritional support.

Symptomatic treatment

Consider the following strategies for symptomatic treatment:

- For nausea that occurs in relation to an event or action (e.g., after taking ARVs) antiemetics may be given preemptively (e.g., 30 minutes beforehand).

- Ginger capsules have proven effective in clinical trials for the management of pregnancy-related and chemotherapy-related nausea. Foods and beverages containing ginger (e.g., tea, cookies, ginger ale, candies) may help provide relief.

- Promethazine (Phenergan) may be given as a 12.5-25 mg PO tablet Q4-6H as needed. For patients unable to tolerate the PO formulation, promethazine suppositories (12.5 or 25 mg) may be used.

- Prochlorperazine (Compazine) may be given as a 5 mg or 10 mg PO tablet, or a 25 mg rectal suppository, Q6-8H as needed. Extended-release spansule, 10 mg Q12H or 15 mg QAM, also can be considered.

- Lorazepam (Ativan) may be given as a 0.5 mg PO tablet 30 minutes before taking medications for symptoms of anticipatory nausea. Patients with anticipatory nausea develop significant nausea or vomiting when even thinking about medications or reaching for the medications.

- Dronabinol (Marinol) may relieve nausea, especially when nausea is accompanied by a loss of appetite. This remedy is best tolerated by patients who have tolerated inhaled marijuana. The starting dosage is 2.5 to 5 mg BID or TID.

- 5-Hydroxytryptamine (5-HT3) receptor antagonists such as dolasetron 50 mg and 100 mg, granisetron 1 mg, and ondansetron 4 mg and 8 mg are highly effective are highly effective in relieving severe nausea and vomiting resulting from chemotherapy and other causes. However, access to these medications is limited by their cost. Their use should be considered a short-term strategy or reserved for cases of nausea/vomiting refractory to other antiemetics.

- Metoclopramide (Reglan) may be used to enhance gastrointestinal motility in patients who experience nausea and vomiting caused by gastroparesis. The typical PO dose is 5-10 mg Q4-6H, or it can be taken TID with meals if the nausea or vomiting is associated with eating.

- H2 antagonists or proton pump inhibitors may be helpful in treating nausea/vomiting related to gastritis or acid reflux (caution: these agents interfere with atazanavir absorption; consult dosing recommendations (see chapter *Esophageal Problems* and Table 15a in the U.S. Department of Health and Human Services *Guidelines for the Use of Antiretroviral Agents in HIV-1-Infected Adults and Adolescents* (see Appendix).

Patient Education

- Nausea and vomiting can have many different causes. Patients should let their health care provider know if they are having these symptoms so that the most likely cause can be determined.

- Patients should stay nourished and well hydrated even if they are experiencing nausea and vomiting. Eating small, frequent meals may be best tolerated, while avoiding dairy products, spicy or greasy foods, and high-fat meals. Taking medications with food may reduce symptoms of nausea (note that some medications must be taken on an empty stomach).

- Patients should not stop taking any of their medications without first discussing it with their health care provider. Many medications must be continued despite nausea. Nausea and vomiting owing to ARVs may resolve or become tolerable over time.

- Many patients wonder whether they should take their medicines again if they vomit after taking a dose. Generally, the medicines are still in the body unless the pills actually come back up. Patients should call their health care provider if they have any questions.

- Ginger may help to relieve nausea. Ginger can be taken in a variety of ways, including ginger ale, tea, cookies, candies, and ginger capsules. Patients can choose the form of ginger that works best for them.

References

Chubineh S, McGowan J. *Nausea and vomiting in HIV: a symptom review.* Int J STD AIDS. 2008 Nov;19(11):723-8.

Hill A, Balkin A. *Risk factors for gastrointestinal adverse events in HIV treated and untreated patients.* AIDS Rev. 2009 Jan-Mar;11(1):30-8.

Sulkowski MS, Chaisson RE. *Gastrointestinal and Hepatobiliary Manifestations of HIV Infection.* In: Mandell GL, Bennett JR, Dolin R, eds. *Principles and Practice of Infectious Diseases,* 6th ed. Philadelphia: Churchill Livingstone, 2005;1575-80.

Neurologic Symptoms

Background

The nervous system may be a site of complications throughout the course of HIV infection, and neurologic complaints are common among HIV-infected individuals. Neurologic symptoms may be caused by many factors, including infections (opportunistic and other), central nervous system (CNS) malignancies, medication toxicities, comorbid conditions (e.g., diabetes, cerebrovascular disease, chronic hepatitis, mental illness), and nervous system injuries related to HIV itself.

The risk of some conditions, such as CNS infection, malignancy, and dementia, increases with advancing immunosuppression, and the CD4 cell count will help to stratify the patient's risk of opportunistic illnesses (see Table 1 in chapter *Risk of HIV Progression/Indications for ART*. This chapter presents a general approach to neurologic symptoms in HIV-infected patients, with reference to other chapters in this manual for more detailed reading. For information on peripheral neuropathy, see chapter *Pain Syndrome and Peripheral Neuropathy*; for information on neurocognitive disease, see *HIV-Associated Dementia and Other Neurocognitive Disorders*.

S: Subjective

The patient, or a friend or family member on his or her behalf, reports new neurologic symptoms such as pain, headache, seizures, altered mental status, or weakness.

Ascertain the following during the history:

- Onset and duration: rapid (hours to days), subacute, chronic
- Characteristics of the symptoms (e.g., location, quality, timing)
- Progression or stability of symptoms
- Constitutional symptoms: fever, night sweats, unintentional weight loss
- Associated symptoms, including other neurologic, muscular, psychiatric, or behavioral symptoms
- Recent trauma to the head or other area
- Visual changes, photophobia
- Dizziness, vertigo
- Mental status changes (including changes in behavior, personality, or cognition; short-term memory loss; mental slowing; reading comprehension difficulties; changes in personal appearance and grooming habits)

- Seizures (description, duration, number)
- Pain
- Sensory symptoms
- Weakness (distinguish weakness from fatigue or pain; determine whether bilateral or focal, proximal or distal)
- Bowel or bladder changes
- Rash or ulcerations
- Medications: current, past, and recently initiated medications, including antiretroviral (ARV) medications
- Alcohol or drug use; date of last use
- Exposures (sexual, environmental), travel history
- Psychiatric history and past psychiatric care
- Most recent CD4 cell count and HIV viral load, previous AIDS-defining illnesses
- Functional impact of the symptoms: social functioning, ability to work and perform activities of daily living

Differentiate delirium from dementia. Delirium presents as acute onset of clouded sensorium, disturbed and fluctuating level of consciousness, disorientation, cognitive deficits, and reduced attention, sometimes with hallucinations. Delirium often is caused by medication toxicities, infections, hypoxia, hypoglycemia, electrolyte imbalances, or mass lesions, and it frequently is correctable. Dementia emerges more gradually and is characterized by cognitive impairment and behavioral, motor, and affective changes. See chapter *HIV-Associated Dementia and Other Neurocognitive Disorders*.

O: Objective

- Check vital signs (temperature, blood pressure, heart rate, respiratory rate, and oxygen saturation) and orthostatic measurements.
- Perform a careful physical examination as guided by the history, with special attention to the following:
  - General appearance: mood, affect, mannerisms
  - Head and neck: signs of trauma, sinus tenderness, lymph node status, neck mobility
  - Eyes, including fundi: lesions, papilledema
  - Lungs, heart: abnormal sounds
  - Extremities: muscle tone and bulk
  - Skin, mucous membranes: rash, lesions
- Conduct a thorough neurologic examination, including cranial nerves, motor function, sensory function, coordination, gait, and deep tendon reflexes.
- Conduct a mental status examination.
- Review recent CD4 measurements, if available, to determine the patient's risk of opportunistic illnesses.

A: Assessment

The differential diagnosis of neurologic abnormalities in patients with HIV infection may be broad, particularly if the CD4 count is low. Both HIV-related and HIV-unrelated causes should be considered; remember that more than one cause of symptoms may be present.

Possible Causes of Neurologic Abnormalities

Causes related to the cerebrum or cranial nerves

- Toxoplasmic encephalitis
- Primary CNS lymphoma
- Cryptococcal meningitis
- Cytomegalovirus (CMV) encephalitis
- Other meningitis (bacterial, tuberculous, fungal, viral)
- Progressive multifocal leukoencephalopathy (PML)
- Neurosyphilis
- CNS coccidioidomycosis, histoplasmosis
- HIV-related dementia
- Cerebrovascular accident; stroke
- Metabolic abnormalities, including hypo- or hyperglycemia, electrolyte abnormalities
- Alcohol or drug intoxication or withdrawal (medications or illicit drugs); chronic alcohol abuse
- Medication adverse effects (e.g., efavirenz, corticosteroids, anticholinergics, many others)
- Depression, mania, anxiety, psychosis

Causes related to the spinal cord, nerve roots, peripheral nerves, and muscle

- Inflammatory demyelinating polyneuropathy (e.g., Guillain-Barré syndrome)
- Polyradiculitis (e.g., CMV, herpes simplex virus)
- Vitamin deficiency
- Myositis
- Myopathy (e.g., owing to zidovudine)
- Myelopathy (e.g., HIV vacuolar myelopathy)
- Epidural abscess or mass
- Mononeuritis multiplex
- Lactic acidosis
- Electrolyte abnormality (e.g., hypokalemia)
- Peripheral neuropathy
- Distal sensory polyneuropathy
- Antiretroviral toxic neuropathy (especially stavudine, didanosine)
- Other neuropathy (e.g., owing to diabetes, alcohol, medications [isoniazid, dapsone, many others])

Note that organic causes of neurologic symptoms must be ruled out before concluding that symptoms are psychiatric in nature.

P: Plan

Diagnostic Evaluation

Unstable or seriously ill patients should be hospitalized for evaluation and treatment. Criteria for hospitalization include acutely altered mental status, fever with focal neurologic findings, and new or unstable seizures.

Perform laboratory work and other diagnostic studies as suggested by the history, physical examination, and differential diagnosis. This may include the following:

- Establish the CD4 count (if not done recently) to help with risk stratification for opportunistic illnesses.
- Determine which laboratory tests are appropriate, depending on the patient's presentation. The initial evaluation often includes a complete blood count with differential and monitoring of electrolyte and glucose levels.

  - In patients with CNS symptoms or signs and low CD4 counts (<100 cells/μL), check serum levels of toxoplasma antibody (IgG) if not previously checked. Check serum cryptococcal antigen (CrAg) titer.
  - In patients with symptoms of neuropathy or dementia, check serum levels of vitamin B12 and thyroid-stimulating hormone (TSH).
  - In patients with cranial nerve abnormalities, meningoencephalitis, symptoms of dementia, or any symptoms of neurosyphilis, check syphilis serology by rapid plasma regain (RPR), Venereal Disease Research Laboratory (VDRL) test, or treponemal enzyme immunoassay (see chapter *Syphilis*).

- When CNS symptoms or signs are present, brain imaging by computed tomography (CT) scan with contrast is usually adequate as the initial test. Magnetic resonance imaging (MRI) is the modality of choice if the neurologic examination is nonfocal or if physical examination suggests a lesion in the posterior fossa.
- For patients with fever and CNS findings, perform lumbar puncture (LP) with cerebrospinal fluid (CSF) sampling. CT or MRI should be performed before the LP, if possible, to rule out a mass lesion that could cause herniation.
- Record the opening pressure, and send CSF for cell count and differential with protein and glucose measurements. Depending on the clinical suspicion, the fluid also should

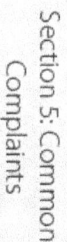

Section 5: Common Complaints

be sent for bacterial culture, India ink stain for fungal organisms (75-85% sensitive), acid-fast bacilli smear and culture, VDRL test, and CrAg titer (95% sensitive).

- If CMV is suspected, perform polymerase chain reaction (PCR) for CMV DNA (62-100% sensitivity; 89-100% specificity).

- If PML is suspected, perform CSF PCR analysis for JC virus DNA (sensitivity approximately 70-90% with patients not taking ART; specificity 92-100%).

- For suspected drug or alcohol use, perform urine or serum toxicology screen. (Note that alcohol usually has been metabolized by the time withdrawal symptoms set in, typically 7-48 hours after the last alcohol intake.)

- For new-onset seizures, perform an electroencephalogram (EEG.)

- Consult with neurology specialists if the workup or the diagnosis is in question.

Treatment

Specific treatment will depend on the cause of neurologic symptoms. Consult relevant chapters in this manual. For complex cases, consult with an HIV-experienced neurologist.

Patient Education

- Inform patients that keeping the CD4 count >200 cells/μL (and preferably higher) with ART is the best way to prevent most HIV-associated neurologic diseases.

- Advise patients to take prophylaxis, as appropriate, to prevent opportunistic infections.

- When an antibiotic treatment is prescribed, advise patients to complete the entire regimen to prevent relapse of symptoms. Long-term treatment (secondary prophylaxis) will be needed to prevent recurrence of certain infections.

- Advise patients who have seizures that driving and other potentially dangerous activities will be prohibited until the condition is stable.

- Counsel patients to avoid substances that impair the nervous system, such as alcohol and recreational drugs.

- If a patient is forgetful, educate other members of the household about the medication regimen and help devise a plan for adherence to medications and appointments.

References

- Cantor CR, McCluskey L. *CNS Complications*. In: Buckley RM, Gluckman SJ, eds. *HIV Infection in Primary Care*. New York: WB Saunders; 2002.

- McArthur JC, Brew BJ, Nath A. *Neurological complications of HIV infection*. Lancet Neurol. 2005 Sep;4(9):543-55.

- McGuire D. *Neurologic Manifestations of HIV*. In: Coffey S, Volberding PA, eds. *HIV InSite Knowledge Base* [textbook online]. San Francisco: UCSF Center for HIV Information; 2003.

- Portegies P, Solod L, Cinque P, et al. *Guidelines for the diagnosis and management of neurological complications of HIV infection*. Eur J Neurol. 2004 May;11(5):297-304.

- Saguil A. *Evaluation of the patient with muscle weakness*. Am Fam Physician. 2005 Apr 1;71(7):1327-36.

Pulmonary Symptoms

Background

Shortness of breath and cough are common manifestations of acute or chronic respiratory diseases, but also may be symptoms of HIV-related opportunistic infections. Further, these symptoms may indicate nonpulmonary conditions such as anemia, cardiovascular disease, and sinusitis, or adverse effects of medications such as angiotensin-converting enzyme inhibitors (ACEIs).

The onset and duration of symptoms, and the presence or absence of other factors such as sputum production, fever, and weight loss, will guide the evaluation. In addition, the patient's CD4 cell count will establish a context for the evaluation, because it will help to stratify the risk of opportunistic infections.

S: Subjective

The patient complains of dyspnea or cough.

Determine the following factors relating to the patient's history:

Recent History

- Onset and duration of symptoms: rapid (hours to days), subacute, chronic
- Progression or stability of symptoms
- Dyspnea at rest or with exertion
- Cough: productive (character of sputum), hemoptysis
- Associated symptoms (e.g., chest pain, pleuritic pain)
- Constitutional symptoms: fever, night sweats, unintentional weight loss
- Sinus congestion, facial tenderness, postnasal discharge, sore throat
- Orthopnea, paroxysmal nocturnal dyspnea (PND), peripheral edema
- Wheezing

Past History

- CD4 nadir, current CD4 count
- If the CD4 count is <200 cells/μL, ask whether the patient is taking *Pneumocystis jiroveci* pneumonia (PCP) prophylaxis (primary or secondary); if taking PCP

prophylaxis and adhering to the regimen, the diagnosis of PCP is less likely

- Tuberculosis (TB): date and result of tuberculin skin test (TST) or interferon-gamma release assay (IGRA), risk factors for *Mycobacterium tuberculosis*
- PCP, bacterial or other pneumonia, bronchitis
- Smoking (and secondhand smoke exposure), pack-years, related symptoms
- Cardiovascular diseases, including congestive heart failure, coronary heart disease, arrhythmia, pulmonary hypertension
- Asthma, emphysema
- Pollen, dander, or dust allergies
- Drug allergies, specifically to penicillins and sulfa drugs
- Medications (e.g., ACEIs)
- Travel history (exposure to regions endemic for particular infections, such as coccidioidomycosis or histoplasmosis)
- Use of inhaled stimulants, injection drugs
- Prolonged exposure (via inhalation) to chemicals or other harmful pulmonary irritants (e.g., asbestos)

O: Objective

Check vital signs, oxygen saturation (resting and after exercise), and weight.

Conduct a thorough physical examination that includes evaluation of the following:

- Ears, nose, oropharynx
- Neck
- Lungs
- Heart
- Extremities

Note: If patients are coughing, strongly consider having them wear a surgical mask in the clinic or office until TB or other transmissible infection is ruled out. Covering both the nose and the mouth should prevent the discharge of infectious particles into the environment.

A: Assessment

The differential diagnosis of pulmonary symptoms is broad (see Table 1). Both HIV-related and HIV-unrelated causes should be considered; the patient's risk of HIV-related causes is strongly influenced by the CD4 count. More than one cause of symptoms may be present.

Table 1. Partial Differential Diagnosis of Pulmonary Symptoms

CD4 Cell Count	Possible Cause
Any Count	• Upper respiratory tract illness • Upper respiratory tract infection (URI) • Sinusitis • Pharyngitis • Acute or chronic bronchitis • Bacterial pneumonia • TB • Influenza • Chronic obstructive pulmonary disease • Reactive airway disease, asthma • Non-Hodgkin lymphoma • Pulmonary embolus • Congestive heart failure • Pulmonary hypertension • Pneumothorax • Bronchogenic carcinoma • Anemia • Gastroesophageal reflux (may cause cough) • Lactic acidosis • Medication adverse effect
≤500 cells/µL	• Bacterial pneumonia (recurrent) • Pulmonary *Mycobacterium* pneumonia (nontuberculous)
≤200 cells/µL	• PCP • *Cryptococcus neoformans* pneumonia or pneumonitis • Bacterial pneumonia (associated with bacteremia or sepsis) • Disseminated or extrapulmonary TB
≤100 cells/µL	• Pulmonary Kaposi sarcoma • Bacterial pneumonia (risk of gram-negative bacilli and *Staphylococcus aureus* is increased) • *Toxoplasma* pneumonitis
≤50 cells/µL	• Disseminated histoplasmosis • Disseminated coccidioidomycosis • Cytomegalovirus pneumonitis • Disseminated *Mycobacterium avium* complex • Disseminated *Mycobacterium* (nontuberculous) • *Aspergillus* pneumonia • *Candida* pneumonia

Adapted from: Huang L. *Pulmonary Manifestations of HIV* (Table 4). In: Coffey S, Volberding PA, eds. *HIV InSite Knowledge Base* [textbook online]; San Francisco: UCSF Center for HIV Information; January 2009. Available at hivinsite.ucsf.edu/InSite?page=kb-04-01-05. Accessed June 30, 2010.

P: Plan

Diagnostic Evaluation

Perform laboratory work and other diagnostic studies as suggested by the history, physical examination, and differential diagnosis. This may include the following:

- Chest X ray, especially if the patient has abnormal findings on chest examination, fever, or weight loss, or if the CD4 count is <200 cells/µL. Consider further imaging such as chest computed tomography (CT) scan or high-resolution chest CT (HRCT) if chest X-ray result is unremarkable in a setting of suspected PCP or persistent symptoms, or if there is question of pulmonary nodules or suspected empyema.

- Arterial blood gas (ABG) on room air, particularly if PCP is suspected, of if the oxygen saturation is low.

- Complete blood count and white blood cell (WBC) count with differential, metabolic panel, and lactate dehydrogenase (LDH).

- If fever is present (especially temperature >38.5°C), obtain routine blood cultures (two specimens) for bacteria. If the CD4 count is <50 cells/µL, obtain blood culture for acid-fast bacilli (AFB); if <100 cells/µL, check the serum level cryptococcal antigen (CrAg) and consider checking urine *Histoplasma* antigen.

- Induced sputum (outside, or in a negative-pressure room or area that is safely vented to the outside, to prevent TB aerosolization) for AFB smear and cultures (three specimens), Gram stain and bacterial cultures, PCP stains, fungal stains and cultures, and cytology, as indicated.

- CD4 count and HIV viral load, if recent values are not known.

- Bronchoscopy with bronchoalveolar lavage (BAL) or biopsy if sputum studies are negative, if the diagnosis is unclear after initial evaluation or if the patient is not responsive to empiric therapy.

- Pulmonary function tests if no infectious or HIV-related pulmonary diagnosis is suspected and symptoms persist.

- Lactate level if lactic acidosis is suspected (e.g., nausea, tachypnea, abdominal pain, fatigue, in the setting of long-term nucleoside analogue therapy).

- Toxicology screen if symptoms are suspected to be related to recent drug use (e.g., crack cocaine pneumonitis).

Treatment

Once the diagnosis is made, appropriate treatment should be initiated. In seriously ill patients, presumptive treatment may be started while diagnostic test results are pending. See the appropriate chapter in section *Comorbidities, Coinfections, and Complications* or relevant guidelines. In some cases, the source of dyspnea or cough cannot be identified. In these cases, consult with an HIV expert or a pulmonologist.

Patient Education

- Shortness of breath and cough can be signs of an opportunistic illness, especially in patients with low CD4 counts. Patients should notify their health care provider if they develop new or worsening symptoms.

- Patients taking antibiotics should be instructed to take their medications exactly as directed and to call their health care provider if they experience worsening fevers, shortness of breath, inability to take the prescribed medications, or other problems.

- Counsel smokers about the importance of smoking cessation; refer to tobacco cessation programs and prescribe cessation supports, as indicated; see chapter *Smoking Cessation*.

- Counsel drug users (particularly those who smoke or inject drugs) regarding the impact of illicit drugs on their overall health and especially their lungs; refer to appropriate cessation programs or rehabilitation programs.

References

- Centers for Disease Control and Prevention. *Guidelines for Prevention and Treatment of Opportunistic Infections in HIV-Infected Adults and Adolescents: Recommendations from CDC, the National Institutes of Health, and the HIV Medicine Association of the Infectious Diseases Society of America.* April 10, 2009. Available at www.aidsinfo.nih.gov/guidelines/.

- Huang L. *Pulmonary Manifestations of HIV* (Table 4). In: Coffey S, Volberding PA, eds. *HIV InSite Knowledge Base* [textbook online]; San Francisco: UCSF Center for HIV Information; January 2009. Available at hivinsite.ucsf.edu/InSite?page=kb-04-01-05. Accessed June 30, 2010.

- Mandell LA, Bartlett JG, Dowell SF, et al. *Update of practice guidelines for the management of community-acquired pneumonia in immunocompetent adults.* Clin Infect Dis. 2003 Dec 1;37(11):1405-33.

Vaginitis/Vaginosis

Background

Vaginitis is defined as inflammation of the vagina, usually characterized by a vaginal discharge containing many white blood cells (WBCs); it may be accompanied by vulvar itching and irritation. Vaginosis presents with increased vaginal discharge without inflammation. Vaginitis usually is caused by an infection, but may be caused by other factors, such as chemicals or irritants. Vaginal infections are common among HIV-infected women. The presence of vaginal infections or inflammation, in the case of bacterial vaginosis in particular, may facilitate acquisition of HIV and other sexually transmitted infections (STIs), and trichomoniasis may facilitate HIV transmission to HIV-uninfected partners. This chapter focuses on two of the most common types of vaginal infections: trichomoniasis and bacterial vaginosis (BV). For information on the topic of vulvovaginal candidiasis, see chapter *Candidiasis, Vulvovaginal.*

S: Subjective

The patient complains of vaginal discharge with or without odor, itching, burning, pelvic pain, vulvar pain, or pain during intercourse.

Take a focused history, including the following:

- Duration of symptoms
- Sexual history, especially recent new partners, unprotected sex
- Relationship of symptoms to sexual contacts
- Contraceptive use, especially:
  - Vaginal contraceptive film
  - Other products containing nonoxynol-9 (N-9)
  - Condoms; type of condoms
- Use of feminine hygiene products (e.g,. sprays, deodorants)
- Douching
- Use of perfumed toiletries (e.g., bath salts, scented toilet tissue, or sanitary napkins)
- Use of any vaginal creams
- Postcoital bleeding
- Vulvar pain
- Pain or burning during urination
- Pain with intercourse
- Recent antibiotic use
- History of STIs, pelvic inflammatory disease (PID)
- Medications, including supplements

O: Objective

Perform a focused physical examination of the external genitalia, including perineum and anal area, for the following:

- Inflammation
- Edema
- Excoriation
- Lesions

Perform speculum examination for:

- Discharge (note color, quality; note that the character of the discharge is not diagnostic)
- Erythema, edema, erosions, lesions
- Cervical friability
- Foreign body

Perform a bimanual examination for masses or tenderness, if indicated.

A: Assessment

A partial differential diagnosis includes the following:

- BV
- Candidiasis
- Trichomoniasis
- PID
- Latex or condom allergy
- Urinary tract infection (UTI)
- Condyloma
- Herpes simplex virus (HSV)
- Contact dermatitis (e.g., from irritants, perfumes)
- Chlamydia
- Gonorrhea
- Normal vaginal discharge

P: Plan

Diagnostic Evaluation

- Obtain a cervical sample for STI testing, if indicated.
- Obtain samples (swabs) from the vaginal wall for wet mounts and pH testing.
- Wet mounts: Perform microscopic examination of saline and potassium hydroxide (KOH) preparations for the following:
  - WBCs, clue cells, motile trichomonads (saline slide)
  - Yeast forms (KOH)
- Perform a whiff test of KOH preparation; if positive, check pH (if >4.5, likely BV or trichomoniasis).

Treatment depends on the specific diagnosis, and in general is the same as for HIV-uninfected women.

Trichomoniasis

Trichomoniasis is caused by the protozoan *Trichomonas vaginalis*. Many infected women have a diffuse, malodorous, yellow-green discharge. Most men who are infected with *T. vaginalis* have no symptoms; others have symptoms of nongonococcal urethritis. The diagnosis usually is made by visualization of motile trichomonads on microscopic examination of wet mounts. Antigen or nucleic acid assays have greater specificity and sensitivity than wet mount preparations, and may be used if microscopy is negative. Culture of vaginal secretions is the most sensitive and specific diagnostic test for *T. vaginalis*, and also may help to rule out other infections.

Treatment: Recommended regimen

- Metronidazole 2 g PO in a single dose
- Tinidazole 2 g PO in a single dose

Treatment: Alternative regimen

- Metronidazole 500 mg PO BID for 7 days

Treatment during pregnancy

- Metronidazole, as in nonpregnant women (see above); the 7-day regimen may be better tolerated.
- Counsel patients about the potential risks and benefits of therapy. In pregnant women with asymptomatic trichomoniasis, may consider deferring therapy until after 37 weeks' gestation; consult with a specialist.

Treatment notes:

Single-dose metronidazole is associated with more side effects than the other treatment regimens.

Sex partners should be treated. Patients should refrain from unprotected intercourse until both partners have resolution of symptoms and have completed treatment; this should be at least 7 days after single-dose therapy.

Sex partners should be treated. Patients must avoid alcohol while taking metronidazole or tinidazole, and for at least 1 day after discontinuing metronidazole and 3 days after discontinuing tinidazole. The combination of alcohol and these drugs may cause a disulfiram-like reaction. Patients taking ritonavir capsules or tipranavir also may experience symptoms because of the small amount of alcohol in the capsules.

Treatment failure

Certain strains of *T. vaginalis* have diminished susceptibility to metronidazole and must be treated with higher dosages. If treatment failure occurs on metronidazole, consider tinidazole as above, or if single-dose metronidazole was used initially, consider metronidazole 500 mg PO BID for 7 days. If this is not effective, consult with a specialist.

Bacterial Vaginosis

BV is a clinical syndrome resulting from loss of the normal vaginal flora, particularly *Lactobacillus*, and replacement with anaerobic and other bacteria such as *Gardnerella vaginalis* and *Mycoplasma hominis*. The diagnosis is made on clinical and laboratory criteria. Usually, three of the following four characteristics should be present (note: only the clue cells are specific to BV):

- Homogeneous, gray-white, noninflammatory discharge on the vaginal walls

- Clue cells on the wet-mount slide

- Vaginal fluid pH level of >4.5

- Fishy odor to the vaginal discharge before or after the addition of KOH (whiff test)

Vaginal culture does not help establish the diagnosis. Rapid diagnostic test cards are available in some settings.

Many studies have documented an association between BV and infections such as endometritis, PID, and vaginal cuff cellulitis after gynecologic procedures. Therefore, the U.S. Centers for Disease Control and Prevention (CDC) recommends screening for and treating BV before invasive gynecologic procedures.

The sex partners of women with BV do not need to be treated.

Treatment: Recommended regimen

- Metronidazole 500 mg PO BID for 7 days

- Metronidazole gel 0.75%, 1 full applicator (5 g) intravaginally QHS for 5 days

- Clindamycin cream 2%, 1 full applicator (5 g) intravaginally QHS for 7 days

Treatment: Alternative regimens

- Tinidazole 2 g PO once daily for 2 days

- Tinidazole 1 g PO once daily for 5 days

- Clindamycin 300 mg PO BID for 7 days

- Clindamycin ovules 100 g intravaginally QHS for 3 days

Treatment during pregnancy

- Symptomatic pregnant women should be treated with oral metronidazole (500 mg BID or 250 mg TID) or oral clindamycin for 7 days.

Treatment notes:

- Patients must avoid alcohol while taking metronidazole or tinidazole, and for at least 1 day after discontinuing metronidazole and 3 days after discontinuing tinidazole. The combination of alcohol and these drugs may cause a disulfiram-like reaction. Patients taking ritonavir capsules or tipranavir also may experience symptoms because of the small amount of alcohol in the capsules.

Treatment failure

Consider re-treatment for 7 days with metronidazole or clindamycin. Consider the possibility of an alternative or second cause of the patient's symptoms, as multiple conditions or pathogens may present concurrently. Perform testing for other conditions as suggested by symptoms, or if symptoms to do not resolve with initial treatment:

- Perform herpes culture if indicated by lesions; see chapter *Herpes Simplex, Mucocutaneous.*

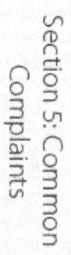

- Test for chlamydia and gonorrhea if indicated; see chapter *Gonorrhea and Chlamydia*.
- Perform urinalysis (with or without culture and sensitivities) if urinary symptoms are prominent.
- If an irritant or allergen is suspected, including N-9, discontinue use.
- If symptoms are related to the use of latex condoms, switch to polyurethane male or female condoms.
- For tenderness on cervical motion or other symptoms of PID, see chapter *Pelvic Inflammatory Disease*.
- Perform workup or obtain referral as needed for other abnormalities found on bimanual examination.

For information on other STIs or related conditions, see the CDC's treatment guidelines at www.cdc.gov/std/treatment.

Patient Education

- Advise patients to avoid any form of alcohol while taking metronidazole or tinidazole and for 24 hours after taking the last dose (72 hours after the last tinidazole dose). Alcohol and metronidazole together can cause severe nausea, vomiting, and other immobilizing symptoms.
- Patients taking ritonavir may experience these symptoms because of the small amount of alcohol in the capsules and should be told to contact their health care provider if nausea and vomiting occur.
- Advise patients that clindamycin cream and ovules are oil based and will weaken latex condoms, diaphragms, and cervical caps. Patients should use alternative methods to prevent pregnancy and HIV transmission.

- Recurrence of BV is common. Patients should contact their health care providers and return for repeat treatment if symptoms recur.
- Instruct patients to avoid douching.
- To avoid being reinfected by *Trichomonas*, patients should bring their sex partners to the clinic for evaluation and treatment.

References

- Abularach S, Anderson J. *Gynecologic Problems*. In: Anderson JR, ed. *A Guide to the Clinical Management of Women with HIV.* Rockville, MD: Health Resources and Services Administration, HIV/AIDS Bureau; 2005.
- Centers for Disease Control and *Prevention. Sexually Transmitted Diseases Treatment Guidelines*, 2010. MMWR 2010 Dec 17; 59 (No. RR- 12):1-110. Available at www.cdc.gov/STD/treatment/2010.
- Cohn SE, Clark RA. *Sexually transmitted diseases, HIV, and AIDS in women.* In: The Medical Clinics of North America, Vol. 87; 2003:971-995.
- Hawkins JW, Roberto-Nichols DM, Stanley-Haney JL. *Protocols for Nurse Practitioners in Gynecologic Settings, 7th Edition.* New York: Tiresias Press, Inc.; 2000.
- Schwebke JR. *Gynecological consequences of bacterial vaginosis.* In: Obstetrics and Gynecology Clinics of North America, Vol. 30; 2003:685-694.

Abnormalities of Body-Fat Distribution

Background

Abnormalities of body-fat distribution are a recognized complication of HIV infection and of antiretroviral therapy (ART), and they are a common concern of patients. They include central fat accumulation (lipohypertrophy) and subcutaneous fat wasting (lipoatrophy). These morphologic changes are often referred to as lipodystrophy, though that term fails to distinguish between the two phenomena. Abnormalities in fat distribution and body shape have been noted in up to 40-50% of patients treated with ART, but the incidence may be much lower with the use of newer, less lipotoxic, antiretroviral (ARV) medications and with earlier initiation of ART. Lipohypertrophy and lipoatrophy are associated with other metabolic abnormalities, such as dyslipidemia and insulin resistance, and visceral fat accumulation (at least in HIV-uninfected persons) is a risk factor for cardiovascular disease.

Research on fat maldistribution has yielded varying results, in part because there are no standard clinical case definitions of lipodystrophy, lipoatrophy, or lipohypertrophy. The pathogenesis of fat abnormalities in HIV-infected individuals is not well understood, but research to date suggests that it is multifactorial and is associated with HIV-related immune depletion and immune recovery, ARV medications, disregulation of fatty acid metabolism, hormonal influences, individual genetic predispositions, and factors that are not related to HIV such as diet and obesity. Lipodystrophy has been associated with lower nadir CD4 count as well as with gender (central lipohypertrophy may be more common in women) and age (more common in older patients), and longer exposure to ART. Lipohypertrophy has not been definitively proven to be related to specific ARVs or to specific ARV classes, but has been variably associated with protease inhibitors (PIs) and with nucleoside reverse transcriptase inhibitors (NRTIs). However, morphologic changes occasionally develop in ARV-naive individuals. Lipoatrophy is most commonly associated with NRTIs, notably stavudine, as well as didanosine and zidovudine.

The most common morphologic changes seen in lipohypertrophy are a firm enlarged abdomen caused by central or visceral fat accumulation, breast enlargement (gynecomastia) in both men and women, development of a dorsocervical fat pad ("buffalo hump"), and neck enlargement. Lipoatrophy most commonly appears as the loss of subcutaneous fat in the face, arms, legs, and buttocks. Lipoatrophy differs from the generalized wasting seen in advanced AIDS, because lean cell mass generally is preserved. When lipohypertrophy and lipoatrophy occur together, the affected individuals show a mixed picture of abdominal obesity with thinning in the face, arms, and legs.

Severe lipoaccumulation can cause discomfort and, in some cases, impairment of breathing or other bodily functions. It may be associated with other metabolic abnormalities, including dyslipidemia, insulin resistance, and the metabolic syndrome. Both lipoaccumulation and lipoatrophy can be disfiguring, can damage self-image and quality of life, and can negatively influence ARV adherence.

S: Subjective

The patient may report any of the following: abdominal fat accumulation with change in waist size, increased neck size, "buffalo hump," enlarged breasts, and reduced range of motion. Women may note an increase in bra size. Alternatively (or in addition), the patient may report sunken cheeks, decreased arm or leg circumference, prominence of veins in the arms or legs, or buttock flattening.

Determine CD4 cell count nadir, ARV medication history with particular attention to past use of thymidine analogues and PIs, and duration of and response to each regimen. Ask about past medical and family history, specifically regarding hyperlipidemia, diabetes or insulin resistance, other metabolic disorders, and cardiovascular disease. Evaluate the effect of body-shape changes on the patient's self-esteem, medication adherence, and interpersonal relationships.

O: Objective

Compare past and current weights. Calculate body mass index (BMI); see chapter *Initial Physical Examination* for information on BMI.

Measure and document waist and hip circumferences. A waist circumference of >102 cm (39 inches) in men and >88 cm (35 inches) in women is the clinical definition of abdominal obesity and is associated with the metabolic syndrome. Waist-to-hip ratios of >0.95 in men and >0.85 in women are associated with an increased risk of coronary heart disease.

Examine the head, neck, back, breasts, and abdomen for fat accumulation, especially looking for dorsocervical fat pad and facial, neck, or breast enlargement. Examine the face and extremities for subcutaneous fat loss (e.g., in the cheeks, temples, limbs, and buttocks).

Review laboratory history (glucose, lipid panel) to identify other metabolic disorders. (See chapters *Dyslipidemia* and *Insulin Resistance,*

Hyperglycemia, and Diabetes on Antiretroviral Therapy.)

A: Assessment

No uniform standard criteria are available for defining or grading lipohypertrophy or lipoatrophy in clinical practice. Clinicians must base their assessment on patient self-report, physical examination (for characteristic body-shape changes), associated symptoms, and psychological consequences.

In research settings, modalities such as dual-energy X-ray absorptiometry (DEXA), computed tomography (CT), and magnetic resonance imaging (MRI) have been used to characterize and quantify lipoaccumulation and lipoatrophy. Anthropometric measurements may be made in the clinic by trained personnel (e.g., nutritionists), but do not measure visceral fat directly. Although measurements such as waist circumference cannot be used to assess lipohypertrophy, they have been validated (in HIV-uninfected individuals) as an assessment of cardiovascular risk (see chapters *Dyslipidemia* and *Coronary Heart Disease Risk*). Bioelectrical impedance analysis (BIA) does not measure regional body composition and thus is not used to measure abnormal body-fat changes.

Differential diagnosis of lipohypertrophy includes obesity or excess weight gain, ascites, and Cushing syndrome.

Differential diagnosis of lipoatrophy includes weight loss and wasting.

P: Plan

Diagnostic Evaluation
Laboratory

Check for other metabolic abnormalities associated with the use of ARVs, such as dyslipidemia and impaired glucose metabolism (check fasting lipids and random or fasting glucose). See chapters *Dyslipidemia* and *Insulin Resistance, Hyperglycemia, and Diabetes on Antiretroviral Therapy* for further information about workup and treatment.

Treatment

Treatments for lipohypertrophy and lipoatrophy have not reliably reversed body shape changes once these changes have occurred. In general, treatment interventions have shown poor results in patients with marked or severe fat maldistribution and inconsistent or limited responses in those with milder conditions. The best approaches to managing lipodystrophy are prevention and early intervention.

Clinicians can help to prevent body fat abnormalities by avoiding, whenever possible, ARV agents known to confer a greater risk of this disorder (particularly stavudine, didanosine, and zidovudine, which particularly are associated with lipoatrophy). All patients who take ARVs should be monitored carefully for the development of fat maldistribution. If abnormalities are noticed, intervention should be initiated, if possible.

The optimal management strategy for established lipoaccumulation or lipoatrophy is not known, although the following approaches can be considered (see below). Also consider referring the patient to clinical studies of lipodystrophy treatment, and for psychological or adherence support and counseling, if indicated. If the patient is distressed enough to consider discontinuing or interrupting ART, review with the patient any gains he or she has made on ART and discuss treatment options (see below). In some cases the patient may insist on discontinuing ARV medications; in this situation, carefully review the risks of treatment interruption as well as the alternatives to discontinuing treatment.

ARV Substitutions

Avoiding thymidine analogue NRTIs, particularly stavudine, and avoiding the NRTI combination stavudine + didanosine have been shown to reduce the risk of lipoatrophy.

In patients with lipoatrophy, modest slow improvement in limb fat has been demonstrated after switching from thymidine analogues (stavudine, zidovudine) to non-thymidine NRTIs (such as abacavir or tenofovir) or to NRTI-sparing regimens. In patients with lipohypertrophy, similar NRTI switch strategies have had little effect on visceral or trunk fat. Studies in which PIs were eliminated from the ART regimen generally have not shown significant effects on body fat measures.

Before switching therapies, carefully assess the potential risk to the patient's long-term HIV management.

Nonpharmacologic Measures
Diet

The effects of diet on lipohypertrophy have not been evaluated thoroughly. If overall weight reduction is needed, recommend dietary changes and exercise. Avoid rapid weight loss plans, as lean body mass often is lost disproportionately. Refer to a dietitian to help the patient decrease intake of saturated fat, simple sugars, and alcohol.

Exercise

Regular, vigorous cardiovascular exercise may help control central fat accumulation, whereas resistance exercises (strength training) will improve the ratio of muscle to fat. Some studies of exercise (done alone or in combination with diet) have shown a reduction in visceral fat accumulation with minimal or no changes in peripheral lipoatrophy. Moderate aerobic exercise should be encouraged for all patients.

Pharmacologic Measures
Insulin-sensitizing agents

In diabetic and non-HIV lipodystrophy,

treatment with thiazolidinediones may decrease visceral fat, increase peripheral fat, and improve glycemic control. In HIV-infected patients with lipoatrophy, studies of thiazolidinediones, specifically rosiglitazone and pioglitazone, have shown mixed results. Some patients have reported improvement in limb fat, particularly those with insulin resistance; however, a larger, 48-week randomized trial of rosiglitazone found no significant increase in limb-fat mass. In patients with visceral fat accumulation, thiazolidinediones have not been found to be effective.

In clinical studies, metformin has been modestly effective in treating visceral adiposity in patients with insulin resistance, but may cause worsening of lipoatrophy. Metformin should be used with caution in patients with chronic liver or renal disease.

Recombinant human growth hormone

Treatment with recombinant human growth hormone (rHGH), 3-6 mg/day for 12 weeks followed by maintenance therapy with lower doses of 1-2 mg/day, has been shown to reduce visceral fat in many patients with minimal impact on peripheral fat wasting; other studies suggest efficacy (and improved tolerability) of lower dosages of rHGH. However, the high cost of rHGH, the high rate of adverse effects (including insulin resistance), and the frequent recurrence of visceral fat accumulation once rHGH is discontinued have resulted in a limited role for this treatment.

Growth hormone-releasing factor

Tesamoralin, a synthetic growth hormone-releasing factor analogue, has been shown in Phase 3 clinical studies to reduce central fat accumulation by about 18% over the course of 12 months, without adverse effects on glucose or lipid parameters. As with rHGH, patients regain visceral fat when tesamoralin is discontinued. Tesamoralin currently is under review for approval by the U.S. Food and Drug Administration (FDA).

Plastic and reconstructive surgery

Various techniques have been investigated, but generally have limited applicability and efficacy. Poly-L-lactic acid (Sculptra, New-Fill) is approved by the FDA as a treatment for facial lipoatrophy. This injectable material has shown good cosmetic results and often significantly improves patients' satisfaction with their appearance. Calcium hydroxylapatite (Radiesse) also has FDA approval for HIV-associated facial lipoatrophy. Treatment effects of both agents typically wane with time and the procedures often must be repeated. Other facial fillers, as well as cheek implants and autologous fat transfer, have been used successfully in some cases. For lipoaccumulation, treatments such as liposuction for focal areas of fat deposition (e.g., dorsocervical) and breast reduction may be effective in the short term, though fat often reaccumulates.

These interventions increasingly are covered by private- and public-payer sources, but still often are deemed to be the financial responsibility of the patient. In some cases, they may be only a temporary solution, because abnormalities may reappear after treatment.

Patient Education

- Instruct patients who are receiving ARV medications to inform their health care provider if they notice changes in the shape or appearance of their bodies.

- Review the importance and benefits of ART and assess adherence to the regimen.

- For patients with lipohypertrophy, recommend aerobic and resistance exercise to reduce fat and build muscle. Assess local resources for safe muscle-strengthening possibilities.

- If weight reduction is needed, refer to a dietitian for consultation. Remind the patient that quick weight-loss diets may result in excessive muscle loss.

- For patients with severe facial lipoatrophy, consider referral to an experienced dermatologist or plastic surgeon for restorative treatment.

References

- Carr A, Workman C, Carey D, et al. *No effect of rosiglitazone for treatment of HIV-1 lipoatrophy: randomised, double-blind, placebo-controlled trial.* Lancet. 2004 Feb 7;363(9407):429-38.

- Chow D, Day L., Souza S, et al. *Metabolic Complications of HIV Therapy.* In: Coffey S, Volberding PA, eds. *HIV InSite Knowledge Base* [online textbook]. San Francisco: UCSF Center for HIV Information; 2006. Available at hivinsite.ucsf.edu/InSite?page=kb-03-02-10. Accessed June 30, 2010.

- Falutz J, Allas S, Blot K, et al. *Metabolic effects of a growth hormone-releasing factor in patients with HIV.* N Engl J Med. 2007 Dec 6;357(23):2359-70.

- Falutz J, Potvin D, Mamputu JC, et al. *Effects of tesamorelin, a growth hormone-releasing factor, in HIV-infected patients with abdominal fat accumulation: a randomized placebo-controlled trial with a safety extension.* J Acquir Immune Defic Syndr. 2010 Mar 1;53(3):311-22.

- Gallant JE, Staszewski S, Pozniak AL, et al.; 903 Study Group. *Efficacy and safety of tenofovir DF vs stavudine in combination therapy in antiretroviral-naive patients: a 3-year randomized trial.* JAMA. 2004 Jul 14;292(2):191-201.

- Haubrich RH, Riddler SA, DiRienzo AG, et al.; AIDS Clinical Trials Group (ACTG) A5142 Study Team. *Metabolic outcomes in a randomized trial of nucleoside, nonnucleoside and protease inhibitor-sparing regimens for initial HIV treatment.* AIDS. 2009 Jun 1;23(9):1109-18.

- Martin A, Smith DE, Carr A, et al.; Mitochondrial Toxicity Study Group. *Reversibility of lipoatrophy in HIV-infected patients 2 years after switching from a thymidine analogue to abacavir: the MITOX Extension Study.* AIDS. 2004 Apr 30;18(7):1029-36.

- Moyle G. *Metabolic issues associated with protease inhibitors.* J Acquir Immune Defic Syndr. 2007 Jun 1;45 Suppl 1:S19-26.

- Pirmohamed M. *Clinical management of HIV-associated lipodystrophy.* Curr Opin Lipidol. 2009 Aug;20(4):309-14.

- Rubenoff R, Schmitz H, Bairos L, et al. *Reduction of abdominal obesity in lipodystrophy associated with human immunodeficiency virus infection by means of diet and exercise: case report and proof of principle.* Clin Infect Dis. 2002 Feb 1;34(3):390-3.

- Schambelan M, Benson CA, Carr A, et al.; International AIDS Society-USA. *Management of metabolic complications associated with antiretroviral therapy for HIV-1 infection: recommendations of International AIDS Society-USA panel.* J Acquir Immune Defic Syndr. 2002 Nov 1;31(3):257-75.

- U.S. Department of Health and Human Services. *Guidelines for the Use of Antiretroviral Agents in HIV-1-Infected Adults and Adolescents.* January 10, 2011. Available at www.aidsinfo.nih.gov/guidelines/.

- Wohl DA. *Diagnosis and management of body morphology changes and lipid abnormalities associated with HIV Infection and its therapies.* Top HIV Med. 2004 Jul-Aug;12(3):89-93.

Dyslipidemia

Susa Coffey, MD

Background

HIV-infected individuals, both those on antiretroviral therapy (ART) and those who are untreated, appear to have higher rates of coronary heart disease (CHD) than HIV-uninfected individuals and higher rates of various risk factors for CHD, including dyslipidemia. As the average lifespan of patients on effective ART lengthens, and as people living with HIV become older, morbidity and mortality from CHD are likely to continue to increase. Thus, identification and reduction of modifiable risk factors for CHD are important aspects of primary care for HIV-infected patients.

HRSA HAB Core Clinical Performance Measures

Percentage of clients with HIV infection on ART who had a **fasting lipid panel** during the measurement year

(Group 2 measure)

Dyslipidemia is a well-described independent risk factor for CHD, and it occurs in a high proportion of persons with HIV infection. Current research suggests that this dyslipidemia is caused by a combination of factors related to HIV disease, ART regimens, and individual patient characteristics. HIV itself causes lipid perturbations, particularly in persons with more advanced immunosuppression; HIV-infected individuals who are not on antiretroviral (ARV) medications often have elevations in triglyceride (TG) levels and decreases in high-density lipoprotein (HDL) as well as in low-density lipoprotein (LDL) cholesterol and total cholesterol (TC). Lipid abnormalities also may be caused by or compounded by ARVs (see chapter *Coronary Heart Disease Risk*). They may appear or worsen within a few weeks to months after starting ART. With some patients, this may, at least in part, represent a return to pre-illness lipid levels, whereas the ARVs cause the abnormality in other cases.

Not all ART-treated patients experience lipid abnormalities to the same degree. Patients with a personal or family history of dyslipidemia, glucose intolerance, diabetes, obesity, or a combination of these health problems may be genetically predisposed to lipid abnormalities that become evident once ART is initiated.

The use of potent combination ART, particularly the use of protease inhibitors (PIs), has increased the prevalence of abnormally high TG, TC, and LDL levels among HIV-infected patients. In fact, dyslipidemia has been associated not only with certain PIs but also with nonnucleoside reverse transcriptase inhibitors (NNRTIs) and some nucleoside reverse transcriptase inhibitors (NRTIs). In the PI class, ritonavir-boosted PIs (with the exception of atazanavir) are particularly likely to cause marked elevations of TG and LDL levels. NNRTIs also may contribute to increases in TC, LDL, and TG levels although the effects, particularly with efavirenz, are more variable (and efavirenz may increase HDL). Of the NRTIs, stavudine, zidovudine, and perhaps abacavir may increase TC and TG levels. To date, available agents from the integrase inhibitor and CCR5 antagonist classes do not appear to have significant adverse impacts on lipid levels.

The largest prospective study of CHD events related to ARVs (the D:A:D study) showed a small but significant increase in the risk of myocardial infarction among HIV-infected patients treated with ARVs; moreover, the effect increased with cumulative years of ARV exposure. This effect was largely but not entirely associated with increases in LDL cholesterol (see chapter *Coronary Heart Disease Risk*).

Identification and management of dyslipidemia in HIV-infected patients is an important part of HIV primary care. For patients with CHD or CHD risk equivalents (see below), ART regimens should, if possible, be selected to minimize the risk of hyperlipidemia.

Guidelines for the evaluation and management of dyslipidemia have been developed by the National Cholesterol Education Program (NCEP). These recommendations are based on studies of HIV-uninfected persons and may not be entirely applicable to HIV-infected persons, in whom HIV itself may increase risk of CHD events. Despite this limitation, expert panels generally recommend similar treatment goals when evaluating and managing dyslipidemia in patients with HIV infection. (For recommendations on screening, see chapter *Initial and Interim Laboratory and Other Tests*.)

S: Subjective

The history should focus on factors that suggest CHD, risk equivalents, or risk factors for CHD. Both CHD risks and CHD equivalents should be the focus of lifestyle modification strategies and lipid-normalizing treatment.

- **CHD** includes the following:
  - A history of myocardial infarction
  - Angina
  - CHD procedures
  - Evidence of clinically significant myocardial ischemia
- **CHD risk equivalents** are considered to be equal in terms of risk level to known CHD. These include the following:
  - Diabetes mellitus
  - Peripheral vascular disease
  - Symptomatic carotid artery disease
  - Abdominal aortic aneurysm
  - Transient ischemic attacks
  - Two or more CHD risk factors with a 10-year risk of CHD >20% (see Appendix "Calculations to Estimate the 10-Year Risk of Cardiac Events for Men and Women," below, or the online risk calculator at hin.nhlbi.nih.gov/atpiii/calculator.asp?usertype=prof.

- **CHD risk factors** are conditions associated with a greater risk of serious cardiac events. These are as follows:
  - Male sex
  - Age (≥45 in men; ≥55 in women)
  - Hypertension
  - Cigarette smoking
  - Low HDL (<40 mg/dL); if >60 mg/dL, subtract one risk factor
  - Family history of premature CHD (first-degree relative aged <55 [men] or <65 [women])
- Assess for causes of secondary dyslipidemias, including insulin resistance, diabetes, hypothyroidism, obstructive liver diseases, chronic renal failure, and medications such as corticosteroids and progestins.
- Screen for other factors that contribute to hyperlipidemia, including obesity, chronic liver diseases, alcohol abuse, high-fat or high-carbohydrate diet, and prothrombotic or proinflammatory states.
- Screen for health behaviors that increase CHD risk, including smoking, high-fat diet, sedentary lifestyle, and use of recreational drugs such as cocaine and methamphetamine.
- Review the patient's family history for premature CHD (as discussed above), obesity (body mass index [BMI] ≥30), diabetes, and lipid abnormalities.

Section 6: Comorbidities, Coinfections, and Complications

- Review the patient's medications, with special attention to ARVs known to increase LDL or TG levels (particularly ritonavir and ritonavir-boosted PIs).

O: Objective

Check vital signs with special attention to blood pressure and weight. Calculate BMI (see chapter *Initial Physical Examination* for information on BMI).

Perform a focused physical examination with particular attention to signs of hyperlipidemia, such as xanthelasma and xanthoma, and to the cardiovascular system.

A: Assessment

Determine whether a specific intervention is appropriate based on the patient's lipid values and identified CHD risks, as indicated in Tables 1 and 2.

LDL is the main indicator for treatment, and the main target for lipid-lowering therapy. Hypertriglyceridemia is associated with CHD risk, but thresholds of risk have not been defined precisely, and targets for intervention are not entirely clear (for persons with triglyceride levels of ≥500 mg/dL the triglycerides usually are treated first; see "Treatment," below). Severe hypertriglyceridemia (e.g., TG >1,000 mg/dL) also increases the risk of pancreatitis.

For patients who do not have diabetes or preexisting CHD and who have two or more CHD risk factors, calculate the "10-year risk of cardiovascular events" by using the Risk Assessment Tool for estimating the 10-year risk of a major CHD event. Use the risk-estimate tool at the end of this chapter or the online risk calculator at the National Institutes of Health website (hin.nhlbi.nih.gov/atpiii/calculator.asp).

Table 1. Low-Density Lipoprotein Cholesterol Goals and Thresholds for Treatment*

Risk Category	LDL Goal*	Initiate Therapeutic Lifestyle Changes	Consider Drug Therapy
Lower risk: No CHD or CHD risk equivalents and <0-1 risk factor	<160 mg/dL (<4.1 mmol/L)	LDL ≥160 mg/dL (≥4.1 mmol/L)	≥190 mg/dL (≥4.9 mmol/L); at 160-189 mg/dL, LDL drug therapy is optional
Moderate risk: No CHD or CHD risk equivalents and ≥2 risk factors, with 10-year estimated risk <10%	<130 mg/dL (<3.4 mmol/L)	LDL ≥130 mg/dL (≥3.4 mmol/L)	≥160 mg/dL (≥4.1 mmol/L)
Moderately high risk: No CHD or CHD risk equivalents and ≥2 risk factors and 10-year estimated risk 10-20%	<130 mg/dL (<3.4 mmol/L) (optional goal of <100 mg/dL)	LDL ≥130 mg/dL (≥3.4 mmol/L)	≥130 mg/dL (≥3.4 mmol/L)
High risk: CHD or CHD risk equivalent (see above)	<100 mg/dL (<2.6 mmol/L) (optional goal of <70 mg/dL#)	LDL ≥100 mg/dL (≥2.6 mmol/L)	≥100 mg/dL (≥2.6 mmol/L)

* Non-HDL cholesterol target levels are 30 mg/dL higher than corresponding LDL cholesterol levels.

\# This goal (LDL <70 mg/dL) is preferred by many cardiologists for persons with CHD or risk equivalents.

Adapted from Adult Treatment Panel III, National Cholesterol Education Program. *Detection, Evaluation, and Treatment of High Blood Cholesterol in Adults.* September 2002; NIH publication 02-5215. Available at www.nhlbi.nih.gov/guidelines/cholesterol/index.htm. Accessed June 30, 2010.

Table 2. Classification of Triglyceride Levels

Risk Category	Triglyceride Measurement	Initiate therapy
Normal triglycerides	<150 mg/dL	
Borderline-high triglycerides	150-199 mg/dL	
High triglycerides	200-499 mg/dL	Start therapeutic lifestyle changes; consider medication if CHD, CHD equivalents, or high risk
Very high triglycerides	≥500 mg/dL	Start therapeutic lifestyle changes; consider medication

Adapted from Adult Treatment Panel III, National Cholesterol Education Program. *Detection, Evaluation, and Treatment of High Blood Cholesterol in Adults.* September 2002; NIH publication 02-5215. Available at www.nhlbi.nih.gov/guidelines/cholesterol/index.htm. Accessed June 30, 2010.

P: Plan

Diagnostic Evaluation

The fasting serum lipid panel should be performed at least 8 hours, but ideally 12 hours, after last food and beverage intake. It measures TC, HDL, TG, non-HDL cholesterol with calculated LDL, and TC/HDL cholesterol ratio.

A fasting lipid panel should be checked at baseline, before patients start ART.

Repeat the fasting lipid panel within 3-6 months after ARVs are started, and sooner for patients who have abnormal values at baseline.

Patients with normal lipid values should be rechecked annually. Those with dyslipidemia may need more intensive monitoring (e.g., every 4-6 weeks) until the LDL goal is met, after which monitoring every 4-6 months is adequate.

Treatment

Treatment of dyslipidemia usually involves a multimodal approach, including diet and exercise in all cases, lipid-modifying medication, and consideration of changes in ARV medication. The primary goal of lipid-lowering therapy is to reduce LDL to target levels. For persons with CHD and CHD risk equivalents, the type and intensity of LDL lowering therapies are adjusted according to LDL baseline levels. Note that other interventions to reduce CHD risk also should be undertaken (e.g., smoking cessation if appropriate).

For patients with serum TG level of >400 mg/dL, the LDL cholesterol calculation is unreliable. In this situation, non-HDL cholesterol (TC minus HDL) can be used as a surrogate target of therapy; the non-HDL goal is 30 mg/dL higher than the LDL goal. For these individuals, dietary intervention is warranted, and drug therapy to decrease LDL (or non-HDL) can be considered if TC is >240 mg/dL or HDL cholesterol is <35 mg/dL. For those with TG levels of 200-500 mg/dL, achieving the LDL cholesterol target is the primary goal, and lowering non-HDL cholesterol levels is a secondary goal (see Table 1 for LDL intervention levels).

The NCEP guidelines recommend that very high TG levels (≥500 ml/dL) be reduced before LDL is treated directly (see "Treatment of hypertriglyceridemia," below).

The LDL levels at which either therapeutic lifestyle change (TLC) or drug therapy should be initiated are shown in Table 1, along with the target goals for LDL cholesterol. The response to therapy should be monitored and therapeutic interventions should be intensified or augmented until lipid targets are met.

Therapeutic lifestyle change

TLC, consisting of diet modification and exercise, is fundamental to the management of dyslipidemia for HIV-infected patients.

Target goals for lipid abnormalities are difficult to achieve without prioritizing these behavioral change efforts. Although TLC is hard to maintain, it can yield significant results in reducing CHD risk and improving quality of life. Effective TLC is best achieved with a multidisciplinary team approach. HIV primary care providers should be instrumental in identifying TLC as a treatment priority and providing referrals to nutritionists for dietary counseling, to mental health professionals for assessment of treatable mood disorders, and to social workers, peer counselors, or clinical nurse specialists for assistance with health-behavior changes, self-care strategies, and identification of resources in the community for smoking cessation support and exercise programs. Specific recommendations for TLC goals and behavior change strategies are contained in the Adult Treatment Panel guidelines, which are available at www.nhlbi.nih.gov/guidelines/cholesterol/index.htm.

Pharmacologic treatment for hypercholesterolemia

All patients with elevated lipid levels should initiate TLC. If pharmacologic intervention is indicated, statins (hydroxymethylglutaryl coenzyme A [HMG-CoA] reductase inhibitors) are the first-line treatment for most patients.

These agents can be effective in reducing TC, LDL, and non-HDL cholesterol levels in HIV-infected patients (see Table 3).

Recommended starting dosages of statins for patients taking PIs are as follows (Note: see "Potential ARV Interactions," below):

- Pravastatin: 20 mg PO once daily

- Atorvastatin: 10 mg PO once daily

Fibrates may be considered as an alternative or adjunct to statins (see "Treatment of hypertriglyceridemia," below, for further information). When given concomitantly, statins and fibrates increase the risk of rhabdomyolysis and must be used cautiously and with careful monitoring). Niacin may be effective as adjunctive therapy, but may worsen insulin resistance and may cause hepatotoxicity. It also causes uncomfortable flushing in some patients; the sustained-release formulations are better tolerated. Ezetimibe (Zetia) appears to be effective in combination with statins for patients whose cholesterol is not controlled adequately with a statin alone, but it has not been shown to decrease CHD events. Bile acid sequestrants generally should be avoided because they may interfere with the absorption of other drugs and may increase TG levels.

Table 3. Drug Treatments for Lipid Abnormalities

Lipid Abnormality	First Choice	Second Choice	Comments
Isolated high LDL, non-HDL cholesterol	Statin	Fibrate	Start with pravastatin* or atorvastatin.* Use low statin dosages and titrate upward; patients taking PIs have increased risk of myopathy.
Isolated high TG	Fibrate	Statin, N-3 (omega-3) fatty acids	Start with gemfibrozil or fenofibrate. Combined statin and fibrate may increase myopathy risk.
High LDL and TG (TG level 200-500 mg/dL)	Statin	Fibrate	Start with pravastatin or atorvastatin. Use fluvastatin,* rosuvastatin,* gemfibrozil, or fenofibrate as alternatives. Combined statin and fibrate may increase myopathy risk.
High LDL and TG (TG level >500 mg/dL)	Fibrate	N-3 (omega-3) fatty acids, niacin, statin	Start with gemfibrozil or fenofibrate. Niacin is associated with insulin resistance. May need to add statin if cholesterol is not controlled adequately.

* May have significant interactions with certain PIs; see Table 4.

Potential ARV Interactions

Clinicians should note that there are clinically significant drug interactions between most statins and both PIs and NNRTIs (see Table 4). PIs can increase serum levels of most statins significantly, thus increasing the risk of severe statin adverse events such as rhabdomyolysis. Of the statin drugs, pravastatin is the least affected by most PIs (darunavir is an exception) and is the recommended statin for most patients with hypercholesterolemia without hypertriglyceridemia. Atorvastatin, if used, should be initiated at low dosage (10 mg) and titrated slowly upward to achieve target lipid levels (note that atorvastatin may lower TG, TC, and LDL levels). Lovastatin and simvastatin are contraindicated for use by patients taking PIs, and pitavastatin is contraindicated for use by patients taking ritonavir-boosted PIs. These can result in severe statin-related adverse events if prescribed. Other available statins include rosuvastatin and fluvastatin. These have not been as well studied but may be used with most PIs. When statins are given concurrently with interacting PIs, the statins should be started at low dosage and increased incrementally, if indicated; in general maximum dosages should not be used.

NNRTIs decrease levels of most statins (however, etravirine increases fluvastatin levels); higher dosages of statins may be needed to overcome this interaction. Be aware that various formulations and combination products contain these statins; check the generic name of components in new or unfamiliar cardiac prescriptions to determine whether they contain lipid-lowering agents.

Other classes of ARV drugs (NRTI, fusion inhibitor, CCR5 antagonist, and integrase inhibitor) do not have recognized interactions with statins. Other types of lipid-lowering medications generally are not metabolized by hepatic cytochrome P450 and are not affected by ARVs (an exception to this is gemfibrozil, whose levels are decreased by lopinavir/ritonavir, by an unknown mechanism).

Table 4. Interactions Between Statin Agents and Antiretroviral Medications

Code:

✓ Generally safe to begin treatment with usual starting dosage

❢ Caution; start with low dosage, monitor effects

☒ Coadministration is contraindicated

	Atorvastatin	Fluvastatin	Lovastatin	Pitavastatin	Pravastatin	Rosuvastatin*	Simvastatin
Protease Inhibitors							
Atazanavir	❢	✓	☒	✓(Unboosted) ☒ (ritonavir boosted)	❢	❢ Rosuvastatin AUC ↑ 213% and ↑ C_{max} 600%	☒
Darunavir/ ritonavir	❢	✓	☒	☒	❢ Pravastatin AUC ↑ up to 500%	❢	☒
Fosamprenavir	❢	✓	☒	☒	✓May need to ↑ pravastatin dosage	❢	☒
Indinavir	❢	✓	☒	☒	❢	❢	☒
Lopinavir/ ritonavir	❢	✓	☒	☒	❢	❢ Rosuvastatin C_{max} ↑ 466%	☒
Nelfinavir	❢	❢ Possible ↓ in nelfinavir levels	☒	No data	❢	❢	☒
Ritonavir	❢	✓	☒	☒	❢	❢	☒
Saquinavir	❢	✓	☒	☒	✓Saquinavir + ritonavir: May need to ↑ pravastatin dosage	❢	☒
Tipranavir	❢ Atorvastatin Cmax ↑ >760%	✓	☒	☒	❢	❢ Rosuvastatin C_{max} ↑ 123%	☒
Nonnucleoside Reverse Transcriptase Inhibitors							
Efavirenz^	✓May need to ↑ atorvastatin dosage	✓May need to ↑ fluvastatin dosage	✓May need to ↑ lovastatin dosage	No data	✓May need to ↑ pravastatin dosage	✓	✓May need to ↑ simvastatin dosage
Etravirine	✓May need to ↑ atorvastatin dosage	❢ May ↑ fluvastatin levels	✓May need to ↑ lovastatin dosage	No data	✓	✓	✓May need to ↑ simvastatin dosage

Notes:

^ Nevirapine in combination with statins has not been well studied; its interactions would be expected to be similar to those of efavirenz. Delavirdine's interactions would be expected to be similar to those of PIs.

* Other risk factors for elevated rosuvastatin levels include Asian or Pacific Islander heritage, renal insufficiency, and concurrent treatment with gemfibrozil; use with extra caution.

Adapted from: Coffey S. *Interactions between ARVs and Statin Medications: Recommendations for Coadministration of PIs and NNRTIs with Statins.* San Francisco: HIV InSite; July 2009. Available at hivinsite.ucsf.edu/InSite?page=md-rr-30. Accessed June 30, 2010.

Treatment of hypertriglyceridemia

Patients with TG levels of 200-500 mg/dL should begin non-drug interventions such as diet modification, reduction in alcohol consumption, aerobic exercise, and smoking cessation. When the TG level is ≥500 mg/dL, a low-fat diet (<15% of caloric intake) is recommended to help prevent pancreatitis, and pharmacologic therapy probably will be required. Patients with CHD or CHD equivalents, those at high risk of CHD, and those with TG levels >200 mg/dL may need pharmacologic therapy.

Fibrates are the first-line drug option for isolated hypertriglyceridemia and are an alternative treatment for combined hypertriglyceridemia and hypercholesterolemia. Fenofibrate or gemfibrozil reduce TG levels effectively in patients on ARVs. Because they are not metabolized by the cytochrome P450 hepatic enzyme system, they do not have significant drug interactions with ARVs. Fibrates are contraindicated for use by patients with renal failure. Recommended dosages of these agents are as follows:

- Fenofibrate: 40-200 mg PO once daily
- Gemfibrozil: 600 mg PO BID, 30 minutes before meals

If a fibrate alone is inadequate in reducing TG levels, several options are possible. A statin (notably atorvastatin, which acts on TGs as well as cholesterol) could be added cautiously, although there is an increased risk of skeletal muscle toxicity with concomitant use of a fibrate and a statin. N-3 (omega-3) fatty acid supplements (e.g., fish oils), administered at 1-2 g BID or TID, have decreased TG levels in patients taking ART. Extended-release niacin at 1,500-2,000 mg/day also decreases both TG and TC levels, although its clinical utility is restricted because of associated insulin resistance and flushing.

Switching antiretroviral therapy

For patients with CHD or CHD equivalents, ARV medications should, if possible, be selected to minimize the risk of hyperlipidemia. In patients with dyslipidemia caused by ARV agents, data suggest that it may be beneficial to discontinue ARVs known to increase lipids if reasonable alternatives exist. Substituting atazanavir or raltegravir in place of a lipogenic PI or replacing stavudine with tenofovir may improve the lipid profile. Before making ARV substitutions, however, consider carefully the possible effect of the substitution on HIV virologic control and the potential adverse effects of new ARVs. In some cases, antihyperlipidemic agents may be necessary even after ARV substitution.

Patient Education

- Review the importance of reducing cardiovascular risk factors. This is of increasing importance for all patients with HIV infection, particularly as they age.

- Educate patients about the benefits of diet and exercise in improving lipid levels and reducing cardiovascular risk.

- If lipid-lowering medications are prescribed, advise patients on possible adverse effects, and advise them to contact their health care provider if these develop.

- Advise patients to talk with their health care provider before starting any new medications so they can be evaluated for possible drug-drug interactions.

Appendix: Calculations to Estimate the 10-Year Risk of Cardiac Events for Men and Women — Framingham Calculator

To calculate the 10-year risk of cardiac events, add up points from the following five tables pertaining to age, HDL, systolic blood pressure, TC, and smoking status (Tables 5.1-5.5). Note that in Tables 5.3-5.5, women's points are in parentheses. After adding points from all of the tables, consult Table 5.6. (Alternatively, an online calculator is available at hin.nhlbi.nih.gov/atpiii/calculator.asp.)

(The Framingham Heart Study risk calculator has not been validated for HIV-positive individuals and may underestimate the risk in this population.)

Table 5.1. Estimate of 10-Year Risk of Cardiac Events: Age

Age (Year)	Points (Men)	Points (Women)
20–34	-9	-7
35–39	-4	-3
40–44	0	0
45–49	3	3
50–54	6	6
55–59	8	8
60–64	10	10
65–69	11	12
70–74	12	14
75–79	13	16

Table 5.2. Estimate of 10-Year Risk of Cardiac Events: High-Density Lipoprotein Cholesterol

HDL (mg/dL)	Points (Men)	Points (Women)
≥60	-1	-1
50–59	0	0
40–49	1	1
<40	2	2

Table 5.3. Estimate of 10-Year Risk of Cardiac Events: Systolic Blood Pressure

Systolic Blood Pressure	Points if Untreated — Men (Women)	Points if Treated — Men (Women)
<120	0 (0)	0 (0)
120–129	0 (1)	1 (3)
130–139	1 (2)	2 (4)
140–159	1 (3)	2 (5)
≥160	2 (4)	3 (6)

Table 5.4. Estimate of 10-Year Risk of Cardiac Events: Total Cholesterol

Total Cholesterol (mg/dL)	Points for Men (Women)				
	Age 20–39	Age 40–49	Age 50–59	Age 60–69	Age 70–79
<160	0 (0)	0 (0)	0 (0)	0 (0)	0 (0)
160–199	4 (4)	3 (3)	2 (2)	1 (1)	0 (1)
200–239	7 (8)	5 (6)	3 (4)	1 (2)	0 (1)
240–279	9 (11)	6 (8)	4 (5)	2 (3)	1 (2)
≥280	11 (13)	8 (10)	5 (7)	3 (4)	1 (2)

Table 5.5. Estimate of 10-Year Risk of Cardiac Events: Smoking Status

Smoking Status	Points for Men (Women)				
	Age 20-39	Age 40-49	Age 50-59	Age 60-69	Age 70-79
Nonsmoker	0 (0)	0 (0)	0 (0)	0 (0)	0 (0)
Smoker	8 (9)	5 (7)	3 (4)	1 (2)	1 (1)

Table 5.6. Estimate of 10-Year Risk of Cardiac Events: Calculating Risk

Men		Women	
Point Total	10-Year Risk (%)	Point Total	10-Year Risk (%)
<0	<1	<9	<1
0	1	9	1
1	1	10	1
2	1	11	1
3	1	12	1
4	1	13	2
5	2	14	2
6	2	15	3
7	3	16	4
8	4	17	5
9	5	18	6
10	6	19	8
11	8	20	11
12	10	21	14
13	12	22	17
14	16	23	22
15	20	24	27
16	25	≥25	≥30
≥17	≥30		

References

- Chow D, Day L, Souza S, et al. *Metabolic Complications of HIV Therapy*. In: Coffey S, Volberding PA, eds. *HIV InSite Knowledge Base* [online textbook]. San Francisco: UCSF Center for HIV Information; May 2006. Available at hivinsite.ucsf.edu/InSite?page=kb-03-02-10. Accessed June 30, 2010.

- Dube MP, Stein JH, Aberg JA, et al. *Guidelines for the evaluation and management of dyslipidemia in human immunodeficiency virus (HIV)-infected adults receiving antiretroviral therapy: recommendations of the HIV Medical Association of the Infectious Disease Society of America and the Adult AIDS Clinical Trials Group*. Clin Infect Dis. 2003 Sep 1;37(5):613-27.

- Expert Panel on Detection Evaluation and Treatment of High Blood Cholesterol in Adults. *Executive summary of the third report of the National Cholesterol Education Program (NCEP) Expert Panel on Detection, Evaluation, and Treatment of High Blood Cholesterol in Adults (Adult Treatment Panel III)*. JAMA. 2001 May 16;285(19):2486-97.

- Fichtenbaum CJ, Berber JG, Rosenkranz SL, et al.; NIAID AIDS Clinical Trials Group. *Pharmacokinetic interactions between protease inhibitors and statins in HV seronegative volunteers: ACTG Study A5047*. AIDS. 2002 Mar 8;16(4):569-77.

- Friis-Moller N, Weber R, Reiss P, et al.; DAD study group. *Cardiovascular disease risk factors in HIV patients—association with antiretroviral therapy. Results from the DAD study*. AIDS. 2003 May 23;17(8):1179-93.

- Grundy SM, Cleeman JI, Merz CN, et al. *Implications of recent clinical trials for the National Cholesterol Education Program Adult Treatment Panel III guidelines*. Circulation. 2004 Jul 13;110(2):227-39.

- Ho JE, Hsue PY. *Cardiovascular manifestations of HIV*. Heart. 2009 Jul;95(14):1193-202.

- McNicholl I. *Database of Antiretroviral Drug Interactions*. In: Coffey S, Volberding PA, eds. HIV InSite. San Francisco: UCSF Center for HIV Information; 2006. Available at hivinsite.ucsf.edu/insite?page=ar-00-02. Accessed June 30, 2010.

- Moyle G. *Metabolic issues associated with protease inhibitors*. J Acquir Immune Defic Syndr. 2007 Jun 1;45 Suppl 1:S19-26.

- Schambelan M, Benson CA, Carr A, et al. *Management of metabolic complications associated with antiretroviral therapy for HIV-1 infection: recommendations of an International AIDS Society-USA panel*. J Acquir Immune Defic Syndr. 2002 Nov 1;31(3):257-75.

- Shor-Posner G, Basit A, Lu Y. *Hypocholesterolemia is associated with immune dysfunction in early human immunodeficiency virus-1 infection*. Am J Med. 1993 May;94(5):515-9.

- Riddler SA, Smit E, Cole SR, et al. *Impact of HIV infection and HAART on serum lipids in men*. JAMA. 2003 Jun 11;289(22):2978-82.

Insulin Resistance, Hyperglycemia, and Diabetes on Antiretroviral Therapy

Background

Diabetes is a substantial risk factor for coronary artery disease, stroke, and peripheral vascular disease, as well as for a number of other conditions including retinopathy and kidney disease. Patients taking antiretroviral (ARV) medications, especially certain protease inhibitors (PIs) and nucleoside reverse transcriptase inhibitors (NRTIs), appear to have an increased risk of hyperglycemia and diabetes mellitus. In particular, the ARVs indinavir and stavudine (now seldom used in the United States) have been shown to induce insulin resistance in short-term studies of healthy HIV-uninfected volunteers, but other ARVs also perturb glucose homeostasis.

Disorders of glucose metabolism may present as the following:

- **Insulin resistance:** a state in which higher concentrations of insulin are required to exert normal effects; blood glucose levels may be normal but fasting insulin levels may be high because of compensatory insulin secretion by the pancreas

- **Impaired glucose tolerance:** glucose 140-199 mg/dL 2 hours after a 75 g oral glucose load

- **Impaired fasting glucose:** glucose 100-125 mg/dL after an 8-hour fast

- **Diabetes mellitus:** any of the following four criteria may be used (results must be confirmed by retesting on a subsequent occasion):

  - Fasting glucose ≥126 mg/dL

  - Glycosylated hemoglobin (HbA1c) level ≥6.5% (note that HbA1c testing has not been validated in HIV-infected persons; see "Diagnostic Evaluation," below)

  - 2-hour glucose level ≥200 mg/dL during glucose tolerance testing

  - Random glucose values ≥200 mg/dL in the presence of symptoms of hyperglycemia

The incidence of new-onset hyperglycemia among HIV-infected patients on ARV therapy (ART) has been reported as about 5%, on average. Even if fasting glucose levels remain normal in patients taking ARVs, up to 40% of those on a PI-containing regimen will show impaired glucose tolerance. The etiology of insulin resistance and hyperglycemia in HIV-infected patients probably is multifactorial, with varying contributions from traditional risk factors (e.g., obesity, family history), comorbid conditions (e.g., hepatitis C virus infection), and ARV-related factors (e.g., direct effects of PIs, cumulative exposure to NRTIs, hepatic steatosis, and fat redistribution).

Patients who have preexisting diabetes should be monitored closely when starting ART; some experts would consider avoiding PIs for these patients, if other options are feasible. Alternatively, PIs with favorable metabolic profiles (e.g., atazanavir) may be preferred for such patients. Patients with no history of diabetes should be advised about the warning signs of hyperglycemia (polydipsia, polyuria, and polyphagia) and the need to use diet and exercise to maintain an ideal body weight.

S: Subjective

Clinicians should consider the potential for abnormal glucose metabolism in the following types of patients:

- Those who are about to begin ART
- Those on an ARV regimen that includes a PI
- Those with extensive exposure to NRTIs
- Those who are obese or overweight
- Those with central fat accumulation or lipoatrophy

Although most patients with hyperglycemia are asymptomatic, some (rarely) may report polydipsia, polyuria, polyphagia, or blurred vision.

When recording the patient's history, ask about the following:

Risk factors:
- Family history of diabetes
- Obesity
- Habitual physical inactivity
- Racial or ethnic heritages (higher risk: African-American, Hispanic, Native American, Asian-Pacific Islander)
- Gestational diabetes or delivery of an infant weighing >9 lb (4.1 kg)
- Current pregnancy
- Hepatitis C virus coinfection
- Polycystic ovary syndrome
- Medications, including PIs, NRTIs, niacin, corticosteroids, antipsychotics

Comorbidities:
- Hypertension
- Low level of high-density lipoprotein (HDL)
- Elevated triglycerides
- Coronary artery disease
- Fat redistribution on ARVs (see chapter *Abnormalities of Body Fat Distribution*)
- Smoking

O: Objective

Perform a physical examination that includes the following:

- Blood pressure, weight, body mass index (BMI) (see chapter *Dyslipidemia*)
- Heart and lung examination
- Peripheral pulses
- Examination of neck, dorsocervical area, breasts, and abdomen for fat accumulation; measurement of waist circumference
- For patients with hyperglycemia or diabetes:
  - Retinal examination (refer to ophthalmologist for dilated examination)
  - Visual inspection of feet (for ulcers)
  - Sensory examination of feet (for neuropathy)

A/P: Assessment and Plan
Diagnostic Evaluation

Determine whether the patient has normal blood glucose, impaired fasting glucose, or diabetes.

Most experts recommend routine checks of fasting blood glucose levels at baseline and within 3-6 months after starting or changing ART, if baseline results are normal. For patients with normal glucose levels, recheck every 6-12 months. Monitoring should be more frequent if abnormalities are detected or if any additional risk factors exist. Patients with risk factors for diabetes must be counseled about prevention of hyperglycemia before starting ART.

The role of 2-hour postprandial glucose measurements or the 75 g oral glucose tolerance test in screening for diabetes is uncertain but may be appropriate for patients with multiple risk factors. The use of HbA1c testing to screen for diabetes has yet to be validated for the HIV-infected population. Of note, HbA1c values may underestimate glycemia in HIV-infected patients, especially in the setting of elevated red blood cell mean corpuscular volume (MCV) (e.g., owing to zidovudine) or anemia.

For patients with diabetes, monitor the following:

- HbA1c, every 3 months for patients who have elevated HbA1c or whose therapy has changed, every 3-6 months for patients with stable and adequate glucose control

- Fasting lipid panel

- Electrolytes, creatinine, estimated glomerular filtration rate (eGFR) (see chapter *Renal Disease*)

- Urine albumin/creatinine ratio (microalbuminuria: 30-299 mg/g)

Treatment
Patients with insulin resistance

For patients with insulin resistance who have normal blood glucose levels, current evidence is inadequate to recommend drug treatment. However, it may be possible to prevent the development of diabetes, and lifestyle modifications can be recommended, including exercise, avoidance of obesity, weight loss if indicated, and diet changes. Weight loss is strongly recommended if the patient is overweight. Refer the patient to a dietitian, if possible. Studies of insulin resistance in HIV-infected individuals are under way, and patients with access to clinical trials may be referred to these studies.

Patients with insulin resistance and hyperglycemia require treatment. A trial of lifestyle modifications may be attempted, including weight loss (if indicated), diet changes, and exercise.

For patients with diabetes and those whose lifestyle changes are not adequate to control blood glucose, specific treatment should be started.

Patients with diabetes

- Treatment should be instituted to control blood sugar and to modify other cardiovascular risk factors, with the aim of preventing heart disease and other end-organ disease.

  - Control glucose: maintain the HbA1c level at <7%, while avoiding hypoglycemia.

  - For hyperglycemia that is associated with the use of PIs, switching to an alternative agent (e.g., a nonnucleoside reverse transcriptase inhibitor or a different PI) may be effective if the HIV treatment history and resistance profile permit.

  - Metformin usually is the initial drug of choice for overweight patients; other options include thiazolidinediones and sulfonylureas.

- Metformin can worsen lipoatrophy and should be avoided in the presence of significant lipoatrophy. Metformin increases risk of lactic acidosis; it should not be used for patients with elevated serum creatinine (>1.5 mg/dL in men or >1.4 mg/dL in women), hepatic impairment, or metabolic acidosis.

- Thiazolidinediones should be avoided in patients with significant liver disease. Rosiglitazone may increase the risk of myocardial infarction and death (study results conflict); both rosiglitazone and pioglitazone have been associated with congestive heart failure and are contraindicated for use by patients with this condition.

- In some cases, insulin may be the safest drug therapy for patients with symptomatic hyperglycemia, although episodes of hypoglycemia are much more common with insulin than with most oral agents.

- Treat dyslipidemia: maintain low-density lipoprotein (LDL) at <100 mg/dL and maintain triglycerides at <150 mg/dL. (Note that diabetes is considered a coronary heart disease equivalent state when evaluating goals for lipid management; see chapter *Dyslipidemia*.)

- Treat hypertension: Maintain systolic blood pressure at <130 mm Hg and diastolic blood pressure at <80 mm Hg.

- Reduce cardiovascular risks through lifestyle modifications such as smoking cessation, exercise, weight loss, nutritional counseling, and moderation of alcohol intake.

- Decrease the risk of end-organ complications:

  - Measure urine microalbumin and creatinine; if the urine albumin/creatinine ratio is >30 mg/g, treat with an angiotensin-converting enzyme inhibitor (ACEI) or angiotensin receptor blocker (ARB) to slow the progression of nephropathy.

  - Schedule annual retinal examination by an ophthalmologist.

  - Perform an annual foot examination.

- Start aspirin therapy (75-162 mg daily) if the patient has evidence of macrovascular disease or a history of vascular events. Consider daily aspirin for those with increased coronary heart disease risk e.g., men >50 years old and women >60 years old with ≥1 coronary heart disease risk factor (e.g., a family history of coronary artery disease, a history of smoking (see chapter *Coronary Heart Disease Risk*).

For further information, see the American Diabetes Association, Clinical Practice Recommendations, Diabetes Care, available online at: care.diabetesjournals.org.

Patient Education

- ART can increase the risk of diabetes in some individuals. Patients should report any difficulty with excessive hunger and thirst and increased urination. Health care providers will monitor blood glucose when doing laboratory work, but it is important for the patient to report the presence of any symptoms.

- Review the patient's eating habits and explain the need to work with a dietitian to keep blood glucose (and triglycerides) within normal limits. Eating a proper diet can reduce the risk of permanent damage to the blood vessels of the eye, the kidney, and the brain, and it can reduce the risk of a heart attack.

- Emphasize other lifestyle modifications, such as weight loss (if appropriate).

- Encourage patients to get regular cardiovascular exercise; work with them to identify activities that might be realistic and acceptable for them.

- Provide medication-specific education, especially if the patient will be taking diabetes medications.

- Consider referral to a diabetes clinic for specialty needs.

References

- Aberg JA, Kaplan JE, Libman H, et al.; HIV Medicine Association of the Infectious Diseases Society of America. *Primary care guidelines for the management of persons infected with human immunodeficiency virus: 2009 update by the HIV medicine Association of the Infectious Diseases Society of America.* Clin Infect Dis. 2009 Sep 1;49(5):651-81.

- American Diabetes Association. *Standards of Medical Care in Diabetes—2010.* Diabetes Care. 2010; 33:S11-61.

- Dubé MP. *Disorders of glucose metabolism in patients infected with human immunodeficiency virus.* Clin Infect Dis. 2000 Dec;31(6):1467-75.

- Kim PS, Woods C, Georgoff P, et al. *Hemoglobin A1c underestimates glycemia in HIV Infection.* Diabetes Care. 2009 Sep;32(9):1591-3.

- Samaras K. *Prevalence and pathogenesis of diabetes mellitus in HIV-1 infection treated with combined antiretroviral therapy.* J Acquir Immune Defic Syndr. 2009 Apr 15;50(5):499-505.

- Schambelan M, Benson CA, Carr A, et al. *Management of metabolic complications associated with antiretroviral therapy for HIV-1 infection: recommendations of an International AIDS Society-USA panel.* J Acquir Immune Defic Syndr. 2002 Nov 1;31(3):257-75.

Coronary Heart Disease Risk

Marshall Glesby, MD

Background

Epidemiologic studies suggest that the incidence of myocardial infarction or hospitalization for coronary heart disease (CHD) is increased up to two- to threefold in HIV-infected individuals compared with age-matched controls without HIV infection. This increased risk of ischemic events likely is attributable to a higher prevalence of certain CHD risk factors that are independent of HIV status, such as smoking, as well as to both HIV infection and antiretroviral (ARV) medications. These various factors may interact in ways that are complex and incompletely understood.

Among the traditional CHD risk factors, dyslipidemia is common among persons with HIV infection, and can be caused both by HIV itself (e.g., resulting in low high-density lipoprotein [HDL] cholesterol) and by ARV therapy (ART); see chapter *Dyslipidemia*. Insulin resistance and diabetes also appear to be more prevalent in HIV-infected patients. (See chapter *Insulin Resistance, Hyperglycemia, and Diabetes on Antiretroviral Therapy*. Visceral fat accumulation, a poorly understood complication of HIV or ART, also may contribute to CHD risk in certain patients (see chapter *Abnormalities of Body Fat Distribution*).

A number of studies suggest that inflammation and immune activation owing to uncontrolled HIV infection also likely contribute to atherosclerosis. For example, in the Strategic Management of Antiretroviral Therapy (SMART) study, CHD events were more common in patients on intermittent ART than in those on continuous ART, possibly because of adverse effects of intermittent HIV viremia on inflammation, coagulation, and lipid parameters. There is even preliminary evidence that so-called elite controllers — patients with undetectable HIV viremia and preserved CD4 counts in the absence of ART — have increased carotid intima-medial thickness (a marker of atherosclerotic burden) compared with HIV-uninfected subjects, after adjusting for other CHD risk factors. Limited data also suggest that initiation of ART leads to improvement of endothelial dysfunction (an early marker of atherosclerosis that is predictive of future CHD events) and to improvement in markers of inflammation and immune activation. Taken together, these observations suggest that earlier initiation of ART could reduce CHD risk.

On the other hand, even patients with virologic suppression on ART appear to have higher levels of various physiologic markers of cardiovascular risk than the HIV-uninfected persons, perhaps owing to persistent immune activation. Additionally, exposure to ARVs has been linked to risk of myocardial infarction in large cohort studies such as the D:A:D study. In particular, the risk has been associated with use of ARV regimens that are based on protease inhibitors (PIs) rather than nonnucleoside reverse transcriptase inhibitors (NNRTIs). The risk is attributable in part to adverse changes in lipid profiles, but there appears to be additional risk associated with PIs that is not accounted for by changes in lipids; this remains poorly understood. Among the nucleoside reverse transcriptase inhibitors (NRTIs), abacavir and didanosine have been associated with increased risk of myocardial infarction in some but not all studies. The mechanism of this potentially increased risk has not been determined.

S: Subjective

Clinicians should ask all patients about CHD, CHD risk equivalents, and CHD risk factors. Assess the following during the history:

- Age (>45 for men, >55 for women)
- History of angina, myocardial infarction, or other heart disease
- Family history of premature CHD in first-degree relatives (men aged <55, women aged <65) and diabetes mellitus
- Smoking history
- Glucose intolerance or diabetes mellitus
- Hypertension
- Dyslipidemia
- CHD risk-equivalent states:
  - Diabetes mellitus
  - Peripheral vascular disease
  - Cerebrovascular disease
  - Abdominal aortic aneurysm
- Use of cocaine or amphetamines
- Physical inactivity

O: Objective

Perform a physical examination to include the following:

- Vital signs, including blood pressure, pulse, weight, and body mass index (BMI); see chapter *Dyslipidemia*
- Jugular venous distention
- Heart and lung examination
- Auscultation for carotid or femoral bruits
- Peripheral pulses and evaluation of extremities for peripheral edema
- Abdominal examination for fat accumulation, ideally with measurement of waist circumference

A: Assessment

- Determine whether the patient has established CHD or a CHD risk-equivalent state (see above).
- Stratify risk based on the number of CHD risk factors and the Framingham risk calculator if two or more major CHD risk factors are present; the risk calculator is available at hp2010.nhlbihin.net/atpiii/ calculator.asp?usertype=prof.
- Check fasting lipids and glucose annually; more frequently if abnormal.
- Patients with established or suspected CHD should undergo standard evaluations such as electrocardiography and exercise stress testing; refer to a cardiologist as appropriate.

P: Plan

- Work closely with patients to reduce their risks of CHD events.
- For patients who smoke, smoking cessation is the single most important intervention to reduce risk of CHD events (see chapter *Smoking Cessation*).
- Manage dyslipidemia according to established guidelines (see chapter *Dyslipidemia*).
- Manage hypertension by lifestyle intervention (e.g., sodium restriction, exercise, weight loss) and pharmacologic therapy as indicated.
- Optimize glycemic control in patients with diabetes mellitus (see chapter *Insulin Resistance, Hyperglycemia, and Diabetes on Antiretroviral Therapy*).
- Encourage weight loss in overweight and obese patients, with referral to a dietitian as appropriate.
- Encourage exercise, ideally 30 minutes at moderate intensity 5-6 times per week.
- Encourage a healthy diet that is low in saturated fats.

- Consider aspirin 81 mg once daily for primary prevention of CHD in patients at moderate to high risk who do not have contraindications to aspirin use.
- For patients who use cocaine or amphetamines, encourage cessation.

Patient Education

- Both HIV infection and ARV medications may contribute to the risk of CHD, and the available data suggest that the risk of CHD is increased in HIV-infected patients relative to the general population.
- Review the benefits of smoking cessation.
- Review exercise possibilities to determine which activities might be realistic and acceptable for the patient.
- Review the patient's eating habits and explain the need to work with a dietitian to optimize lipid levels and keep blood glucose within normal ranges.
- Emphasize the importance of other lifestyle modifications, such as weight loss (if appropriate).
- Educate patients about any pharmacologic therapy that is indicated.

References

- Aberg JA. *Cardiovascular complications in HIV management: past, present, and future.* J Acquir Immune Defic Syndr. 2009 Jan 1;50(1):54-64.
- Currier JS, Lundgren JD, Carr A, et al.; *Working Group 2. Epidemiological evidence for cardiovascular disease in HIV-infected patients and relationship to highly active antiretroviral therapy.* Circulation. 2008 Jul 8;118(2):e29-35.
- Dube MP, Stein JH, Aberg JA, et al. *Guidelines for the evaluation and management of dyslipidemia in human immunodeficiency virus (HIV)-infected adults receiving antiretroviral therapy: recommendations of the HIV Medical Association of the Infectious Disease Society of America and the Adult AIDS Clinical Trials Group.* Clin Infect Dis. 2003 Sep 1;37(5):613-27.
- El Sadr WM, Lundgren JD, Neaton JD, et al.; *Strategies for Management of Antiretroviral Therapy (SMART) Study Group. CD4+ count-guided interruption of antiretroviral treatment.* N Engl J Med. 2006 Nov 30;355(22):2283-96.
- Friis-Moller N, Reiss P, Sabin CA, et al.; D:A:D Study Group. *Class of antiretroviral drugs and the risk of myocardial infarction.* N Engl J Med. 2007 Apr 26;356(17):1723-35.
- Glesby M. *HIV and Cardiovascular Risk* (Oxford American Pocket Notes). In press, Oxford University Press.
- Stein JH, Hadigan CM, Brown TT, et al.; *Working Group 6. Prevention strategies for cardiovascular disease in HIV-infected patients.* Circulation. 2008 Jul 8;118(2):e54-60.
- Triant VA, Lee H, Hadigan C, et al. *Increased acute myocardial infarction rates and cardiovascular risk factors among patients with human immunodeficiency virus disease.* J Clin Endocrinol Metab. 2007 Jul;92(7):2506-12.

Renal Disease

Alfredo Tiu, DO

Background

The prevalence of renal complications among patients with HIV infection has increased as more patients with HIV are living longer as a result of effective antiretroviral therapy (ART) and opportunistic infection prophylaxis. More widespread access to and earlier initiation of ART has decreased the incidence of HIV-associated nephropathy (HIVAN), but other causes of renal disease persist, and in some cases are increasing in prevalence. These may be infections and other conditions related to HIV infection, other comorbidities (e.g., hypertension, diabetes), or medication adverse effects, including those caused by some antiretroviral (ARV) medications (see "Kidney disease associated with HIV infection" and Table 2, below).

Risk factors for renal disease in HIV-infected patients include the following:

- CD4 count <200 cells/µL

- HIV viremia, particularly RNA levels >4,000 copies/mL

- African-American race

- Family history of kidney disease

- Use of nephrotoxins (including medications; see Table 2, below)

- Comorbidities

  - Diabetes mellitus

  - Hypertension

  - Hepatitis C

Renal disease in HIV-infected individuals can occur as a primary disease, as a secondary disease in the setting of other systemic illness, or as an adverse effect of medications. In the United States, the most common causes of end-stage renal disease in the general population are diabetes mellitus and hypertension. HIV-infected patients are at a fourfold higher risk of developing diabetes mellitus and a threefold higher risk of developing hypertension compared with seronegative individuals. Chronic hepatitis C, seen in 30-40% of HIV-infected individuals in the United States, is associated with several types of chronic kidney disease, including progressive secondary glomerulonephropathy, membranoproliferative glomerulonephropathy, and mixed cryoglobulinemia.

Note that ART should be given to HIV-infected individuals with renal disease, according to usual criteria for ART initiation; however, some ARVs must be avoided and some should be given at modified dosages according to the degree of renal dysfunction (see Table 3). Additionally, for patients with HIVAN, ART is the primary treatment.

Screening

Screening for kidney disease in HIV-infected persons is an important aspect of primary care, as patients typically have no symptoms until very late. High-risk patients (see list of risk factors, above) should be identified and monitored. Early identification of patients with renal dysfunction allows early intervention targeted at reversing the process of renal injury or slowing down its progression. Current guidelines of the U.S. Department of Health and Human Services (DHHS) and the Infectious Diseases Society of America recommend screening at entry to care, with subsequent screening as indicated by the patient's risk factors.

Screening consists of three tests:

- Serum creatinine (Cr) and calculated estimate of renal function (eGFR); the eGFR usually is provided by the laboratory but may be calculated as follows:

  - eGFR by the Modification of Diet in Renal Disease (MDRD) equation:

    GFR (mL/min/1.73 m2) = 186 × [serum Cr (mg/dL)]$^{-1.154}$ × [age (years)]$^{-0.203}$ × [0.742 if female] × [1.212 if African-American]

    Normal GFR: ≥90 mL/min/1.73 m^2

    Chronic kidney disease (CKD): GFR <60 mL/min/1.73 m^2

    An online eGFR calculator is available at:
    www.nkdep.nih.gov/professionals/gfr_calculators/orig_con.htm

  - The creatinine clearance (CrCl) can be used as a surrogate for eGFR but is considered to be less accurate. Note that CrCl is used in determining medication dosages.

    CrCl (Cockroft-Gault equation):

    $$\frac{(140 - age) \times (weight\ in\ kilograms)}{72 \times serum\ Cr\ (mg/dL)}; multiply\ by\ 0.85\ for\ females$$

- Urinalysis, for proteinuria, hematuria
- Quantitative test for proteinuria (if eGFR <60 mL/min/1.73m2 or ≥1+ protein on dipstick):
  - Random urinary protein to urinary Cr ratio (U Pr/U Cr)
  - This estimates 24-hour protein excretion; correlates well with grams per day of proteinuria; for example, a random U Pr/U Cr of 1.0 correlates with 1 g/day of proteinuria (normal is ≤0.2)

Suggested follow up for patients with normal screening test results is shown in Figure 1; suggested follow up of abnormal screening test results is shown in "Diagnostic Evaluation."

Figure 1. Follow-Up for Patients with Normal Screening Test Results

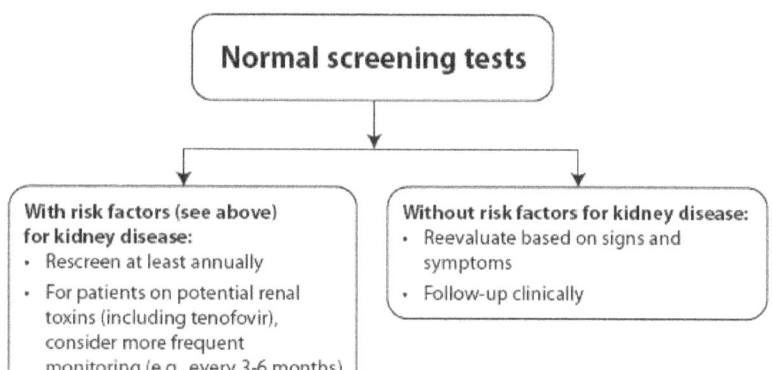

S: Subjective

As noted above, patients usually have no symptoms until late in the course of kidney disease and are diagnosed on the basis of laboratory abnormalities.

In symptomatic patients, presenting signs or symptoms are nonspecific. Patients with renal failure may present with fatigue, weakness, anorexia, nausea, pruritus, vomiting, edema, diminished urine output, discolored urine, altered mental status, and seizures. Those with renal disease associated with systemic illnesses may present with fever, arthralgias, respiratory symptoms, flank pain, abdominal pain, and diarrhea.

For patients with renal disease suspected on the basis of laboratory abnormalities (e.g., elevated serum Cr [azotemia], electrolyte disturbances, acid-base disorders, proteinuria, hematuria, and anemia), and for symptomatic patients with known kidney disease, ask about the risk factors and symptoms described above, and about the following:

- Systemic illness
  - Night sweats, fever, weight lost
  - Shortness of breath, cough, hemoptysis, nasal congestion, rhinorrhea

- Diarrhea, hematochezia, melena
- Dysuria, frequency, urgency, polyuria, decreased urine output, discoloration of urine
- Skin rash or skin lesions
- Edema, arthralgias, painful swollen joints, myalgias
- Family history of kidney disease, hypertension, diabetes mellitus
- Recent radiographic imaging with IV dyes

Review the patient's medication list (see Table 1).

- Include over-the-counter medications, nonsteroidal antiinflammatory drugs, phosphate-containing enemas

O: Objective

Check blood pressure, temperature, and weight. Compare these with values from previous readings. Perform a physical examination, including evaluations of the following:

- Volume status (blood pressure, pulse, skin turgor, mucous membrane moistness, edema)

- Optic fundi (signs of retinopathy)

- Cardiovascular system (peripheral pulses, bruits), to assess for peripheral vascular disease

- Abdomen (auscultate for unilateral bruit [renal artery stenosis], distention, mass, organomegaly, tenderness)

- Musculoskeletal system (bruises, muscle pain, muscle weakness, swollen joints)

- Skin (rash to help evaluate for drug reaction, vasculitis)

- Rectum (enlarged prostate, if obstruction is suspected)

Review previous laboratory values (e.g., serum Cr, blood urea nitrogen [BUN], electrolytes, urinalysis) to determine whether the kidney disease is acute or chronic.

- Acute kidney injury (AKI) is assumed if there are no previous serum Cr values.

The presence of an abnormal GFR (≤60 mL/min for at least 3 months) suggests chronic kidney disease (CKD).

Review the CD4 cell count and HIV viral load.

A: Assessment

Once the duration of the elevated serum Cr is assessed, a differential diagnosis can be made.

The causes of renal failure are classified traditionally based on the area of the renal anatomy where the injury occurred: prerenal, renal, and postrenal (obstructive uropathy). Acute tubular necrosis (ATN) is the most common cause of acute kidney injury.

Table 1. Causes of Renal Failure

Prerenal	Renal	Postrenal
Laboratory Data		
• Urine sodium (Na) <30 mEq/L • Fractional excretion of Na (FeNa) <1% (see below) • Fractional excretion of urea <35% • Serum BUN:serum Cr ratio ≥20	• Urine Na >30 mEq/L • FeNa >1% (see below) • Fractional excretion of urea >50 • Serum BUN:serum Cr ratio ≥10	Hematuria Imaging showing obstruction

Prerenal	Renal	Postrenal
	Partial Differential Diagnosis	

Decreased renal perfusion
• Volume depletion
• Effective volume depletion
  • Heart failure
  • Cirrhosis
  • Shock
Vascular disease
• Renal artery stenosis
Medication induced
• Prostaglandin inhibition (NSAID)
• ACE inhibitors and angiotensin receptor blockers
	Acute Tubular Necrosis
	Ischemia leading to ATN
	• Prolonged hypotension due to any cause
	  • Sepsis syndrome
	  • Volume depletion (gastrointestinal bleeding)
	• Atheroembolism and thromboembolism
	• Systemic vasculitis
	• Thrombotic microangiopathy (TTP, HUS)
	Endogenous toxins
	• Myoglobin (rhabdomyolysis)
	• Uric acid and calcium-phosphate complexes (tumor lysis syndrome)
	Exogenous-induced ATN
	• Aminoglycosides
	• Amphotericin B
	• Foscarnet
	• Ganciclovir
	• Intravenous pentamidine
	• Tenofovir
	• Chemotherapeutic agents (methotrexate, cisplatinum)
	Glomerulonephropathy*
	• Many specific types; some associated with HIV (including HIVAN) or associated infections and other conditions
	Other intrarenal lesions
	• Acute interstitial nephritis (AIN)
	• Drug induced
	• Infections associated with AIN
	  • Bacterial (*Streptococcus*, *Mycobacteria*, *Legionella*, *Pneumococcus*)
	  • Viral (Epstein-Barr, herpes simplex type 1, cytomegalovirus, BK virus)
	  • Fungal (histoplasmosis, candidiasis)
	  • Other infections (toxoplasmosis, syphilis, schistosomiasis, malaria, leptospirosis)
	• Infectious
	  • Granulomatous (mycobacterial disease, coccidioidomycosis, histoplasmosis)
	• Tumors
	  • Multiple myeloma
	  • Lymphoma
	• Nephrolithiasis
	  • Intratubular obstruction
	    • Drug-induced crystalluria
	    ⊳ Antiviral (acyclovir, indinavir, atazanavir)
	    ⊳ Antibiotic (trimethoprim/sulfamethoxazole)
		Prostate hypertrophy
		
		Tumors
		
		Stones or crystal deposition

Abbreviations: ACE = angiotensin-converting enzyme; HUS = hemolytic uremic syndrome; NSAID = nonsteroidal antiinflammatory drug; TTP = thrombotic thrombocytopenic purpura

Kidney disease associated with HIV infection

A discussion of glomerulonephropathy is beyond the scope of this chapter, but HIV and associated comorbidities (e.g., infections such as hepatitis C, hepatitis B, and cytomegalovirus, along with malignancies, heroin use, nephrotoxic medications, diabetes mellitus, and hypertension) are among the many causes of glomerulonephropathy. The condition most closely associated with HIV is HIVAN. This is a collapsing focal segmental glomerulosclerosis (FSGS) that usually occurs in persons of African heritage, and particularly those with a low CD4 count or high HIV RNA level. The clinical presentation includes the following:

- Nephrotic syndrome or nonnephrotic proteinuria

- Normal blood pressure

- Elevated Cr, often with rapid progression to endstage renal disease (<6 months)

- Renal ultrasound usually reveals normal size or slightly enlarged echogenic kidneys

- Renal biopsy shows a collapsing FSGS

In addition, several conditions may be caused by ARV medications. Tenofovir may cause, though rarely, AKI with type 2 renal tubular acidosis (RTA) and Fanconi syndrome. Alternatively, it may cause a gradual increase in serum Cr; this perhaps is seen more commonly in persons on ritonavir-boosted PIs. Patients who take tenofovir should have renal function monitored every 3-6 months. Indinavir can cause crystalluria, nephrolithiasis, and acute interstitial nephritis, and atazanavir can cause nephrolithiasis.

Some other medications commonly used in the treatment of patients with HIV infection and associated conditions may cause acute or chronic kidney injury. See "Causes of Renal Failure," above, and Table 2, below.

Table 2. Selective Drugs Causing Acute or Chronic Kidney Injury in HIV-Infected Patients

Drugs	Acute Tubular Necrosis	Acute Interstitial Nephritis	Other Associated Abnormalities
Antiretroviral Medications			
Abacavir		+/-	
Atazanavir		+	Nephrolithiasis
Indinavir		+	Crystalluria
Tenofovir	+		Fanconi syndrome (hypokalemia, non-gap metabolic acidosis, hypophosphatemia, glycosuria) May cause a slow increase in Cr
Other Medications			
TMP-SMX (Bactrim, Septra)		+++	Hyperkalemia, crystalluria
Beta-lactams		++	
Sulfonamides		++	
Fluoroquinolones		+	
Aminoglycosides (e.g., streptomycin, gentamycin, amikacin)	+++		
Rifampin	+	+	
INH		+	Overdose leads to high anion gap metabolic acidosis
Dapsone	+/-		Papillary necrosis
Amphotericin B	+++		Hypokalemia, hypernatremia (nephrogenic diabetes insipidus)
Pentamidine	+++		Crystalluria
Foscarnet	+++		
Gancyclovir	+		
Acyclovir	+		Crystalluria
NSAIDs		+	Proteinuria, secondary minimal change disease, papillary necrosis

P: Plan

Diagnostic Evaluation

Figure 2. Workup of Abnormal Screening Test Results

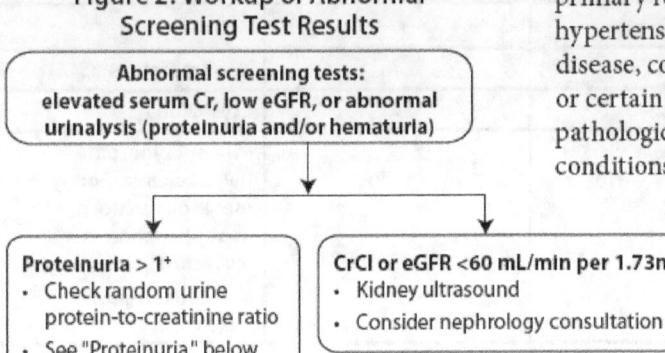

Determine whether the renal disease is acute or chronic, as above (see "O: Objective").

Perform a targeted laboratory evaluation, depending on results of initial tests, history, and physical examination.

- Urinalysis with microscopy and examination of urine sediment (e.g., hematuria, pyuria, casts) can help in identifying etiologies such as nephritic syndrome, ATN, or infection.

- Quantify the proteinuria by obtaining a random urine protein-to-urine creatinine ratio (U Pr/U Cr), if not done already; this correlates well with grams per day of proteinuria, as discussed above.

- Fractional excretion of sodium (FeNa) may be helpful in distinguishing causes of acute kidney injury.

  - $\text{FeNa} = \dfrac{\text{Urine sodium} \div \text{Serum sodium}}{\text{Urine Cr} \div \text{Serum Cr}}$

  - FeNa <1 is highly suggestive of prerenal state

  - FeNa >1 is suggestive of intrinsic renal injury

- Urine culture, if urinary tract infection is suspected

Further workup will depend on the findings and the suspected cause.

Proteinuria

Proteinuria can be present in patients with primary renal disease, and also in those with hypertension, diabetes mellitus, vascular disease, collagen vascular disease, malignancy, or certain infections. Proteinuria is not always pathologic and may be caused by transient conditions such as pregnancy, strenuous exercise, fever, seizure, or congestive heart failure; in some cases, it may be benign. However, proteinuria should be evaluated if it persists. If present with hematuria, proteinuria is highly suspicious for a glomerular disease.

The major classifications of persons with proteinuria are as follows:

Nephrotic syndrome:

- >3.5 g/day proteinuria

- "Bland" sediment, with no or few red or white blood cells

- Edema

- Hyperlipidemia

- Hypoalbuminemia

- Check serum complements (C3 and C4):

  - Low complements: glomerulonephritis associated with subacute bacterial endocarditis, infection (postinfectious), lupus, membranoproliferative glomerulonephritis, and mixed cryoglobulinemia

Glomerulonephritis:

- Proteinuria

- "Active" sediment, with white and red blood cells; may see red blood cell casts

- Further categorized into those with normal renal function and those with abnormal renal function

Hematuria

For asymptomatic isolated microscopic hematuria, obtain a follow-up urinalysis. If hematuria is persistent, obtain a renal ultrasound. If the result is normal, the eGFR is normal, and there are no other urine abnormalities, conduct routine follow-up with urinalysis and serum Cr testing. Refer patients aged ≥40 with persistent hematuria to a urologist for formal evaluation. Consider checking urine cytology, though that test is not sensitive enough to rule out genitourinary malignancy.

Red blood cell casts

Red blood cell casts strongly suggest glomerulonephritis, which can progress rapidly.

ATN

ATN is the most common cause of AKI. A history of certain medication exposures, recent IV contrast, and concurrent illness may provide important clues to ATN. Laboratory findings that are consistent with ATN include increasing serum Cr and a characteristic urine sediment that shows "muddy brown" casts, which are casts that contain densely packed tubular cells.

AIN

During AIN, the classic triad of AKI, fever, and rash are not always present. Laboratory findings suggestive of AIN in the setting of AKI include sterile pyuria and eosinophiluria.

Sterile pyuria

Sterile pyuria also may occur in malignancy (e.g., renal, bladder), and in genitourinary tuberculosis. If tuberculosis is suspected, further testing usually requires three first-void urine specimens sent for acid-fast bacilli culture.

Crystalluria and nephrolithiasis

Usual causes of nephrolithiasis should be considered in patients with hematuria, particularly if symptoms consistent with nephrolithiasis are present. Other causes in persons with HIV infection include some medications, including the ARVs indinavir and (rarely) atazanavir; see Table 2 above.

Obtain radiographic imaging (see below) as part of the initial evaluation, and send the passed renal calculus, if available, for analysis in order to provide more specific recommendations for management. If there is suspicion that the condition is caused by a medication, order specific chemical analysis (e.g., for atazanavir).

In patients with multiple renal stones, active renal stone formation, and recurrent kidney stones, a metabolic evaluation should be done. This includes a serum intact parathyroid hormone measurement and 24-hour urine collection for Cr, sodium, calcium, oxalate, uric acid, and citrate.

Imaging

Radiographic imaging of the kidneys is important in the evaluation of renal disease. The size and echogenicity of the kidneys may help differentiate acute and chronic kidney disease. Small and echogenic kidneys are consistent with CKD, though HIV, diabetes, and some other chronic conditions are associated with normal size or large kidneys. Imaging also helps identify obstruction (though the absence of hydronephrosis does not completely rule that out), malignancy, and other conditions.

Both spiral computed tomography (CT) scan and renal ultrasound are acceptable radiographic imaging studies for nephrolithiasis. The advantage of spiral CT scan is its ability to localize stones and assess their size without the use of contrast. Gallium renal scan may be helpful in AIN.

Renal biopsy

Biopsy is not always indicated for patients

with renal disease, but it can be very helpful in establishing some diagnoses and determining treatment options.

Treatment

Patients with proteinuria will benefit from angiotensin-converting enzyme inhibitors (ACEIs) or angiotensin receptor blockers (ARBs). Follow the serum potassium and Cr during treatment with an ACEI or ARB (check 1 week after initiation, then periodically). Follow the JNC VII (Joint National Committee on Prevention, Detection, Evaluation and Treatment of Blood Pressure) guidelines for blood pressure control. For patients with hypertension and proteinuria, the target blood pressure is <125/80 mm Hg.

The cornerstone of HIVAN management is fully suppressive ART, and this should be quickly initiated or optimized in all patients, if possible. An ACEI or ARB also should be used to treat proteinuria. A trial of corticosteroids can be considered for patients with deteriorating kidney function while on effective ART plus an ACEI or ARB; consult with a specialist.

For ATN and AIN, discontinue the offending medications and provide supportive care, which may include gentle volume repletion, replacement of bicarbonate deficit, and management of electrolyte abnormalities (e.g., hyperkalemia); consult with a renal specialist.

Other modalities of treatment such as steroids or immunomodulators may be needed, depending on the specific glomerular disease diagnosed by renal biopsy.

Uncomplicated nephrolithiasis can be managed with hydration and pain control. Oral fluid intake should be titrated to produce ≥2 liters of urine output per day. Recommendations for dietary modifications should be based on the 24-hour urine metabolic evaluation. A low-calcium diet usually is not helpful for patients with normal serum calcium and may be detrimental

to patients with oxalate renal stones. If the crystalluria is caused by medications, discontinue the offending medications, if possible (in the case of ARVs, make substitutions to maintain optimal virologic suppression).

Patients with complicated nephrolithiasis or pyelonephritis require urgent urologic evaluation.

Follow-Up

- Acute kidney injury
  - Monitor serum electrolytes, BUN and Cr
  - After these normalize, perform routine follow-up
- Acute interstitial nephritis
  - Avoid offending medications
- Chronic kidney disease
  - Follow blood pressure closely
    - If hypertensive, consider an ACEI or ARB as first-line medication, as above
    - Target blood pressure is <130/80 mm Hg
    - If evidence of nephropathy, target blood pressure is <125/75 mm Hg
- For patients with diabetes, optimize blood glucose control
- Address other risk factors for cardiovascular disease (see chapter *Coronary Heart Disease Risk*)
  - Dyslipidemia
  - Cigarette smoking
  - Obesity
  - Physical inactivity
- Monitor serum electrolytes, BUN, Cr, and hemoglobin
- Risk of secondary hyperparathyroidism:
  - Serum calcium <9.5 mg/dL
  - Parathyroid hormone level >35 pg/mL

- Management
  - Low phosphate diet
  - Phosphate binders with meals
  - 1,25-dihyroxyvitamin D3 or its analogues
- Anemia
  - Consider recombinant human erythropoietin and iron supplement (consult with a nephrologist)
  - Target hemoglobin 11-12 g/dL
- Avoid nephrotoxins, if possible
- Adjust medication dosages based on renal function (eGFR); see below

Patients with severe or chronic renal disease should be referred to Nephrology for further evaluation and assistance with the following:

- Management
- Education
- Evaluation for renal replacement therapy
  - Peritoneal dialysis
  - Hemodialysis
- Kidney transplant evaluation

Medication Dosage Adjustment

Dosages of many medications, including most nucleoside analogues (NRTIs), must be adjusted for patients with CKD, and for those on hemodialysis; see Table 3, below.

Table 3. Dosing of Antiretroviral Drugs in Adults with Chronic Kidney Disease and Hemodialysis

Drug	Standard Dosage	Dosing in Chronic Kidney Disease and Hemodialysis		
Abacavir	300 mg PO BID	Dosage adjustment for CKD does not appear necessary		
Didanosine (enteric-coated capsules)	250 mg to 400 mg PO once daily, depending on weight	CrCl (mL/min)	Weight ≥60 kg	Weight <60 kg
		≥60	400 mg once daily	250 mg once daily
		30-59	200 mg once daily	125 mg once daily
		10-29	125 mg once daily	125 mg once daily
		<10	125 mg once daily	Formulation not suitable
		HD	125 mg once daily	Formulation not suitable
Emtricitabine	200 mg PO once daily	CrCl (mL/min)		
		≥50	200 mg once daily	
		30-49	200 mg Q48H	
		15-29	200 mg Q72H	
		<15	200 mg Q96H	
		HD	200 mg Q96H, give dosage after dialysis	

Drug	Standard Dosage	Dosing in Chronic Kidney Disease and Hemodialysis		
Lamivudine	150 mg PO BID or 300 mg PO once daily	CrCl (mL/min)		
		≥50	150 mg BID or 300 mg once daily	
		30-49	150 mg once daily	
		15-29	150 mg first dose, then 100 mg once daily	
		5-14	150 mg first dose, then 50 mg once daily	
		<5	50 mg first dose, then 25 mg once daily	
Stavudine	20 mg to 40 mg PO BID, depending on weight	CrCl (mL/min)	Weight ≥60 kg	Weight <60 kg
		>50	40 mg BID	30 mg BID
		26-50	20 mg BID	15 mg BID
		10-25	20 mg once daily	15 mg once daily
		HD	20 mg once daily	15 mg once daily
Tenofovir	300 mg PO once daily	Experience in patients with CrCl <60 mL/min is limited. Preliminary data suggest the following:		
		CrCl (mL/min)		
		≥50	300 mg once daily	
		30-49	300 mg Q48H	
		10-29	300 mg twice weekly (i.e., Q 3-4 days)	
		HD	300 mg once weekly	
Zidovudine	300 mg PO BID	CrCl (mL/min)		
		<15	100 mg Q6-8H (or 300 mg once daily)	
		HD	100 mg TID (or 300 mg once daily)	

Fixed-Dose Combinations

Drug	Standard Dosage	Dosing in Chronic Kidney Disease and Hemodialysis	
Atripla (efavirenz/ emtricitabine/ tenofovir)	1 tab PO QHS	Substitute component drugs, adjusting dosage of each drug for CrCl	
Combivir (zidovudine/ lamivudine)	1 tab PO BID	Substitute component drugs, adjusting dosage of each drug for CrCl	
Epzicom or Kivexa (abacavir/ lamivudine)	1 tab PO once daily	Substitute component drugs, adjusting dosage of each drug for CrCl	
Trizivir (zidovudine/ lamivudine/ abacavir)	1 tab PO BID	Substitute component drugs, adjusting dosage of each drug for CrCl	
Truvada (emtricitabine/ tenofovir)	1 tab PO once daily	CrCl (mL/min)	
		≥50	1 tablet once daily
		30-49	1 tablet Q48H
		<30	Substitute component drugs, adjusting dosage of each drug for CrCl

Abbreviations: CrCl = creatinine clearance; HD = hemodialysis; Wt = weight

Adapted from McNicholl I, Rodriguez R. *Dosing of Antiretroviral Drugs in Adults with Chronic Kidney Disease and Hemodialysis.* In: HIV InSite, Coffey S, Volberding P, eds. San Francisco: UCSF Center for HIV Information; October 2009. Available at hivinsite.ucsf.edu/InSite?page=md-rr-18. Accessed June 30, 2010.

Protease inhibitors (PIs) and nonnucleoside reverse transcriptase inhibitors (NNRTIs) do not appear to require dosage adjustment in persons with CKD. Some PIs and NNRTIs, however, do require changes in dosing strategy for patients on hemodialysis. (It should be noted that most PIs have not been studied in the setting of hemodialysis.) The CCR5 antagonist maraviroc should not be used for certain patients with CKD. Available recommendations for hemodialysis patients include the folowing:

Atazanavir
- Unboosted atazanavir should not be used.
- Treatment-naive patients: atazanavir must be boosted by ritonavir.
- Treatment-experienced patients: atazanavir (boosted or unboosted) is not recommended.

Lopinavir/ritonavir
- Once-daily dosing should not be used
- In patients with PI resistance, lopinavir/ritonavir levels may be subtherapeutic.

Maraviroc
- Should not be used in patients with severe renal impairment or end-stage renal disease who are taking a potent CYP 3A inhibitor or inducer.

Nevirapine
- An additional dose (200 mg) should be given after each dialysis session.

Available agents in the integrase inhibitor and fusion inhibitor classes do not appear to require dosage adjustment for patients with CKD.

Patient Education
- Early diagnosis of kidney disease is important. Acute kidney injury usually is reversible but may take time and may require temporary hemodialysis support.
- Advise patients to report all the medications they take, including over-the-counter medications and herbs or supplements.
- Risk factors for kidney disease are uncontrolled HIV infection (viral load above 4,000 copies/mL and CD4 count <200 cells/µL), coexisting conditions (diabetes mellitus, hypertension, hepatitis C), and ethnicity (African-Americans, Hispanic Americans, Asians, Pacific Islanders, and American Indians). Advise patients that it is important to reduce any modifiable risks, including optimizing HIV control and diabetes mellitus and/or hypertension management.
- Advise patients that control of blood pressure is important in slowing the progression of renal disease. Hypertension control can be maximized by both lifestyle modifications (e.g., weight lost, exercise, avoiding excessive alcohol intake) and antihypertensive medications. ACEIs or ARBs are the drugs of choice for patients with hypertension and kidney disease. Target blood pressure is <125/75 mm Hg for patients with proteinuric kidney disease.
- Educate patients that management of chronic kidney disease helps avoid or control complications such as high blood pressure, weak bones (osteodystrophy), anemia, and nerve damage (neuropathy).
- When the kidney disease progress to end-stage renal disease, several options can be explored. These are dialysis, kidney transplant, or palliative care. There are two modes of dialysis, hemodialysis and peritoneal dialysis. A nephrologist and the patient can decide which option is best. HIV control (suppressed viral load, optimal CD4) is required if kidney transplant is to be considered.

Section 6: Comorbidities, Coinfections, and Complications

References

- Aberg JA, Kaplan JE, Libman H, et al.; HIV Medicine Association of the Infectious Diseases Society of America. *Primary care guidelines for the management of persons infected with human immunodeficiency virus: 2009 update by the HIV medicine Association of the Infectious Diseases Society of America.* Clin Infect Dis. 2009 Sep 1;49(5):651-81.

- Atta MG, Gallant JE, Rahman H, et al. *Antiretroviral therapy in the treatment of HIV-associated nephropathy.* Nephrol Dial Transplant. 2006 Oct;21(10):2809-13.

- Berliner AR, Fine DM, Lucas GM, et al. *Observations on a cohort of HIV-infected patients undergoing native renal biopsy.* Am J Nephrol. 2008;28(3):478-86.

- Brown TT, Cole SR, Li X, et al. *Antiretroviral therapy and the prevalence and incidence of diabetes mellitus in the multicenter AIDS cohort study.* Arch Intern Med. 2005 May 23;165(10):1179-84.

- Brown TT, Li X, Cole SR, et al. *Cumulative exposure to nucleoside analogue reverse transcriptase inhibitors is associated with insulin resistance markers in the Multicenter AIDS Cohort Study.* AIDS. 2005 Sep 2;19(13):1375-83.

- Campbell LJ, Ibrahim F, Fisher M, et al. *Spectrum of chronic kidney disease in HIV-infected patients.* HIV Med. 2009 Jul;10(6):329-36.

- McNicholl I, Rodriguez R. *Dosing of Antiretroviral Drugs in Adults with Chronic Kidney Disease and Hemodialysis.* In: HIV InSite, Coffey S, Volberding P, eds. San Francisco: UCSF Center for HIV Information; October 2009. Available at hivinsite.ucsf.edu/InSite?page=md-rr-18. Accessed June 30, 2010.

- Moore J, Carome MA. *Proteinuria.* Clin Lab Med. 1993 Mar;13(1):21-31.

- National Kidney Foundation. *K/DOQI clinical practice guidelines for chronic kidney disease evaluation: evaluation, classification, and stratification.* Am J Kidney Dis. 2002 Feb;39(2 Suppl 1):S1-266.

- Post FA, Campbell LJ, Hamzah L, et al. *Predictors of renal outcome in HIV-associated nephropathy.* Clin Infect Dis. 2008 Apr 15;46(8):1282-9.

- Szczech LA, Gupta SK, Habash R, et al. *The clinical epidemiology and course of the spectrum of renal diseases associated with HIV infection.* Kidney Int. 2004 Sep;66(3):1145-52.

- Verdecchia P, Staessen J, Angeli F, et al. *Usual versus tight control of systolic blood pressure in non-diabetic patients with hypertension (Cardio-Sis): an open-label randomized trial.* Lancet. 2009 Aug 15;374(9689):525-33.

- U.S. Department of Health and Human Services. *Guidelines for the Use of Antiretroviral Agents in HIV-1-Infected Adults and Adolescents.* January 10, 2011. Available at www.aidsinfo.nih.gov/guidelines/.

- U.S. Department of Veterans Affairs. *Renal Disease.* In: Ross D, Coffey S, eds. *Primary Care of Veterans with HIV.* Washington: U.S. Department of Veterans Affairs, Veterans Health Administration; April 2009;211-25. Available at www.hiv.va.gov/vahiv?page=pcm-212_renal . Accessed June 30, 2010.

- Zietse R, Zoutendijk R, Hoorn EJ. *Fluid, electrolyte and acid-base disorders associated with antibiotic therapy.* Nat Rev Nephrol. 2009 Apr;5(4):193-202.

Immune Reconstitution Inflammatory Syndrome

Background

For most patients, initiating antiretroviral therapy (ART) improves immune responses to a wide range of opportunistic pathogens. The process of ART-induced immune reconstitution typically is uneventful. However, a small percentage of patients develop inflammatory disease in response to specific opportunistic pathogens within a few weeks or months after initiating therapy. This exuberant inflammatory response has been called the immune reconstitution inflammatory syndrome (IRIS), also known as immune reconstitution syndrome (IRS) or immune reconstitution disease (IRD).

The term IRIS is used to describe two distinct entities:

- An exacerbation of a partially or successfully treated opportunistic infection (OI), referred to as paradoxical IRIS
- A previously undiagnosed (subclinical) OI, referred to as unmasking IRIS

IRIS may occur in response to many pathogens, including *Mycobacterium tuberculosis*, *Mycobacterium avium* complex (MAC), cytomegalovirus (CMV), *Cryptococcus, Pneumocystis, Toxoplasma,* hepatitis B, and varicella-zoster virus.

Many of the IRIS cases described in the medical literature occurred within a few months after initiating ART and in the context of a rapid and marked rise in CD4 cell count from very low pretreatment levels (often <50-100 cells/μL). IRIS also can occur in the absence of ART, as has been reported during tuberculosis (TB) treatment. The specific mechanisms involved in the pathogenesis of IRIS are not well understood and may vary from one infection to another. However, experts believe that IRIS is caused by an enhanced immune response to disease-specific antigens, which leads to an overproduction of inflammatory mediators.

IRIS may be difficult to identify in clinical practice because the clinical presentation is nonspecific and, currently, there are no laboratory markers to identify the syndrome. To make the diagnosis of IRIS, the following must be excluded:

- Presence of a new OI or concomitant illness
- Failure of treatment for HIV infection (e.g., owing to poor adherence or drug resistance)
- Failure of treatment for a known OI (e.g., owing to drug resistance, inadequate treatment, or poor adherence)

The severity of IRIS varies widely, from mild to life-threatening. Treatment varies according to the specific pathogen and clinical situation, but typically includes continuing ART if possible, treating the OI as indicated, and adding antiinflammatory therapy as needed.

Clinical Presentation

IRIS is largely a clinical diagnosis, and other conditions must be excluded, as indicated above. To consider IRIS in the differential diagnosis, clinicians must recognize the clinical findings (typical or atypical) of a specific OI and the temporal association with treatment (usually after ART initiation, but IRIS may occur with treatment of the OI alone). For example, for a patient with TB who has recently initiated ART after responding to treatment of TB, the "red flags" for a diagnosis of IRIS (rather than progression of the TB) would include new or worsening fever, new effusions, and new or worsening lymphadenopathy, in the absence of poor adherence to TB treatment and the absence of drug-resistant TB.

The clinical manifestations of IRIS associated with some common OIs are described below. (This is not an exhaustive list, but it includes most of the important IRIS manifestations seen in patients with HIV infection.)

Tuberculosis

The signs and symptoms of TB IRIS may include high fevers, new or worsening pulmonary symptoms and infiltrates, and new or increasing pleural effusions. Nonpulmonary presentations may include expanding central nervous system (CNS) lesions, lymphadenopathy (mediastinal or peripheral), skin or visceral abscesses, bone lesions, and hypercalcemia. In a patient who is receiving therapy for active TB, the onset of TB IRIS typically occurs within 3-6 months after the patient begins ART and is more common among patients with low CD4 cell counts at the time of ART initiation (see chapter *Mycobacterium tuberculosis*).

Mycobacterium avium Complex

Lymphadenitis and fever are the characteristic symptoms of MAC IRIS, but pulmonary and other symptoms may develop. These and the other signs and symptoms of MAC IRIS may be clinically indistinguishable from active MAC. In contrast to disseminated MAC, MAC IRIS is associated with a rapid and striking increase in CD4 count (usually from <50 cells/µL to ≥100 cells/µL), and bacteremia usually is absent. MAC IRIS can be mild and localized or it can be severe, requiring systemic antiinflammatory therapy in addition to anti-MAC therapy.

Cytomegalovirus
CMV retinitis

CMV retinitis may occur in patients with a history of CMV retinitis or in patients with no previous evidence of retinitis. In those with a previous diagnosis of CMV retinitis, a new opacified retinal lesion develops, frequently at the site of an earlier lesion. CMV retinitis IRIS is identical to active CMV retinitis on ophthalmologic examination. Clinical information, therefore, will guide the diagnosis, and patients should be monitored closely. As with other IRIS reactions, symptoms often are associated temporally with initiation of ART. For patients who were adequately treated for CMV and who experience IRIS, serial ophthalmologic examinations will reveal that the lesions clear without a new or different therapy for CMV. This clinical picture differs from that of retinal lesions caused by active CMV infection and uncontrolled CMV replication, in which lesions will increase in size or new lesions will appear, if CMV therapy has not been introduced or changed (see chapter *Cytomegalovirus*).

CMV vitreitis and CMV uveitis

CMV vitreitis and CMV uveitis are seen exclusively in patients with previous CMV retinitis infection who responded to ART:

CMV vitreitis

CMV vitreitis IRIS is an alarming syndrome,

but a benign one. Patients who are receiving anti-CMV therapy typically present with acute onset of blurred vision and "floaters" caused by posterior segment inflammation. Ophthalmologic examination reveals numerous inflammatory cells in the vitreous humor. Symptoms usually resolve in 1 month without specific treatment and without any lasting visual effects.

CMV uveitis

In patients with a history of CMV retinitis, CMV uveitis IRIS may occur within months of ART initiation, but typically is a late complication, occurring about 3 years after patients begin ART. Uveitis is painless and primarily involves inflammation in the iris, the ciliary body, and the choroid layers. However, CMV uveitis may have serious sequelae. It often results in macular edema, epiretinal membrane formation, or cataracts, which can lead to permanent vision loss. Because of the risk of vision loss, clinicians should have a high index of suspicion for CMV uveitis.

Cryptococcal Meningitis

In patients with or without previously diagnosed cryptococcal meningitis, presentation of cryptococcal IRIS typically includes fever, headache, and meningeal signs and symptoms. Onset has been reported between 1 week and 11 months after initiation of ART. Lymphadenitis also has been reported (see chapter *Cryptococcal Disease*).

Pneumocystis jiroveci Pneumonia

Pneumocystis jiroveci pneumonia (PCP) IRIS may occur in patients with current or recent PCP who are starting ART in the early weeks after initiation of PCP treatment. IRIS may present as worsening pulmonary symptoms and high fever in patients who had been improving on PCP therapy or in patients with recent successful treatment of PCP. Chest X rays may show worsening lung involvement, and oxygen saturation or arterial blood gas measurements may show worsening hypoxia

or alveolar-arterial oxygen gradient. PCP IRIS sometimes causes severe acute respiratory failure (see chapter *Pneumocystis Pneumonia*).

S: Subjective

Symptoms of IRIS will vary according to the specific illness.

Include the following in the history:

- Specific symptoms and time course of symptoms
- History of OIs, including recently diagnosed OIs
- Treatment of OIs, including date of initiation, medication adherence, duration of therapy, and clinical response
- ART initiation date, specific antiretroviral regimen, medication adherence, and previous history of ART
- CD4 cell count and HIV viral load before ART initiation
- Current CD4 cell count and HIV viral load, if known
- Other medications, especially new medications, including over-the-counter and herbal preparations

O: Objective

Obtain vital signs, including temperature, heart rate, blood pressure, respiratory rate, and oxygen saturation.

Perform a thorough physical examination based on symptoms and suspicion of systems involved.

A: Assessment

In the appropriate clinical setting (especially in patients with advanced AIDS who recently initiated ART), IRIS should be considered in the differential diagnosis of patients who present with new or worsening symptoms. In these patients, the differential is broad, and causes other than IRIS should be considered carefully, including:

- Worsening or progression of a known OI despite treatment (e.g., owing to drug resistance or inadequate therapy)
- A new infection or illness
- Drug toxicity (e.g., hypersensitivity reaction)
- Failure of ART; progression of AIDS

Perform the appropriate diagnostic tests to exclude other etiologies. Consider consulting with an HIV specialist if the diagnosis is in question.

P: Plan

Diagnostic Evaluation

It is important to rule out new, incompletely treated, or untreated infections; malignancy; and other illnesses before concluding the patient has IRIS.

The workup of the patient with possible IRIS will depend on the specific clinical presentation. Perform laboratory tests, blood cultures, and other diagnostic tests as appropriate for the individual patient. These may include the following:

- Complete blood count (CBC) with differential, electrolytes and creatinine, liver function tests
- CD4 cell count and HIV viral load
- Blood cultures for bacteria, acid-fast bacteria (MAC), fungi
- Chest X ray; other radiographic studies
- Sputum stain and culture
- Biopsy or culture of skin or other lesions
- Lumbar puncture and cerebrospinal fluid studies
- Ophthalmologic examination
- Drug resistance testing for the OI being treated, if indicated

Treatment

Prevention and treatment recommendations from randomized prospective trials are lacking for most IRIS syndromes. However, the majority of cases of IRIS reported in the medical literature are not life-threatening and appear to have resolved within a matter of weeks to months with the following:

- Continuing the current ART regimen (unless the clinical presentation was life-threatening)
- Treating any newly identified, untreated OI
- If indicated, administering antiinflammatory medications (nonsteroidal drugs or systemic corticosteroids) to suppress the inflammatory process (prednisone was shown in one study to decrease hospital days and improve symptoms in TB IRIS in sub-Saharan Africa)

For patients with recent OIs that resolved with a full course of appropriate therapy, it is not always necessary to resume antimicrobial therapy or to change maintenance therapy. For example, if a patient with TB IRIS has finished a full course of treatment for TB, repeat treatment is not indicated. If a patient with previously treated cryptococcal meningitis is receiving maintenance therapy and IRIS develops, the therapy does not need to be altered. However, if IRIS reveals a new, untreated OI, that infection should be treated appropriately. For instance, if new cryptococcal meningitis presents as IRIS, the cryptococcus should be treated as indicated. If treatment is in question, consult with an HIV specialist.

Timing of ART initiation

The risk of IRIS is highest for patients who start ART with low CD4 counts (<50-100 cells/µL) and those for whom ART is initiated soon after OI treatment is begun. The optimal time for ART initiation in the setting of an OI is not known, but one randomized controlled trial suggests a mortality benefit to early ART initiation in patients with newly diagnosed OIs. Decisions about the timing of ART initiation may depend on a number of variables, including the specific pathogen, the severity of the OI, whether the CNS is involved (IRIS in the CNS may be life-threatening), the medication burden, and the potential for drug toxicity or drug interactions. In most cases, ART initiation should be considered within 1-2 weeks after initiation of OI therapy. For patients with cryptococcal or mycobacterial disease who are otherwise stable and for whom ART can be deferred temporarily, many specialists would recommend delaying ART until they have received appropriate OI treatment for 2-6 weeks. Ongoing trials will better define timing of ART in patients with TB and cryptococcal meningitis.

For decisions about initiating ART in patients with active OIs, consult with an HIV specialist.

IRIS in resource-limited settings

As access to ART improves in resource-limited countries, IRIS increasingly is being recognized in patients receiving ART. Clinicians should include IRIS in the differential diagnosis when evaluating patients who recently have begun ART and present with new or worsening symptoms of an OI. However, limited diagnostic testing resources may make it difficult to establish IRIS and other diagnoses.

Given that coinfection with HIV and TB is epidemic in many countries, and because IRIS is not uncommon in patients with TB, clinicians should be particularly vigilant about symptoms that may signal IRIS. As in resource-sufficient countries, consultation with a clinician trained in caring for patients with HIV is recommended if diagnosis or treatment is in question.

Patient Education

- Patients starting ART who have CD4 counts of <100 cells/µL or known concomitant OIs should be counseled about the possibility of IRIS.

- All patients starting ART should be advised to contact the clinic promptly if they experience new or worsening symptoms.

- Advise patients to take their medications for HIV and for the treatment or prevention of OIs exactly as prescribed.

References

- Centers for Disease Control and Prevention. *Guidelines for Prevention and Treatment of Opportunistic Infections among HIV-Exposed and HIV-Infected Children.* April 10, 2009. Available at www.aidsinfo.nih.gov/guidelines/.

- DeSimone JA, Pomerantz RJ, Babinchak TJ. *Inflammatory reactions in HIV-1-infected persons after initiation of highly active antiretroviral therapy.* Ann Intern Med. 2000 Sep 19;133(6):447-54.

- Egger M, May M, Chene G, et al. *Prognosis of HIV-1-infected patients starting highly active antiretroviral therapy: a collaborative analysis of prospective studies.* Lancet. 2002 Jul 13;360(9327):119-29.

- French MA. *HIV/AIDS: immune reconstitution inflammatory syndrome: a reappraisal.* Clin Infect Dis. 2009 Jan 1;48(1):101-7.

- Jacobson MA. *Clinical Implications of Immune Reconstitution in AIDS.* In: Coffey S, Volberding PA, eds. *HIV InSite Knowledge Base* [textbook online]. San Francisco: UCSF Center for HIV Information; 2006. Available at hivinsite.ucsf.edu/InSite?page=kb-03-04-03. Accessed June 30, 2010.

- Lawn SD, Wilkinson RJ, Lipman MC, et al. *Immune reconstitution and "unmasking" of tuberculosis during antiretroviral therapy.* Am J Respir Crit Care Med. 2008 Apr 1;177(7):680-5.

- Meintjes G, Lawn SD, Scano F, et al.; International Network for the Study of HIV-associated IRIS. *Tuberculosis-associated immune reconstitution inflammatory syndrome: case definitions for use in resource-limited settings.* Lancet Infect Dis. 2008 Aug;8(8):516-23.

- Meintjes G, Rabie H, Wilkinson RJ, et al. *Tuberculosis-associated immune reconstitution inflammatory syndrome and unmasking of tuberculosis by antiretroviral therapy.* Clin Chest Med. 2009 Dec;30(4):797-810.

- Ratnam I, Chiu C, Kandala NB, et al. *Incidence and risk factors for immune reconstitution inflammatory syndrome in an ethnically diverse HIV type 1-infected cohort.* Clin Infect Dis. 2006 Feb 1;42(3):418-27.

- Shelburne SA, Montes M, Hamill RJ. *Immune reconstitution inflammatory syndrome: more answers, more questions.* J Antimicrob Chemother. 2006 Feb;57(2):167-70.

- Shelburne SA, Visnegarwala F, Darcourt J, et al. *Incidence and risk factors for immune reconstitution inflammatory syndrome during highly active antiretroviral therapy.* AIDS. 2005 Mar 4;19(4):399-406.

- Shelburne SA 3rd, Darcourt J, White AC, et al. *The role of immune reconstitution inflammatory syndrome in AIDS-related Cryptococcus neoformans disease in the era of highly active antiretroviral therapy.* Clin Infect Dis. 2005 Apr 1;40(7):1049-52.

- Zolopa A, Andersen J, Powderly W, et al. *Early antiretroviral therapy reduces AIDS progression/death in individuals with acute opportunistic infections: a multicenter randomized strategy trial.* PLoS One. 2009;4(5):e5575.

Anal Dysplasia

Background

Anal cancer is a squamous cell cancer associated with human papillomavirus (HPV), the same virus that is associated with cervical cancer (see chapter *Cervical Dysplasia*). The anal canal and cervical canal share a common embryologic origin: both have a squamocolumnar transition zone and are prone to infection with HPV, a sexually transmitted virus. HPV infection, in combination with cofactors, may stimulate dysplastic changes in the cervix or anus that may develop through precursor stages into squamous cell cancer. In the United States, the current incidence of anal cancer in the general population is approximately 1:100,000 per year. In HIV-infected men and women, the incidence of anal cancer and the prevalence of its precursors are significantly higher than in the general population.

Rates of anal cancer also are higher among men who have sex with men (MSM), whether HIV infected or uninfected, compared with the general population. Before the HIV epidemic, the anal cancer incidence among MSM was estimated to be as high as 37:100,000. This incidence is comparable to the incidence of cervical cancer in women before the introduction of screening using Papanicolaou (Pap) tests. Current rates in an HIV-infected MSM population are estimated to be as high as 70-144 per 100,000.

Although most studies have examined anal dysplasia and cancer among MSM, the prevalence of anal intraepithelial neoplasia (AIN), a precursor to anal cancer, also is high among HIV-infected women. A recent study found a significantly increased rate of AIN (16%) in a group of HIV-infected women when compared with a control group having similar risk factors. In some studies of HIV-infected women, anal dysplasia has been seen more frequently than cervical dysplasia, and it has not been exclusive to those with behavioral risk factors (e.g., history of anal intercourse).

Some studies have shown that, among HIV-infected individuals, anal HPV infection is present in 93% of MSM and 76% of women, and anal dysplasia (any grade) is present in 56% of MSM and 26% of women. Receptive anal intercourse (RAI) may increase the likelihood of anal HPV infection, but is not a prerequisite for anal HPV or dysplasia. It is posited that HPV can spread throughout the anogenital region in the absence of sexual contact. In a study of HIV-infected heterosexual men with no history of RAI, anal HPV infection was found in 46% and anal dysplasia in 32%. Patients with lower CD4 cell counts appear to be at higher risk of developing anal dysplasia.

Screening strategies for anal dysplasia and cancer and the optimal management of abnormal test results are controversial areas in which questions remain unanswered. The rationale for screening for anal cancer and its precursors is based on the success of cervical Pap screening in reducing cervical cancer incidence and mortality. Because of the similarities between cervical and anal dysplasia, many experts postulate that many of the paradigms of managing cervical cytologic abnormalities may be translated to management of anal dysplasia. However, there are no randomized clinical trials that document the value of screening for anal precancers.

Currently, there are no national recommendations that call for routine screening for anal cancer, but many experts recommend screening all HIV-infected individuals for anal dysplasia, if adequate diagnostic and treatment resources and referral networks exist. The New York State Department of Health AIDS Institute recommends that an anal Pap test be done at baseline and annually thereafter for MSM, patients with a history of anogenital warts, and women with abnormal cervical or vulvar histology, and many HIV clinics elsewhere do routine screening. Further investigations are ongoing to define appropriate screening intervals, diagnostic approaches, indications for therapy, and modalities of treatment.

ART and subsequent immune reconstitution does not appear to alter the prevalence or distribution of anal cancers and anorectal disease nor does it appear to reduce the progression of AIN and other cancer precursors.

For information on prevention of HPV infection, see "Prevention," below.

S: Subjective

Patients with anal dysplasia usually are asymptomatic, and the condition cannot be identified without screening tests. Exophytic anal condylomata may cause itching, discomfort, or bleeding, but are usually associated with low-risk phenotypes of HPV and low-grade dysplasia (note, however, that oncogenic HPV types also may be present). Anal cancer may cause nonspecific symptoms such as pain (with defecation or after intercourse), itching, bleeding, or sensation of a rectal mass.

Risk factors for anal dysplasia and cancers include the following:

- HIV infection
- CD4 count of <200 cells/μL
- RAI
- HPV infection
- Genital warts (or history of genital warts)
- Immunosuppression
- High-grade cervical or vulvar dysplasia
- Cigarette smoking
- Multiple sex partners

Ask patients about these risk factors, about previous history of anal dysplasia or cancer, and about previous screening.

O: Objective

Examine the genital and perianal region, and perform a digital anorectal examination. Look and feel for masses, condylomata, and other abnormalities such as hypo- or hyperpigmented plaques or lesions, and lesions that bleed. Note that simple visual examination may not reveal abnormalities. In women, also examine the vulva, vagina, and cervix. Examine the inguinal lymph nodes.

If the digital examination is performed in conjunction with an anal Pap test, the Pap specimen should be obtained before the introduction of lubrication.

Anoscopic examination with the naked eye may not reveal any abnormality because dysplastic tissue tends to be flat and difficult to differentiate from normal anal tissue; application of 3% acetic acid is required (see below for a description of how high-resolution anoscopy [HRA] is performed).

A: Assessment

HIV-infected individuals with anal dysplasia have an increased risk of progression to anal cancer. If the history or physical examination reveals abnormalities suggestive of anal dysplasia or anal cancer, an appropriate evaluation should be undertaken. Because most patients with anal dysplasia have no symptoms, anal cancer screening using a Pap test can be considered if follow-up evaluation of an abnormal cytologic result (ASCUS or higher, see Bethesda 2001 grading system, below) by high-resolution anoscopy is available either on-site or by referral.

P: Plan

Screening

As mentioned above, there are no national guidelines for anal cancer screening in people with HIV infection. However, some experts recommend that anal Pap tests and digital anal examination be part of the initial evaluation of both male and female HIV-infected patients. The intervals for screening have not been established, but (based on recommendations for cervical cancer screening) if the first test result is normal, the anal Pap usually is repeated in approximately 6 months. If both results are normal, then anal Pap tests can be performed annually. Some clinicians would consider more frequent screening in patients with genital warts, cervical dysplasia, or a history of treatment for anal dysplasia. Any patients with positive results should be referred for further evaluation; see below.

An anal Pap test is done using a standard Pap kit. The swab or cytobrush should be inserted into the anal canal, past the anorectal junction, and withdrawn while rotating it against the anal walls to collect cells. The sample should then be handled according to the kit manufacturer's instructions. (See "References," below, for information about a video on how to conduct an anal Pap screen that is available from the Johns Hopkins University Local Performance Site of the Pennsylvania/MidAtlantic AIDS Education and Training Center.)

As with cervical cytology, anal cytology is graded using the Bethesda 2001 system, which categorizes disease in increasing order of severity as follows:

- Negative for intraepithelial lesion or malignancy
- Atypical squamous cells of undetermined significance (ASCUS)
- Atypical squamous cells — cannot exclude HSIL (ASC-H)
- Low-grade squamous intraepithelial lesion (LSIL)
- High-grade squamous intraepithelial lesion (HSIL)
- Squamous cell carcinoma (SCC)

Other abnormalities, such as atypical glandular cells (AGC), may be noted.

All individuals with abnormal anal cytology, defined as ASCUS or higher, should be referred for HRA and biopsy to grade the lesion. HRA typically is performed at specialty anal cancer practices or clinics, colorectal surgery and gastrointestinal specialty facilities, and some academic medical centers.

Evaluation of Cytologic Abnormalities

HRA of the anal canal should be performed using a colposcope for magnification (16×) and the application of 3% acetic acid with or without Lugol iodine solution to aid in visualization of dysplastic lesions. Abnormal areas should be examined by biopsy. Anoscopic features of high-grade disease are similar to those seen in the cervix; these include coarse punctation, mosaicism, and the presence of ring glands.

Treatment

The goal of treatment is to prevent progression to anal cancer. Treatment of HSIL to prevent anal cancer is biologically plausible, following the model of cervical dysplasia treatment. However, the indications for treatment of anal dysplasia, the efficacy of treatment, and the most effective treatments have not been optimally defined.

The focus of treatment is on high-grade, premalignant dysplasia. For patients with HSIL, refer to an anal dysplasia specialty clinic, if possible. The optimal treatment for high-grade dysplasia is not known, and it should be individualized in consultation with a specialist. Specific treatment may vary depending on the size, location, extent of the lesions, and histological grade. Therapies include topical 5-fluorouracil, cryotherapy, infrared coagulation, laser therapy, and surgical excision. Infrared coagulation, an in-office procedure, has been shown to be effective in treating HIV-infected patients with high-grade dysplasia. With some therapies, treatment-associated pain and other complications may occur, and recurrence of dysplastic lesions is common.

LSIL is not considered premalignant, but it frequently progresses to high-grade dysplasia. Some specialists do not treat LSIL but monitor regularly instead with HRA, whereas others choose to treat LSIL to prevent progression.

Prevention

Prevention of HPV infection can be challenging. Latex or plastic barriers may block transmission of HPV in areas covered by these barriers, but infection may occur through bodily contact outside the area covered by the barriers. Nonetheless, their use is recommended to prevent transmission or acquisition of HPV.

There are no data on the efficacy of HPV vaccines in preventing anal HPV; studies are under way. A quadrivalent vaccine against certain oncogenic (types 16 and 18) and wart-causing (types 6 and 11) types of HPV is FDA approved for prevention of cervical dysplasia and cancer and for prevention of genital warts in females. It also is FDA approved for prevention of genital warts in males. A second vaccine against HPV types 16 and 18 has been approved for females (see chapter *Cervical Dysplasia*).

The HPV vaccines have not been thoroughly studied in HIV-infected persons and thus are not specifically recommended for them; studies to evaluate efficacy, safety, immunogenicity, and tolerability are under way. The vaccines are not contraindicated for use by HIV-infected persons, and many clinicians do provide them.

Patient Education

- All HIV-infected men and women should be encouraged to use condoms during vaginal, anal, and oral sex to prevent the spread of HPV. However, condoms do not offer complete protection from HPV.

- All patients should be counseled on how to reduce or avoid unprotected anal receptive intercourse.

- Both women and men who are HIV infected have an increased risk of developing anal dysplasia and cancer. MSM are at higher risk than other men of developing anal dysplasia.

- Emphasize the importance of keeping follow-up appointments to allow for early detection of precancerous lesions, further grading of abnormalities by HRA, and appropriate monitoring and treatment of abnormalities.

- Patients who have anal dysplasia should be informed about anal cancer symptoms, such as new-onset anal pain, bleeding, or the development of a mass. Patients should call their health care provider if these symptoms develop.

- If an anal Pap test is being performed, advise patients to avoid having anal sex, douching, or using enemas before the test.

References

- Centers for Disease Control and Prevention. *Guidelines for Prevention and Treatment of Opportunistic Infections in HIV-Infected Adults and Adolescents: Recommendations from CDC, the National Institutes of Health, and the HIV Medicine Association of the Infectious Diseases Society of America.* April 10, 2009. Available at www.aidsinfo.nih.gov/guidelines/.

- Chiao EY, Giordano TP, Palefsky JM, et al. *Screening HIV-infected individuals for anal cancer precursor lesions: a systematic review.* Clin Infect Dis. 2006 Jul 15;43(2):223-33.

- Chin-Hong PV, Palefsky JM. *Natural history and clinical management of anal human papillomavirus disease in men and women infected with human immunodeficiency virus.* Clin Infect Dis. 2002 Nov 1;35(9):1127-34.

- Diamond C, Taylor TH, Aboumrad T, et al. *Increased incidence of squamous cell anal cancer among men with AIDS in the era of highly active antiretroviral therapy.* Sex Transm Dis. 2005 May;32(5):314-20.

- Hessol NA, Holly EA, Efird JT, et al. *Anal Intraepithelial neoplasia in a multisite study of HIV-infected and high-risk HIV-uninfected women.* AIDS. 2009 Jan 2;23(1):59-70.

- Palefsky JM, Cranston RD. *Anal Intraepithelial Neoplasia: Diagnosis, Screening, and Treatment* [online resource]. Waltham, MA: Up to Date; May 2009. Available at www.uptodate.com/index.asp. [Fee required.]

- Palefsky JM, Holly EA, Efirdc JT, et al. *Anal intraepithelial neoplasia in the highly active antiretroviral therapy era among HIV-positive men who have sex with men.* AIDS. 2005 Sep 2;19(13):1407-14

- Piketty C, Darragh TM, Da Costa M, et al. *High prevalence of anal human papillomavirus infection and anal cancer precursors among HIV-infected persons in the absence of anal intercourse.* Ann Intern Med. 2003 Mar 18;138(6):453-9.

- Wright TC Jr, Cox JT, Massad LS, et al. *2001 consensus guidelines for the management of women with cervical cytological abnormalities.* JAMA. 2002 Apr 24;287(16):2120-9.

- A video titled *Anal Pap Smear: A Simple, Fast and Easy Procedure* is available on CD-ROM at-cost to health care professionals ($12.00 for 1-4 copies) by calling the Johns Hopkins University Local Performance Site of the Pennsylvania Mid/Atlantic AIDS Education and Training Center to order: 888-333-2855 (toll free) by or downloading the order form on the AETC NRC website. Available at www.aids-ed.org/aidsetc?page=etres-display&resource=etres-229. Accessed June 30, 2010.

Candidiasis, Oral and Esophageal

Background

Oropharyngeal candidiasis ("thrush"), a fungal disease of the oral mucosa and tongue, is the most common intraoral lesion among persons infected with HIV. In the absence of other known causes of immunosuppression, oral thrush in an adult is highly suggestive of HIV infection. Although thrush in the absence of esophageal disease is not an AIDS-defining condition, it usually occurs with CD4 counts of <200 cells/μL. Three clinical presentations of thrush are common in people with HIV: pseudomembranous, erythematous, and angular cheilitis. *Candida* also may infect the esophagus in the form of esophageal candidiasis, which causes dysphagia (difficulty with swallowing) or odynophagia (pain with swallowing). Esophageal candidiasis is an AIDS-defining condition, generally occurring in individuals with CD4 counts of <200 cells/μL. It is the most common cause of esophageal infection in persons with AIDS.

Oropharyngeal and esophageal candidiasis are caused most commonly by *Candida albicans*, although non-*albicans* species increasingly may cause disease and may be resistant to first-line therapies.

S: Subjective

Oropharyngeal Candidiasis

The patient may complain of painless white patches on the tongue and oral mucosa, smooth red areas on the dorsal tongue, burning or painful areas in the mouth, a bad or unusual taste, sensitivity to spicy foods, or decreased appetite.

Esophageal Candidiasis

The patient complains of difficulty or pain with swallowing, or the sensation that food is "sticking" in the retrosternal chest. Weight loss is common, and nausea and vomiting may occur. Fever is not common with candidal esophagitis and suggests another cause. The patient may note symptoms of oral candidiasis (as above).

O: Objective

Perform a thorough oropharyngeal examination. Patients presenting with oral candidiasis may be totally asymptomatic, so it is important to inspect the oral cavity thoroughly. Patients with esophageal candidiasis usually have oral thrush and often experience weight loss.

Lesions can occur anywhere on the hard and soft palates, under the tongue, on the buccal mucosa or gums, or in the posterior pharynx.

Pseudomembranous oral candidiasis appears as creamy white, curdlike plaques on the buccal mucosa, tongue, and other mucosal surfaces. Typically, the plaques can be wiped away, leaving a red or bleeding underlying surface. Lesions may be as small as 1-2 mm, or they may form extensive plaques that cover the entire hard palate.

Erythematous oral candidiasis presents as one or more flat, red, subtle lesions on the dorsal surface of the tongue or the hard or soft palate. The dorsum of the tongue may show loss of filiform papillae.

Angular cheilitis causes fissuring and redness at one or both corners of the mouth and may appear alone or in conjunction with another form of oral *Candida* infection.

A: Assessment

A partial differential diagnosis for the two conditions is as follows:

Oropharyngeal Candidiasis

- Oral hairy leukoplakia
- Abrasion of the mucosa or a topical burn
- Bacterial gingivitis
- Periodontitis

Esophageal Candidiasis

- GERD
- Cytomegalovirus (CMV)
- Herpes simplex virus (HSV)
- Aphthous ulceration

P: Plan

Diagnostic Evaluation

Oropharyngeal candidiasis

Clinical examination alone usually is diagnostic. If the diagnosis is unclear, organisms may be detected on smear or culture if necessary.

- On a potassium hydroxide (KOH) preparation of a smear collected by gentle scraping of the affected area with a wooden tongue depressor, visible hyphae or blastospheres on KOH mount indicate *Candida* infection.

- Culture is diagnostic and may detect non-albicans species in cases resistant to first-line therapies. Sensitivities also may be needed in such cases to diagnose azole-resistant infections.

Esophageal candidiasis

A presumptive diagnosis usually can be made with a recent onset of typical symptoms, especially in the presence of thrush, and empiric antifungal therapy may be started as a diagnostic trial. If the patient fails to improve clinically after 3-7 days of therapy, endoscopy should be performed for a definitive diagnosis.

Treatment

Treatment of oropharyngeal candidiasis

- Oral therapy is convenient and very effective as first-line treatment. Note that azole antifungal drugs are not recommended for use during pregnancy.

- Fluconazole 100 mg PO once daily for 7-14 days

- Alternative topical therapy is less expensive, safe for use during pregnancy, and effective for mild to moderate disease. Such therapies include 7-14 days of the following:
  - Clotrimazole troches 10 mg dissolved in the mouth 5 times daily
  - Nystatin oral suspension 5 mL "swish and swallow" QID
  - Miconazole mucoadhesive tablet PO daily

- Other alternatives include 7-14 day therapy with the following (Note: These agents may present a greater risk of drug interactions [see "Potential ARV Interactions," below] and hepatotoxicity than do fluconazole or topical treatments, so these typically are reserved for use in cases of documented azole resistance or in cases clinically refractory to azole therapy):
  - Itraconazole oral solution 200 mg PO once daily
  - Posaconazole oral solution 400 mg PO BID for 1 day, then 400 mg PO once daily

Treatment of esophageal candidiasis

- Fluconazole 200 mg PO as an initial dose, then 100 mg PO once daily for 14-21 days (fluconazole dose can range from 100-400 mg, as tolerated by the patient). IV therapy can be given if the patient is unable to swallow pills.

- Itraconazole PO solution 200 mg PO once daily for 14-21 days

- Alternative options: IV therapy with an echinocandin (caspofungin, micafungin, anidulafungin), voriconazole, or amphotericin, if the patient is unable to tolerate PO therapy; or PO voriconazole or posaconazole. (Note: Treatment with echinocandins is associated with a higher rate of relapse. See "Potential ARV Interactions," below, regarding potential drug-drug interactions between voriconazole or posaconazole and ARVs.)

Treatment of refractory candidiasis

Oral or esophageal candidiasis that does not improve after at least 7-14 days of appropriate antifungal therapy can be considered refractory to treatment. The primary risk factors for development of refractory candidiasis are CD4 counts of <50 cells/µL and prolonged, chronic antifungal therapy (especially with azoles). In such cases, it is important to confirm the diagnosis of candidiasis. As noted, other infections such as HSV, CMV, and aphthous ulcerations can cause similar symptoms. Once refractory candidiasis is confirmed, several treatment options are available, including the following:

Preferred options:
- Itraconazole oral solution ≥200 mg PO once daily
- Posaconazole 400 mg PO BID

Alternative options:
- Voriconazole 200 mg PO or IV BID (see "Potential ARV Interactions," below)
- For patients who are unable to tolerate PO therapy: IV therapy with an echinocandin (caspofungin 50 mg once daily; micafungin 150 mg once daily; anidulafungin 100 mg for one dose, then 50 mg once daily), voriconazole 200 mg once daily, or amphotericin B deoxycholate 0.3 mg/

kg IV once daily. (Note: Treatment with echinocandins is associated with a higher rate of relapse. See "Potential ARV Interactions," below, for information on potential drug interactions.)

The choice of treatment depends upon anticipated drug-drug interactions, the patient's preferences and tolerability, availability of medications, and the provider's experience. Consult with an HIV or infectious disease expert for advice about treatment regimens.

Maintenance therapy

Use caution when considering chronic maintenance therapy, because it has been associated with refractory and azole-resistant candidiasis, as noted above. Fluconazole 100 mg PO daily or TIW or itraconazole oral solution 200 mg PO daily can be effective for patients who have had multiple or severe recurrences of oral disease (azole sensitive). Fluconazole 100-200 mg PO daily or posaconazole 400 mg PO BID (see "Potential ARV Interactions," below) can be considered for patients who have had frequent or severe recurrent esophageal candidiasis.

There are no data to guide this decision; it is reasonable to discontinue maintenance therapy in patients who achieve immunologic responses on fully suppressive ART (i.e., with an increase in CD4 count to ≥200 cells/µL). Patients with fluconazole-refractory oropharyngeal or esophageal disease who respond to IV echinocandins are recommended to take posaconazole or voriconazole suppression until they achieve immune reconstitution on ART, because of high relapse rates.

Potential ARV Interactions

There may be significant drug-drug interactions between certain systemic antifungals, particularly itraconazole, voriconazole, and posaconazole, and ritonavir-boosted protease inhibitors (PIs), nonnucleoside reverse transcriptase inhibitors (NNRTIs), or maraviroc. Some combinations are contraindicated and others require dosage adjustment of the ARV, the antifungal, or both. Check for adverse drug interactions before prescribing. For example, voriconazole use is not recommended for patients taking ritonavir-boosted PIs, and dosage adjustment of both voriconazole and NNRTIs may be required when voriconazole is used concurrently with NNRTIs. See Tables 15a-e of the U.S. Department of Health and Human Services *Guidelines for the Use of Antiretroviral Agents in HIV-1-Infected Adults and Adolescents* or consult with an expert.

Patient Education

- Patients should maintain good oral hygiene by brushing teeth after each meal.

- A soft toothbrush should be used to avoid mouth trauma.

- Advise patients to rinse the mouth of all food before using lozenges or liquid medications.

- Tell patients to avoid foods or liquids that are very hot in temperature or very spicy

- Patients who have candidiasis under a denture or partial denture should remove the prosthesis before using topical agents such as clotrimazole or nystatin. When not in use, the prosthesis should be stored in a chlorhexidine solution.

- Pregnant women and women who may become pregnant should avoid azole drugs (e.g., fluconazole, itraconazole, voriconazole) during pregnancy because they can cause skeletal and craniofacial abnormalities in infants.

- Patients should be informed of proper storage of oral solutions (i.e., refrigeration requirements, etc.)

References

- Centers for Disease Control and Prevention. *Guidelines for Prevention and Treatment of Opportunistic Infections in HIV-Infected Adults and Adolescents: Recommendations from CDC, the National Institutes of Health, and the HIV Medicine Association of the Infectious Diseases Society of America.* April 10, 2009. Available at www.aidsinfo.nih.gov/guidelines/.

- de Wet N, Llanos-Cuentas A, Suleiman J, et al. *A randomized, double-blind, parallel-group, dose-response study of micafungin compared with fluconazole for the treatment of esophageal candidiasis in HIV-positive patients.* Clin Infect Dis. 2004 Sep 15;39(6):842-9.

- Klein RS, Harris CA, Small CB, et al. *Oral candidiasis in high-risk patients as the initial manifestation of the acquired immunodeficiency syndrome.* N Engl J Med. 1984 Aug 9;311(6):354-8.

- Krause DS, Simjee AE, van Rensburg C, et al. *A randomized, double-blind trial of anidulafungin versus fluconazole for the treatment of esophageal candidiasis.* Clin Infect Dis. 2004 Sep 15;39(6):770-5.

- Pappas PG, Kauffman CA, Andes D, et al.; Infectious Diseases Society of America. *Clinical practice guidelines for the management of candidiasis: 2009 update by the Infectious Diseases Society of America.* Clin Infect Dis. 2009 Mar 1;48(5):503-35.

- Skiest DJ, Vazquez JA, Anstead GM, et al. *Posaconazole for the treatment of azole-refractory oropharyngeal and esophageal candidiasis in subjects with HIV infection.* Clin Infect Dis. 2007 Feb 15;44(4):607-14.

- U.S. Department of Health and Human Services. *Guidelines for the Use of Antiretroviral Agents in HIV-1-Infected Adults and Adolescents.* January 10, 2011. Available at www.aidsinfo.nih.gov/guidelines/.

Candidiasis, Vulvovaginal

Background

Vulvovaginal candidiasis is a yeast infection caused by several types of *Candida*, typically *Candida albicans*. This disease is common in all women, but may occur more frequently and more severely in immunocompromised women.

Although refractory vaginal *Candida* infections by themselves should not be considered indicators of HIV infection, they may be the first clinical manifestation of HIV infection and can occur early in the course of disease (at CD4 counts of >500 cells/μL). The frequency of vaginal candidiasis tends to increase as CD4 counts decrease; however, this may be attributable in part to increased use of antibiotics among women with advanced HIV infection.

Risk factors for candidiasis include diabetes mellitus and the use of oral contraceptives, corticosteroids, or antibiotics.

S: Subjective

The patient may complain of itching, burning, or swelling of the labia and vulva; a thick white or yellowish vaginal discharge; painful intercourse; and pain and burning on urination.

The most important elements in the history include the following:

- Type and duration of symptoms
- Previous vaginal yeast infection
- Oral contraceptive use
- Recent or ongoing broad-spectrum antibiotic therapy
- Recent corticosteroid therapy
- Sexual exposures (to evaluate for sexually transmitted infections)
- Diabetes history
- Cushing syndrome
- Obesity
- Hypothyroidism
- Pregnancy
- Use of douches, vaginal deodorants, or bath additives

O: Objective

Perform a focused physical examination of the external genitalia, vagina, and cervix. This may reveal inflammation of the vulva with evidence of discharge on the labial folds and vaginal opening. Speculum examination usually reveals a thick, white discharge with plaques adhering to the vaginal walls and cervix. Bimanual examination should not elicit pain or tenderness and otherwise should be normal.

A: Assessment

Rule out other causes of vaginal discharge and pruritus:

- Bacterial vaginosis
- Atrophic vaginitis
- Chemical or mechanical causes
- Trichomoniasis
- Gonorrhea, chlamydia, and other sexually transmitted infections
- Scabies
- Pediculosis

P: Plan

Diagnostic Evaluation

A presumptive diagnosis is made on the basis of the clinical presentation and potassium hydroxide (KOH) preparation:

- Perform microscopic examination of a KOH preparation of vaginal secretions. This usually reveals pseudohyphae and *Candida* spores (presumptive diagnosis).

- Definitive diagnosis rarely is needed, but may be made by analysis of a culture of vaginal secretions; this may be useful if azole-resistant or non-*albicans* species are suspected.

- In the presence of urinary tract symptoms (beyond external vulvar burning), perform urinalysis, culture, or both on a clean-catch urine specimen.

- Consider testing for gonorrhea and chlamydia in patients with a history of possible sexual exposure.

Treatment

Uncomplicated infections

Topical medications

- Prescribe topical vaginal antifungal agents in the form of cream or suppositories, including the following: butoconazole, clotrimazole, miconazole, nystatin, terconazole, and tioconazole. Treat for 3-7 days and offer refills depending on the time to the next scheduled clinic visit. The creams also may be used on the vulva for treatment of pruritus.

Note that the mineral-oil base in topical vaginal antifungal preparations may erode the latex in condoms, diaphragms, and dental dams. Advise the patient to use alternative methods to prevent HIV transmission or conception, or to discontinue intercourse while using these medications. Nonlatex condoms (plastic and polyethylene only) or "female" condoms (polyurethane) can be used.

Oral medications

- Fluconazole 150 mg PO, single dose (see "Treatment notes," below)

- Itraconazole 200 mg PO BID for 1 day, or 200 mg PO once daily for 3-7 days (see "Treatment notes," below)

Complicated infections

Severe or recurrent candidiasis

Severe or recurrent candidiasis is defined as four or more episodes within 1 year. Consider the following treatments:

- Topical therapy as described above, for 7-14 days

- Fluconazole 150 mg PO every 3 days for 3 doses (see "Treatment notes," below)

For severe cases that recur repeatedly, secondary prophylaxis can be considered (e.g., fluconazole 150 mg PO weekly, or clotrimazole vaginal suppository 500 mg once weekly).

Non-*albicans* candidiasis

- Non-fluconazole azole (posaconazole, voriconazole) for 10-14 days (see "Treatment notes," below)

- Boric acid 600 mg intravaginal gelatin capsules once daily for 2 weeks for refractory cases

- Consult with a specialist

Treatment notes

- Systemic azole drugs are not recommended for use during pregnancy, and women taking azoles should use effective contraception. Topical azoles are recommended for the treatment of pregnant women.

- Resistance to azole medications may develop, especially with prolonged use of oral agents.

- Itraconazole should not be used by pregnant women or women considering pregnancy.

- Avoid ketoconazole: Case reports have associated ketoconazole with a risk of fulminant hepatitis (1 in 12,000 courses of treatment with oral ketoconazole). Experts agree that the risks may outweigh the benefits for women with vulvovaginal candidiasis. Ketoconazole interacts with many other drugs, including some antiretroviral drugs.

Potential ARV Interactions

There may be significant drug-drug interactions between certain systemic antifungals, particularly itraconazole, voriconazole, and posaconazole, and ritonavir-boosted protease inhibitors (PIs), nonnucleoside reverse transcriptase inhibitors (NNRTIs), or maraviroc. Some combinations are contraindicated and others require dosage adjustment of the ARV, the antifungal, or both. Check for adverse drug interactions before prescribing. For example, voriconazole use is not recommended for patients taking ritonavir-boosted PIs, and dosage adjustment of both voriconazole and NNRTIs may be required when voriconazole is used concurrently with NNRTIs. See Table 15a-e of the U.S. Department of Health and Human Services *Guidelines for the Use of Antiretroviral Agents in HIV-1-Infected Adults and Adolescents*, or consult with an expert.

Patient Education

- Advise patients to wash external genitals daily with a fresh washcloth or water-soaked cotton balls and to wipe the vulva and perirectal area from front to back after toileting. Women should not use baby wipes on inflamed vulval tissue because they may increase irritation.

- Women should avoid the use of perfumed soaps, bubble baths, feminine hygiene or vaginal deodorant products, and bath powders.

- Advise women not to douche.

- Women should wear cotton underwear and avoid tight, constrictive clothing, particularly pantyhose.

- If patients are prescribed medication for vaginal candidiasis, they should take the medication exactly as prescribed and finish the medicine even during a menstrual period.

- Women who continue to have symptoms can purchase Monistat or Gyne-Lotrimin medication over the counter. Advise patients to start using these as soon as symptoms return and to contact the clinic if symptoms worsen while they are taking these medicines.

- Women taking fluconazole or ketoconazole must avoid pregnancy. Some birth defects have been reported.

- The mineral-oil base in topical vaginal antifungal preparations may erode the latex in condoms, diaphragms, and dental dams. Advise patients to use alternative methods to prevent HIV transmission or conception or to discontinue intercourse while using these medications. Nonlatex condoms (plastic and polyethylene only) or "female" condoms (polyurethane) can be used.

- Sex toys, douche nozzles, diaphragms, cervical caps, and other items can reinfect patients if not properly cleaned and thoroughly dried after use.

- Some studies have suggested that eating yogurt with live cultures (check labels) can reduce the occurrence of vaginal yeast infections.

References

- Abularach S, Anderson J. *Gynecologic Problems*. In: Anderson JR, ed. *A Guide to the Clinical Care of Women with HIV/AIDS, 2005.* Rockville, MD: Health Resources and Services Administration, HIV/AIDS Bureau; 2005. Available at hab.hrsa.gov/publications/womencare05/. Accessed June 30, 2010.

- Centers for Disease Control and Prevention. *Guidelines for Prevention and Treatment of Opportunistic Infections in HIV-Infected Adults and Adolescents: Recommendations from CDC, the National Institutes of Health, and the HIV Medicine Association of the Infectious Diseases Society of America.* April 10, 2009. Available at www.aidsinfo.nih.gov/guidelines/.

- Centers for Disease Control and Prevention. *Sexually Transmitted Diseases Treatment Guidelines,* 2010. MMWR 2010 Dec 17; 59 (No. RR- 12):1-110. Available at www.cdc.gov/STD/treatment/2010.

- Cohn SE, Clark RA. *Sexually transmitted diseases, HIV, and AIDS in women.* In: The Medical Clinics of North America, Vol. 87; 2003:971-995.

Cervical Dysplasia

Background

Cervical dysplasia and cancer are associated with human papillomavirus (HPV), a sexually transmitted virus. Carcinogenic strains of HPV, in conjunction with other factors, may cause dysplasia and cancer not only of the cervix, but also of the vulva, vagina, anus, and oropharynx. HIV-infected women have a higher prevalence of HPV infection than do HIV-uninfected women, and a higher prevalence of oncogenic HPV types. They are about 10 times more likely to develop cervical dysplasia, or squamous intraepithelial lesions (SIL), precursors to cervical cancer. Unfortunately, they also have a higher risk of invasive cervical cancer and tend to have more aggressive forms of cervical cancer and poorer responses to treatment. Invasive cervical cancer is an AIDS-defining illness.

> **HRSA HAB Core Clinical Performance Measures**
>
> Percentage of women with HIV infection who had a **Papanicolaou screening** in the measurement year
>
> (Group 2 measure)

The risk of high-grade cervical lesions appears to be higher for women with advanced immunodeficiency than for women with preserved CD4 cell counts. Other risk factors for dysplasia and cervical cancer include African-American ethnicity, a history of smoking, younger age at onset of sexual intercourse, and multiple sex partners. Effective antiretroviral therapy (ART) with immune reconstitution has not been shown to prevent the progression of dysplasia.

Screening for cervical dysplasia and appropriate intervention in women with high-grade dysplasia are effective in preventing cervical cancer. Frequent monitoring and careful follow-up in women with low-grade lesions are essential for preventing progression to invasive disease. Papanicolaou (Pap) testing should be performed routinely for all HIV-infected women, with testing initiated at the time of HIV diagnosis, repeated 6 months after the first test, then performed annually thereafter if the results are normal. (See chapter *Initial and Interim Laboratory and Other Tests.*)

Because the risk of anal dysplasia also is increased among HIV-infected women (in some studies, rates of anal dysplasia were higher than rates of cervical dysplasia), many experts recommend concurrent screening for anal dysplasia. For further information, see chapter *Anal Dysplasia.*

For information on prevention of HPV infection, see "Prevention," below.

S: Subjective

Patients with cervical dysplasia or early cervical cancer usually are asymptomatic and disease will not be diagnosed unless screening is performed. Genital condylomata (warts) indicate infection with HPV and typically are associated with low-risk types of HPV; however, a mixture of HPV types may be present, and women with genital warts may have concurrent dysplasia.

The classic symptom of early invasive cervical neoplasia is intermittent, painless bleeding between menstrual periods, which may present initially as postcoital spotting. Late symptoms of invasive cervical carcinoma include flank and leg pain, dysuria, hematuria, rectal bleeding, and obstipation.

Ask all female patients about risk factors for, previous history of, and preventive measures against cervical dysplasia and cancer, including the following:

- Genital warts; previous or current HPV infection
- Previous abnormal cervical Pap test result
- Previous abnormal anal Pap test result
- Previous cervical cancer; when and how treated
- Sexual activity before age 20
- History of multiple sex partners
- Cigarette smoking
- CD4 count of <200 cells/µL
- Pregnancy
- Oral contraceptive use
- History of HPV vaccination

O: Objective

Perform a focused examination of the abdomen and pelvis. Examine the external genital and perianal region. Perform speculum and bimanual examinations to evaluate the vagina and cervix. Look for lesions, masses, warts, and cervical inflammation or discharge, as well as exophytic or ulcerative cervical lesions with or without bleeding. Note that simple visual examination may not reveal abnormalities.

A: Assessment

HIV-infected women have an increased risk of cervical dysplasia with progression to cervical cancer. If abnormalities of cervical disease are suspected, an appropriate evaluation should be performed. Because most women with cervical dysplasia have no symptoms, routine screening should be performed for all women.

P: Plan

Screening

Perform screening Pap test for all HIV-infected women. The initial test should be conducted at the time of HIV diagnosis, a second (if the first is normal) should be performed 6 months later. Screening should be repeated annually thereafter if all results are normal. (For HIV-uninfected women, recent guidelines from the American Congress of Obstetricians and Gynecologists recommend increasing the screening interval to 3 years if both Pap and HPV test results are negative; this screening strategy has not been shown to be safe and effective for HIV-infected women and is not recommended). If a Pap result is abnormal, see below. Also consider screening for anal dysplasia with an anal Pap test (see chapter *Anal Dysplasia*).

Cervical (and anal) cytology is graded using the Bethesda 2001 system (see "References," below), which categorizes disease in increasing order of severity as follows:

- Negative for intraepithelial lesion or malignancy
- Atypical squamous cells of undetermined significance (ASCUS)
- Atypical squamous cells, cannot exclude HSIL (ASC-H)
- Low-grade squamous intraepithelial lesion (LSIL)
- High-grade squamous intraepithelial lesion (HSIL)
- Squamous cell carcinoma (SCC)

Other abnormalities may be noted, including the following:

- Atypical glandular cells (AGCs), including the following subcategories:
  - AGC NOS (includes endocervical, endometrial, or glandular cells not otherwise specified)
  - AGC favor neoplasia (includes endometrial or glandular cells)
  - AIS (endocervical adenocarcinoma in situ)
- Infectious organisms such as *Trichomonas*

Evaluation of Cytologic Abnormalities

Atypical squamous cells of undetermined significance

If ASCUS is present without inflammation or suspected neoplastic process, several options for management exist.

- Most experts recommend that all women with ASCUS be referred for colposcopy and directed biopsy, regardless of their degree of immunodeficiency. If the biopsy result shows no dysplasia (and the examination is adequate), the patient should be monitored by annual Pap tests.

- As an alternative, patients who are considered reliable for follow-up may be monitored closely with repeat Pap tests every 4-6 months for 2 years until three consecutive results have been negative. If a follow-up test shows ASCUS (or higher-grade abnormalities), colposcopy with directed biopsy should be performed. If the biopsy result does not show dysplasia, the patient should be monitored as usual with Pap tests at 6 months and 12 months.

- There are limited and conflicting data to support utilizing HPV DNA testing as part of the management of HIV-infected women with ASCUS. By this strategy, colposcopic examination is performed if HPV DNA testing shows an oncogenic HPV type. This approach is recommended by American Society for Colposcopy and Cervical Pathology (ASCCP) guidelines but is not favored by most experts on HPV infection in HIV-infected persons.

Atypical squamous cells, cannot exclude HSIL

Women with abnormalities suggestive of high-grade dysplasia should be referred for colposcopy.

Low-grade squamous intraepithelial lesion

Women with LSIL should be referred for colposcopy and directed biopsy.

High-grade squamous intraepithelial lesion or squamous cell carcinoma

Women with HSIL are at high risk of high-grade intraepithelial neoplasia or cervical cancer and should undergo colposcopy with endocervical assessment and directed biopsy as soon as possible. Refer to an oncology specialist for treatment.

Atypical glandular cells

Because of the high rate of significant lesions in patients with AGS, colposcopy with endocervical sampling is recommended for all subcategories, including AIS. In women over age 35, endometrial sampling is recommended in addition to colposcopy and endocervical sampling. Refer to an appropriate specialist for evaluation.

Treatment

The optimal management of precancerous cervical lesions has not been identified clearly for all classes of SIL. Consult with an HIV-experienced gynecologist, oncologist, or other dysplasia specialist.

Prevention

Latex or plastic barriers may block transmission of HPV in areas covered by these barriers, but infection may occur through bodily contact outside the area covered by the barriers. Nonetheless, their use is recommended to prevent transmission or acquisition of HPV.

Two vaccines have been approved by the U.S. Food and Drug Administration for the prevention of certain HPV strains in women:

- **Gardasil:** includes HPV types 16 and 18 (which cause about 70% of cervical cancer, as well as vaginal and vulvar cancer), and types 6 and 11 (which cause most anogenital warts); approved for females of age 9-26

- **Cervarix**: includes HPV types 16 and 18; approved for females of age 10-25.

Gardasil also has been approved for use with males of age 9-26 for prevention of genital warts; no data are available to evaluate efficacy in preventing cervical dysplasia or cancer in female partners.

These vaccines are not effective against HPV types other than those covered by the vaccine, and they may not be protective against a covered type to which a patient has been exposed previously.

The HPV vaccines have not been thoroughly studied in HIV-infected persons and thus are not specifically recommended for such patients; studies to evaluate efficacy, safety, immunogenicity, and tolerability are under way. The vaccines are not contraindicated for HIV-infected persons, and many clinicians do provide them. There are no data on the efficacy of the vaccines in preventing anal HPV; studies are under way.

Patient Education

- Recommend the use of latex or polyurethane male or female condoms for vaginal or anal intercourse and plastic or latex barriers for oral sex to reduce the risk of transmitting HPV (the usual cause of cervical cancer) to partners. Barriers also reduce the risk of exposure to other sexually transmitted pathogens.

- Patients who smoke should be advised to quit. Cigarette smoking appears to heighten the risk of cervical cancer and makes HPV more difficult to treat. Discuss options for smoking cessation (see chapter *Smoking Cessation*), and refer patients to the American Lung Association if local programs are available.

- Emphasize the importance of keeping follow-up appointments for Pap screening or colposcopy to allow early detection of precancerous lesions and appropriate monitoring of abnormalities.

- For women with dysplasia who require treatment, emphasize that early treatment is essential for managing the disease and preventing the development of cancer. Advise patients to keep all medical appointments.

References

- Aberg JA, Kaplan JE, Libman H, et al.; HIV Medicine Association of the Infectious Diseases Society of America. *Primary care guidelines for the management of persons infected with human immunodeficiency virus: 2009 update by the HIV Medicine Association of the Infectious Diseases Society of America.* Clin Infect Dis. 2009 Sep 1;49(5):651-81.

- Abularach S, Anderson J. *Gynecological Problems.* In: Anderson JR, ed. *A Guide to the Clinical Care of Women with HIV.* Rockville, MD: Health Services and Resources Administration; 2001:153. Available online at hab.hrsa.gov/publications/womencare05/. Accessed June 30, 2010.

- Centers for Disease Control and Prevention. *Guidelines for Prevention and Treatment of Opportunistic Infections in HIV-Infected Adults and Adolescents: Recommendations from CDC, the National Institutes of Health, and the HIV Medicine Association of the Infectious Diseases Society of America.* April 10, 2009. Available at www.aidsinfo.nih.gov/guidelines/.

- Ellerbrock TV, Chiasson MA, Bush TJ, et al. *Incidence of cervical squamous intraepithelial lesions in HIV-infected women.* JAMA. 2000 Feb 23;283(8):1031-7.

- Massad LS, Ahdieh L, Benning L, et al. *Evolution of cervical abnormalities among women with HIV-1: evidence from surveillance cytology in the women's interagency HIV study.* J Acquir Immune Defic Syndr. 2001 Aug 15;27(5):432-42.

- Solomon D, Davey D, Kruman R, et al. *The 2001 Bethesda System: terminology for reporting results of cervical cytology.* JAMA. 2002 Apr 24;287(16):2114-9.

- Wright TC, Massad LS, Dunton CJ, et al.; 2006 American Society for Colposcopy and Cervical Pathology-sponsored Consensus Conference. *2006 Consensus Guidelines for the management of women with cervical intraepithelial neoplasia or adenocarcinoma in situ.* J Low Genit Tract Dis. 2007 Oct;11(4):223-39.

Cryptococcal Disease

Background

Cryptococcosis is a systemic or central nervous system (CNS) fungal infection caused by the yeast *Cryptococcus neoformans.* The organism is ubiquitous, and is particularly plentiful in soils enriched with bird droppings. It also may be present in fruit skins or juices, and in unpasteurized milk. In immunocompetent patients, cryptococcal infection usually is asymptomatic, self-limited, and confined to the lungs. In persons with advanced HIV infection (e.g., those with CD4 counts of <100 cells/μL), *Cryptococcus* may cause life-threatening illness, either from a new exposure or through reactivation of a previously acquired latent infection.

In HIV-infected patients, *Cryptococcus* can infect almost all organs in the body, but most commonly causes meningitis or meningoencephalitis. Disseminated disease, pneumonia, and skin lesions also may be seen.

S: Subjective

Symptoms depend upon the locus of infection. In the case of meningitis, the patient typically experiences subacute onset of fever, headaches, and malaise, which worsen over the course of several weeks. These symptoms may be accompanied by nausea with or without vomiting. Classic meningeal signs, nuchal rigidity, and photophobia are present in only about 25% of cases. Cryptococcal meningitis may cause confusion, personality or behavior changes, blindness, deafness, and, if left untreated, coma and death. If the disease involves the lungs, patients may experience cough or shortness of breath, pleuritic chest pain, and fever. Skin lesions may be present.

O: Objective

Perform a thorough physical examination with particular attention to the following:

- Vital signs, hydration status
- Funduscopic findings
- Neck (for nuchal rigidity, which is uncommon)
- Lungs, especially if respiratory symptoms are present
- Neurologic evaluation, including cranial nerves, visual acuity, and mental status
- Skin

Cryptococcal Meningitis

Physical examination may reveal papilledema with loss of visual acuity and cranial nerve deficits (particularly in cranial nerves III and VI).

Cryptococcal Pulmonary Disease

Examination may reveal tachypnea or fine rales.

Cutaneous Infection

Skin lesions are variable and may appear as papules, nodules, or ulcers; they often resemble molluscum lesions.

A: Assessment

The differential diagnosis for cryptococcal meningitis or meningoencephalitis is broad and includes other infectious causes of meningitis (fungal, mycobacterial, bacterial, viral), syphilis, lymphoma, mass lesions, intoxication, HIV encephalopathy, and trauma. (See chapter *Neurologic Symptoms.*)

The differential diagnosis for cryptococcal pneumonia is broad and includes other infectious causes of pneumonia (fungal, mycobacterial, bacterial, viral), malignancy, and congestive heart failure. (*See* chapter *Pulmonary Symptoms*.)

P: Plan

Diagnostic Evaluation

The workup should include serum cryptococcal antigen (CrAg), which usually is very sensitive, and blood cultures, including bacterial, acid-fast bacilli (AFB), and fungal cultures. Patients with symptoms of disseminated or pulmonary infection should be evaluated by chest X ray (which may show diffuse or focal infiltrates, sometimes appearing as nodular or miliary; intrathoracic adenopathy; or pleural effusions), sputum culture (including fungal and AFB cultures), and AFB stain. Bronchoscopy and bronchoalveolar lavage may be necessary for diagnosis. For cutaneous lesions, consider biopsy and histopathologic evaluation or culture. As part of the general fever workup, urinalysis and urine cultures should be checked.

Patients with a positive serum CrAg, another positive test for *Cryptococcus*, or signs or symptoms of meningitis should undergo analysis of the cerebrospinal fluid (CSF). If neurologic symptoms or signs are present, obtain a computed tomography (CT) scan of the brain before performing a lumbar puncture (LP) to rule out a mass lesion or increased intracranial pressure (ICP), which could cause herniation upon LP. Always measure the CSF opening pressure; a high ICP contributes to morbidity and mortality and determines the need for serial LP to manage the increased ICP. Send the CSF for the following:

- CrAg (usually positive at high titer in meningitis)
- Fungal culture

- India ink stain (less sensitive than CSF CrAg; perform if CSF CrAg is not available)
- Cell count
- Glucose
- Protein

For exclusion of other etiologies, perform CSF Venereal Disease Research Laboratory (VDRL) test, bacterial culture, AFB smear and culture, or polymerase chain reaction (PCR), if tuberculosis is suspected, and other tests as indicated by the patient's symptoms and exposures.

Treatment

Cryptococcal meningitis

Acute treatment of cryptococcal meningitis consists of two phases: induction and consolidation. Acute treatment is followed by chronic maintenance (suppressive) therapy.

Induction

Patients with cryptococcal meningitis should be hospitalized to start 2 weeks of induction therapy with amphotericin B (0.7 mg/kg/day) IV plus flucytosine (25 mg/kg) PO Q6H.

Amphotericin B causes many adverse effects, including fever, rigors, hypotension, nausea, nephrotoxicity and electrolyte disturbances, anemia, and leukopenia. The patient's hemoglobin, white blood cell (WBC) count, platelets, electrolytes, magnesium, and creatinine must be monitored closely during treatment. Note that liposomal forms of amphotericin (AmBisome and Abelcet) cause fewer adverse effects and appear to be effective, although data on use for treatment of cryptococcal meningitis are limited. These liposomal forms should be considered for patients who have difficulty tolerating standard amphotericin B and for those who are at high risk of renal failure. Flucytosine is associated with bone marrow toxicity, and complete blood counts should be monitored during induction therapy. If available, flucytosine levels can be evaluated 3-5 days after the start of therapy, with a target 2 hour post-dose level of 30-80 mg/mL; a level of >100 mg/mL should be avoided. Note that the dosage of flucytosine must be adjusted for patients with renal insufficiency.

If amphotericin is not available, is contraindicated, or is not tolerated by the patient, alternative induction therapies may be considered. The primary alternative to amphotericin-based therapy is high-dose fluconazole (800-1,200 mg PO once daily), with or without flucytosine. Among the newer antifungal agents, echinocandins have no activity against *Cryptococcus*. Voriconazole and posaconazole have good in vitro activity and may be considered for treatment of relapsed disease but not as first-line agents. The efficacy of alternative regimens is not well defined. See "Potential ARV Interactions," below, regarding drug-drug interactions between these antifungals and ARVs.

Resistance testing may be considered for patients who have relapsed and for those for whom fluconazole failed to sterilize the CSF.

Consolidation

After clinical improvement with 2 weeks of induction therapy, and a negative CSF culture on repeat LP, treatment can be switched to fluconazole (400 mg PO once daily to complete 8 weeks of acute treatment). Itraconazole (200 mg PO BID) sometimes is used as an alternative for patients who cannot take fluconazole. It should be noted that itraconazole is less effective than fluconazole and has significant drug interactions with commonly used medications.

Maintenance

After completing acute treatment, the patient should receive chronic maintenance therapy with fluconazole (200 mg PO once daily) to prevent recurrence of cryptococcosis. An alternative treatment is itraconazole (200 mg

PO once daily or BID) — with the caution indicated above.

Maintenance therapy should be continued for life, unless the patient has sustained CD4 cell recovery in response to effective antiretroviral therapy (ART) (CD4 count >200 cells/μL for at least 6 months during ART). Maintenance therapy should be restarted if the CD4 count declines to <200 cells/μL.

Management of elevated ICP

Elevated ICP significantly increases the morbidity and mortality of cryptococcal meningitis and should be treated by the removal of CSF. The CSF opening pressure should be checked on the initial LP. If the initial opening pressure is >250 mm H_2O, remove up to 30 mL of CSF to lower the ICP by 50%, if possible. LP and CSF removal should be repeated daily as needed for ICP reduction. A lumbar drain or ventriculoperitoneal shunt may be needed if the initial opening pressure is >400 mm H_2O, or in refractory cases. There is no role for acetazolamide, mannitol, or steroids in the treatment of elevated ICP.

A repeat LP is not required for patients who did not have elevated ICP at baseline and are responding to treatment. If new symptoms develop, a repeat LP is indicated. Serum CrAg titers are not useful in monitoring response to treatment.

Cryptococcal pulmonary disease, with negative CSF CrAg and culture results

After CSF cryptococcal disease has been excluded, treat with fluconazole if symptoms are mild or moderate, 400 mg PO once daily for 6-12 months, then 200 mg once daily for maintenance. Otherwise, consider amphotericin induction, as described above with CNS disease. Monitor fungal blood cultures and CrAg to verify the effectiveness of therapy. Itraconazole may be used as an alternative (200 mg PO BID for capsules; 100-200 mg once daily for oral suspension). Therapy should be continued for life, unless the patient has sustained CD4 cell recovery in response to effective ART (CD4 count of >200 cells/µL for at least 6 months during ART) and with a minimum of 12 months of antifungal therapy. Therapy should be restarted if the CD4 count declines to <200 cells/µL.

Cutaneous infection, with negative CSF CrAg and culture results

Treat with fluconazole 400 mg PO once daily for 6-12 months, then continue with 200 mg once daily for chronic maintenance therapy, as discussed above.

Asymptomatic antigenemia

Data are limited for management of asymptomatic antigenemia, which can be associated with development of subsequent disease. Fungal cultures of CSF and blood should be obtained; if either result is positive for cryptococcal growth, treatment should be initiated for symptomatic meningoencephalitis or disseminated disease. If no meningoencephalitis is found, fluconazole 400 mg PO once daily should be given until immune reconstitution occurs; treatment may be discontinued per maintenance guidelines described above.

Cryptococcus IRIS

Immune reconstitution through ART is effective for preventing recurrence of cryptococcal infections. However, initiating ART within the first 1-2 months after cryptococcal infection may result in worsening or recurrence of symptoms because of immune reconstitution inflammatory syndrome (IRIS). IRIS can be life-threatening in cryptococcal meningeal disease. IRIS and relapse of cryptococcal disease (e.g., treatment failure) must be differentiated; in IRIS, the serum and CSF cultures are negative. (See chapter *Immune Reconstitution Inflammatory Syndrome*.)

Optimal timing of ART initiation in cryptococcal CNS disease is unknown. Some experts recommend treating cryptococcosis

with effective antifungal therapy for 1-2 months before starting ART, to decrease the risk of IRIS.

Other treatment notes

Pregnancy: Fluconazole and other azole drugs are not recommended for use during pregnancy, especially in the first trimester. During the first trimester, pregnant women should be treated with amphotericin for both induction and consolidation therapy. Flucytosine is teratogenic at high doses in rats and class C in humans; it should be used during pregnancy only if the benefits clearly outweigh the risks.

Preventive therapy: Studies have suggested that routine primary prophylaxis for cryptococcal disease in patients with CD4 counts of <100 cells/µL is effective at preventing cryptococcal infection but is not cost efficient. Therefore, it is not routinely recommended.

Potential ARV Interactions

There may be significant drug-drug interactions between certain systemic antifungals, particularly itraconazole, voriconazole, and posaconazole, and ritonavir-boosted protease inhibitors (PIs), nonnucleoside reverse transcriptase inhibitors (NNRTIs), or maraviroc. Some combinations are contraindicated and others require dosage adjustment of the ARV, the antifungal, or both. Check for adverse drug interactions before prescribing. For example, voriconazole use is not recommended for patients taking ritonavir-boosted PIs, and dosage adjustment of both voriconazole and NNRTIs may be required when voriconazole is used concurrently with NNRTIs. See Tables 15a-e of the U.S. Department of Health and Human Services *Guidelines for the Use of Antiretroviral Agents in HIV-1-Infected Adults and Adolescents*, or consult with an expert.

Patient Education

- Cryptococcosis is not curable in persons with low CD4 cell counts and may require lifelong treatment. Patients should be instructed to take their treatment without interruptions.

- Even with therapy, disease may recur. Patients should report fevers or recurrence of other symptoms immediately.

- Patients should avoid pregnancy while taking any oral antifungal drug. Fetal craniofacial and skeletal abnormalities have been reported.

References

- Bicanic T, Harrison TS. *Cryptococcal meningitis.* Br Med Bull. 2005 Apr 18;72:99-118.

- Brouwer AE, Rajanuwong A, Chierakul W, et al. *Combination antifungal therapies for HIV-associated cryptococcal meningitis: a randomised trial.* Lancet. 2004 May 29;363(9423):1764-7.

- Centers for Disease Control and Prevention. *Guidelines for Prevention and Treatment of Opportunistic Infections in HIV-Infected Adults and Adolescents: Recommendations from CDC, the National Institutes of Health, and the HIV Medicine Association of the Infectious Diseases Society of America.* April 10, 2009. Available at www.aidsinfo.nih.gov/guidelines/.

- McNicholl I. *Database of Antiretroviral Drug Interactions.* In: Coffey S, Volberding PA, eds. HIV InSite. San Francisco: UCSF Center for HIV Information. Available at hivinsite.ucsf.edu/insite?page=ar-00-02. Accessed June 30, 2010.

- Nussbaum JC, Jackson A, Namarika D, et al. *Combination flucytosine and high-dose fluconazole compared with fluconazole monotherapy for the treatment of cryptococcal meningitis: a randomized trial in Malawi.* Clin Infect Dis. 2010 Feb 1;50(3):338-44.

- Perfect JR, Dismukes WE, Dromer F, et al. *Clinical practice guidelines for the management of cryptococcal disease: 2010 update by the Infectious Diseases Society of America.* Clin Infect Dis. 2010 Feb 1;50(3):291-322.

Cryptosporidiosis

Background

Cryptosporidiosis is caused by a species of protozoan parasite that typically infects the mucosa of the small intestine, causing watery diarrhea. Diarrhea may be accompanied by nausea, vomiting, abdominal cramping, and occasionally fever. The infection is spread by the fecal-oral route, usually via contaminated water, and is highly contagious. The course of infection depends on the immune status of the host. In immunocompetent individuals, cryptosporidiosis usually is self-limited and can cause a mild diarrheal illness. However, in HIV-infected patients with advanced immunosuppression, cryptosporidiosis can cause severe chronic diarrhea, electrolyte disturbances, malabsorption, and profound weight loss. Infection also can occur outside the intestinal tract and can cause cholangitis, pancreatitis, and hepatitis. In severe cases, cryptosporidiosis can be life-threatening without aggressive fluid, electrolyte, and nutritional support. Patients at greatest risk of acquiring cryptosporidiosis are those with CD4 counts of <100 cells/μL. Immune reconstitution inflammatory syndrome (IRIS) has not been described in association with cryptosporidiosis.

S: Subjective

The patient may complain of some or all of the following: watery diarrhea (can be profuse), abdominal pain or cramping, flatulence, nausea, vomiting, anorexia, fever, and weight loss.

The history should include questions about the presence and characteristics of the symptoms listed above, as well as the following:

Stool frequency (typically 6-26 bowel movements daily)

- Stool volume (up to 10 liters per day and can be described as "cholera-like" in some patients with AIDS)

- Duration of symptoms (subacute or acute onset)

- Associated symptoms

- Exposures: recent travel to areas with unsafe water supply; ingestion of possibly contaminated water while swimming, boating, or camping; oral-anal contact, fecal exposures during sexual contact

- Recent CD4 cell count (highest risk is in patients with CD4 counts of <100 cells/μL)

O: Objective

Perform a thorough physical examination with particular attention to the following:

- Vital signs

- Hydration status (e.g., orthostatic vital signs, mucous membrane moistness, skin turgor)

- Weight (compare with previous values; document weight loss)

- Signs of malnourishment (e.g., cachexia, wasting, thinning hair, pallor)

- Abdominal examination for bowel sounds (usually hyperactive), tenderness (can be diffuse), rebound

- Recent CD4 count

A: Assessment

In HIV-infected patients with advanced immunosuppression, the differential diagnosis includes other infectious causes of subacute or chronic diarrhea or cholangitis, such as microsporidia, *Isospora*, *Giardia*, cytomegalovirus (CMV), and *Mycobacterium avium* complex (MAC), as well as lymphoma.

P: Plan

Diagnostic Evaluation

- Test the stool for ova and parasites, including *Cryptosporidium*. Diagnosis is made by microscopic identification of the *Cryptosporidium* oocysts in stool.

  - Be sure to ask the laboratory to look for *Cryptosporidium*; certain labs do not look for these parasites or their precursor, the oocyst, unless requested.

  - Test for fecal leukocytes. The result usually is negative in cryptosporidiosis; if positive, consider the possibility of a second enteric infection, especially if the CD4 count is low, or a different infection.

- Among persons with profuse diarrhea, a single stool specimen usually is adequate for diagnosis.

- For patients with milder disease, repeat stool sampling is recommended.

- If stool is negative for ova and parasites, consider a referral for biopsy of the gastrointestinal mucosa or flexible sigmoidoscopy.

- If cholangitis is suspected, consider abdominal ultrasound to look for biliary ductal dilatation, and endoscopic retrograde cholangiopancreatography (ERCP).

- Check electrolytes; conduct liver function studies including alkaline phosphatase and bilirubin to check for possible biliary or hepatic infection.

- If fever is present, obtain blood cultures.

- Conduct other diagnostic testing as indicated by the history and physical examination (e.g., evaluation for CMV, MAC, and other infectious causes of diarrhea or cholangitis) (see chapter *Diarrhea*).

Treatment

- Effective antiretroviral therapy (ART) with immune reconstitution (and CD4 count >100 cells/μL) can resolve cryptosporidiosis, and it is the primary treatment. All patients with cryptosporidiosis should be offered ART (see chapter *Antiretroviral Therapy*). Patients who are on incompletely suppressive ART should have their regimens optimized.

- Provide supportive care and symptomatic relief (this may require hospitalization in cases of severe dehydration), including the following:

  - Aggressive fluid and electrolyte replacement as needed

  - Oral rehydration (solutions containing glucose, sodium bicarbonate, potassium, magnesium, and phosphorus); in severe cases, IV hydration may be required

  - Antidiarrheal agents: atropine/diphenoxylate (Lomotil), loperamide (Imodium), tincture of opium (Paregoric)

  - Antispasmodics

  - Antiemetics

  - Topical treatment for the anorectal area, as needed (witch hazel pads [e.g., Tucks]), sitz baths)

- No antiparasitic therapy has been proven to consistently and effectively cure cryptosporidiosis if used without ART.

  - Nitazoxanide is approved for use in children and adults with diarrhea caused by *Cryptosporidium parvum*, the most common strain of *Cryptosporidium*. It may increase the likelihood of clinical response. It should be given in conjunction with ART, but never instead of ART.

    - Usual adult dosage: 500-1,000 mg PO BID for 14 days

- Adverse events associated with nitazoxanide are limited and typically mild; there are no important drug-drug interactions

  - Paromomycin with or without azithromycin does not appear to be effective, especially for patients with CD4 counts of <100 cells/μL. Current data do not support a recommendation for use.

- For patients with weight loss, nutritional supplementation is a critical aspect of treatment. In some cases, partial or total parenteral nutrition may be necessary while patients are awaiting clinical improvement in response to ART or other therapies. Consult or refer to a dietitian or nutritionist, if available. If not, assess food intake and counsel the patient about increasing caloric and nutritional intake.

Cryptosporidiosis in Resource-Limited Settings

Cryptosporidium infection in HIV-uninfected populations is more common in countries with overcrowding and poor sanitary conditions. The disease is also associated with rainy seasons and is frequent among children <2 years of age.

The prognosis for HIV-infected patients with cryptosporidiosis who lack access to ART is poor. In one study, the mean survival time of coinfected patients was 25 weeks.

Prevention of Disease and Exposure

- Rifabutin or clarithromycin, when taken for MAC prophylaxis, have been found to protect against cryptosporidiosis. However, current data are insufficient to warrant a recommendation of their use as prophylaxis.

- Scrupulous handwashing can prevent the spread of cryptosporidiosis, and HIV-infected patients should be advised to wash their hands after potential contact with human feces (diapering small children, handling pets, gardening, and before and after sex).

- HIV-infected patients should avoid sexual practices that could lead to direct (e.g., oral-anal) or indirect (e.g., penile-anal) contact with feces and should be advised to use barrier methods during sex (e.g., condoms and dental dams).

- HIV-infected persons should avoid drinking water from lakes or rivers. Waterborne infection also can result from recreational activities such as boating, fishing, and swimming.

- HIV-infected patients should avoid raw oysters as the cryptosporidial oocysts can survive in oysters for >2 months.

Patient Education

- Recommend scrupulous handwashing for the patient and all contacts, especially household members and sex partners.

- Explain that effective ART is the best treatment for alleviating symptoms and helping the immune system eradicate the parasite.

- Advise the patient to increase fluid intake (not alcohol), and avoid foods that aggravate diarrhea. A lactose-free diet may improve symptoms.

- Educate the patient about healthful food choices that increase calorie intake and nutrition.

- Provide supportive counseling; discuss how to manage symptoms and the isolation that may accompany chronic diarrhea.

References

- Abubakar I, Aliyu SH, Arumugam C, et al. *Treatment of cryptosporidiosis in immunocompromised individuals: systematic review and meta-analysis.* Br J Clin Pharmacol. 2007 April;63(4);387-393.

- Centers for Disease Control and Prevention. *Guidelines for Prevention and Treatment of Opportunistic Infections in HIV-Infected Adults and Adolescents: Recommendations from CDC, the National Institutes of Health, and the HIV Medicine Association of the Infectious Diseases Society of America.* April 10, 2009. Available at www.aidsinfo.nih.gov/guidelines/.

- Leder K, Weller PF. *Cryptosporidiosis* [online resource]. Waltham, MA: Up to Date; May 2009. Available online at www.uptodate.com/index.asp. [Fee required.] Accessed June 30, 2010.

- Pantenburg B, Cabada MM, White AC. *Treatment of cryptosporidiosis.* Expert Rev Anti Infect Ther. 2009 May;7(4):385-91.

Cytomegalovirus Disease

Background

Although chronic infection with cytomegalovirus (CMV) rarely causes disease among immunocompetent persons, it is a major cause of morbidity and mortality in HIV-infected patients with CD4 counts of <50 cells/μL. CMV infection causes disease in several organ systems, including the central nervous system (CNS) (chorioretinitis, encephalitis, polyradiculopathy, myelopathy) and the gastrointestinal (GI) tract (oral ulcers, esophagitis, hepatitis, colitis, intestinal perforation), as well as life-threatening adrenalitis and pneumonitis. The prevalence of chronic infection with CMV, a member of the human herpesvirus family, is high among sexually active adults (40-60% in resource-rich countries and 80-90% in resource-poor countries). CMV is spread by sexual or other types of close personal contact, blood-to-blood contact (via transfusion or needle sharing), organ transplantation, and perinatal transmission. As with other herpesviruses, CMV is not cleared from the body, but is kept in a state of latency by an intact immune system. Symptomatic disease represents either primary infection or reactivation of latent infection that has escaped immunologic control. Effective antiretroviral therapy (ART) greatly reduces the risk of CMV reactivation and disease.

Immune reconstitution inflammatory syndrome:

Although effective ART greatly reduces the risk of CMV reactivation and disease, patients on effective ART may experience CMV-related visual changes.

- Patients without a previous history of CMV disease will occasionally present with full-blown CMV retinitis after starting ART. This is thought to reflect delayed restoration of CMV-specific immunity. It is diagnosed and treated in an identical manner as for patients diagnosed with CMV disease who are not taking effective ART.

- Approximately 20% of patients with previously treated CMV retinitis may experience CMV-related immune reconstitution uveitis (IRU) after starting successful ART. Symptoms include floaters and moderate, occasionally severe, vision loss. The most common causes of vision loss are posterior disease, specifically cystoid macular edema (CME) and epiretinal membrane formation (ERM), although inflammation of the anterior region and cataract formation also can occur. It is not clear whether treatment with steroids or anti-CMV antivirals is effective. (See chapter *Immune Reconstitution Inflammatory Syndrome*.)

S: Subjective

The patient may present with symptoms involving various organ systems, including the following:

CNS, including the eye:

- Floaters, scotomata (blind spots), "flashing lights," loss of peripheral or field vision (chorioretinitis)

- Headache, difficulty concentrating, sleepiness, personality changes (encephalitis, dementia)

- Bilateral lower extremity weakness, urinary retention, incontinence, spasticity (polyradiculopathy)

- Low back pain, especially radiating to the perianal area (polyradiculopathy, myelitis)

- Family members or caregivers may report confusion, apathy, lethargy, somnolence, withdrawal, or personality changes in the patient (CMV encephalitis, dementia)

GI tract disease:

- Mouth ulcerations
- Dysphagia or odynophagia (esophagitis)
- Abdominal pain and bloody diarrhea, weight loss, rectal ulcers, fever (colitis)

Disease outside the CNS or GI tract:

- Persistent fever, fatigue, weight loss (adrenalitis)
- Shortness of breath, dyspnea on exertion, dry cough (pneumonia; rare in patients with advanced HIV infection)
- Pancytopenia (bone marrow infection)

The history should include questions about the presence and characteristics of the symptoms listed above, as well as the following:

- Duration of symptoms
- Associated symptoms
- Recent CD4 count; nadir CD4 count (risk is highest when count is <50 cells/μL)
- Whether the patient is taking ART; if so, date initiated, specific medications, and CD4 and HIV RNA responses

O: Objective

Perform a thorough physical examination, with particular attention to the following:

- Vital signs: Document fever.
- Weight: Compare with previous values; document weight loss.
- Eyes: Funduscopic examination in patients with CMV retinitis may show pathognomonic "cottage cheese in ketchup" yellow-white lesions, representing vascular hemorrhages and exudates.
- Nervous system: Evaluate mental status and perform a complete neurologic examination, including cranial nerves, sensation (sensory deficits may occur with preserved vibratory sense and proprioception), motor, deep tendon reflexes, coordination, and gait.

A: Assessment

For HIV-infected patients with advanced immunosuppression, the differential diagnosis includes the following:

- For suspected CMV retinitis: consider cotton-wool spots, HIV retinopathy, and progressive outer or acute retinal necrosis.
- For suspected CMV encephalitis: consider other causes of neurologic deterioration such as progressive multifocal leukoencephalopathy, toxoplasmosis, CNS lymphoma, and other mass lesions.
- For suspected CMV enteritis: consider gastrointestinal pathogens such as *Mycobacterium avium* complex, *Cryptosporidium*, other parasites, and lymphoma.
- For suspected CMV pneumonitis: consider *Pneumocystis jiroveci* and other respiratory pathogens.

P: Plan

Diagnostic Evaluation

CMV can be detected by serology, culture, antigen testing, nucleic acid amplification, or examination of tissue samples. However, serologic tests are not reliable for diagnosing CMV disease because most adults are seropositive and because patients with advanced AIDS may serorevert while remaining infected. Furthermore, for HIV-infected patients, demonstration of CMV in the blood, urine, semen, cervical secretions, or bronchoalveolar lavage (BAL) fluid does not necessarily indicate active disease, although patients with end-organ disease usually are viremic.

Diagnosis of end-organ disease generally requires demonstration of tissue invasion. The recommended evaluation is as follows:

CMV retinitis

Dilated retinal examination should be performed emergently by an ophthalmologist experienced in the diagnosis of CMV retinitis. The diagnosis usually is based on the identification of typical lesions. Diagnosis and monitoring should include serial examinations with photography to assess and follow response to treatment and to detect failure to respond early enough to change therapy.

Other sites

Detection of CMV at other sites requires visualization of typical lesions (e.g., on endoscopy or BAL) and tissue biopsy. Viral inclusions ("owl's eye cells") in tissue biopsy samples demonstrate invasive disease (as opposed to colonization). **Because retinitis is the most common manifestation of CMV disease, patients with CNS, gastrointestinal, or pulmonary disease should undergo ophthalmologic evaluation to detect subclinical retinal disease.**

Neurologic CMV disease

- Encephalitis: Magnetic resonance imaging (MRI) of the brain should be done to rule out mass lesions. CMV effects may appear as periventricular or meningeal enhancement. Lumbar puncture should be performed; cerebrospinal fluid (CSF) should be analyzed for CMV (by PCR, which is sensitive and specific), cell count (may show lymphocytic or mixed lymphocytic or polymorphonuclear pleocytosis), glucose (may be low), and protein (may be high). A brain biopsy may be performed if the diagnosis is uncertain after imaging and CSF evaluation.

- Polyradiculopathy: Spinal MRI should be done to rule out mass lesions. In CMV disease, nerve root thickening may be present. Lumbar puncture with CSF analysis should be performed, as described above.

- Myelitis: Spinal MRI should be done to rule out mass lesions. Cord enhancement may be present. Lumbar puncture with CSF analysis should be performed, as described above.

Gastrointestinal CMV disease (esophagitis or colitis)

- Perform endoscopy with visualization of ulcers and obtain tissue biopsy to look for inclusion bodies.

Pulmonary CMV disease

- Perform chest radiography showing interstitial pneumonia and obtain lung biopsy to look for inclusion bodies.

Treatment

Ganciclovir, valganciclovir, foscarnet, and cidofovir may be effective for treating CMV end-organ disease. The choice of therapy depends on the site and severity of the infection, the level of underlying immunosuppression, the patient's ability to tolerate the medications and adhere to the treatment regimen, and the potential medication interactions.

Immune reconstitution through ART is a key component of CMV treatment and relapse prevention. The optimal timing of ART initiation in relation to the treatment of CMV is not clear. CMV flares may occur if patients develop immune reconstitution inflammatory syndrome (see chapter *Immune Reconstitution Inflammatory Syndrome*), but in most cases of nonneurologic disease, ART probably should not be delayed.

CMV retinitis

Treatment consists of two phases: initial therapy and chronic maintenance therapy.

Initial therapy

Before the advent of valganciclovir, the preferred strategy for treating CMV retinitis involved ganciclovir intraocular implants and systemic therapy. Because implants deliver a higher dose of drug to the retina than any other modality (1.4 mcg/hour for up to 8 months), many experts still prefer them for patients with sight-threatening (zone 1) disease. About half of patients treated with implants develop disease in the contralateral eye, and one third experience systemic disease, within 3 months of implantation. Therefore, patients with implants also should be treated systemically with valganciclovir (900 mg once daily; some experts increase this to 900 mg BID for patients with vision-threatening disease).

For patients with peripheral retinitis (beyond zone 1), oral valganciclovir alone (see below) is the preferred treatment because it is easy to administer and is not associated with the surgery- or catheter-related complications seen with intraocular treatments and IV therapies. This formulation quickly converts to ganciclovir in the body and has good bioavailability. Valganciclovir should be used only if the patient is thought to be capable of strict adherence. Other possible IV treatments include ganciclovir, ganciclovir followed by oral valganciclovir, foscarnet, and cidofovir. See below for dosing recommendations.

- For sight-threatening disease: treat with ganciclovir intraocular implants plus valganciclovir 900 mg PO once daily or BID.
- For peripheral disease: treat with valganciclovir 900 mg PO BID for 14-21 days.

Alternatives for initial therapy:

- IV ganciclovir 5 mg/kg Q12H for 14-21 days
- IV foscarnet 60 mg/kg Q8H or 90 mg/kg Q12H for 14-21 days
- IV cidofovir 5 mg/kg weekly for 2 weeks, then every other week (must be given with probenecid [2 g PO 3 hours before, 1 g PO 2 hours after, and 1 g PO 8 hours after the cidofovir infusion] and IV saline to decrease

the risk of renal toxicity)

- Intraocular injections with antiviral agents

Note: Valganciclovir, ganciclovir, and foscarnet require dosage adjustment in patients with renal insufficiency. Cidofovir is contraindicated for use by patients with renal insufficiency or proteinuria.

Monitor patients closely to gauge the response to therapy. Repeat the dilated retinal examination after completion of induction therapy, 1 month after initiation of therapy, and monthly during anti-CMV therapy, with photography to document progression or resolution of disease. Consult with a specialist if the response to therapy is suboptimal.

Note: Retinal detachment may occur in up to 50-60% of patients in the first year after diagnosis. Regular follow-up with an ophthalmologist is required for all patients. Patients should be instructed to report any vision loss immediately.

Chronic maintenance therapy

After initial CMV treatment, lifelong maintenance therapy with valganciclovir or IV foscarnet should be given to prevent recurrence, and patients need regular reevaluation by an ophthalmologist. Recommended dosages for maintenance therapy are as follows:

- Valganciclovir 900 mg PO once daily
- IV foscarnet 90-120 mg/kg once daily

Discontinuation of maintenance therapy can be considered for patients with inactive CMV and sustained immune reconstitution on ART (CD4 count of >100-150 cells/μL for at least 6 months). However, the decision should be guided by factors such as the extent and location of the CMV lesions and the status of the patient's vision. An ophthalmologist who is experienced in caring for HIV-infected patients with CMV should be involved in making any decision to discontinue therapy, and patients should receive regular ophthalmologic follow-up. Maintenance therapy should be resumed if the CD4 count drops below 100-150 cells/μL or the patient develops other signs of HIV progression.

Neurologic CMV disease

The optimal treatment for neurologic disease has not been determined. Prompt initiation of dual therapy with IV ganciclovir and foscarnet may be effective for some patients.

Gastrointestinal and pulmonary CMV disease

These infections are usually treated with IV ganciclovir or foscarnet for 21-28 days unless the patient is able to absorb oral medications, in which case valganciclovir PO is an option (refer to the dosing suggestions above). Some specialists recommend a follow-up endoscopy to verify regression of lesions before discontinuing therapy. Many experts do not recommend maintenance therapy for gastrointestinal CMV infections unless the disease recurs.

Immune reconstitution inflammatory syndrome retinitis or uveitis

Urgent consultation with experts is recommended.

Monitoring CMV therapies

The medications used to treat CMV have several important potential adverse effects, and monitoring for these is required. Valganciclovir and ganciclovir have been associated with bone marrow suppression, neutropenia, anemia, thrombocytopenia, and renal dysfunction. Foscarnet has been associated with cytopenia, renal insufficiency, electrolyte abnormalities, and seizures. For patients taking these medications, perform complete blood count with differential and check electrolytes and creatinine twice weekly during initial therapy and once weekly during maintenance therapy. Cidofovir has been associated with renal insufficiency and ocular hypotony. For patients taking cidofovir, check creatinine and blood urea nitrogen and

perform urinalysis (for proteinuria) before each dose. Intraocular pressure must be checked at least every 6 months.

Patient Education

- Educate patients about the importance of ART in treating CMV. Urge patients to start ART if they have not done so already.

- Patients with CMV retinitis may have to remain on suppressive therapy for life to prevent blindness. Patients with CMV esophagitis or enteritis usually see improvements within 2-4 weeks after starting therapy.

- Treatment of CMV retinitis halts progression of the infection but does not reverse the damage already done to the retina. Warn patients that vision will not return to pre-CMV status.

- Advise patients to report any visual deterioration immediately. Retinal detachment or progression of CMV must be treated immediately to avoid further vision loss.

- For patients who experience significant vision loss, offer referral to education, training, and support services to help them adjust.

- With gastrointestinal disease, recurrence of symptoms warrants repeat endoscopy. Advise patients to report any recurrence of symptoms.

- Adverse reactions to current therapies are common. Educate patients about these and advise them to promptly report any adverse reactions.

- Help patients cope with the possibility of therapeutic failure, and, in the case of CMV retinitis, permanent loss of vision.

- Teach patients how to maintain indwelling venous access lines, if used. Have patients demonstrate these techniques before discharge.

Section 6: Comorbidities, Coinfections, and Complications

References

- Centers for Disease Control and Prevention. *Guidelines for Prevention and Treatment of Opportunistic Infections in HIV-Infected Adults and Adolescents: Recommendations from CDC, the National Institutes of Health, and the HIV Medicine Association of the Infectious Diseases Society of America.* April 10, 2009. Available at www.aidsinfo.nih.gov/guidelines/.

- Drew WL, Lalezari JP. *Cytomegalovirus and HIV.* In: Coffey S, Volberding PA, eds. *HIV InSite Knowledge Base* [textbook online]. San Francisco: UCSF Center for HIV Information; May 2006. Accessed June 30, 2010.

- Goldberg DE, Smithen LM, Angelilli A, et al. *HIV-associated retinopathy in the HAART era.* Retina. 2005 Jul-Aug;25(5):633-49.

- Jacobsen MA. AIDS Related *Cytomegalovirus Gastrointestinal Disease.* In: UpToDate v14.1. Available at www.uptodate.com/home/index.html. Accessed June 30, 2010. [Registration required.]

- Jacobsen MA. AIDS Related *Cytomegalovirus Neurologic Disease.* In: UpToDate v14.1. Available at www.uptodate.com/home/index.html. Accessed June 30, 2010. [Registration required.]

- Jacobsen MA. *AIDS Related Cytomegalovirus Retinitis.* In: UpToDate v14.1. Available at www.uptodate.com/home/index.html. Accessed June 30, 2010. [Registration required.]

- Kempen JH, Min YI, Freeman WR, et al.; Studies of Ocular Complications of AIDS Research Group. *Risk of immune recovery uveitis in patients with AIDS and cytomegalovirus retinitis.* Ophthalmology. 2006 Apr;113(4):684-94.

Gonorrhea and Chlamydia

Background

Gonorrhea, caused by *Neisseria gonorrhoeae* (GC), and chlamydia, caused by *Chlamydia trachomatis* (CT), are sexually transmitted infections (STIs). These infections may be transmitted during oral, vaginal, or anal sex; they also can be transmitted from a mother to her baby during delivery and cause significant illness in the infant.

Both organisms can infect the urethra, oropharynx, and rectum in women and men; the epididymis in men; and the cervix, uterus, and fallopian tubes in women. Untreated GC or CT infection in women may lead to pelvic inflammatory disease (PID), which can cause scarring of the fallopian tubes and result in infertility or ectopic pregnancy (tubal pregnancy). The organisms also can affect other sites; *N. gonorrhoeae* can cause disseminated infection involving the skin, joints, and other systems. Infection with GC or CT may facilitate transmission of HIV to HIV-uninfected sex partners.

Certain strains of CT can cause lymphogranuloma venereum (LGV). This infection is common in parts of Africa, India, Southeast Asia, and the Caribbean. Outbreaks among men who have sex with men (MSM) have been reported in recent years in Europe and the United States. LGV may cause genital ulcers, followed by inguinal adenopathy; it also can (as seen in the recent cases among MSM) cause gastrointestinal symptoms, notably anorectal discharge and pain.

Patients with symptoms of gonorrhea or chlamydia should be evaluated and treated as indicated below. Although GC or CT urethritis in men typically causes symptoms, urethral infection in women and oral or rectal infections in both men and women often cause no symptoms. In fact, a substantial number of individuals with GC or CT infection have no symptoms. Thus, sexually active individuals at risk of GC and CT exposure should receive regular screening for these infections as well as for syphilis and other STIs. Patients frequently are infected with both GC and CT, so they should be tested and treated for both.

HRSA HAB Core Clinical Performance Measures

Percentage of clients with HIV infection at risk of sexually transmitted infections who had a **test for gonorrhea** within the measurement year

Group 3 measure)

Percentage of clients with HIV infection at risk of sexually transmitted infections who had a **test for chlamydia** within the measurement year

(Group 3 measure)

S: Subjective

Symptoms will depend on the site of infection (e.g., oropharynx, urethra, cervix, rectum). Symptoms are not present in all patients.

If symptoms are present, **women** may notice the following:

- Vaginal discharge
- Urinary hesitancy
- Pain with sexual intercourse
- Pain or burning on urination
- Abdominal or pelvic pain

- Sore throat
- Mouth sores
- Rectal discharge
- Anal discomfort

If symptoms are present, **men** may notice the following:

- Increased urinary frequency or urgency
- Urethral discharge
- Red or swollen urethra
- Incontinence

- Pain on urination
- Testicular tenderness or pain
- Rectal discharge
- Anal discomfort

During the history, ask the patient about the following:

- Any of the symptoms listed above, and their duration
- Previous diagnosis of gonorrhea or chlamydia
- New sex partner(s)
- Unprotected sex (oral, vaginal, anal)
- For women: last menstrual period, and whether the patient could be pregnant; use of an intrauterine device

O: Objective

Physical Examination

During the physical examination, check for fever and document other vital signs.

For **women**, focus the physical examination on the mouth, abdomen, and pelvis. Inspect the oropharynx for discharge and lesions; check the abdomen for bowel sounds, distention, rebound, guarding, masses, and suprapubic or costovertebral angle tenderness; perform a complete pelvic examination for abnormal discharge or bleeding; check for uterine, adnexal, or cervical motion tenderness; and search for pelvic masses or adnexal enlargement. Check the anus for discharge and lesions; perform anoscopy if symptoms of proctitis are present. Check for inguinal lymphadenopathy.

For **men**, focus the physical examination on the mouth, genitals, and anus/rectum. Check the oropharynx for discharge and lesions, the urethra for discharge, the external genitalia for other lesions, and the anus for discharge and lesions; perform anoscopy if symptoms of proctitis are present. Check for inguinal lymphadenopathy.

A: Assessment

A partial differential diagnosis includes the following:

- Urinary tract infection
- Dysmenorrhea
- Appendicitis
- Cystitis
- Proctitis
- PID
- Irritable bowel syndrome
- Pyelonephritis

P: Plan

Diagnostic Evaluation

Test for oral, urethral, or anorectal infection, according to symptoms and possible exposures. Perform concurrent testing for both gonorrhea and chlamydia. The availability of the various testing methods varies according to the specific clinic site. Consider the following:

- Culture (oropharynx, endocervix, urethra, rectum)
- Nucleic acid amplification test (NAAT): urine specimens (first stream) and urethral (men), vaginal, and endocervical swab specimens; also used with pharyngeal and rectal swab specimens (although not yet FDA approved for this use)
- Nucleic acid hybridization assay (DNA probe): endocervical and male urethral swab specimens; not approved for rectal or pharyngeal swabs
- Gram stain (pharyngeal, cervical, or urethral discharge), for evidence of GC
- Serologic tests (microimmunofluorescence test or complement fixation test) for suspected LGV

Treatment

Treatments for gonorrhea and chlamydia are indicated below. Fluoroquinolone-resistant GC is widespread in the United States, Pacific Islands, Asia, and Britain. Thus, the U.S. Centers for Disease Control and Prevention (CDC) recommends that fluoroquinolones not be used for treatment of GC in MSM or in any infected patient in the areas listed above, unless antimicrobial susceptibility test results are used to guide therapy. Similarly, resistance of GC to azithromycin is emerging, and azithromycin should be used to treat GC only in select patients in whom other treatments should be avoided.

Because dual infection is common, *patients diagnosed with either GC or CT should receive empiric treatment for both infections, unless the other infection has been ruled out.* Reinfection is likely if reexposure occurs. Any sex partners within the last 60 days, or the most recent sex partner from >60 days before diagnosis, also should receive treatment. Patients should abstain from sexual activity for 7 days after a single-dose treatment or until a 7-day treatment course is completed.

Adherence is essential for treatment success. Single-dose treatments maximize the likelihood of adherence and are preferred. Other considerations in choosing the treatment include antibiotic resistance, cost, allergies, and pregnancy. For further information, see the CDC STI treatment guidelines (see "References," below).

Treatment of Gonorrhea

Treatment options include the following (see the full CDC STI treatment guidelines, referenced below); the current guidelines emphasize that ceftriaxone should be used, if possible, for GC infection at any anatomic site and that azithromycin or doxycycline also should be given, to improve likelihood of cure and decrease risk of emergent cephalosporin resistance. Note that GC infection of the pharynx is more difficult to cure than GC infection at other sites. Patients who report possible oral sexual exposures should be treated with ceftriaxone 250 mg, if possible (see below).

Recommended regimens

- Ceftriaxone 250 mg IM injection in a single dose, plus azithromycin 1 g PO in a single dose or doxycycline 100 mg PO BID for 7 days (for pharyngeal GC, this is the only recommended regimen)
If ceftriaxone is not an option; for GC of the urethra, cervix, and rectum ONLY:

  - Cefixime 400 mg PO in a single dose (tablet or oral suspension), plus azithromycin or doxycycline as above; cefixime is NOT sufficiently effective to treat pharyngeal GC

  - Single-dose injectable cephalosporin plus azithromycin or doxycycline as above; efficacy for pharyngeal GC is uncertain

Alternative regimens *(for GC infection of the urethra, cervix, and rectum ONLY; inadequate for pharyngeal GC)*

- Cefpodoxime 400 mg PO in a single dose

- Cefuroxime axetil 1 g PO

- Spectinomycin 2 g IM injection in a single dose (currently not available in the United States)

- Azithromycin 2 g PO in a single dose (concern for possible emergence of resistance; use other agents if possible)

If penicillin allergy:

- Cephalosporins are contraindicated only in patients with a history of severe reaction to penicillin.

- Consultation with an infectious disease specialist is recommended.

- Spectinomycin can be used for urogenital or rectal infection (inadequate for pharyngeal GC).

- Azithromycin 2 g PO; use caution owing to concerns over emerging resistance to macrolides.
- Consider cephalosporin treatment following desensitization.

Note: Fluoroquinolones are not recommended for treatment of gonococcal infection because of widespread resistance in the United States.

Please see full CDC STI treatment guidelines regarding treatment of PID, epididymitis, and disseminated gonococcal infection.

Treatment of Chlamydia

(See the full CDC STI treatment guidelines, referenced below.)

Recommended regimens

- Azithromycin 1 g PO in a single dose
- Doxycycline 100 mg PO BID for 7 days

Alternative regimens

- Erythromycin base 500 mg PO QID for 7 days
- Erythromycin ethylsuccinate 800 mg PO QID for 7 days
- Ofloxacin 300 mg PO BID for 7 days (see Note above)
- Levofloxacin 500 mg PO once daily for 7 days (see Note above)

Treatment of LGV

Recommended regimens

- Doxycycline 100 mg PO BID for 21 days

Alternative regimens

- Erythromycin base 500 mg PO QID for 21 days
- Azithromycin 1 g PO once weekly for 3 weeks (limited data)

For recent sex partners (within 6 days of the onset of patient's symptoms), test for urethral or cervical CT, treat with azithromycin 1 g PO in a single dose or doxycycline 100 mg PO BID for 7 days.

Treatment During Pregnancy

Use of fluoroquinolones and tetracyclines should be avoided during pregnancy.

Recommended GC regimens

- A recommended cephalosporin or azithromycin 2 g PO (see above)

Recommended CT regimens

- Azithromycin 1 g PO in a single dose
- Amoxicillin 500 mg PO TID for 7 days

Alternative CT regimens

- Erythromycin base 500 mg PO QID for 7 days
- Erythromycin base 250 mg PO QID for 14 days
- Erythromycin ethylsuccinate 800 mg PO QID for 7 days
- Erythromycin ethylsuccinate 400 mg PO QID for 14 days

Follow-up

- Evaluate the patient's sex partners; treat them empirically if they had sexual contact with the patient during the 60 days preceding the patient's onset of symptoms. (Some clinics provide empiric treatment for partners via "partner packs," or a treatment regimen that the patient takes to the partner(s); this approach does not require the partner to present for evaluation and may be effective if the partner(s) is/are unlikely to come to the clinic.)
- Most recurrent infections come from sex partners who were not treated.
- If symptoms persist, evaluate for the possibility of reinfection, treatment failure, or a different cause of symptoms. If treatment failure is suspected, perform culture and antimicrobial sensitivity testing.
- The CDC recommends rescreening male patients 3 months after treatment.

- For pregnant women with chlamydia, retest (by culture) 3 weeks after completion of treatment.

- Screen for gonorrhea, chlamydia, syphilis, and other STIs at regular intervals according to the patient's risk factors. The sites of sampling (e.g., pharynx, urethra, endocervix, anus/rectum) will be determined according to the patient's sexual exposures.

- Evaluate each patient's sexual practices with regard to the risk of acquiring STIs and of transmitting HIV; work with the patient to reduce sexual risks.

Patient Education

- Instruct patients to take all of their medications. Advise patients to take medications with food if they are nauseated and to call or return to clinic right away if they experience vomiting or are unable to take their medications.

- Sex partners from the previous 60 days need to be tested for sexually transmitted pathogens, and treated as soon as possible with a regimen effective against GC and CT, even if they have no symptoms. Advise patients to inform their partner(s) that they need to be tested and treated. Otherwise, patients may be reinfected.

- Advise patients to avoid sexual contact until the infection has been cured (at least 7 days).

- Provide education about sexual risk reduction. Instruct patients to use condoms with every sexual contact to prevent reinfection with GC or CT, to prevent other STIs, and to prevent transmission of HIV to sex partners.

References

- Abularach S, Anderson J. *Gynecologic Problems.* In: Anderson JR, ed. *A Guide to the Clinical Management of Women with HIV.* Rockville, MD: Health Resources and Services Administration, HIV/AIDS Bureau; 2005. Available at hab.hrsa.gov/publications/womencare05/. Accessed June 30, 2010.

- Centers for Disease Control and Prevention. *Gonorrhea — CDC Fact Sheet.* Available at www.cdc.gov/std/gonorrhea/. Accessed June 30, 2010.

- Centers for Disease Control and Prevention. *Increases in fluoroquinolone-resistant Neisseria gonorrhoeae among men who have sex with men — United States, 2003, and revised recommendations for gonorrhea treatment, 2004.* MMWR. 2004 Apr 30;53(16):335-8.

- Centers for Disease Control and Prevention. *Lymphogranuloma venereum among men who have sex with men — Netherlands, 2003-2004.* MMWR. 2004 Oct 29;53(42):985-8.

- Centers for Disease Control and Prevention. *Male Chlamydia Screening Consultation — Review and Guidance. May 25, 2007.* Available at www.cdc.gov/std/chlamydia/.

- Centers for Disease Control and Prevention. *Sexually Transmitted Diseases Treatment Guidelines, 2010.* MMWR 2010 Dec 17; 59 (No. RR- 12):1-110. Available at www.cdc.gov/STD/treatment/2010.

- Centers for Disease Control and Prevention. *Update of sexually transmitted diseases treatment, 2006: fluoroquinolones no longer recommended for treatment of gonococcal infections.* MMWR. 2007 Apr; 56(14):332-336.

Hepatitis B Infection

Rena Fox, MD

Background

Hepatitis B virus (HBV) is the most common cause of chronic liver disease worldwide. Chronic HBV can cause necroinflammation and over time can cause hepatic fibrosis and eventually cirrhosis, end-stage liver disease, and hepatocellular carcinoma (HCC). It is estimated that 350 million people have chronic HBV infection, with approximately 1.25 million of them in the United States. HBV is a DNA virus that is spread through exposure to infected blood and body fluids. It typically is transmitted by parenteral, sexual, and vertical exposures, but may be transmitted through person-to-person contacts among household members, especially because HBV can survive outside the body for long periods of time. Because HIV and HBV share transmission routes, up to 90% of HIV-infected patients have evidence of HBV exposure. In the United States, chronic HBV infection has been identified in 6-15% of HIV-infected persons.

HRSA HAB Core Clinical Performance Measures

Percentage of clients with HIV infection who completed the **vaccination series for hepatitis B**

(Group 2 measure)

Percentage of clients with HIV infection and hepatitis B or C who received **alcohol counseling** in the measurement year

(Group 3 measure)

The epidemiology of HBV infection varies by geographic region. In Southeast Asia and sub-Saharan Africa, HBV is highly prevalent and almost all infections occur perinatally or during early childhood. In the United States and Western Europe, most infections occur through sexual exposure or high-risk injection drug use behavior.

To identify patients with HBV coinfection, and to identify and vaccinate susceptible individuals, all HIV-infected persons should be tested for HBV (see chapters *Initial and Interim Laboratory and Other Tests* and *Immunizations for HIV-Infected Adults and Adolescents*). In addition, all patients with chronic HBV infection should be tested for HIV and all patients with evidence of prior resolved HBV infection should be strongly considered for HIV testing.

It is universally recommended that HBV vaccination should be given to all HIV-infected persons who test negative for all HBV seromarkers (see "Interpreting HBV test results," below, and chapter *Immunizations for HIV-Infected Adults and Adolescents*). If possible, it is recommended that the vaccine series be given when CD4 counts are >200 cells/μL, as doing so is associated with higher rates of vaccine response. For patients with CD4 counts of <200 cells/μL, it is recommended that they first receive antiretroviral therapy (ART) and then be vaccinated when the CD4 count rises to >200 cells/μL. HBV vaccination also is recommended for persons who test negative for HBV seromarkers but are at high risk (e.g., men who have sex with men [MSM], persons who are infected with hepatitis C virus [HCV], and persons who are in close contact with someone who has HBV infection).

The natural history of HBV infection is complex. The likelihood of developing chronic HBV after exposure varies with age, mode of infection, and immunocompromised status. Among newborns born to HBV-infected mothers, 90% develop chronic hepatitis B, whereas 30% of exposed infants and young children and <5% of exposed adults develop chronic infection. Most adults who become infected with HBV are able to clear the virus without treatment, and they subsequently become immune to HBV. Progressive HBV can lead to cirrhosis and then to decompensated liver disease including ascites, portal hypertension, esophageal varices, coagulopathy, thrombocytopenia, and hepatic encephalopathy. HCC can develop in patients with or without cirrhosis; in fact, 30-50% of HCC cases attributable to HBV occur in the absence of cirrhosis.

Factors associated with increased rates of cirrhosis include the following:

- Longer duration of infection
- HBV genotype C
- High levels of HBV DNA
- Alcohol consumption
- Smoking
- Aflatoxin exposure
- Coinfection with HIV
- Coinfection with hepatitis D virus
- Coinfection with HCV

Factors associated with increased rates of HCC include the following:

- Male gender
- Family history of HCC
- Older age
- Presence of HBV envelope antigen (HBeAg); history of reversion from anti-HBe to HBeAg
- High levels of HBV DNA
- Presence of cirrhosis
- HBV genotype C
- Core promoter mutation
- Coinfection with HCV

Among individuals who are not taking ART, HIV infection significantly modifies the natural history of HBV infection. HIV infection appears to increase the risk of developing chronic HBV infection after acute HBV, and it is associated with a higher level of HBV DNA replication and lower rates of spontaneous HBeAg seroconversion. In patients with chronic HBV, HIV coinfection is associated with faster progression of liver disease and cirrhosis and increased rates of liver-related deaths. Although HIV coinfection itself is not known to increase the risk of HCC development, it does increase the risk of cirrhosis, which in turn increases the risk of HCC.

Treatment of HIV infection with effective ART has increased the life expectancy of HIV-infected patients in recent years, and paradoxically has given HIV/HBV-coinfected patients a longer lifespan during which cirrhosis may develop. Partly for this reason, the relative proportion of deaths attributable to liver disease among HIV-infected patients is rising. On the other hand, ART can positively impact the natural history of HBV infection. Effective ART can improve patients' immune responses against HBV. ART also may be used to treat HBV in coinfected patients. Several of the nucleoside analogues (NRTIs) used against HIV also are active against HBV, and these should be included in an ART regimen to treat both HIV and HBV for coinfected persons (see "Antiviral Treatment of Chronic HBV Infection," below). Withdrawal of NRTIs with anti-HBV activity can precipitate a reactivation of HBV. ART that contains anti-HBV NRTIs also may prevent acute infections in patients who are receiving them.

S: Subjective

Persons with acute HBV infection may have symptoms including fatigue, nausea, vomiting, arthralgias, fever, right upper quadrant pain, jaundice, dark urine, and clay-colored stools. Some patients may have no symptoms at all.

Persons with chronic HBV, even with early cirrhosis, may be asymptomatic or may experience only fatigue or mild right upper quadrant tenderness. Patients with decompensated cirrhosis may experience increased abdominal girth, easy bruising, telangiectasis, pruritus, gastrointestinal bleeding, or altered mentation. Patients with early or small HCC may have no additional symptoms or may develop significant abdominal pain, weight loss, nausea, or bone pain.

Ask patients with known HBV infection about symptoms that suggest complications of HBV such as cirrhosis, decompensation, risk factors for worsening liver disease, and hepatotoxins. Questions should address the symptoms listed above, and the following:

- Fatigue
- Weight loss
- Impaired concentration
- Chronic HCV
- Alcohol intake
- Substance use
- Antiretroviral (ARV) medications that may cause hepatotoxicity (e.g., didanosine, protease inhibitors, nevirapine, maraviroc)
- Medications with potential for hepatotoxicity or accumulation in persons with liver disease (e.g., acetaminophen, benzodiazepines, opiates)

O: Objective

Measure vital signs.

Perform a physical examination to include evaluation of the following:

- Head, ears, eyes, nose, throat (HEENT): temporal wasting, icterus, gum bleeding
- Heart and lungs: signs of congestive heart failure
- Chest: gynecomastia
- Abdomen: caput medusa, venous prominence, distention, signs of ascites, hepatomegaly, splenomegaly
- Extremities: edema
- Neurologic: alertness, mental status, asterixis
- Skin: jaundice, palmar erythema, petechiae, ecchymoses, spider angiomata

P: Plan
HBV Testing

As discussed above, all HIV-infected persons should be screened for HBV surface antigen (HBsAg), HBs antibody (HBsAb), and HBV core antibody (total) (HBcAb-total) and be vaccinated if not immune (see chapter *Immunizations for HIV-Infected Adults and Adolescents*).

Nonimmune persons with elevated transaminases or signs or symptoms of acute or chronic liver disease should be retested for HBV and HCV infection.

Interpreting HBV test results

Routine baseline HBV serologic screening tests for HIV-infected individuals are outlined in Table 1.

Markers of chronic hepatitis B can manifest in a number of patterns (see Table 1).

Table 1. Interpreting HBV Laboratory Tests

	Acute Hepatitis B	Recovery from Acute Hepatitis B	Chronic HBeAg+ Disease	Chronic HBeAg- Disease	Occult Hepatitis B	Successful Vaccination	Isolated HBcAb
HBsAg	X (may clear)		X	X			
Anti-HBs		X				X	
Anti-HBc IgM	X (may be the only marker during window period)						
Anti-HBc	X	X	X	X	X		X
HBeAg	X		X		X		
Anti-HBe		X (in some cases)		X			X (in some cases)
DNA* (PCR if required)	X		X	X	X		(in rare cases may be +)

* Absence of detectable HBV DNA does not rule out chronic HBV infection in patients who are on ARVs with anti-HBV activity.

Because of the complexity of HBV diagnosis and test interpretation, it is important to test for HBsAg, HBcAb, and HBsAb. If the result for either HBsAg or HBcAb is positive, then test for HBV DNA. The presence of HBsAg for >6 months indicates chronic HBV infection, but detectable HBV DNA is required for the diagnosis. HBV DNA should be tested before initiation of ART, if possible, as NRTIs with anti-HBV activity may suppress HBV viremia and interfere with diagnosis. Some persons with HIV infection can have chronic HBV infection with high HBV DNA levels and hepatic inflammation while testing negative for HBsAg and positive only for HBcAb. This sometimes is termed "occult hepatitis B infection." Patients with chronic HBV may test either positive or negative for HBeAg. Patients with inactive chronic HBV are positive for HBsAg but have persistently normal alanine aminotransferase (ALT) levels, low-level or no detectable HBV DNA, and negative HBeAg results. Ongoing viral replication and infectiousness is indicated by the presence of HBV DNA or a positive result for HBeAg.

Markers of immunity or previous exposure to HBV also can manifest in a number of patterns (see Table 1). Successful vaccination to HBV (in someone who has never been infected) will result in positive HBsAb but negative HBcAb results. Prior exposure to HBV may result in positive HBcAb and HBsAb findings, indicating the development of immunity. However, prior exposure may present as positive HBcAb only, with negative results for HBsAb, HBsAg, and HBV DNA. This pattern shows that the patient was previously infected with hepatitis B but did not develop chronic infection, and lost the HBsAb. This sometimes is termed "isolated core Ab," and it is seen more commonly in patients coinfected with HIV or HCV. It is not known whether patients who display this pattern would have sufficient immunity to ward off another HBV infection if they were reexposed. Some experts recommend vaccinating such patients so that they do mount an HBsAb response whereas others do not believe that vaccination for these patients is necessary.

In acute HBV infection, HBV DNA will be detectable before HBsAg, if highly sensitive nucleic acid testing is used. Otherwise, HBsAg (which takes an average of 30 days to develop) is the only marker detected during the first 3-5 weeks after infection. HBcAb develops at approximately 6 weeks after infection and both immunoglobulin M (IgM) and immunoglobulin G (IgG) will be evident. The IgM will decline within 6 months but the IgG will persist for life. Among individuals who recover from acute HBV infection, HBeAg typically seroconverts to HBeAb at approximately 3 months whereas, for those who develop chronic HBV infection, HBeAg typically persists for years.

Diagnostic Evaluation of Acute HBV infection

When approaching the diagnosis of a patient with acute hepatitis B infection, the following steps should be taken:

1. Obtain history and perform physical examination.

   Determine the time and route of infection if possible. Take a complete history, including HIV disease course and treatment, and other medical history. Perform physical examination, focusing on evidence of acute liver dysfunction.

2. Assess HBV replication serially.

   As soon as acute infection is suspected, check HBsAg, HBV DNA, HBeAg, HBeAb, ALT, HBcAb-IgM, and HBsAb. Recheck each every 4 weeks to track the serologic course of infection.

3. Assess liver function serially.

   When ALT is abnormal and rising, additional tests of liver function should be serially evaluated until it is clear that ALT is trending back down. Tests should include albumin, total bilirubin, prothrombin time, and platelet count.

4. Determine whether HBV infection resolves or persists as chronic HBV infection.

   If the HBsAg is still present at 6 months after acute infection, the HBV infection has persisted and patient has chronic hepatitis B infection.

Initial Diagnostic Evaluation of Chronic HBV Infection

When approaching the diagnosis of a patient with chronic HBV infection, the following steps should be taken:

- Take a complete history, including family history of HBV or HCC, and HIV disease course and treatment. Perform physical examination.

- Assess HBV replication to determine HBV DNA level, HBeAg and HBeAb serostatus, and ALT level. Note that HBV DNA levels may be difficult to interpret in patients who are on ARVs that have anti-HBV activity (HBV may be low or undetectable because of these medications).

- Assess liver disease — check complete blood cell count with platelet count, albumin, total bilirubin, transaminases (especially ALT), and prothrombin time.

- Assess for possible overlying liver diseases (e.g., HCV, alcoholic liver disease, fatty liver disease).

- Consider liver biopsy to assess histological degree of inflammation and fibrosis, especially if the result would affect the decision to use treatment.

- Screen for HCC at baseline via ultrasound.

- Test for hepatitis A antibodies (IgG) and vaccinate against hepatitis A if not immune.

Long-Term Monitoring of Chronic HBV Infection

For patients who are not on treatment for HBV, regular monitoring of HBV replication and liver function should be performed.

For patients with the following seromarkers, recommendations are as indicated:

Negative HBeAg, low ALT, and low-level DNA (<2,000 IU/mL) (inactive HBV):

HBV DNA, HBeAg, and ALT testing should be performed every 3 months for the first year to determine whether the virus is truly inactive. If it remains inactive (with, negative HBeAg, normal ALT, and low-level DNA), monitoring can continue every 6-12 months; some specialists recommend more frequent monitoring.

Negative HBeAg, elevated ALT, and high HBV DNA (>20,000 IU/mL):

Biopsy should be considered, and treatment should be considered. If treatment is not started, monitoring should occur every 3 months.

Negative HBeAg, moderately elevated ALT, and moderately elevated DNA (2,000-20,000 IU/mL):

Follow-up should be performed every 3-6 months if treatment is not started.

Positive HBeAg, moderately elevated ALT:

Monitoring should be performed every 3 months and, if ALT is persistently elevated, a biopsy should be considered to guide the decision regarding initiation of HBV treatment.

Positive HBeAg, high HBV DNA (>20,000 IU/mL) but low-level ALT:

Monitoring should be performed every 3-6 months to check for changes in ALT. If ALT rises significantly, treatment should be considered.

Cirrhosis:

Treatment should be considered. If not treated, monitoring should be performed every 3-6 months.

Antiviral Treatment of Chronic HBV Infection

The goals and markers of HBV treatment for HIV/HBV-coinfected patients are the same as for HBV-monoinfected patients.

The goals of treatment are as follows:

- To decrease progression of liver disease
- To prevent development of cirrhosis
- To prevent development of HCC

Treatment endpoints for the HBV/HIV-coinfected population are not well defined but efficacy is determined by the following measures:

- HBeAg seroconversion to HBeAb (this is harder to achieve for coinfected patients than for HBV-monoinfected persons)
- HBV DNA suppression
- ALT normalization, which usually follows the changes in HBV DNA

The optimal duration of treatment is not clearly known; it generally is considered to be long-term, with the primary risks being the development of drug resistance and a subsequent reactivation of HBV.

The timing of treatment and choice of treatment for HBV/HIV-coinfected patients are important. Determine the patient's need for anti-HIV treatment (see chapters *Risk of HIV Progression/Indications for ART* and *Antiretroviral Therapy*).

- If treatment for HIV is indicated, HBV should be treated concurrently with the HIV by using an ART regimen that includes two NRTIs that are active against both viruses (tenofovir + emtricitabine or tenofovir + lamivudine), if possible. In this situation, liver biopsy to stage disease is not necessary because HBV treatment will be undertaken (incorporated into the HIV regimen). Note that treatment of HBV with a single NRTI is not recommended, because of the risk of HBV resistance; if tenofovir cannot be used, entecavir (plus combination ART) is the preferred alternative (see Table 2).

- If treatment for HIV is deferred, the hepatitis B should be treated if the patient otherwise meets criteria for HBV treatment (see below). ALT, HBeAg, and HBV DNA results, and possibly a liver biopsy, should be used to determine whether HBV should be treated.

  - Inactive chronic hepatitis B (HBV DNA is <2,000 IU/mL, HBeAg is negative and ALT is not elevated: the HBV can be monitored and does not require treatment.

  - HBeAg positive, ALT is more than two times the upper limit of normal (ULN), and HBV DNA >20,000 IU/mL: consider HBV treatment.

  - HBeAg negative, ALT is more than two times the ULN and HBV DNA >2,000 IU/mL: consider HBV treatment.

  - HBeAg positive, HBV DNA >20,000 IU/mL, but ALT is less than two times the ULN: can use a biopsy to determine the need for HBV treatment.

  - HBeAg negative, DNA >2,000 IU/mL, but ALT is less than two times the ULN: can use a biopsy to determine the need for HBV treatment.

  - Any patient with cirrhosis (if not decompensated) and a detectable DNA level: should be considered for HBV treatment, regardless of HBeAg status and regardless of ALT level.

- Patients with decompensated cirrhosis should not be treated for HBV but should be referred for transplant.

- Some specialists recommend HBV treatment for all patients with detectable HBV DNA, particularly if ALT is elevated or inflammation or fibrosis is seen on liver biopsy.

- If HBV treatment is indicated, HIV infection should be treated concurrently, if possible. As stated above, the recommended treatment is a potent ARV regimen that includes two dual-acting (anti-HIV and anti-HBV) drugs (i.e., tenofovir + emtricitabine or lamivudine). If tenofovir is contraindicated, entecavir or another anti-HBV drug should be used (with emtricitabine or lamivudine) to construct a two-drug therapy for HBV, and the HIV ART regimen should be designed for complete HIV suppression (see Table 2).

- If a decision is made to treat HBV but not HIV, HBV treatment should *not* include agents that are dually active, as that could lead to early HIV resistance. This limits choices to pegylated interferon alfa-2a (although it has not been studied in HBV/HIV-infected patients) or adefovir dipivoxil. Data on possible anti-HIV activity of telbivudine are conflicting but it is recommended that telbivudine not be used in this setting. Tenofovir, lamivudine, emtricitabine, and entecavir should not be used as monotherapy for HIV/HBV-coinfected patients, because HIV (and HBV) resistance may develop (see Table 2).

Table 2. Antiviral Therapies for Chronic HBV Infection

	Lamivudine	Emtricitabine	Tenofovir	Adefovir	Entecavir	Telbivudine	Pegylated Interferon
Dual activity against HBV and HIV	Yes	Yes	Yes	No (at the low HBV treatment dosage)	Yes	Uncertain	No
Recommended for use in HIV/HBV coinfection	With tenofovir, as part of fully suppressive ART	With tenofovir, as part of fully suppressive ART	With lamivudine or emtricitabine, as part of fully suppressive ART	If HIV is not being treated, or in combination with a lamivudine- or emtricitabine-containing ART regimen, if tenofovir is not used	With fully suppressive ART	With fully suppressive ART	If HIV is not being treated
Loss of HBV DNA	40-44%		76%	21%	67%	60%	25%
HBeAg seroconversion	16-21%		21%	12%	21%	22%	27–32%
Class	Nucleoside analogue	Nucleoside analogue	Nucleoside analogue	Nucleotide analogue	Nucleoside analogue	Nucleotide analogue	Interferon

Additional points about treatment for HIV/HBV-infected patients:

- When lamivudine is used as a single agent, HBV resistance develops in many patients by 1-2 years. Although combination therapy has not been well studied, specialists recommend using dual-NRTI combinations that have activity against HBV (lamivudine + tenofovir, or emtricitabine + tenofovir [Truvada]) as part of the ARV regimen, to treat HBV and to prevent HBV resistance.

- For patients infected with HCV as well as HBV and HIV, evaluate the need for HIV therapy first. If ART is not required, consider treating HCV first, because interferon therapy is active against both HCV and HBV (see chapter *Hepatitis C Infection*). Also consider consultation with an expert if optimal timing for treatment of the three infections is not clear. If interferon-based therapy for HCV has failed, consider treating chronic HBV with an oral agent.

- Some patients treated with ART may experience worsening of HBV symptoms and laboratory markers in the weeks after ART initiation, because of immune reconstitution inflammatory reactions. Hepatic decompensation owing to immune reconstitution must be distinguished from other causes, such as medication toxicity, or other infection. Liver function tests should be monitored closely for patients starting ART.

- Some ARV medications are hepatotoxic and should be avoided or used cautiously. These include nevirapine, tipranavir, and high-dose ritonavir. Numerous other medications (e.g., fluconazole, isoniazid) are hepatotoxic and can pose problems for patients with impaired liver function.

- Discontinuation of HBV medications in patients with HIV/HBV coinfection may cause a flare of liver disease. Be very cautious when discontinuing HBV-active medications from an anti-HIV ART regimen. If the HBV DNA is suppressed, options include continuing the HBV-active ARVs, even if there is HIV resistance (modify the ART regimen for maximal HIV suppression) or substituting other HBV-active medications to avoid rebound liver inflammation and decompensation. For example, if it is decided to discontinue lamivudine/tenofovir-containing ART in an HIV/HBV-coinfected patient on ART, consider starting adefovir or interferon to maintain activity against HBV. If HBV therapy is discontinued and a flare occurs, consider reinstating HBV therapy as soon as possible.

Screening for HCC in patients with chronic HBV infection

Persons with chronic HBV are at increased risk of developing HCC. Note that HCC may occur even in the absence of cirrhosis. HCC screening should be performed every 6-12 months using ultrasound (computed tomography [CT] is an alternative); alpha-fetoprotein should be monitored if ultrasound reliability is low.

HBV-infected patients who should be screened for HCC include the following:

- Anyone with cirrhosis
- Anyone over age 40 with elevated ALT or HBV DNA >2,000 copies/mL
- Asian men aged >40
- Asian women aged >50
- Persons of African descent aged >20
- Anyone with a family history of HCC

Interventions to slow progression and prevent complications

Persons with HCV infection should be counseled to avoid exposure to hepatotoxins, including alcohol and hepatotoxic medications (e.g., acetaminophen in large doses, fluconazole, isoniazid). Heavy alcohol use is a risk factor for increasing rate of fibrosis. It is not clear what degree of alcohol consumption is safe, so many experts recommend complete abstinence from alcohol.

- No specific dietary measures are recommended.
- Patients who are not already immune to hepatitis A should be vaccinated against hepatitis A.
- Patients should be counseled on ways to avoid infection with hepatitis C.

Preventing transmission

All patients with HBV infection should receive individualized counseling on ways to reduce the risk of HBV transmission (including by sexual or needle-sharing behavior, perinatal routes, or household exposure), as appropriate.

Household members and sexual contacts should be vaccinated against HBV.

Women who are pregnant or considering pregnancy should consult with a specialist in both HBV and HIV to discuss ways of decreasing the infection risk for the fetus; this may include treatment for HBV and HIV. Infants born to coinfected women should receive HBV immune globulin and start the

HBV vaccine series within 12 hours after birth (with subsequent vaccine doses per usual protocol).

Patient Education

- Advise patients that most people with HBV will remain asymptomatic for several years. However, ongoing injury to the liver occurs during this time and can culminate in liver failure. Patients can slow the damage by avoiding alcohol and any medications (including over-the-counter drugs and recreational drugs) that may damage the liver. Patients should contact their pharmacist or health care provider if they have questions about a specific medication or supplement.

- As with HIV, patients must avoid passing HBV to others. Instruct patients not to share toothbrushes, dental appliances, razors, sex toys, tattoo equipment, injection equipment, or personal care items that may have blood on them. Emphasize to patients the importance of safer sex to protect themselves and their partners.

- Tell patients to discuss HBV with their sex partners, and suggest that partners be tested for HBV.

- Nonimmune sex partners and individuals in close contact with persons with chronic hepatitis B (e.g., family and household members) should be vaccinated.

- Pregnant women have a high risk of transmitting HIV or HBV to the fetus because each virus makes it easier to transmit the other. Women who are pregnant or considering pregnancy should talk with a specialist in HIV and HBV to discuss ways of decreasing the infection risk for the fetus.

- Advise patients who are on treatment for HBV that abrupt discontinuation of HBV treatment can cause a flare of HBV; they should not stop treatment without medical supervision.

- Certain ARV drugs are more likely than others to cause hepatotoxicity. Advise patients that their liver function should be monitored carefully if they start an ARV regimen, in order to determine whether the body is able to process the medicines.

References

- Benhamou Y. *Hepatitis B in the HIV-coinfected patient.* J Acquir Immune Defic Syndr. 2007 Jul 1;45 Suppl 2:S57-65; discussion S66-7.

- Centers for Disease Control and Prevention. *Guidelines for Prevention and Treatment of Opportunistic Infections in HIV-Infected Adults and Adolescents: Recommendations from CDC, the National Institutes of Health, and the HIV Medicine Association of the Infectious Diseases Society of America.* April 10, 2009. Available at www.aidsinfo.nih.gov/guidelines/.

- Lok A, McMahon B. *Chronic hepatitis B: update 2009.* Hepatology. 2009 Sep;50(3):661-2.

- U.S. Department of Health and Human Services. *Guidelines for the Use of Antiretroviral Agents in HIV-1-Infected Adults and Adolescents.* January 10, 2011. Available at www.aidsinfo.nih.gov/guidelines/.

- Weinbaum CM, Williams I, Mast EE, et al.; Centers for Disease Control and Prevention. *Recommendations for identification and public health management of persons with chronic hepatitis B virus infection.* MMWR Recomm Rep. 2008 Sep 19;57(RR-8):1-20.

Hepatitis C Infection

Rena Fox, MD

Background

Liver disease owing to hepatitis C virus (HCV) infection has become a leading cause of death among HIV-infected patients, as the widespread availability of antiretroviral therapy (ART) has led to a decrease in AIDS-related causes of death. HCV is common among patients with HIV infection in the United States. It is estimated that 30-40% of the HIV-infected population in the United States is coinfected with HCV, but the prevalence varies with risk factor for transmission. Among HIV-infected injection drug users and hemophiliacs in the United States, 70-95% may be coinfected with HCV; among HIV-infected men who have sex with men, 1-12% are coinfected with HCV.

> ### HRSA HAB Core Clinical Performance Measures
>
> Percentage of clients for whom **hepatitis C screening** was performed at least once since the diagnosis of HIV infection
>
> *(Group 2 measure)*
>
> Percentage of clients with HIV infection and hepatitis B or C who received **alcohol counseling** in the measurement year
>
> *(Group 3 measure)*

HCV is a single-stranded RNA virus that is transmitted primarily through blood exposure and, less commonly, through sexual or vertical transmission. HCV/HIV coinfection is common because of these shared risk factors. However, HCV is more likely than HIV to be transmitted via a bloodborne route; there is an approximately 10-fold greater risk of HCV transmission after needlestick exposure compared with the risk of HIV transmission, and the concentrations of HCV in a given volume of blood are greater than those of HIV. Women who are coinfected with HIV and HCV have a higher risk of transmitting HIV to their infants than do women with HIV infection alone. Coinfected women also are more likely than HCV-monoinfected women to pass HCV to their infants. Approximately 20% of babies born to HIV/HCV-coinfected mothers acquire HCV, compared with 5-6% of infants born to HCV-infected women without HIV. Breast-feeding is not known to transmit HCV, although HIV-infected women are advised against breast-feeding because of the risk of transmitting HIV.

Coinfection with HIV adversely impacts the natural history of HCV infection. HIV/HCV-coinfected patients have lower rates of spontaneous HCV clearance, increased HCV viral loads, decreased rates of successful virologic response to HCV treatments, faster progression to cirrhosis, and increased risk of developing liver decompensation, end-stage liver disease, and hepatocellular carcinoma (HCC). HCV coinfection does not appear to increase HIV- and AIDS-related complications or decrease rates of successful HIV antiretroviral (ARV) treatment.

Acute HCV Infection

Acute infection can be symptomatic and severe but rarely is fulminant. Patients who do present with onset of jaundice, weakness, anorexia, abdominal pain, or malaise without a known cause should be tested for acute HCV infection. Symptoms usually subside after several weeks. Patients who present after a potential exposure, such as a needlestick injury, should be tested for acute infection whether or not they are symptomatic. Overall, approximately 25% of patients acutely infected with HCV will clear the virus spontaneously, but there are few prospective studies on the natural history of acute HCV infection with preexisting HIV infection. Because it is difficult to establish the precise timing of HCV infection, prospective natural history studies are difficult to perform.

Chronic HCV Infection

For the majority of HCV patients, other than laboratory abnormalities, there are no clinical manifestations of infection until the development of cirrhosis. Cirrhosis develops in approximately 20% of HCV-monoinfected patients, usually 20 years or more from the time of infection. More than 20% of HIV/HCV-coinfected patients are thought to develop cirrhosis, and at a faster rate. Once patients have developed cirrhosis, approximately 50% will decompensate within the first 5 years. Typically, the first sign of decompensation is the development of ascites. Of patients with cirrhosis, approximately 1-4% per year will develop HCC, or approximately 20% of cirrhotic patients in total. The median survival time from the onset of HCC is approximately 5 months and, the 1-year survival rate is 29%.

S: Subjective

Patients with HCV infection, whether acute or chronic, often have no symptoms, and the infection is discovered via screening tests or on workup of an abnormal liver test result.

Patients with acute HCV infection typically are asymptomatic but may present with symptoms such as jaundice, abdominal pain, and malaise. If symptoms from acute infection develop, they usually do so within 4 weeks after infection has occurred. Most patients with chronic HCV cannot recall a time when they were acutely symptomatic, and HCV is detected because of an incidental finding of abnormal transaminases or through a screening test.

Ask patients with known HCV infection about symptoms that suggest complications of HCV, such as cirrhosis, decompensation, risk factors for worsening liver disease, and hepatotoxins, and about drugs whose metabolism may be affected by liver disease.

- Fatigue
- Weight loss
- Impaired concentration
- Chronic hepatitis B
- Alcohol intake
- Substance use
- ARVs that may cause hepatotoxicity (didanosine, protease inhibitors, nevirapine, maraviroc)
- Medications with potential for hepatotoxity, or accumulation in persons with liver disease (e.g., acetaminophen, benzodiazepines, opiates)

O: Objective

Measure vital signs. Calculate body mass index (see chapter *Initial Physical Examination*).

Perform physical examination to include evaluation of the following:

- Head, eyes, ears, nose, and throat (HEENT): temporal wasting, icterus
- Heart and lungs: signs of congestive heart failure
- Chest: gynecomastia
- Abdomen: caput medusa, venous prominence, distension, signs of ascites, hepatomegaly, splenomegaly
- Extremities: edema
- Neurologic: alertness, mental status, asterixis
- Skin: jaundice, palmar erythema, petechiae, ecchymoses, spider angiomata

P: Plan

Diagnostic Evaluation

Acute HCV infection

After initial exposure, HCV RNA can be detected in blood within 1-3 weeks and is present at the onset of symptoms. Antibodies to HCV can be detected in only 50-70% of patients at the onset of symptoms, but in >90% after 3 months. Within an average of 4-12 weeks, liver cell injury is manifested by elevation of serum alanine aminotransferase (ALT). It is important to understand the timeline of these diagnostic tests in order to appropriately diagnose acute infection and follow for potential resolution versus persistent infection.

In patients with suspected acute HCV infection, check HCV antibody (IgG), HCV RNA, and ALT immediately and then weekly until the ALT has begun to decline and HCV antibody has seroconverted to positive status. The seroconversion of HCV antibody establishes the diagnosis of acute infection. At that point, check the HCV RNA every 2-4 weeks for the following 3 months. If HCV RNA is still present at 3 months, strongly consider starting treatment for acute HCV promptly. If treatment is not initiated and RNA is still present at 6 months after infection, the likelihood of spontaneous clearance is extremely low, and the patient is diagnosed with chronic infection.

Chronic HCV infection

HCV antibodies

All HIV-infected patients should be tested for HCV infection with the HCV antibody test. Patients with risk factors for HCV infection should be retested at regular intervals. In HIV-infected patients, the HCV antibody test result sometimes is falsely negative; therefore, if HCV infection is suspected (e.g., because of a history of high-risk behavior, unexplained elevated ALT, or evidence of cirrhosis), the HCV RNA should be tested even if the HCV antibody test result is negative. A false-negative HCV RNA result is very unlikely in chronic infection.

HCV RNA

All patients who test positive for HCV antibody should have HCV RNA testing performed. As noted above, if patients have negative results on HCV antibody tests but persistently abnormal transaminases or suspected acute or chronic infection, HCV RNA testing should be performed.

The definition of chronic HCV infection is the presence of HCV RNA 6 months after the estimated time of infection. If a patient is HCV antibody positive but HCV RNA negative, the patient has cleared the HCV and does not have chronic HCV infection.

There are quantitative RNA tests and qualitative RNA tests. Although both types of RNA tests are highly sensitive and specific, the qualitative tests can detect lower levels of viremia than the quantitative tests. The choice of RNA test can be important.

The quantitative RNA tests will be reported as a value, with a measured number of international units per milliliter (IU/mL). Quantitative tests are useful for determining the prognosis of HCV treatment and then monitoring while on HCV treatment. Qualitative RNA tests will be reported as a present or absent value, but without a numerical value. They are useful for serial testing during suspected acute infection and for determining whether spontaneous viral clearance has occurred, a sustained virological response has occurred during treatment, or a relapse has occurred after treatment.

Genotyping

The HCV genotype is the strongest predictor of response to HCV treatment and also is a critical determinant of the dosage and duration of treatment. HCV genotyping should be performed once for all patients with detectable HCV RNA; it does not need to be repeated.

Alanine aminotransferase

Monitoring of ALT can be useful to assess acute infection, chronic liver inflammation, and response to HCV treatment. However, ALT does not always correlate with the degree of fibrosis and in addition, ALT can be persistently normal in 25% of HCV patients, including patients with cirrhosis or advanced liver disease. Small fluctuations in ALT usually are not clinically significant in HCV, though trends can be significant during or following HCV treatment.

Additional tests

Check complete blood cell count with platelet count, albumin, total bilirubin, and prothrombin time.

Test all patients for hepatitis B (HBsAg, anti-HBsAb, and anti-HBcAb). For those with a positive HBsAg or a positive anti-HBcAb result (absent anti-HBsAb), test for active HBV infection (HBV DNA and HBeAg) (see chapter *Hepatitis B Infection*). Patients with a negative HBsAg and negative anti-HBsAb result should be vaccinated against HBV.

Test for hepatitis A virus (HAV) antibodies (total). All patients with a negative HAV antibody result should be vaccinated against HAV.

Imaging

Ultrasonography can be performed to screen for cirrhosis or focal hepatic masses. Computed tomography (CT), magnetic resonance imaging (MRI), and single-photon emission computed tomography (SPECT) are more expensive and generally are reserved for further evaluation of liver masses detected by ultrasound.

Liver biopsy

Liver biopsy is used to define the degree of inflammation (the grade) and degree of fibrosis (the stage) to determine the need for HCV treatment. Unless there is clear evidence of cirrhosis, laboratory tests and radiology studies are unable to quantitate the degree of fibrosis in the liver. Liver biopsy carries some risk, primarily from bleeding (the risk of significant bleeding or fatality is approximately 1/10,000). Patients with severe thrombocytopenia or coagulopathy should not undergo liver biopsy. Fibrosis is scored from 0 to 4, with 0 indicating no fibrosis and 4 indicating cirrhosis.

Biopsy can be useful in making management decisions for some HCV patients, for example when determining whether to treat a patient, particularly those with genotype 1 virus (see below). If the biopsy reveals only mild-to-moderate fibrosis, it may be preferable to defer treatment and monitor the patient. Conversely, if the biopsy reveals more advanced fibrosis, treatment should be considered more urgently. With genotype 2 or 3 patients, some providers consider biopsy to be unnecessary because treatment outcomes are sufficiently high that findings from a biopsy would not necessarily change the management strategy. For HIV/HCV-coinfected patients, a biopsy may be particularly useful in determining the stage of disease and in planning whether or when to initiate HCV treatment, as the course of liver disease may accelerate. Overall, deciding whether to conduct a biopsy largely is a matter of individual choice. It is not a requirement for treatment of any patient, but may be useful for helping the provider and patient make a decision about whether or when to undergo treatment.

Treatment

Treatment of acute HCV

The presence of HIV infection is not a contraindication to treatment of acute HCV infection. With HIV/HCV-coinfected patients, as with HCV-monoinfected patients, early treatment of acute HCV infection yields a much higher rate of sustained virological response (SVR) than does treatment of chronic HCV infection. In three prospective trials of treatment for acute HCV in HIV-coinfected patients, using pegylated interferon (PEG-IFN) alpha-2a and ribavirin for 24 or 48 weeks, the SVR for genotype 1 HCV was 55-75%, compared with 100% for genotype 3. By contrast, in the largest study of in chronic HCV treatment in HIV-coinfected patients (n = 868), the SVR was about 29% for genotype 1 and 62% for genotype 2 or 3.

As mentioned above, RNA should be tested repeatedly for 12 weeks from the time of infection to ascertain whether spontaneous clearance will occur. If RNA is still present at 12 weeks, treatment should be strongly considered.

Treatment of chronic HCV

HIV coinfection is a strong indication for treatment of chronic HCV infection, because the risk of accelerated fibrosis and cirrhosis is higher for coinfected patients. Treatment of chronic HCV infection in HIV/HCV-coinfected patients has lower rates of SVR than treatment in monoinfected patients (see below), but HIV-coinfected patients should be strongly considered for HCV treatment. HIV-infected patients with low CD4 cell counts should not be excluded from HCV treatment on the basis of CD4 count alone; this is particularly true for patients already on ART. For timing of HCV treatment, see "Timing of HCV treatment and HIV treatment," below.

Patients with a high risk of progression to cirrhosis, including coinfected patients, should receive higher priority for treatment. For patients with minimal fibrosis, especially those with genotype 1 virus, treatment can be deferred. Patients who have developed cirrhosis but remain compensated should be

treated as soon as possible if they are otherwise candidates. Patients with decompensated liver disease should not receive HCV treatment (risks outweigh benefits); appropriate candidates can be considered for liver transplantation.

The most effective treatment for HCV in patients with or without HIV is combination therapy with pegylated interferon-alfa (PEG-IFN) plus ribavirin. Among HIV-uninfected patients, approximately 45% with genotype 1 achieve HCV viral clearance using this combination. HCV/HIV-coinfected patients have much lower rates of response, from 14-44%, varying by genotype, duration of treatment, and dosage. Several novel drugs, including HCV-specific protease inhibitors, are being investigated as adjuncts to standard therapy.

Data suggest that early virologic response (EVR), defined as a $\geq 2 \log_{10}$ decrease in HCV viral load 12 weeks into treatment, predicts SVR; treatment may be stopped if patients do not demonstrate EVR. The recommended duration of treatment in patients with HCV genotype 1 and EVR is 48 weeks. For genotype 2 or 3, the optimal duration of treatment is not clear; some guidelines state that treatment can be limited to 24 weeks, whereas others recommend 48 weeks of treatment for any HIV/HCV-coinfected patient.

Adverse effects of treatment

HCV therapy may cause significant adverse effects. IFN reduces total white blood cell counts, and can cause neutropenia. It also decreases CD4 cell counts, although the CD4 percentage usually does not change. IFN can reduce HIV RNA somewhat (by approximately $0.5 \log_{10}$ copies/mL). IFN also may produce flulike symptoms, depression, peripheral neuropathy, and other symptoms. Ribavirin can cause anemia and other adverse effects. Zidovudine and didanosine should be avoided, if possible, with patients taking ribavirin, because of the risk of compounded toxicities (anemia with zidovudine, neuropathy, lactic acidosis, liver toxicity, and pancreatitis with didanosine).

HCV treatment should not be given during pregnancy, and women receiving HCV treatment should avoid pregnancy. IFN may cause fetal growth abnormalities, and it is abortifacient in animals. Ribavirin is teratogenic, and both women and men must use contraception consistently during treatment with ribavirin and for 6 months after discontinuation of treatment.

Timing of HCV treatment and HIV treatment

The decision of whether and when to treat HCV among people infected with HIV must be determined individually. When coinfected patients require treatment for both infections, some experts begin with HIV treatment in hope that improved CD4 cell counts will enhance the response to HCV therapy, even though CD4 counts by themselves are not firmly associated with increased likelihood of an SVR. With patients who are not considered to require ART (e.g., because their CD4 counts are very high), many experts recommend treating HCV first, with ART delayed until after completion of HCV treatment. This strategy is intended to simplify treatment and improve the tolerability of both therapies. Patients already on ART generally should remain on ART throughout HCV treatment. Consult with an HCV treatment expert to determine the appropriateness and timing of HCV treatment.

Some patients with HCV will experience worsening of hepatic function during ART, and liver function tests should be monitored closely. Some ARV medications are hepatotoxic and should be avoided or used cautiously; these include nevirapine, tipranavir, and high-dose ritonavir. Numerous other medications (e.g., fluconazole and isoniazid) are hepatotoxic and can pose problems for patients with impaired liver function.

Other Care Issues

Acute HAV or HBV infection in persons with chronic HCV can cause fulminant liver disease. All patients with HCV infection should be tested for immunity to HAV and HBV; patients who are not immune should be vaccinated.

Persons with HCV infection should be counseled to avoid exposure to hepatotoxins, including alcohol and hepatotoxic medications (e.g., acetaminophen in large doses, fluconazole, and isoniazid).

As appropriate, all persons with hepatitis C should receive individualized counseling on ways to reduce the risk of HCV transmission to others (including by unprotected sex, sharing of injection drug equipment, other blood exposures (e.g., from sharing razors or tattoo equipment), and via perinatal exposure).

Patient Education

- Advise patients that most people with HCV will remain asymptomatic for several years. However, ongoing injury to the liver occurs during this time and can culminate in liver failure. Patients can slow the damage by avoiding alcohol and any medications (including over-the-counter drugs and recreational drugs) that may damage the liver. Patients should contact their pharmacist or health care provider if they have questions about a specific medication or supplement.

- As with HIV, patients must avoid passing HCV to others. Instruct patients not to share toothbrushes, dental appliances, razors, sex toys, tattoo equipment, injection equipment, or personal care items that may have blood on them. Emphasize the importance of safer sex to protect themselves and their partners.

- Tell patients to discuss HCV with their sex partners, and suggest that partners be tested for HCV.

- Pregnant women have a high risk of transmitting HIV or HCV infection to the fetus because each virus makes it easier to transmit the other. Women who are pregnant or considering pregnancy should talk with a specialist in HIV and HCV to discuss ways to decrease the infection risk for the fetus.

- HCV medications (ribavirin and interferon) should not be given during pregnancy. Both men and women who are taking ribavirin should use contraception consistently during ribavirin therapy and for 6 months after completion of treatment.

- For children who are born after their mothers were infected with HCV, consider having them tested as well. Even though their risk is low, they should be screened for HCV.

- Certain ARV drugs are more likely to cause problems with the liver because of HCV. Advise patients that their liver function should be watched carefully if they start an ARV regimen in order to determine whether the body is able to process the medicines.

- HAV can cause severe illness, liver damage, or even death in people with HCV. Patients who are not immune to HAV need to receive two vaccinations 6 months apart.

- HBV also can worsen liver function greatly if it is acquired in addition to HCV. Patients who are not immune to HBV should complete the vaccine series, which consists of three shots. If patients have been vaccinated in the past, they should have the anti-HBV titer checked to make sure that they are protected.

- Patients who are not immune to HBV should use safer sex (latex barriers) to avoid exposure. Patients who use injection drugs should not share needles or injection equipment.

- HCV-infected patients who use injection drugs should consider entering a treatment program. Quitting drug use will reduce strain on the liver, protect against other bloodborne illnesses that can affect the liver, and help prevent transmission of HCV to others. Patients who are not ready to stop injection drug use should let their providers know so that they can try to find a source for clean, single-use needles.

- HCV is not spread by coughing, sneezing, hugging, sharing food and water, or other casual contact.

- The HCV treatments interferon-alfa and ribavirin can cause flulike symptoms, body aches, fevers, anemia, neuropathy, and depression. Most of these adverse effects are treatable with medications. Patients should contact their medical provider right away if they experience depression. Antidepressant medications can help to relieve depression, but they take a couple of weeks to become effective.

References

- Carrat F, Bani-Sadr F, Pol S, et al., ANRS HCO2 RIBAVIC Study Team. *Pegylated interferon alfa-2b vs standard interferon alfa-2b, plus ribavirin, for chronic hepatitis C in HIV-infected patients: a randomized controlled trial.* JAMA. 2004 Dec 15;292(23):2909-13.

- Centers for Disease Control and Prevention. *Guidelines for Prevention and Treatment of Opportunistic Infections in HIV-Infected Adults and Adolescents: Recommendations from CDC, the National Institutes of Health, and the HIV Medicine Association of the Infectious Diseases Society of America.* April 10, 2009. Available at www.aidsinfo.nih.gov/guidelines/.

- Chung RT, Andersen J, Volberding P, et al. *Peginterferon Alfa-2a plus ribavirin versus interferon alfa-2a plus ribavirin for chronic hepatitis C in HIV-coinfected persons.* N Engl J Med. 2004 Jul 29;351(5):451-9.

Section 6: Comorbidities, Coinfections, and Complications

- Dominguez S, Ghosn J, Valantin MA, et al. *Efficacy of early treatment of acute hepatitis C infection with pegylated interferon and ribavirin in HIV-infected patients.* AIDS. 2006 May 12;20(8):1157-61.

- Fried MW. *Advances in therapy for chronic hepatitis C.* Clin Liver Dis. 2001 Nov;5(4):1009-23.

- Gonzalez SA, Talal AH. *Hepatitis C virus in human immunodeficiency virus-infected individuals: an emerging comorbidity with significant implications.* Semin Liver Dis. 2003 May;23(2):149-66.

- Heller B, Rehermann T. *Acute hepatitis C: a multifaceted disease.* Semin Liver Dis. 2005 Feb;25(1):7-17.

- Jaeckel E, Cornberg M, Wedemeyer H, et al. *Treatment of acute hepatitis C with interferon alfa-2b.* N Engl J Med. 2001 Nov 15;345(20):1452-7.

- National Institutes of Health. *NIH Consensus Development Conference Statement: Management of Hepatitis C: 2002.* Available at consensus.nih.gov/2002/2002H epatitisC2002116html.htm. Accessed June 30, 2010.

- Sulkowski MS, Thomas DL, Chaisson RE, et al. *Hepatotoxicity associated with antiretroviral therapy in adults infected with human immunodeficiency virus and the role of hepatitis C or B virus infection.* JAMA. 2000 Jan 5;283(1):74-80.

- Talal AH, Shata MT, Markatou M, et al. *Virus dynamics and immune responses during treatment in patients coinfected with hepatitis C and HIV.* J Acquir Immune Defic Syndr. 2004 Feb 1;35(2):103-13.

- Torriani FJ, Rodriguez Torres M, Rockstroh JK, et al. *Peginterferon alfa-2a plus ribavirin for chronic hepatitis C virus infection in HIV-infected patients.* N Engl J Med. 2004 Jul 29;351(5):438-50.

- van de Laar T, Pybus O, Bruisten S, et al. *Evidence of a large, international network of HCV transmission in HIV-positive men who have sex with men.* Gastroenterology. 2009 May;136(5):1609-17.

- Zeremski M, Talal AH. *Noninvasive markers of hepatic fibrosis: are they ready for prime time in the management of HIV/HCV co-infected patients?* J Hepatol. 2005 Jul;43(1):2-5.

Herpes Simplex, Mucocutaneous

Background

Herpes simplex virus (HSV) types 1 and 2 cause both primary and recurrent oral and genital disease. HSV usually appears as a vesicular eruption of the mucous membranes of the oral or perioral area, vulva, perianal skin, rectum, and occasionally the inguinal or buttock areas. The eruption develops into tender or painful ulcerated lesions that frequently are covered with a clear yellow crust. In some patients, however, the typical painful vesicular or ulcerative lesions may be absent. Persons with HIV disease and low CD4 cell counts have more frequent recurrences of HSV and more extensive ulcerations than do HIV-uninfected people. Persistent HSV eruption (lasting >1 month) is an AIDS-indicator diagnosis.

S: Subjective

The patient may complain of eruption of red, painful vesicles or ulcers ("fever blisters") with or without an exudate in the mouth, on the lips (and occasionally in nares), on the genitals, or in the perianal area. The patient may complain of burning, tingling, or itching before eruption of the lesions.

The vesicles will rupture and ulcerate, generally crusting over and healing in approximately 7-14 days. The lesions may be pruritic and are often painful. As immunosuppression progresses, the lesions may recur more frequently, grow larger or coalesce, and become chronic and nonhealing.

Perform a history, asking the patient about the symptoms described above, duration, associated symptoms, and history of HSV or similar infection.

O: Objective

Look for grouped vesicular or ulcerative lesions on an erythematous base on the mouth, anus, or external genitals, or ones that are visible on speculum or anoscopic examination. When immunosuppression is severe, lesions may coalesce into large, painful, and nonhealing ulcerations that spread to the skin of the thighs, lips, face, or perirectal region. These chronic erosive lesions may be confused with a chronic bacterial infection or decubitus ulcer, and should prompt consideration of acyclovir-resistant HSV infection. Recurrent lesions may start atypically, first appearing as a fissure, pustule, or abrasion.

A: Assessment

A partial differential diagnosis includes the following:

- Oral aphthous ulcers
- Chancroid
- Syphilis
- Cytomegalovirus
- Candidiasis
- Drug-related eruption

P: Plan

Diagnostic Evaluation

A clinical diagnosis of HSV often can be made on the basis of the patient's symptoms and clinical appearance, but symptoms and signs may be variable. Also, HSV-1 (rather than HSV-2) is increasingly the cause of initial episodes of anogenital herpes. For these reasons, current guidelines recommend laboratory testing to establish the diagnosis of HSV and to determine its type.

For cell culture or polymerase chain reaction (PCR), obtain a specimen from a freshly opened vesicle or the base of an ulcer for culture confirmation. Note that lesions that are >72 hours old or are beginning to resolve may not show HSV in culture.

PCR is more sensitive for detection of herpes DNA in ulcerative lesions, but is more expensive to perform and is less widely available than viral culture. If virologic test results are positive, typing should be performed to determine the type of HSV. Negative results do not rule out the possibility of HSV infection.

If cultures are negative and there is a high suspicion of HSV infection, skin may be taken from the edge of an ulcer for biopsy. Biopsy material also may be cultured. Tzanck smears are not sensitive or specific.

Type-specific serologic tests may be useful in the evaluation of patients in whom a diagnosis of genital HSV is not clear. Current guidelines also recommend that serologic testing be considered for HIV-infected individuals, for MSM, and for those who present for STI evaluation. Glycoprotein G (gG)-based serologic assays are recommended, as older assays do not reliably differentiate HSV-1 antibody from HSV-2 antibody.

Strongly consider checking for syphilis with a rapid plasma regain (RPR) or Venereal Disease Research Laboratory (VDRL) test in any patient who presents with genital, anal, or oral ulceration.

Treatment

Empiric treatment for suspicious lesions often is initiated in the absence of laboratory confirmation. In some instances, treatment can be started empirically and, if no response is seen within 7-10 days, laboratory studies can be undertaken.

Episodic outbreak

- Acyclovir 400 mg PO TID
- Valacyclovir 1,000 mg PO BID
- Famciclovir 500 mg PO BID

Note: Dosage must be adjusted for patients with renal impairment.

Duration of treatment: 5-10 days. Short-course therapy (1-3 days) usually is not recommended for persons with HIV infection.

Symptomatic treatment helps the healing of lesions but does not prevent recurrences. Large, extensive ulcers may need to be treated for a longer period of time.

Severe disease

Treat initially with acyclovir 5 mg/kg IV Q8H (10 mg/kg for encephalitis).

Acyclovir-resistant HSV

The diagnosis of acyclovir-resistant HSV should be suspected if lesions fail to respond to 7-10 days of standard therapy and should be confirmed with culture and sensitivities. Cross-resistance to valacyclovir and ganciclovir will be present, and cross-resistance to famciclovir is likely. The usual alternative treatment is foscarnet (40 mg/kg IV Q8H); other possibilities include IV cidofovir, topical imiquimod, and topical cidofovir. An HIV specialist should be consulted.

Chronic suppressive therapy

Consider suppressive therapy with acyclovir (400 mg PO BID), famciclovir (500 mg PO BID), or valacyclovir (500 mg PO BID) for patients with frequent or severe recurrences and those with HSV-2. Acyclovir dosage may need to be increased to 800 mg BID or TID for individuals whose HSV episodes are not adequately suppressed by 400 mg BID. Treatment may be continued indefinitely. Note that suppressive therapy also reduces the risk of transmission of HSV. Effective antiretroviral therapy (ART) also may reduce the frequency of HSV outbreaks.

HSV During Pregnancy

Acyclovir appears to be safe and effective for use by pregnant women and remains the drug of choice. Few data are available on the use of valacyclovir and famciclovir during pregnancy.

It is important to avoid peripartum transmission of HSV. For women with recurrent or new genital HSV late in pregnancy, obstetric or infectious disease specialists should be consulted. All women should be evaluated carefully for symptoms and signs of genital HSV.

Patient Education

- Patients should be told that HSV has no cure, and outbreaks may occur at intervals for the rest of their lives.

- HSV is spread easily through kissing (if mouth or lips are infected) and sexual contact (oral, anal, or vaginal). HSV can be transmitted when no lesions are present, so it is important that patients inform their sex partners of their herpes infection before sexual activity. Patients must avoid all sexual contact when lesions are visible, because a high volume of virus is present at those times. Condom use at each sexual encounter offers the best chance of preventing HSV transmission. If HSV is transmitted, sex partners also will have it for life.

- Instruct patients to avoid use of occlusive dressings or ointments, which can prevent healing of sores.

- Treatment is most effective when taken early in the outbreak, so patients not taking suppressive therapy should keep medication on hand and start treatment at the first signs of eruption.

- Genital HSV in a pregnant woman around the time of delivery can cause severe illness in the newborn. Women should inform their obstetrician and pediatrician if they have a history of HSV or are exposed to or infected with HSV during pregnancy. Pregnant women who do not have HSV should avoid having sex with partners who have HSV, and men who have HSV should avoid having sex with pregnant women who do not have HSV.

References

- Centers for Disease Control and Prevention. *Guidelines for Prevention and Treatment of Opportunistic Infections in HIV-Infected Adults and Adolescents: Recommendations from CDC, the National Institutes of Health, and the HIV Medicine Association of the Infectious Diseases Society of America.* April 10, 2009. Available at www.aidsinfo.nih.gov/guidelines/.

- Centers for Disease Control and Prevention. *Sexually Transmitted Diseases Treatment Guidelines,* 2010. MMWR 2010 Dec 17; 59 (No. RR- 12):1-110. Available at www.cdc.gov/STD/treatment/2010.

- Cernik C, Gallina K, Brodell RT. *The treatment of herpes simplex infections: an evidence-based review.* Arch Intern Med. 2008 Jun 9;168(11):1137-44.

- Lingappa JR, Celum C. *Clinical and therapeutic issues for herpes simplex virus-2 and HIV co-infection.* Drugs. 2007;67(2):155-74.

- Strick LB, Wald A, Celum C. *Management of herpes simplex virus type 2 infection in HIV type 1-infected persons.* Clin Infect Dis. 2006 Aug 1;43(3):347-56.

- Wald A, Langenberg AG, Krantz E, et al. *The relationship between condom use and herpes simplex virus acquisition.* Ann Intern Med. 2005 Nov 15;143(10):707-13.

Herpes Zoster/Shingles

Background

Shingles is a skin or mucosal infection caused by the varicella-zoster virus (VZV) that occurs along a dermatome and represents a reactivation of varicella (chickenpox). Zoster is common in patients with HIV infection, including apparently healthy individuals before the onset of other HIV-related symptoms. The incidence may be higher among patients with low CD4 cell counts and during the four months after initiating potent antiretroviral therapy.

Zoster may be particularly painful or necrotic in HIV-infected individuals. Disseminated infection, defined as outbreaks with >20 vesicles outside the primary and immediately adjacent dermatomes, usually involves the skin and the visceral organs. Neurologic complications of zoster include encephalitis, aseptic meningitis, cranial nerve palsies, optic neuritis, transverse myelitis, and vasculitic stroke.

S: Subjective

The patient complains of painful skin blisters or ulcerations along one side of the face or body. Loss of vision may accompany the appearance of facial lesions. Pain in a dermatomal distribution may precede the appearance of lesions by many days (prodrome).

Assess the following during the history:

- Duration of pain or blisters (average of 2-3 weeks if untreated)
- Location of pain or blisters; severity of pain
- History of chickenpox (usually in childhood)

O: Objective

Perform a skin and neurologic examination to include the following:

- Vesicular lesions with erythematous bases in a dermatomal distribution; may be bullous or hemorrhagic
- Necrotic lesions; may persist for as long as 6 weeks
- Dermatomal scarring (particularly in dark-skinned individuals)
- Lesions in the eye area or tip of nose, along the trigeminal nerve; these represent ophthalmic nerve involvement, which requires immediate evaluation and IV treatment (see below)

A: Assessment

- Rule out other causes of vesicular skin eruptions (e.g., herpes simplex virus, severe drug reactions).
- Assess contact exposures (see below).

P: Plan

Diagnostic Evaluation

The diagnosis usually is clinical and is based on the characteristic appearance and distribution of lesions. If the diagnosis is uncertain, perform viral cultures or antigen detection by direct fluorescent antibody from a freshly opened vesicle or biopsy from the border of a lesion.

Treatment

- Treatment ideally should begin within 72 hours of an outbreak or while new lesions are appearing and should be continued for 7-10 days. Early treatment may attenuate a herpes zoster attack.

- Valacyclovir 1 g PO TID

- Famciclovir 500 mg PO TID

- Acyclovir 800 mg PO five times per day

- Dosage reductions of these drugs are required for patients with renal impairment.

- If new blisters are still appearing at the end of treatment, repeat course of PO therapy or consider IV treatment. Adjunctive corticosteroids aimed at preventing postherpetic neuralgia are not recommended.

- Consult an ophthalmologist immediately if lesions appear in the eye area or on the tip of the nose, or if the patient complains of visual disturbances, because VZV-related retinal necrosis can cause blindness. Because of the rapid progression associated with this diagnosis, hospitalization for administration of IV acyclovir and possibly foscarnet is recommended.

- VZV from zoster lesions is contagious, and contact or airborne spread from vesicle fluid may cause chickenpox in nonimmune people. If a zoster patient's household includes a pregnant woman (HIV infected or uninfected) or an HIV-infected child, consult with a specialist immediately for advice on management of exposed household members. (See "Postcontact Chickenpox Prevention," below.)

- Give analgesics for pain; narcotics may be required.

- Postherpetic neuralgia (PHN) is a common sequela of zoster. Antiviral therapy may reduce the risk of PHN, but PHN often requires special treatment for pain control. Treatment options include:

  - Nortriptyline 10-25 mg. To be taken QHS and increased by 25 mg every 3-5 days to a maximum dosage of 150 mg daily until pain is controlled, assuming adverse effects remain tolerable. Other tricyclics may be used.

- Gabapentin 100-300 mg PO BID; this may be increased by 300 mg every 3 days until reaching 3,600 mg total daily dosage. Adjust gabapentin dosage in patients with kidney disease.

- Pregabalin 75 mg BID (or 50 mg TID) in patients with estimated creatinine clearance of >60 mL/minute; this may be increased to 300 mg total daily dosage over the course of a week as needed.

- Lidocaine 5% patches provide good local relief with minimal systemic absorption. Up to 3 patches may be applied simultaneously to the affected area for up to 12 hours in a 24-hour period.

- Capsaicin cream may be applied to the affected area TID or QID. Patients should wear gloves to apply the cream and wash their hands with soap and water afterward.

- Sustained-release opiates may be required.

(See chapter *Pain Syndrome and Peripheral Neuropathy* for more options and specific recommendations.)

Severe or unresponsive cases

- IV acyclovir may be indicated if:

  - The patient is severely immunocompromised

  - The ophthalmic branch of the trigeminal nerve is affected (as noted above)

  - Dissemination has occurred

  - Lesions are not responsive to oral therapy

  - Pain is intractable in the setting of active skin lesions

- The usual adult dosage is 10-15 mg/kg Q8H for 7-14 days; dosage reduction is required for patients with renal impairment. Refer to an infectious disease specialist.

- Acyclovir resistance may occur in patients previously treated with acyclovir or related drugs, and foscarnet may be required for effective treatment. Resistance should be suspected if lesions are not resolving after 10 days of therapy or if they develop a verrucous appearance. Such lesions should be cultured and drug sensitivities should be obtained.

Prevention

The vaccine for prevention of herpes zoster (Zostavax) currently is not recommended for HIV-infected patients but is under study.

Postcontact Chickenpox Prevention

All susceptible persons, including pregnant women, who have close contact with a patient who has chickenpox or zoster must be treated to prevent chickenpox. Exposed individuals who have no history of chickenpox or shingles or no detectable antibody against VZV should be administered varicella zoster immune globulin (VariZIG) as soon as possible, but at least within 96 hours after contact. Some experts also would recommend varicella vaccination for exposed patients with CD4 counts of ≥200 cells/µL, or preemptive treatment with acyclovir; these approaches have not been studied in HIV-infected persons. Even immunocompetent adults with primary VZV (chickenpox) can develop viral dissemination to the visceral organs. HIV-infected patients may develop encephalitis, pneumonia, or polyradiculopathy during primary varicella (chickenpox) or reactivated zoster (shingles).

Patient Education

- Patients should bathe the skin lesions in mild soap and water. For necrotic lesions, use warm, moist compresses 2-3 times a day to remove debris.

- Antibiotic ointments may help prevent secondary infection and keep dressings from sticking.

- Advise patients to take their medications as directed, and to contact the clinic if symptoms worsen.

References

- Centers for Disease Control and Prevention. *Guidelines for Prevention and Treatment of Opportunistic Infections in HIV-Infected Adults and Adolescents: Recommendations from CDC, the National Institutes of Health, and the HIV Medicine Association of the Infectious Diseases Society of America.* April 10, 2009. Available at www.aidsinfo.nih.gov/guidelines/.

- Fishman S. *Post-Herpetic Neuralgia* (Oxford American Pocket Notes). Oxford University Press; 2008.

- Gebo KA, Kalyani R, Moore RD, et al. *The incidence of, risk factors for, and sequelae of herpes zoster among HIV patients in the highly active antiretroviral therapy era.* J Acquir Immune Defic Syndr. 2005 Oct 1;40(2):169-74.

- Harpaz R, Ortega-Sanchez IR, Seward JF; Advisory Committee on Immunization Practices (ACIP) Centers for Disease Control and Prevention (CDC). *Prevention of herpes zoster: recommendations of the Advisory Committee on Immunization Practices (ACIP).* MMWR Recomm Rep. 2008 Jun 6;57(RR-5):1-30; quiz CE2-4.

Histoplasmosis

Background

Histoplasmosis is caused by *Histoplasma capsulatum*, a fungus that thrives in soil contaminated by droppings from birds and bats. In the United States, *H. capsulatum* is found most often along the Ohio and Mississippi River Valleys, in the central, mid-Atlantic, and south-central states, and from Alabama to southwest Texas. In highly prevalent areas, such as Indianapolis and Kansas City, more than 80% of the population has been exposed to *Histoplasma* through inhalation of airborne infectious elements. Histoplasmosis also is found in the Canadian provinces of Quebec and Ontario, Puerto Rico, Mexico, Central and South America, Africa, East Asia, and Australia.

The initial infection in most cases either produces no symptoms or manifests only as a mild flulike illness. However, immunosuppressed individuals may develop disseminated disease. Progressive disseminated histoplasmosis often represents a reactivation of latent infection, occurs late in the course of HIV disease (the CD4 count usually is <150 cells/µL), and is an AIDS-defining illness. Pulmonary histoplasmosis (without dissemination) may occur in people with higher CD4 counts. Within endemic areas, histoplasmosis accounts for 5% of opportunistic infections among patients with AIDS. In hyperendemic areas, the prevalence of histoplasmosis may reach 25% among AIDS patients. The incidence of histoplasmosis in the United States has declined with the use of effective antiretroviral therapy (ART).

Common clinical features that may be associated with histoplasmosis are shown in Table 1.

S: Subjective

Histoplasmosis may be difficult to diagnose because the symptoms are nonspecific. In addition, clinicians may not suspect this diagnosis in low-prevalence areas.

Patients may experience fever, weight loss, fatigue, cough, and shortness of breath. They also may develop skin lesions, adenopathy, central nervous system (CNS) changes, oropharyngeal ulcers, nausea, diarrhea, and abdominal pain. Symptoms usually begin several weeks before patients present for care. On occasion, histoplasmosis presents abruptly as a sepsis-like syndrome.

Ask the patient about possible exposures, but note that absence of reported exposures does not rule out histoplasmosis. The following activities are associated with significant risk of exposure:

- Residence or travel in endemic areas (see above); in the United States, particularly the Ohio and Mississippi River Valleys

O: Objective

Measure vital signs and document fever.

Perform a complete physical examination, with special attention to the lymph nodes, lungs, abdomen, skin, and neurologic system.

Common findings include enlargement of the liver, spleen, and lymph nodes. Skin lesions and oropharyngeal ulcers may be seen.

Table 1. Common Clinical Manifestations of Histoplasmosis

Symptom Group	Percentage of Cases	Examples	
Constitutional	95%	• Weight loss • Fever	• Fatigue
Gastrointestinal	>10%	• Splenomegaly • Hepatomegaly	• Diarrhea • Abdominal pain
Respiratory	50-60%	• Pneumonia	• Pneumonitis
Hematologic	>50%	• Anemia • Leukopenia	• Thrombocytopenia
Neurologic	15-20%	• Meningitis, cerebritis • Encephalopathy	• Focal parenchymal lesions
Septic	10-20%	• Hypotension • Respiratory insufficiency • Renal or hepatic failure	• Disseminated intravascular coagulopathy • High fever
Dermatologic	<10%	• Follicular, pustular, maculopapular, or erythematous lesions	

- Occupational history of farming or construction/remodeling
- Hobbies that involve contact with caves, bird roosts or nests, or farm areas
- Contact with soil having a high organic content and undisturbed bird droppings, such as that found around old chicken coops and bird roosts

A: Assessment

A partial differential diagnosis includes the following:

- Other deep-seated fungal infections, such as cryptococcosis and coccidioidomycosis
- Mycobacterial disease (*Mycobacterium tuberculosis* or *Mycobacterium avium* complex)
- *Pneumocystis* pneumonia
- Lymphoma

P: Plan

Diagnostic Evaluation

- The *H. capsulatum* antigen test is sensitive and specific. The test is most sensitive for urine samples (95% in disseminated disease), but can be used on serum (85% sensitive in disseminated disease), bronchial fluids, or cerebrospinal fluid (CSF) specimens. Results may be obtained in a few days' time. Urine antigen levels can be used to monitor the response to therapy.

- Cultures of blood, bone marrow, and specimens from other sources have reasonable sensitivity (about 85%), but obtaining results may take several weeks.

- Wright stain of the buffy coat of a blood specimen may reveal intracellular organisms.

- Biopsies of lymph nodes, liver, cutaneous lesions, and lungs may be diagnostic in up to 50% of cases; bone marrow can be stained with methenamine silver to show the organism within macrophages.

- Meningitis can be challenging to diagnose. Diagnostically, *Histoplasma* antigen or anti-*Histoplasma* antibodies can be detected in CSF in up to 70% of cases, whereas results for cultures are often negative. Nonspecific findings in the CSF include elevated protein and low glucose as well as a lymphocytic pleocytosis. A diagnosis of *Histoplasma* meningitis should be considered if the patient has known disseminated disease and other more common etiologies of meningitis have been ruled out.

- Lactate dehydrogenase (LDH) and ferritin, although not specific, may be markedly elevated in disseminated disease.

- Complete blood count and chemistry panels may show pancytopenia, elevated creatinine, or abnormal liver function.

Treatment

Treatment consists of two phases: induction and chronic maintenance. Treatment should be continued for at least 12 months.

Mild to moderate disseminated histoplasmosis without CNS involvement

- Induction and maintenance therapy: itraconazole 200 mg PO TID or 300 mg PO BID for 3 days followed by itraconazole 200 mg BID to complete 12 months of therapy. Liquid formulation of itraconazole is preferred.

Severe disseminated histoplasmosis

Severe infection requires IV induction therapy with a lipid formulation of amphotericin; standard amphotericin is less effective and is associated with more adverse effects, but may be used as an alternative.

- **Induction therapy:**
  - **Preferred:** liposomal amphotericin B lipid formulation 3 mg/kg IV daily
  - **Alternatives:** amphotericin B 0.7 mg/kg IV daily or amphotericin B lipid complex 5 mg/kg IV daily

- **Maintenance therapy:** After ≥2 weeks of therapy or improvement of the patient's clinical status, therapy may be switched to itraconazole 200 mg PO TID for 3 days, then BID to complete 12 months of therapy. Liquid formulation of itraconazole is preferred.

Histoplasma meningitis

Amphotericin B must be used because itraconazole has poor penetration into the CNS:

- **Induction therapy:** liposomal amphotericin B 5 mg/kg daily for 4-6 weeks

- **Maintenance therapy:** itraconazole 200 mg PO BID or TID for ≥12 months and until abnormal CSF findings resolve

Pulmonary histoplasmosis in patients with CD4 counts of >350 cells/μL

Manage as for non-immunocompromised patients.

See "Potential ARV Interactions," below, regarding azoles.

Long-term suppressive therapy

Long-term therapy must be given to prevent relapse after 12 months of initial treatment; this typically consists of itraconazole 200 mg PO once daily. Fluconazole 800 mg once daily is less effective but can be used as an alternative for patients who cannot tolerate or cannot obtain itraconazole. Voriconazole and posaconazole appear to be effective. (See "Potential ARV Interactions," below, regarding azoles.)

Few data support the discontinuation of chronic maintenance therapy. One small study sponsored by the AIDS Clinical Trials Group demonstrated safety in discontinuing suppressive itraconazole therapy for patients who met the following criteria: had completed >1 year of itraconazole therapy, negative blood cultures, *Histoplasma* serum antigen <2 units, CD4 counts >150 cells/μL, and had been on ART for ≥6 months. Therefore, per U.S. Centers for Disease Control and Prevention (CDC) guidelines, discontinuing suppressive therapy for any patient who meets these criteria can be considered.

Monitoring and relapse

Monitor either serum or urine *Histoplasma* antigen, as well as clinical status, to evaluate response to therapy; a rise in the antigen level suggests relapse of histoplasmosis. A drug level of itraconazole should be measured at least once during therapy as absorption of this drug can be erratic.

In cases of treatment failure, both voriconazole and posaconazole have been successful in a few case reports; if treatment failure is suspected, an infectious disease specialist should be consulted.

Primary Prophylaxis

Currently, there are no studies that prove any survival benefit in using primary prophylaxis; however, for patients with CD4 counts of <150 cells/μL, prophylaxis with itraconazole 200 mg PO once daily can be considered for high-risk patients (e.g., those with occupational exposure and those who reside in hyperendemic regions). HIV-infected patients with CD4 counts of ≤150 cells/μL should be educated about precautions for avoiding exposure.

Primary prophylaxis can be discontinued if the CD4 count remains >150 cells/μL for 6 months on effective ART; prophylaxis should be restarted if the CD4 count drops to ≤150 cells/μL.

Potential ARV Interactions

Note that azoles (particularly itraconazole, posaconazole, and voriconazole) may interact with certain protease inhibitors, nonnucleoside reverse transcriptase inhibitors, and other medications); some combinations are contraindicated.

Patient Education

- Histoplasmosis is not transmitted from person to person, so isolation is not necessary.

- Patients should take all their medications exactly as prescribed by their health care provider.

- Even with maintenance therapy, relapses can occur. Patients should contact their provider immediately if symptoms worsen.

- The azoles may cause birth defects. Women who are taking azole medications should avoid pregnancy. In addition, itraconazole and other azoles interact with some antiretrovirals and other medications; patients should tell their provider if they begin taking any new medications while receiving itraconazole.

References

- Centers for Disease Control and Prevention. *Guidelines for Prevention and Treatment of Opportunistic Infections in HIV-Infected Adults and Adolescents: Recommendations from CDC, the National Institutes of Health, and the HIV Medicine Association of the Infectious Diseases Society of America.* April 10, 2009. Available at www.aidsinfo.nih.gov/guidelines/.

- Deepe GS Jr. *Histoplasma Capsulatum.* In: Mandell G, Bennett JE, Dolin R, eds. *Principles and Practice of Infectious Diseases,* 6th ed. Philadelphia: Elsevier; 2005:3012-26.

- Goldman M, Zackin R, Fichtenbaum CJ, et al. *Safety of discontinuation of maintenance therapy for disseminated histoplasmosis after immunologic response to antiretroviral therapy.* Clin Infect Dis. 2004 May 15;38(10):1485-9.

- McKinsey DS, Wheat LJ, Cloud GA, et al. *Itraconazole prophylaxis for fungal infections in patients with advanced human immunodeficiency virus infection: randomized, placebo-controlled, double-blind study.* Clin Infect Dis. 1999 May;28(5):1049-56.

- Wheat J. Histoplasmosis. In: Dolin R, Masur H, Saag M, eds. *AIDS Therapy, 2nd Edition.* Philadelphia: Churchill Livingstone; 2003:511-521.

- Wheat J, Sarosi G, McKinsey D, et al. *Practice guidelines for the management of patients with histoplasmosis. Infectious Diseases Society of America.* Clin Infect Dis. 2000 Apr;30(4):688-95.

Kaposi Sarcoma

Background

Kaposi sarcoma (KS) is an endothelial neoplasm that usually occurs as skin or oral lesions but may involve the internal organs. It is the most common AIDS-associated neoplasm and is an AIDS-defining disease. AIDS-associated KS is one of four types of KS, along with classic, endemic, and organ transplant-associated KS. Although the types vary in epidemiology and clinical presentation, all are associated with human herpesvirus type 8 (HHV-8), also known as KS-associated herpesvirus. The clinical manifestations of AIDS-associated KS (sometimes called epidemic KS) range in severity from mild to life-threatening. The progression of disease may be rapid or slow, but the overall prognosis is poor in the absence of treatment. The skin lesions of KS, even when they do not cause medical morbidity, may cause significant disfigurement and emotional distress.

AIDS-associated KS usually occurs in HIV-infected persons with advanced immunosuppression (CD4 count of <200 cells/μL), but may occur at any CD4 count. In the United States and Europe, KS occurs in all HIV risk groups, but most frequently among men who have sex with men (MSM). Risk factors for MSM include multiple sexual partners and a history of sexually transmitted infections (STIs); risk factors for other groups have not been clearly identified. The transmission of HHV-8 is not well understood. Although experts believe HHV-8 is transmitted sexually, it apparently also passes from person to person by other routes.

The incidence of KS in resource-abundant countries has declined markedly since the early 1990s, in part because of the widespread availability of effective combination antiretroviral therapy (ART). In parts of sub-Saharan Africa, where endemic KS has long existed in people with normal immune function, the incidence of KS has risen sharply in people with HIV. ART appears to be effective in reducing the risk of AIDS-associated KS, particularly when initiated before the development of advanced immunosuppression.

S: Subjective

Skin Lesions

The cutaneous presentation of KS is the most common, occurring in 95% of cases. Lesions may occur anywhere on the skin. Common sites include the face (particularly under the eyes and on the tip of the nose), behind the ears, and on the extremities and torso. Lesions may be macules, papules, plaques, or nodules. At first, the lesions are small and may be flat. Their color may vary from pink or red to purple or brown-black (the latter particularly in dark-skinned individuals), and they are nonblanching, nonpruritic, and painless (lesions may become painful in the setting of immune reconstitution inflammatory syndrome [IRIS] associated with KS). Over time, the lesions often increase in size and number, darken, and rise from the surface; they may progress to tumor plaques (e.g., on the thighs or soles of the feet), or to exophytic tumor masses, which can cause bleeding, necrosis, and extreme pain.

Oral Lesions

Oral lesions may be flat or nodular and are red or purplish. They usually appear on the hard palate, but may develop on the soft palate, gums, tongue, and elsewhere. Oral lesions, if extensive, may cause tooth loss, pain, and ulceration.

Lymphedema

Lymphedema associated with KS usually appears in patients with visible cutaneous lesions, and edema may be out of proportion to the extent of visible lesions. Lymphedema also may occur in patients with no visible skin lesions. Common sites include the face, neck, external genitals, and lower extremities. A contiguous area of skin usually is involved. Lymph nodes may be enlarged.

Pulmonary KS

Pulmonary KS may be asymptomatic or cause intractable cough, bronchospasm, hemoptysis, chest pain, and dyspnea. The patient may exhibit difficulty breathing, bronchospasm, cough (sometimes with hemoptysis), and hypoxemia.

Gastrointestinal KS

Gastrointestinal KS may arise anywhere in the gastrointestinal tract. Patients usually are asymptomatic except in cases of intestinal obstruction or bleeding. KS may cause protein-losing enteropathy. Visceral disease is uncommon in the absence of extensive cutaneous disease.

During the history, ask about the symptoms noted above and associated characteristics, including the following:

- Duration of lesions
- Pain
- Frequency of new lesions
- Respiratory or gastrointestinal symptoms
- Edema or swelling

O: Objective

Physical Examination

Perform a careful physical examination, with particular attention to the following:

- Vital signs

- Skin (examine the entire skin surface including the scalp and conjunctiva)
- Oropharynx
- Extremities and external genitals (look for lesions, edema)
- Lymph nodes

Examine the lungs, abdomen, rectum, and other systems as indicated.

A: Assessment

The partial differential diagnosis depends on the type of symptoms present.

For cutaneous, oral, and lymph node presentations, consider the following:

- Bacillary angiomatosis
- Lymphoma
- Dermatofibromas
- Bacterial or fungal skin infections
- Venous stasis

For pulmonary symptoms, consider the following:

- *Pneumocystis jiroveci* pneumonia (PCP)
- Cytomegalovirus (CMV) pneumonia
- Pulmonary lymphoma (rare)

P: Plan

Diagnostic Evaluation

For cutaneous or oral KS, a presumptive diagnosis often can be made by the appearance of skin or mucous membrane lesions. Biopsy of a lesion (or a suspect lymph node) is strongly recommended to verify the diagnosis and rule out infectious or other neoplastic causes. Biopsy is particularly important if the lesions are unusual in appearance or if the patient has systemic or atypical symptoms.

If respiratory symptoms are present, obtain chest X rays or computed tomography (CT) studies. The chest X ray typically shows diffuse interstitial infiltrates, often accompanied by nodules or pleural effusion. Radiographic findings may be suggestive of KS, but cannot provide a definitive diagnosis. Bronchoscopy with visualization of characteristic endobronchial lesions usually is adequate for diagnosis.

For patients with gastrointestinal symptoms and suspected KS, perform endoscopy.

If the patient has fever or respiratory, gastrointestinal, or constitutional symptoms, evaluate for other infectious and malignant causes (e.g., by culture or biopsy) as suggested by the history and physical examination.

Treatment

Treatment of KS is not considered curative, and no single therapy is completely efficacious. ART is a key component of the treatment of KS and should be initiated (or optimized to achieve complete HIV RNA suppression) for all persons with KS, unless contraindicated (for further information, see chapter *Antiretroviral Therapy*). KS often regresses and sometimes resolves in patients treated with effective ART. Some data suggest that protease inhibitors may have an anti-KS effect; however, non-PI-containing regimens also lead to KS regression. The role of specific antiretroviral agents beyond HIV control in KS remains unclear, although some experts prefer to use PIs for patients with active KS.

KS-associated IRIS has been described, and patients may experience painful enlarged lesions or progression of KS lesions during the first months of ART; they should be advised of this possibility.

Specific treatment of KS depends on various factors such as the number, extent, severity, and location of lesions; cosmetic considerations; and presence of visceral involvement. The goals of therapy may vary according to the clinical presentation and may include controlling symptoms, improving cosmetic appearance, reducing edema, eliminating pain, and clearing lesions.

Local treatment (preferably in conjunction with ART) usually is given to patients who have a few small lesions causing only minor symptoms. Systemic therapy (in conjunction with ART) is needed for more extensive or more severe disease, including symptomatic visceral disease, widespread skin involvement, significant edema, and rapidly progressive KS. Consultation with a KS-experienced oncologist or dermatologist is recommended.

Local treatment of limited disease
Options for local treatment of limited disease include the following:

- ART with observation for response (limited, stable cutaneous disease may require no specific treatment)
- Topical treatment with alitretinoin gel (Panretin) 0.1%
- Intralesional chemotherapy (e.g., vinblastine)
- Radiation therapy, for localized or facial lesions (may cause mucositis when used for oropharyngeal lesions)
- Cryotherapy
- Laser therapy

Treatment of extensive or rapidly progressing disease
Extensive or rapidly progressing disease may include lymphedema, intraoral or pharyngeal disease that interferes with eating, painful or bulky lesions, and symptomatic pulmonary or visceral disease. Options for treatment include the following:

- Intralesional chemotherapy (e.g., vinblastine)
- Systemic chemotherapy (e.g., liposomal formulations of doxorubicin or daunorubicin, paclitaxel, or vinorelbine)

- Numerous experimental agents are under evaluation

- Consultation with an oncologist is recommended for optimal treatment of extensive disease

Patient Education

- KS often responds to treatment. Educate patients that ART is a cornerstone of treatment; encourage them to start and adhere to ART.

- Swollen or edematous lesions increase the risk of cellulitis, whereupon lesions can become infected and progress rapidly. Advise patients to avoid injuring swollen or edematous lesions, to keep them clean, and to call their health care provider if lesions appear to be spreading or if swelling worsens.

- Advise patients to return to the clinic if respiratory or gastrointestinal symptoms develop.

- Patients may use cosmetic preparations to cover facial lesions. Refer patients to support groups or counseling services if they are having difficulty coping with their physical appearance.

References

- Centers for Disease Control and Prevention. Guidelines for Prevention and Treatment of Opportunistic Infections in HIV-Infected *Adults and Adolescents: Recommendations from CDC, the National Institutes of Health, and the HIV Medicine Association of the Infectious Diseases Society of America.* April 10, 2009. Available at www.aidsinfo.nih.gov/guidelines/.

- Gill J, Bourboulia D, Wilkinson J, et al. *Prospective study of the effects of antiretroviral therapy on Kaposi sarcoma-associated herpesvirus infection in patients with and without Kaposi sarcoma.* J Acquir Immune Defic Syndr. 2002 Dec 1;31(4):384-90.

- Jones JL, Hanson DL, Dworkin MS, et al. *Incidence and trends in Kaposi's sarcoma in the era of effective antiretroviral therapy.* J Acquir Immune Defic Syndr. 2000 Jul 1;24(3):270-4.

- Leidner RS, Aboulafia DM. *Recrudescent Kaposi's sarcoma after initiation of HAART: a manifestation of immune reconstitution syndrome.* AIDS Patient Care STDS. 2005 Oct;19(10):635-44.

- Martinez V, Caumes E, Gambotti L, et al. *Remission from Kaposi's sarcoma on HAART is associated with suppression of HIV replication and is independent of protease inhibitor therapy.* Br J Cancer. 2006 Apr 10;94(7):1000-6.

- Paparizos VA, Kyriakis KP, Papastamopoulos V, et al. *Response of AIDS-associated Kaposi sarcoma to highly active antiretroviral therapy alone.* J Acquir Immune Defic Syndr. 2002 Jun 1;30(2):257-8.

- Tam HK, Zhang ZF, Jacobson LP, et al. *Effect of highly active antiretroviral therapy on survival among HIV-infected men with Kaposi sarcoma or non-Hodgkin lymphoma.* Int J Cancer. 2002 Apr 20;98(6):916-22.

Molluscum Contagiosum

Background

Molluscum contagiosum is a viral infection of human epidermal keratinocytes, caused by a double-stranded DNA virus of the Poxviridae family. Molluscum appears as papules or nodules and sometimes is called "molluscum warts." It is seen most frequently in HIV-uninfected children (up to 5% of children in the United States), in sexually active young adults, and in immunocompromised persons. It occurs in 5-18% of HIV-infected persons. Molluscum is benign but may cause extensive and cosmetically bothersome lesions, particularly in persons with advanced HIV infection.

Transmission occurs by person-to-person skin-to-skin contact (e.g., sexual activity, contact sports [especially wrestling], or simply touching) or via fomites (towels, bedclothes, clothing [including underwear], soft toys, shaving utensils, electrolysis equipment, tattooing tools, and sponges). The virus may be spread to other areas via self-inoculation (e.g., scratching, shaving, or touching a lesion).

In immunocompetent persons, the infection usually resolves spontaneously after 6-12 months, though genital lesions may remain longer. In HIV-infected persons, the lesions may be more extensive and persistent. There is a strong correlation between the degree of immunosuppression and the risk of molluscum infection, the number of lesions, and the ability of lesions to resist treatment.

S: Subjective

Patients complain of new papules on the trunk, axillae, antecubital and popliteal fossae, face, or genital/crural area. Papules of molluscum contagiosum may cause no symptoms but also can be intensely pruritic or tender to the touch. Ask patients whether others in the home (especially children and adolescents) or their sex partners have similar papules. Genital lesions are transmitted sexually; patients may recall seeing such lesions on the genitals of a previous partner.

Ask about fever or other systemic symptoms to evaluate for other causes of the papules.

O: Objective

Perform a thorough evaluation of the skin, genitals, and mouth. Molluscum commonly presents as multiple grouped lesions. The lesions are white, pink, or flesh colored; shiny, smooth surfaced, firm, pearly, and spherical (dome-shaped) papules (2-5 mm) or nodules (6-10 mm), with umbilicated, or dimpled, centers. Patients with HIV infection may develop giant lesions (>1 cm) or clusters of hundreds of small lesions. Occasionally, molluscum will have a polyp-like appearance. Lesions are usually found on the head, face, or neck or in the genital area, but may affect every part of the body except the palms and soles. Molluscum may occur inside the mouth, vagina, and rectum, and around the eyes. Lesions on the eyelids can cause conjunctivitis.

A: Assessment

A partial differential diagnosis includes the following:

- Disseminated cryptococcosis
- Histoplasmosis skin lesions
- Other fungal skin lesions
- Folliculitis

- Syphilis, condyloma acuminata, vulvar syringoma for multiple small molluscum genital lesions

- Squamous or basal cell carcinoma

P: Plan

Diagnostic Evaluation

The diagnosis of molluscum usually is based on the characteristic appearance of the lesions. Perform histologic or other laboratory testing to confirm the diagnosis or to exclude other infections or malignancies. Special staining will show keratinocytes containing eosinophilic cytoplasmic inclusion bodies. Electron microscopy will show poxvirus particles.

Treatment

Because molluscum does not cause illness and rarely causes symptoms, the treatment usually is undertaken primarily for cosmetic purposes. For individuals with large or extensive lesions, molluscum may be disfiguring or stigmatizing, and treatment may be important for their well being. Treatment (particularly of genital lesions) can be considered to prevent transmission to others.

In HIV-infected patients, molluscum is difficult to eradicate and lesions often recur, particularly if immune suppression persists. Effective antiretroviral therapy may achieve resolution of lesions or significant improvement in the extent or appearance of molluscum.

Lesions that remain after weeks of antiretroviral therapy should be treated to prevent further spread. Refer complex cases to a dermatologist.

Choice of treatment modality is based on age, likelihood of compliance, number and size of lesions, and potential adverse effects of treatment. Therapeutic options include the following:

- Local excision: may be done by curettage, electrocautery, evisceration, or cryotherapy. Adverse effects include pain, irritation, soreness, and mild scarring. Repeated treatments are necessary. Curettage appears to be most efficacious (even for children) but is painful and requires anesthesia and a large time commitment over the course of several visits; it also has a risk of scarring. Relapse is common.

- Imiquimod 5% (Aldara): an immune response modifier; stimulates production of interferon-alfa and other proinflammatory cytokines, inducing a tissue reaction associated with viral clearance from the skin. Apply TIW for up to 16 weeks or QPM for 4 weeks. Clearing can take up to 3 months. Limited studies; painless.

- Tretinoin (Retin-A) 0.1% cream: can be applied to lesions BID. Adverse effects include drying, peeling, irritation, and soreness.

- Podophyllum resin (podophyllin): can be administered by a health care provider and washed off after 1-4 hours. This treatment is caustic, may cause significant irritation, and has limited effectiveness. It is contraindicated for use during pregnancy. Patient-administered podophyllotoxin (Podofilox) may be a safer alternative to podophyllum. Adverse effects include burning, pain, inflammation, erosion, and itching.

- Trichloroacetic acid: can be administered by a health care provider. Controlling the depth of acid penetration is difficult. Adverse effects include pain and irritation; mild scarring is common.

- A combination of salicyclic and lactic acid: response is highly variable and recurrence is common.

- Laser therapy: safe, efficient, tolerable, and efficacious.

- Cidofovir 1-3% topical cream: applied BID for 2 weeks, followed by a 30-day rest period and then two additional cycles. This treatment has been shown to be effective in several small studies and case reports, but it is expensive and difficult to compound. No systemic adverse effects are noted.

- Silver nitrate paste may be used to burn each lesion individually.

- Cantharidin 0.7%: can be applied by a health care provider. One study of 300 children found that lesions cleared after two visits. This treatment may cause allergic reactions, stinging, and blistering. Do not use cantharidin around the eyes.

Patient Education

- Molluscum infection is benign but may be distressing.

- Molluscum infection may be transmitted both sexually and nonsexually, through direct contact with lesions. Molluscum also can be transmitted indirectly by contact with infected objects.

- Latex condoms or barriers may not prevent transmission of genital molluscum.

- To prevent the spread of molluscum, instruct patients to take the following precautions:
  - Avoid close contact between their molluscum lesions and the skin, mouth, and genitals of other people.
  - Avoid picking at, squeezing, or puncturing the lesions, as a lesion's central plug is full of viral particles that can be spread easily by coming into contact with other parts of the body. In addition, lesions may become secondarily infected.
  - Wash hands frequently.
  - Keep fingernails short.
  - Avoid shaving in areas with lesions because shaving could result in lesions spreading to other areas.
  - Avoid sharing towels, bedclothes, clothing, shaving utensils, bathing equipment, or other objects that have been in contact with molluscum lesions.
  - Wash all contaminated items in very hot, but not scalding, water.
  - Cover lesions with clothing, if possible.

Section 6: Comorbidities, Coinfections, and Complications

References

- Binder B, Weger W, Komericki P, et al. *Treatment of molluscum contagiousum with a pulsed-dye laser: pilot study with 19 children.* J Dtsch Dermatol Ges. 2008 Feb;6(2):121-5.

- Calista D. *Topical cidofovir for severe cutaneous human papillomavirus and molluscum contagiosum infections in patients with HIV/AIDS: a pilot study.* J Eur Acad Dermatol Venereol. 2000 Nov;14(6):484-8.

- Connell CO, Oranje A, Van Gysel D, et al. *Congenital molluscum contagiosum: Report of four cases and review of the literature.* Pediatr Dermatol. 2008 Sep-Oct;25(5):553-6.

- Fornatora ML, Reich RF, Gray RG, et al. *Intraoral molluscum contagiosum: a report of a case and a review of the literature.* Oral Surg Oral Med Oral Pathol Oral Radiol Endod. 2001 Sep;92(3):318-20.

- Gould D. *An overview of molluscum contagiosum: a viral skin condition.* Nurs Stand. 2008 Jun 18-24;22(41):45-8.

- Isaacs SN. *Molluscum contagiosum.* UpToDate. In: UpToDate v14.1. Available at www.uptodate.com/patients/content/. Accessed June 30, 2010. [Registration required.]

- Ku JK, Kwon HJ, Kim MY, et al. *Expression of toll-like receptors in verruca and molluscum contagiosum.* J Korean Med Sci. 2008 Apr;23(2):307-14.

- Moiin A. *Photodynamic therapy for molluscum contagiosum infection in HIV-coinfected patients: review of 6 patients.* J Drugs Dermatol. 2003 Dec;2(6):637-9.

- Simonart T, De Maertelaer V. *Curettage treatment for molluscum contagiosum: a follow-up survey study.* Br J Dermatol. 2008 Nov;159(5):1144-7.

- Strauss RM, Doyle EL, Mohsen AH, et al. *Successful treatment of molluscum contagiosum with topical imiquimod in a severely immunocompromised HIV-positive patient.* Int J STD AIDS. 2001 Apr;12(4):264-6.

- Toro JR, Wood LV, Patel NK, et al. *Topical cidofovir: a novel treatment for recalcitrant molluscum contagiosum in children infected with human immunodeficiency virus 1.* Arch Dermatol. 2000 Aug;136(8):983-5.

Mycobacterium avium **Complex**

Background

Mycobacterium avium complex (MAC) is an opportunistic infection caused by species of *Mycobacterium* that can produce severe illness in people with advanced AIDS but rarely affects others. The risk of disseminated MAC (DMAC) is directly related to the severity of immunosuppression. DMAC typically occurs in persons with CD4 counts of <50 cells/μL, and its frequency increases as the CD4 count declines. In the absence of antibiotic prophylaxis, DMAC occurs in up to 40% of AIDS patients with CD4 counts of <50 cells/μL. Antimicrobial therapy, especially if given in conjunction with antiretroviral therapy (ART) that achieves immune reconstitution, can be successful in treating MAC disease. Specific antimicrobial prophylaxis and effective ART also may be used to prevent MAC in patients with advanced AIDS (see chapter *Opportunistic Infection Prophylaxis*).

Mycobacterium organisms are common in the environment. They are found worldwide and have been isolated from soil, water, animals, birds, and foods. They usually enter the body through the respiratory or gastrointestinal tract and disseminate to cause multisystem infection, typically manifested by nonspecific symptoms and signs such as fever, sweats, weight loss, abdominal pain, fatigue, chronic diarrhea, and anemia and other cytopenias. MAC also can cause local disease such as central nervous system infection, lymphadenitis, soft-tissue or bone infections, and rarely, isolated pulmonary disease. Focal MAC disease is more common among patients on ART, whereas DMAC is the more common manifestation among those with low CD4 cell counts who are not on ART. Unlike *Mycobacterium tuberculosis, M. avium* is not thought to be transmitted via person-to-person contact. In patients with subclinical or incompletely treated MAC who have recently started ART, an immune reconstitution inflammatory syndrome (IRIS) may occur with localized lymphadenitis or paradoxically worsening symptoms (see chapter *Immune Reconstitution Inflammatory Syndrome*).

S: Subjective

The patient complains of one or more of the following symptoms:

- Persistent or cyclic fever
- Night sweats
- Unintentional weight loss
- Anorexia
- Chronic diarrhea
- Weakness
- Fatigue
- Abdominal pain
- Lymph node enlargement

When taking the history, ask about the following:

- Any symptoms as described above, including duration and intensity; other symptoms of infection
- Whether the patient is taking MAC prophylaxis or ART

O: Objective

Perform a full physical examination with particular attention to the following:

- Vital signs (temperature, heart rate, blood pressure, respiratory rate)
- Weight (compare with previous measurements)

- General appearance (cachexia, wasting, signs of chronic illness, jaundice, pallor)
- Lymph nodes (lymphadenopathy)
- Abdomen (hepatosplenomegaly, tenderness)

Review previous laboratory values, particularly the CD4 count (usually <50 cells/μL).

A: Assessment

Rule out other infectious or neoplastic causes of constitutional symptoms, anemia, or organomegaly. A partial differential diagnosis would include the following:

- *M. tuberculosis* infection
- Cytomegalovirus infection
- Lymphoma
- Bartonellosis
- Disseminated fungal infection
- Pyogenic abscess
- Other septicemia

P: Plan

Diagnostic Evaluation

A definitive diagnosis requires isolation of MAC from the blood or other normally sterile body fluids or tissues (*M. avium* cultured from sputum, bronchial washing, or stool may represent colonization rather than infection). Send blood for acid-fast bacilli (AFB) culture (sensitivity of a single blood culture for MAC bacteremia is 91%, sensitivity increases to 98% if two samples [drawn at different times] are sent). Because MAC may take weeks to grow in culture, ancillary studies should be performed. The following are not specific, but may be helpful in reaching a presumptive diagnosis:

- Complete blood count (CBC) for anemia, lymphopenia, and thrombocytopenia
- Serum alkaline phosphatase (often elevated in DMAC)

- Computed tomography (CT) scan of the chest and abdomen (intraabdominal and mediastinal lymphadenopathy or hepatosplenomegaly often are present)

If blood cultures are negative and MAC is suspected (or if results of blood cultures are pending), consider biopsy of the lymph nodes, bone marrow, liver, or bowel (via endoscopy) to detect DMAC by microscopic examination for AFB and culture. If the evidence suggests pulmonary MAC, consider bronchoscopy and bronchoalveolar lavage. Note that in MAC IRIS, MAC bacteremia usually is absent and a tissue-based diagnosis is required.

Perform additional studies as indicated to rule out other causes of the patient's symptoms, including bacterial blood cultures, sputum for *M. tuberculosis*, *Bartonella* studies, lymph node cytology for lymphoma, and stool cultures.

Treatment

Because antimicrobial resistance develops quickly with single-drug therapy, multidrug regimens must be administered for DMAC.

Recommended regimen:
- Clarithromycin 500 mg BID + ethambutol 15 mg/kg once daily

Clarithromycin is the preferred cornerstone of MAC therapy, as it has been studied more extensively and is associated with more rapid clearance of MAC bacteremia. If clarithromycin cannot be tolerated or if there is concern regarding drug interactions, azithromycin 500-600 mg once daily may be substituted for clarithromycin. Clarithromycin dosages should not exceed 1 g per day, as high-dose clarithromycin has been associated with excess mortality.

Ethambutol is the recommended second agent, to be given with a macrolide.

Some experts recommend including a third agent for more advanced disease and for patients who are not receiving effective ART. The addition of rifabutin (300 mg daily) has been associated with a mortality benefit in one study and with reduced emergence of mycobacterial resistance in two other trials. A fluoroquinolone (e.g., ciprofloxacin, levofloxacin) or amikacin may be used instead of rifabutin as a third agent, or in addition to rifabutin as a fourth agent; however, studies have not confirmed the clinical benefit of these medications.

Because immune reconstitution is essential for controlling MAC, all patients who are not already receiving ART should begin ART, if possible. Patients who are receiving suboptimal ART should be evaluated for enhancement of their regimens. The optimal timing of ART initiation in relation to MAC treatment is unclear. Because immune reconstitution from effective ART may cause a paradoxical inflammatory response if started during active DMAC infection, some experts recommend treating DMAC for at least 2 weeks before adding antiretroviral (ARV) medications (see chapter *Immune Reconstitution Inflammatory Syndrome*). This strategy also helps to avoid or forestall interactions between DMAC and ARV drugs and the additive toxicities of those medications.

Potential ARV Interactions

Clarithromycin and rifabutin have a number of significant drug interactions, including interactions with some commonly prescribed ARVs. These interactions should be reviewed prior to initiation of MAC therapy. Dosage adjustments or alternative medications may be required. Interactions of concern include the following:

- **Atazanavir** may raise clarithromycin levels by 50% while decreasing levels of clarithromycin's active metabolite; some experts recommend using azithromycin in place of clarithromycin, dosage reduction of clarithromycin by 50%, or an alternative ARV regimen.

- **Darunavir** may increase clarithromycin levels; dosage reduction of clarithromycin is recommended for patients with renal impairment.

- **Tipranavir** decreases levels of clarithromycin's active metabolite; also, tipranavir levels may be increased.

- **Efavirenz** may lower clarithromycin levels; some experts recommend use of azithromycin in place of clarithromycin.

- **Etravirine** may lower clarithromycin levels, while clarithromycin may in turn increase etravirine levels. Avoid this combination, if possible.

- **Nevirapine** may decrease clarithromycin levels and increase levels of its active metabolite.

Protease inhibitor-based ART (e.g., lopinavir or darunavir) or integrase inhibitor-based ART may be the preferred HIV treatment for patients on MAC therapy, because of limited drug interactions associated with those ARV classes.

Rifabutin has significant interactions with many drugs, including nonnucleoside reverse transcriptase inhibitors and protease inhibitors, and therefore dosage adjustments or alternative agents may be needed (for further information, see chapter *Mycobacterium Tuberculosis*.

The patient should show clinical improvement within the first weeks of treatment. If there is not a response to treatment after 2-4 weeks, assess adherence, consider adding one or more drugs, and consider evaluation for other or additional causes of the patient's symptoms. Consider repeating a blood culture with antimicrobial sensitivities for patients whose clinical status has not improved after 4-8 weeks of treatment. Interpretation of MAC drug susceptibility testing should be undertaken in consultation with an infectious disease or HIV specialist, because laboratory evidence of drug resistance does not always correlate with clinical drug resistance.

If immune reconstitution inflammatory reactions are suspected, consider adding antiinflammatory medications, including corticosteroids if MAC IRIS is moderate to severe (see chapter *Immune Reconstitution Inflammatory Syndrome*).

Treatment of MAC generally is required for the remainder of the patient's life in the absence of immune reconstitution with effective ART. It may be reasonable to discontinue MAC therapy if patients complete at least 12 months of MAC treatment, have no further symptoms, and demonstrate immune restoration in response to ART (an increase in CD4 counts to >100 cells/µL for at least 6 months). If MAC treatment is discontinued, the patient must be monitored carefully for any decrease in CD4 cell count or recurrence of MAC symptoms. Some clinicians verify negative AFB cultures before discontinuing therapy. Treatment should be resumed if the CD4 count drops to <100 cells/µL or if symptoms recur.

Prevention

Primary prevention using azithromycin or clarithromycin should be initiated in persons with CD4 cell counts <50 cells/µL. See chapter *Opportunistic Infection Prophylaxis*.

Patient Education

- Advise patients that antimycobacterial therapy alone will not eradicate MAC infection, but should decrease symptoms and improve quality of life. A response to treatment may take up to 4 weeks. If medications are discontinued, the disease almost always recurs, unless the CD4 count has increased to >50-100 cells/µL in response to ART.

- Patients must take all medicines exactly as prescribed. If doses are missed, or if the medication is stopped and restarted, MAC can develop resistance to the medications. If patients are having trouble taking the medications on schedule, they should contact their health care provider promptly.

- Advise patients that MAC IRIS is a common complication of effective ART and MAC therapy, and its occurrence in the course of treatment should be anticipated.

- Urge patients to contact the clinic immediately if they notice worsening of existing symptoms or the development of new symptoms.

- DMAC is an opportunistic infection of late-stage HIV and it is indicative of profound immunosuppression. Some patients may not respond to MAC treatment or to ART. Because this is a life-threatening disease, clinicians should discuss advance directives and durable power of attorney with patients. Referral to a social worker, mental health clinician, or chaplain experienced in such issues may facilitate the discussion.

References

- Benson CA, Williams PL, Currier JS, et al.; AIDS Clinical Trials Group 223 Protocol Team. *A prospective, randomized trial examining the efficacy and safety of clarithromycin in combination with ethambutol, rifabutin, or both for the treatment of disseminated Mycobacterium avium complex disease in persons with acquired immunodeficiency syndrome.* Clin Infect Dis. 2003 Nov 1;37(9):1234-43.

- Cabié A, Abel S, Brebion A, et al. *Mycobacterial lymphadenitis after initiation of highly active antiretroviral therapy.* Eur J Clin Microbiol Infect Dis. 1998 Nov;17(11):812-3.

- Centers for Disease Control and Prevention. *Guidelines for Prevention and Treatment of Opportunistic Infections in HIV-Infected Adults and Adolescents: Recommendations from CDC, the National Institutes of Health, and the HIV Medicine Association of the Infectious Diseases Society of America.* April 10, 2009. Available at www.aidsinfo.nih.gov/guidelines/.

- Gordin FM, Sullam PM, Shafran SD, et al. *A randomized, placebo-controlled study of rifabutin added to a regimen of clarithromycin and ethambutol for treatment of disseminated infection with Mycobacterium avium complex.* Clin Infect Dis. 1999 May;28(5):1080-5.

- Horsburgh CR Jr, Gettings J, Alexander LN, et al. *Disseminated Mycobacterium avium complex disease among patients infected with human immunodeficiency virus, 1985-2000.* Clin Infect Dis. 2001 Dec 1;33(11):1938-43.

- Phillips P, Bonner S, Gataric N, et al. *Nontuberculous mycobacterial immune reconstitution syndrome in HIV-infected patients: spectrum of disease and long-term follow-up.* Clin Infect Dis. 2005 Nov 15;41(10):1483-97.

- Race EM, Adelson-Mitty J, Kriegel GR, et al. *Focal mycobacterial lymphadenitis following initiation of protease-inhibitor therapy in patients with advanced HIV-1 disease.* Lancet. 1998 Jan 24;351(9098):252-5.

Mycobacterium tuberculosis

Background

In HIV-infected individuals, tuberculosis (TB) causes more deaths worldwide than any other condition. A biologic synergy exists between HIV and TB such that HIV-induced immunosuppression increases susceptibility to TB infection, whereas active TB infection enhances HIV replication through immunologic stimulation. The populations infected by these two pathogens overlap in many respects, creating epidemiologic synergy. Poverty, crowded living conditions, and inadequate efforts to reduce transmission combine to enhance the transmission of both organisms.

In the United States, most cases of TB occur among immigrants, and TB is a relatively infrequent AIDS-defining illness. Nevertheless, TB remains important to HIV clinicians in the United States because it is highly infectious, though curable with proper treatment, and because improper treatment leads to drug resistance both in the infected patient and in those to whom that patient transmits. Although other conditions increase the risk of TB disease (e.g., malnutrition, diabetes, end-stage renal disease, pulmonary silicosis, and iatrogenic immunosuppressive drugs [especially inhibitors of tumor necrosis factor]), HIV infection is by far the most important risk factor.

TB is an infection caused by organisms in the *Mycobacteria* genus. These organisms grow slowly and can be identified only with special staining techniques, a trait that led to the name "acid-fast bacteria." This chapter focuses on disease caused by *Mycobacterium tuberculosis* (MTB); other chapters describe diagnosis and management of latent MTB infection (see chapter *Latent Tuberculosis*) and diagnosis and management of disease caused by *Mycobacteria avium* (see chapter *Mycobacterium avium Complex*).

MTB most often causes a chronic pneumonia, but it can affect organs other than the lungs as well. The lung destruction caused by MTB may create cavities, similar to abscesses; these contain huge numbers of organisms. TB is transmitted almost always by persons with active pulmonary TB who release large numbers of organisms in their sputum. The organisms remain suspended in the air for hours or days, making TB among the most easily transmitted respiratory pathogens. Organisms are inhaled and infect the lung. In most people, the initial lung infection is contained by an effective immune response. It usually is asymptomatic but leads to foci in the lung (and sometimes in other organs) of latent TB, which may reactivate and cause disease years later. Shortly after the onset of infection with MTB, before its containment in the lung by the immune system, organisms can spread to other organs and establish latent infection in those areas as well. Reactivation in these other organs can lead to local disease (e.g., in the lymph nodes, meninges, bone, pericardium, peritoneum or intestine, and urogenital tract).

Persons with limited immunity, such as persons with HIV-associated immunosuppression and very young children, are at high risk of developing progressive primary TB at the time of initial MTB infection. Primary progressive MTB usually causes pulmonary disease, but also can cause meningitis or disseminated disease (blood, liver, spleen, lung, and other organs). Persons who have latent TB infection and then develop immunodeficiency are at high risk of developing reactivation disease. For example, compared with the 10% lifetime risk of developing active TB in immunologically normal persons, an HIV-infected person with latent TB has about a 10% chance each year of developing active disease.

Classical pulmonary tuberculosis, with upper lobe infiltrates and cavitary lesions, may occur in HIV-infected persons with relatively intact immunity. As the CD4 count decreases (particularly to <200 cells/µL), TB is more likely to manifest atypically in the chest (without cavitary disease, or with lower lobe disease, adenopathy, pleural effusions, or interstitial or military infiltrates), and as extrapulmonary or multiorgan disease (particularly in lymph nodes, peritoneum, pericardium, and meninges), and disseminated infection. Granulomas may be seen in the tissues; in persons with advanced immunodeficiency, these may be poorly formed and non-caseating. Bone, joint, and urogenital TB are less commonly associated with HIV-induced immunosuppression. Symptoms and signs in HIV-infected persons therefore can vary widely.

Before an effective treatment for TB was developed, one half of persons with TB died within a period of about 5 years; others recovered, but relapses sometimes occurred. Appropriate use of modern chemotherapy applied to drug-susceptible MTB disease cured at least 95% of persons in the pre-HIV era. Nowadays, drug-susceptible TB remains highly curable, even for persons with HIV infection. However, drug resistance seriously reduces the cure rate. Drug resistance usually is caused by improper or erratic treatment, and is spreading rapidly and becoming more severe. Effective diagnosis and cure of drug-susceptible TB not only reduces the disease burden in the individual and reduces further transmission, it also is crucial to avoiding drug resistance.

MTB resistance to a single drug may extend or complicate treatment but usually does not prevent successful treatment of TB. Resistance to several drugs (**polydrug resistance or PDR**) requires a longer course of therapy using medications that are less potent and have more side effects, and it markedly reduces the chance of cure. Resistance to both isoniazid and rifampin, with or without resistance to other first-line drugs, is called **multidrug resistance (MDR)**, and it makes treatment especially difficult. **Extreme drug resistance (XDR)** occurs when, in addition to isoniazid and rifampin resistance, there is resistance to specific second-line drugs: a fluoroquinolone plus an injectable agent (either kanamycin, amikacin, or capreomycin). Treatment of drug-resistant TB should be managed by experts or in consultation with experts.

Effective antiretroviral treatment (ART) is a critical component of the care of persons with TB, and ART should be initiated or optimized in all persons with active TB.

This chapter will discuss the evaluation and management of TB in the United States and other high-income settings. For management of TB in resource-limited settings, see the relevant World Health Organization guidelines and other resources.

S: Subjective

Persons with TB generally describe an illness lasting several weeks to months, associated with systemic features such as high fevers, night sweats, loss of appetite, and weight loss. These symptoms are nonspecific, but should raise the possibility of TB.

- Pulmonary TB presents with a chronic productive cough and sometimes with hemoptysis; shortness of breath occurs late in the disease course.

- TB adenitis presents with enlarged lymph nodes (usually asymmetric involvement in one region) that may suppurate and drain but usually are not painful, hot, or erythematous.

- TB meningitis presents with headache, gradual change in mental status, and at times with cranial nerve abnormalities such as double vision or decreased hearing.

- Disseminated TB may occur with only systemic manifestations such as fever, sweats, and weight loss, with no localizing features.

The diagnosis is more probable when a patient has a likelihood of both TB infection and a clinical state permissive for MTB disease. Risk factors for TB infection include known prior contact with an active case, exposure in congregate settings (such as homeless shelters and prisons, but also in health care facilities), or travel or residence in countries with high rates of endemic TB. In the United States, persons with active or past substance use disorders and persons of color are more likely than others to have had exposure to TB. History of a prior positive tuberculin skin test (TST) or interferon-gamma releasing assay (IGRA) result provides evidence of TB infection (see chapter *Latent Tuberculosis*). Risks for active TB disease include any degree of HIV-associated immunosuppression, immunosuppression associated with other diseases (e.g., leukemia, lymphoma) or caused by medical therapies, and malnutrition.

O: Objective

- Measure vital signs, including oxygen saturation.

- Measure weight; compare with previous values.

- Perform thorough physical examination with particular attention to the lungs, heart, abdomen, lymph nodes, and neurologic system.

Systemic signs of chronic disease and inflammation are common, including fever, night sweats (which may occur without awareness of the high fever that precedes them), and weight loss.

In patients with pulmonary TB, the breath sounds may be normal or focally abnormal; tachypnea and hypoxia occur only with extensive lung damage.

Extrapulmonary TB may present with focal adenopathy without local signs of inflammation, but perhaps with a draining sinus.

TB meningitis presents as subacute or chronic meningitis, with neck stiffness and changes in mental status. Symptoms may include cranial nerve palsies owing to inflammation at the base of the brain or increased intracranial pressure.

Pericardial disease can cause the pain and friction rub of pericarditis or signs of pericardial tamponade.

Infiltration of the bone marrow can produce pancytopenia.

Disseminated TB may cause diffuse adenopathy, hepatic or splenic enlargement, and abnormal liver function, although hepatic failure is rarely attributable to TB alone. Infection of the adrenal glands can cause adrenal insufficiency.

A: Assessment

The differential diagnosis of TB is extensive and depends in part on the degree of immunosuppression (as indicated by the CD4 cell count) of the individual. It includes a broad range of bacterial, mycobacterial, viral, and fungal infections in addition to noninfectious causes. A partial differential diagnosis of pulmonary TB includes the following:

- Bacterial pneumonia
- Pulmonary *Mycobacterium* pneumonia (nontuberculous)
- *Pneumocystis jiroveci* pneumonia (PCP)
- *Cryptococcus neoformans* pneumonia/ pneumonitis
- Pulmonary Kaposi sarcoma
- *Toxoplasma* pneumonitis
- Disseminated histoplasmosis
- Disseminated coccidioidomycosis
- Cytomegalovirus pneumonia
- Bronchogenic carcinoma
- Non-Hodgkin lymphoma
- Influenza
- Pulmonary embolus
- Chronic obstructive pulmonary disease
- Reactive airway disease
- Congestive heart failure
- Lactic acidosis

P: Plan

Diagnostic Evaluation

Initial evaluation

Suspected TB should be evaluated aggressively.

- During the initial evaluation, check complete blood count (CBC) and differential, sputum gram stain, sputum acid-fast bacilli (AFB) stain, culture and nucleic acid amplification (NAA) (see below), blood cultures, and chest X ray.

- For patients with lymphadenopathy, consider fine-needle aspiration biopsy for bacterial and AFB stains and culture, and cytologic evaluation.

- For patients with meningitis or central nervous system abnormalities, perform lumbar puncture (LP) and cerebral spinal fluid (CSF) analysis including cell count, protein, glucose, AFB smear and culture, and bacterial and fungal cultures.

- If focal neurologic abnormalities are present, obtain computed tomography (CT) scan of the head to rule out mass lesion before doing the LP.

- Perform other diagnostic tests as suggested by the clinical presentation.

Imaging

Pulmonary TB can be associated with any chest X-ray appearance, including a normal X-ray image. However, the chest X ray classically demonstrates upper-lobe infiltrates with or without cavities. Patients with HIV infection (especially advanced HIV) are more likely to have atypical chest X-ray presentations, including absence of cavities, presence of lower-lobe disease, hilar or mediastinal adenopathy, and pleural effusions.

In disseminated TB, the chest X ray may show a miliary pattern with small nodules ("millet seeds") scattered throughout both lungs.

AFB testing

TB should be diagnosed by identification of the organism in stained sputum smears or stains of tissue by biopsy and confirmed by culture or NAA test. All positive cultures should undergo drug susceptibility testing. Proof of the diagnosis is important because other opportunistic diseases can mimic TB, and mycobacterial infections other than TB can occur; these require different treatment. Drug susceptibility testing is necessary because improper treatment of drug-resistant TB will lead to treatment failure, more severe drug resistance within the patient, and increased risk of transmission of drug-resistant TB.

Three specimens of expectorated sputum should be sent for acid-fast staining and mycobacterial culture on each of three days or at least 8 hours apart, including at least one first-morning specimen. A presumptive diagnosis of pulmonary TB can be made if acid-fast bacilli are seen, but confirmation is required. Sputum induction with nebulized saline (e.g., by respiratory therapists) can be used for patients who do not have spontaneous sputum production. (Young children cannot produce sputum, so gastric lavage on three successive mornings can be performed to obtain swallowed sputum for smear [although false-positive results can occur] and culture.)

Many laboratories will perform nucleic acid hybridization on acid-fast-positive sputum to identify the species of infecting *Mycobacteria*, and probes are available to confirm MTB and certain non-TB *Mycobacteria*. Two NAA tests are licensed in the United States, and some U.S. clinical laboratories use "in-house" NAA tests. Other NAA tests are licensed and available in other countries. These tests confirm *M. tuberculosis* in sputum smear-positive patients with a specificity of >95%, and results can be available within 24 hours of obtaining a positive smear. The rapid identification of MTB facilitates appropriate respiratory infection control precautions, contact tracing, and immediate treatment of MTB. NAA tests also are useful in making a presumptive diagnosis in smear-negative patients who are suspected to have active pulmonary TB, pending culture results. However, these tests can yield false-positive results, particularly with persons in whom pulmonary TB is unlikely. Also, false negatives can occur in both smear-positive and smear-negative patients. Other NAA tests

can be used to diagnose non-TB *Mycobacteria*. If a non-TB *Mycobacterium* is diagnosed, respiratory precautions can be discontinued, and treatment for the specific or suspected organism can be started.

Patients with suspected pulmonary TB and negative sputum microscopy or NAA should undergo bronchoscopy and transbronchial biopsy (which is more sensitive than bronchoalveolar lavage for TB). The Gen-Probe AMPLIFIED MTD Test also is approved by the U.S. Food and Drug Administration (FDA) for smear-negative cases but sensitivity in this scenario is as low as 66%, whereas specificity remains close to 100%. If the NAA test result is negative, diagnosis of TB may not be excluded, and decisions about treatment must be based on clinical assessment.

A diagnosis of extrapulmonary TB generally requires an examination of infected tissue or body fluid by microscopy and culture. NAA for MTB and some other atypical *Mycobacteria* also can be performed on tissue and body fluids (such as CSF); specimens that are fresh or frozen generally are preferable to specimens preserved in formalin or a similar chemical. Specimens of organs with suspected TB can be obtained by peripheral lymph node aspiration, CT-guided or other guided aspiration and biopsy, liver biopsy, bone marrow biopsy, or thoracoscopy- or laparoscopy-guided biopsies of pleura or peritoneum. In some cases, surgery is required to obtain appropriate specimens. Blood cultures for *Mycobacteria* (using appropriate mycobacterial media rather than standard blood culture media) may be positive in disseminated TB; the technique is the same as in culturing blood for *M. avium* complex organisms. Urine culture is used to diagnose renal TB, although this condition is rare among HIV-infected persons.

Initial growth of MTB on culture may occur within 3-8 weeks. A nucleic acid probe can confirm a positive culture as MTB within few days of culture growth; otherwise, speciation may take several weeks. Susceptibility testing generally takes 3-4 weeks after the initial culture growth, depending on what laboratory procedures are used. NAA tests for diagnosis of drug resistance are in development and early use internationally but are not yet approved for use in the United States. These are most efficient at testing for resistance against drugs for which a single mutation (e.g., rifampin) or a few mutations (e.g., isoniazid) are responsible for most clinically important drug resistance. Rapid assays to detect mutations that confer resistance to other first- and second-line drugs are in development.

Note that a positive TST or IGRA result confirms TB infection but does not prove active disease (see chapter *Latent Tuberculosis*). Similarly, a negative result may occur in up to 25% of HIV-infected persons with active TB and does not rule out TB disease. When a specific microbiologic diagnosis cannot be made or may be delayed (as with TB meningitis testing, for which CSF culture results may take weeks to obtain or may be negative), a positive TST or IGRA result can help support the diagnosis and implementation of therapy; however, a negative result on these tests does not rule out active TB.

Respiratory Precautions

Respiratory infection control precautions should be implemented for HIV-infected patients with an undiagnosed chronic cough or undiagnosed inflammatory infiltrate on chest X ray. Individual institutions have specific guidelines that should be followed; patients usually are housed in single negative-pressure rooms and persons entering the rooms are required to wear protective respirators. If three sputum smears yield negative results on AFB staining, or if a single deep specimen (bronchial lavage or tracheal aspirate) is smear negative, infectious TB is unlikely and respiratory precautions can be discontinued. Patients who are highly suspect

for MTB and lack an alternate diagnosis may be kept on precautions and empiric treatment may be started. Persons who have responded to treatment for an alternative diagnosis (e.g., bacterial pneumonia), and those who cannot produce the requisite three sputum samples, may be released from the TB precautions.

The impact of TB transmission is greater in a health care setting, where immunosuppressed persons may be exposed, than at home, where exposure has already occurred prior to the TB evaluation. Of course, children younger than age 5 and immunosuppressed persons in the home are at increased risk.

Treatment

Treatment for TB should be instituted promptly when TB is considered likely and the proper specimens to prove the diagnosis have been obtained. It is ideal to have a positive smear result (and confirmation by NAA) prior to initiating treatment, but empiric treatment can be started while the initial specimens are collected from patients in whom the suspicion of TB is high, in severely ill persons, or in circumstances in which positive smear results are unlikely (e.g., the cerebrospinal fluid smears).

Randomized trials have demonstrated that ART decreases mortality in HIV-infected persons with active TB; thus, effective ART should be initiated or optimized in everyone with TB/HIV coinfection; see "Coordinating with Antiretroviral Therapy," below.

Adherence is the most important treatment issue once the decision to treat is made and an appropriate regimen is selected. *It is the responsibility of the treating clinician to ensure that the patient completes a full course of therapy.* Therefore, it is strongly recommended that patients be referred to public health departments for TB treatment. Health departments usually can provide free TB treatment and have specific resources and systems to promote adherence. It is recommended that all patients receive directly observed therapy (DOT), an approach by which the taking of every dose of anti-TB medication is observed and documented. The intermittent therapies shown in Table 1 (regimens 1b, 2, and 3) were designed to simplify DOT; however, twice-weekly regimens should not be used for persons with CD4 counts of <100 cells/μL and once-weekly regimens with rifapentine should not be used for anyone with HIV infection.

Clinical trials have documented that DOT with enhancements to maximize adherence not only improves the rate of completion of therapy but also reduces mortality among HIV-infected TB patients. If a health department manages the TB treatment, the HIV clinician must coordinate with the health department for the following reasons: 1) to coordinate TB and HIV treatment regimens; 2) to avoid or adjust for drug interactions; 3) to assist the health department in avoiding diagnostic or treatment confusion in the event of immune reconstitution inflammatory syndrome (IRIS) or incident opportunistic diseases; and 4) to maximize adherence with the TB medications, ART, opportunistic infection treatment or prophylaxis, and any other medications.

U.S. guidelines for TB treatment in HIV-infected persons are shown in Table 1; dosages are given in Table 2.

Recommended (drug-susceptible TB):

- **Initial Phase:** Isoniazid + rifampin (or rifabutin) + pyrazinamide + ethambutol once daily for 8 weeks

- **Continuation Phase:** isoniazid + rifampin or rifabutin

Four anti-TB drugs are administered for the first 2 months, then two drugs are administered for an additional 4 months (if the organism is susceptible to standard medications). The initial phase of TB treatment usually consists of isoniazid, rifampin or rifabutin (see below), pyrazinamide, and ethambutol; the continuation phase typically is simplified to isoniazid and rifampin. Pyridoxine (vitamin B6) at a dosage of 10-50 mg per day usually is included to minimize the risk of isoniazid-induced peripheral neuropathy. If drug resistance or MDR is suspected, more drugs can be used initially, and treatment should be directed by experts. Resistance may be suspected among persons exposed to TB in countries with high rates of endemic resistance, those for whom previous treatment has failed, those who have been on and off treatment erratically, those who may have had a specific exposure to drug-resistant TB, and those who have been diagnosed during an outbreak.

In certain circumstances treatment duration is extended. In cavitary TB or TB in an HIV-infected person that remains sputum culture positive after 2 months of treatment, the two-drug continuation phase should be extended to 7 months for a total treatment course of 9 months. For extrapulmonary TB in HIV-infected persons, a 6- to 9-month course of treatment is recommended. Exceptions include meningeal TB and bone or joint TB, which are treated for 9-12 months. If cultures obtained prior to treatment demonstrate drug resistance, the regimen and the duration of therapy may need to be changed.

For TB meningitis or pericarditis, a course of corticosteroids may be given in addition to specific anti-TB therapy: dexamethasone 0.3-0.4 mg/kg/day tapered over the course of 6-8 weeks or prednisone 1 mg/kg/day for 3 weeks followed by a taper over the course of 3-5 weeks. For adrenal insufficiency, replacement corticosteroids should be given.

Section 6: Comorbidities, Coinfections, and Complications

Table 1. Regimens for Treatment of Tuberculosis Among HIV-Infected Persons in the United States

Initial Phase		Continuation Phase			Complete Therapy
Drugs	Interval and Dosages (minimum duration)	Regimen	Drugs	Interval and Dosages (minimum duration)	Range of Total Doses (minimum duration)
1. Preferred Regimen					
Isoniazid Rifampin* Pyrazinamide Ethambutol	7 days/week for 56 doses or 5 days/week for 40 doses (8 weeks)	For any CD4 count	Isoniazid Rifampin*	7 days/week for 126 doses or 5 days/week for 90 doses (18 weeks)#	182-130 doses (26 weeks)
		Alternative if CD4 count >100 cells/µL	Isoniazid Rifampin*	Twice weekly for 36 doses (18 weeks)***#	92-76 doses (26 weeks)
2. Acceptable Alternatives if CD4 >100 cells/µL					
Isoniazid Rifampin* Pyrazinamide Ethambutol	7 days/week for 14 doses (2 weeks) followed by twice weekly for 12 doses (6 weeks) OR 5 days/week for 10 doses (2 weeks) followed by twice weekly for 12 doses (6 weeks)		Isoniazid Rifampin*	Twice weekly for 36 doses (18 weeks)***#	62-58 doses (26 weeks)
OR					
Isoniazid Rifampin* Pyrazinamide Ethambutol	3 times weekly for 24 doses (8 weeks)		Isoniazid Rifampin*	3 times weekly for 54 doses (18 weeks)#	72 doses (26 weeks)

* See Table 2 for dosages. See Table 3 for contraindications, substitutions, and dosage adjustments of rifampin. Rifampin should not be used with etravirine, nevirapine, maraviroc, or with protease inhibitors other than ritonavir; rifabutin may be substituted with appropriate dosage adjustments (see U.S. Department of Health and Human Services. *Guidelines for the Use of Antiretroviral Agents in HIV-1-Infected Adults and Adolescents*; Tables 15a-e. January 10, 2011. Available at www.aidsinfo.nih.gov/guidelines/).

** In HIV-infected persons with a CD4 count ≤100 cells/µL, twice-weekly regimens should not be used. For these patients, most experts recommend daily treatment during the induction phase.

\# For patients who experience slow responses, and those in whom sputum cultures are still positive after the initial 2 months of treatment, the continuation phase may be extended to 7 months, for a total of 9 months of treatment. Pediatric patients should be treated for 7 months in the continuation phase, for a total of 9 months of treatment. TB meningitis caused by susceptible organisms should be treated for 9-12 months. Bone and joint TB should be treated for 9-12 months; the longer time may be prudent when multiple bones and joints are involved or when it is difficult to document a response to treatment. Extrapulmonary disease in other sites should be treated for 6-9 months.

Adapted from American Thoracic Society, CDC, and Infectious Disease Society of America. *Treatment of Tuberculosis*. Morb Mort Weekly Rpts Recommendations and Reports. June 20, 2003, 52(RR11);1-77.

Table 2. Dosages of First-Line Anti-TB Drugs: U.S. Formulary

Agent	Daily or 5 Times/Week Dosage (maximum)		2 Times/Week Dosage (maximum)			3 Times/Week Dosage (maximum)
	Adults	Children	Adults	Children	Adults	Children
Isoniazid* (tablets: 100 and 300 mg)	5 mg/kg (300 mg maximum)	10-15 mg/kg (300 mg max)	15 mg/kg (900 mg maximum)	20-30 mg/kg (900 mg maximum)	15 mg/kg (900 mg maximum)	NA
Rifampin** (capsules: 150 and 300 mg)	10 mg/kg (600 mg maximum)	10-20 mg/kg (600 mg max)	10 mg/kg (600 mg maximum)	10-20 mg/kg (600 mg maximum)	10 mg/kg (600 mg maximum)	NA
Pyrazinamide (tablets: 500 mg)		10-30 mg/kg (2 g max)		10-30 mg/kg (2 g maximum)		NA
40-55 kg body weight	1,000 mg		2,000 mg		1,500 mg	
56-75 kg body weight	1,500 mg		3,000 mg		2,500 mg	
>75 kg body weight	2,000 mg		4,000 mg		3,500 mg	
Ethambutol (tablets: 100 and 400 mg)		10-20 mg/kg (1 g max)		10-20 mg/kg (1 g maximum)		NA
40-55 kg body weight	800 mg		2,000 mg		1,200 mg	
56-75 kg body weight	1,200 mg		2,800 mg		2,000 mg	
>75 kg body weight	1,600 mg		4,000 mg		2,400 mg	
Rifamate# (capsules: isoniazid 150 mg, rifampin 300 mg)	2 capsules daily	NA	NA	NA	NA	NA
Rifater## (tablets: isoniazid 50 mg, rifampin 120 mg, pyrazinamide 300 mg)	≤44 kg: 4 tablets 45-54 kg: 5 tablets 55-90 kg: 6 tablets	NA	NA	NA	NA	NA

Typical daily dosage for a 60 kg patient is as follows: isoniazid 300 mg (2 tablets), rifampin 600 mg (2 capsules), pyrazinamide 1,500 mg (3 tablets), ethambutol 1,200 mg (3 tablets).

* Add pyridoxine 10-25 mg per dose of isoniazid.
** See Table 3 for dosage adjustments or rifabutin substitution based on combination with antiretroviral therapy.
\# Suitable for daily dosing during continuation phase.
\## May be part of daily initial phase combined with ethambutol tablets.

Adapted from: Table 3. Centers for Disease Control and Prevention. *Guidelines for prevention and treatment of opportunistic infections in HIV-infected adults and adolescents. Recommendations from the Centers for Disease Control, the National Institutes of Health, and the HIV Medicine Association of the Infectious Diseases Society of America.* April 10, 2009. Available at www.aidsinfo.nih.gov/guidelines.

Considerations during pregnancy

Pyrazinamide has not been formally proven safe for use during pregnancy; however, it is used during pregnancy in many countries and there have been no reports of problems. Some health departments in the United States avoid the use of pyrazinamide for pregnant women and extend the continuation phase to 7 months, whereas others prescribe the standard regimens shown in Table 1 during pregnancy. Streptomycin and certain second-line drugs should be avoided during pregnancy. HIV-infected women in the United States are instructed not to breast-feed, so there usually are no issues regarding TB treatment of HIV-infected women during breast-feeding. ART should be started as early as possible; consult with an expert.

Coordinating with Antiretroviral Therapy

ART and TB treatment must be coordinated for both to be successful. ART is indicated for all adults and adolescents with active TB, and both metaanalyses and randomized trials have demonstrated reduction in mortality when ART is combined with anti-TB chemotherapy.

The optimal timing of ART initiation in relation to TB therapy is not well established, but recent studies have shown that the risk of death is substantially lower if ART is initiated early, particularly in patients with low CD4 cell counts. Recent recommendations for the timing of ART initiation are based on CD4 thresholds. Adults and adolescents with active TB and CD4 counts of <200 cells/μL should start ART within 2-4 weeks of starting TB

treatment. Those with CD4 counts of 200-350 cells/μL should start ART within 2-4 weeks, or at least within 8 weeks of starting TB therapy, and those with CD4 counts >500 cells/μL should start ART within 8 weeks of starting TB therapy. In all cases, TB treatment should be started immediately.

Although paradoxical immune responses (i.e., IRIS, see below) may be more common in patients who start ART earlier in the course of TB treatment, IRIS generally is not fatal.

Drug-Drug Interactions

Drug interactions between TB medications and ARVs may require dosage adjustments or modifications in treatment (see Table 3). Rifampin is a potent inducer of cytochrome P450 enzymes and has many clinically important drug interactions. It reduces the blood levels of nonnucleoside reverse transcriptase inhibitors (NNRTIs), protease inhibitors (PIs), the integrase inhibitor raltegravir, and the CCR5 antagonist maraviroc, but does not affect nucleoside/nucleotide reverse transcriptase inhibitors (NRTIs) or the fusion inhibitor enfuvirtide. Triple nucleoside regimens can be administered safely during rifampin treatment but are less potent than first-line ARV combinations and generally are not recommended. The safest ARV combination to use with rifampin is a two-drug NRTI backbone with efavirenz (see Table 3). Some clinicians increase the efavirenz dosage to 800 mg/day because efavirenz blood levels may be reduced 25% by concomitant rifampin. Limited clinical data support the use of nevirapine at standard dosages in combination with rifampin. This is not a favored approach because nevirapine levels are reduced up to 50% when combined with rifampin. In one study, 20% of patients on ARV and TB treatment with rifampin had trough nevirapine levels that were below target, although they achieved the same rates of HIV RNA suppression as patients on efavirenz.

To avoid rifampin-ARV interactions, rifabutin typically is used in place of rifampin. Rifabutin has fewer marked effects on the pharmacokinetics of other drugs, although its own blood concentrations can be affected by certain ARVs. Dosing recommendations for rifabutin with ARVs are found in Table 3. Rifabutin is expensive; some public

health systems do not provide rifabutin as part of TB treatment and it generally is not available in resource-limited countries. The FDA characterizes rifabutin in pregnancy category B: it has been safe in animal studies of pregnancy but has not been proven safe for humans. For pregnant women who require both TB and ARV therapy, the use of rifabutin rather than rifampin allows the use of non-efavirenz-based ARV regimens.

Persons who are already on ART when TB treatment is begun must have their ARV regimens reassessed; the appropriate dosages of rifampin or rifabutin must be chosen or the ARV regimen must be modified, at least until completion of TB treatment.

Table 3. Interactions Between Antiretroviral Medications and Rifampin or Rifabutin: Contraindicated Combinations and Dosage Adjustments

Antiretroviral Agent	Rifampin	Rifabutin* (Preferred in combination with PIs, boosted or unboosted)
Nonnucleoside Reverse Transcriptase Inhibitors		
Delavirdine	Never combine	Never combine
Efavirenz** (Preferred in combination with rifampin, see exceptions)	Rifampin dosage unchanged; efavirenz dosage 600-800 mg daily	Use standard efavirenz dosage. Increase rifabutin to 450-600 mg daily or 600 mg TIW.
Etravirine	Never combine	Etravirine without ritonavir-boosted PI: dose rifabutin at 300 mg daily. Etravirine with a boosted PI: DO NOT use with rifabutin.
Nevirapine	Do not combine; 25-50% reduction in nevirapine levels	Use standard dosage of nevirapine. Dose rifabutin at 300 mg daily or TIW.
Protease Inhibitors, Nonboosted		
Atazanavir	Never combine	Use atazanavir at standard dosage. Dose rifabutin at 150 mg QOD or TIW.
Fosamprenavir	Never combine	Use PIs at standard dosage. Dose rifabutin 150 mg daily or 300 mg TIW.
Indinavir	Never combine	Increase indinavir dosage to 1,000 mg Q8H. Dose rifabutin at 150 mg daily or 300 mg TIW.
Nelfinavir	Never combine	Increase nelfinavir dosage to 1,000 mg Q8H. Dose rifabutin at 150 mg daily or 300 mg TIW.
Ritonavir	May be used at standard dosages; limited clinical experience	Use ritonavir at standard dosage. Dose rifabutin at 150 mg QOD or TIW.
Protease Inhibitors, Ritonavir-Boosted		
Lopinavir/ritonavir (Kaletra)	Lopinavir/ritonavir must be supplemented with additional ritonavir 300 mg BID; high rates of hepatotoxicity; should not be used	Use standard dosage of lopinavir/ritonavir. Usual rifabutin dosage: 150 mg QOD or TIW.***
Saquinavir/ritonavir	Owing to high rates of hepatotoxicity, this combination should not be used	Use standard dosage of saquinavir/ritonavir. Usual rifabutin dosage: 150 mg QOD or TIW.***
All other ritonavir-boosted PIs	Should not be used (adequate dosing regimens not defined)	Use standard dosage of PI/ritonavir. Usual rifabutin dosage: 150 mg QOD or TIW.***
Integrase Inhibitors		
Raltegravir	Increase raltegravir dosage to 800 mg BID; monitor for virologic response	No dosage adjustment.

Antiretroviral Agent	Rifampin	Rifabutin* (Preferred in combination with PIs, boosted or unboosted)
CCR5 Receptor Antagonists		
Maraviroc	Not recommended; if used without a strong CYP 3A4 inhibitor: 600 mg BID; if used with a strong CYP 3A4 inhibitor: 300 mg BID	Without a strong CYP 3A4 inhibitor: 300 mg BID. With a strong CYP 3A4 inhibitor: 150 mg BID.
Fusion Inhibitors		
Enfuvirtide	No dosage adjustment	No dosage adjustment

Note: NRTIs are given in standard dosages with either rifampin or rifabutin.

* If available, rifabutin may be substituted for rifampin when TB treatment and ART are combined.

** Avoid use of efavirenz during pregnancy and with women who may become pregnant while on therapy. Both rifampin and rifabutin significantly reduce estrogen and progestin levels for women on hormonal contraceptives; efavirenz raises estrogen levels moderately. Two forms of birth control including one barrier method and either a mid-to-high-dose hormonal contraceptive or an intrauterine device are recommended most often. Barrier methods are recommended for women who are infertile, in order to reduce HIV transmission.

*** Cases of inadequate rifabutin levels and rifamycin resistance in patients on rifabutin 150 mg QOD or TIW and ritonavir-boosted PIs. Consider rifabutin 150 mg QD or 300 mg TIW. Monitor rifabutin drug levels, if possible.

Adapted from U.S. Centers for Disease Control and Prevention. *Managing Drug Interactions in the Treatment of HIV-Related Tuberculosis.* Available at www.cdc.gov/tb/TB_HIV_Drugs/default.htm; and U.S. Department of Health and Human Services. *Guidelines for the Use of Antiretroviral Agents in HIV-1-Infected Adults and Adolescents.* January 10, 2011. Available at www.aidsinfo.nih.gov/guideline.

Monitoring for efficacy

Ideally, every dose of anti-TB therapy is observed and documented by a health care agent or responsible individual. Patients' adherence should be evaluated by a health care team member at least weekly during the initial phase of treatment and at least weekly or monthly during the continuation phase. If gaps in medication use occur, the cause must be evaluated and a plan to improve adherence must be implemented.

In treatment of pulmonary TB, monthly sputum specimens should be obtained for smear and culture until two sequential specimens are sterile on culture. Patients with extrapulmonary and disseminated TB usually are monitored clinically and with imaging studies. Biopsies are not repeated but other specimens (CSF and other body fluids) may be obtained for repeat AFB smear and culture. Monitoring of patients with extrapulmonary and disseminated TB should be done in consultation with an expert.

Immune reconstitution inflammatory syndrome

Patients on treatment for active TB who begin ART may experience a paradoxical increase in signs and symptoms of TB (fever, dyspnea, increased cough, enlarging lymph nodes, worsening chest X-ray findings, increased inflammation at other involved sites, or enlargement of central nervous system tuberculomas). These often are attributable to an enhanced immune response against remaining MTB organisms that occurs because of immunologic improvement from ART. IRIS may occur at any point from within 2 weeks up to several months after ART is initiated, and usually is accompanied by a sharp drop in HIV viral load and at least a twofold increase in the CD4 lymphocyte count. TB treatment failure (potentially owing to an inappropriate treatment regimen, inadequate adherence, or drug resistance) must be ruled out, and the possibility of drug toxicity should be considered. If IRIS is diagnosed, TB and HIV treatment should be continued and symptoms managed with nonsteroidal antiinflammatory drugs or, in severe cases, with a short course of corticosteroids. (See chapter *Immune Reconstitution Inflammatory Syndrome.*)

Adverse effects of anti-TB medications

Anti-TB medications may have significant adverse effects. The most important adverse reactions reported for the commonly used anti-TB medications are listed in Table 4. The most frequent toxicities of first-line TB medications include hepatic enzyme elevations. Before initiating TB treatment, conduct a complete blood count with platelet count, serum creatinine count, liver function tests (aspartate aminotransferase [AST], alanine aminotransferase [ALT], bilirubin, alkaline phosphatase), and hepatitis B and C serology. Newly diagnosed TB patients with unknown HIV status should be tested for HIV infection.

Patients should be monitored monthly with a symptom review to assess possible toxicity, and laboratory tests should be performed if symptoms suggest adverse effects. For patients with liver disease, it may be prudent to perform routine laboratory monitoring after 1 month on treatment and every 3 months thereafter. Persons with symptoms and aminotransferase elevations ≥3 times the upper limit of normal, and asymptomatic persons with aminotransferase elevations ≥5 times the upper limit of normal, should have therapy interrupted and should be managed thereafter in consultation with an expert.

Patients should be monitored for isoniazid-induced peripheral neuropathy; this adverse effect is rare if pyridoxine is administered with isoniazid, as recommended. Testing of visual acuity and red-green color vision is recommended at the start of therapy with ethambutol. Persons on standard ethambutol dosages with normal baseline examinations should be asked monthly about visual disturbances. Patients on higher ethambutol dosages and those who have been on ethambutol for more than 2 months should have periodic eye examinations for acuity and color discrimination.

Table 4. Adverse Events Associated with Common Anti-TB Medications

Medication	Common Toxicity	Rare Toxicity
First-Line Agents		
Isoniazid	Transient aminotransferase elevation, hepatitis, positive antinuclear antibody (ANA)	Peripheral neurotoxicity, lupus-like syndrome, central nervous system effects, hypersensitivity, rash, monoamine poisoning
Rifampin	Transient bilirubin elevation, anorexia, nausea, vomiting, hepatitis, red-orange discoloration of urine and tears	Acute renal failure, shock, thrombocytopenia, rash, "flu" syndrome from intermittent doses, pseudomembranous colitis, pseudoadrenal crisis, osteomalacia, hemolytic anemia
Rifabutin	Elevated liver function tests, nausea, red-orange discoloration of urine and tears	Cytopenias, uveitis, rash
Ethambutol	Optic neuritis	Skin rash, joint pains, peripheral neuropathy
Pyrazinamide	Joint pains, gout, hepatitis	Gastrointestinal symptoms, skin rash, sideroblastic anemia
Streptomycin	Auditory and vestibular nerve damage, renal injury	Rash
Second-Line Agents		
Moxifloxacin	Nausea, diarrhea, dizziness	Tendon rupture, hepatotoxicity, renal damage, prolonged QT interval, skin reactions
Amikacin/ Kanamycin	Auditory, vestibular, renal injury	

Adapted from American Thoracic Society; CDC; Infectious Diseases Society of America. *Treatment of Tuberculosis.* MMWR Recomm Rep. 2003 Jun 20;52(RR-11):1-77; and Harries A, Maher D, Gramm S; World Health Organization. *HIV/TB: A Clinical Manual, 2nd Edition.* Geneva: World Health Organization; 2004:131-2.

Patient Education

- All patients with TB-positive sputum or bronchoscopy specimens can infect others with TB. All close contacts, especially children, should be screened for TB as soon as possible and given medication to prevent (or treat) active disease.

- The health department will be notified of each TB case and will provide the required follow-up care.

- Patients must take all medicines exactly as prescribed. If doses are missed, or if the medication is stopped and restarted, the TB bacteria can develop resistance to even the best medications and become even more dangerous. If patients are having trouble taking the medication on schedule, they should contact their health care provider immediately.

- If patients become ill, if their skin or eyes turn yellow, or if their urine darkens to a cola color, they should contact their health care provider immediately.

- Patients must keep all follow-up appointments. Blood tests will be done regularly to ensure that the liver is working well, and patients will be checked for medication adverse effects. They should show their health care provider all medications, vitamins, and supplements they are taking so that the provider can check for drug interactions.

- Rifampin and rifabutin will make urine, sweat, and tears turn orange; this is not harmful. They will cause staining of plastic contact lens; patients should avoid wearing contact lenses if they are taking rifamycins.

- Rifampin and rifabutin will cause birth control pills to become ineffective. An alternative method of contraception should be used when the patient is undergoing treatment.

- The use of alcohol should be avoided during treatment with TB drugs to avoid the risk of liver damage.

References

- Abdool Karim SS, Naidoo K, Grobler A, et al. *Timing of initiation of antiretroviral drugs during tuberculosis.* N Engl J Med. 2010 Feb 25;362(8):697-706.

- American Thoracic Society; Center for Disease Control and Prevention; Infectious Diseases Society of America. *Treatment of Tuberculosis.* MMWR Recomm Rep. 2003 Jun 20;52(RR-11):1-77. Available at www.aidsinfo.nih.gov/guidelines. Accessed June 30, 2010.

- Blumberg HM, Leonard MK Jr, Jasmer RM. *Update on the treatment of tuberculosis and latent tuberculosis infection.* JAMA. 2005 Jun 8;293(22):2776-84.

- Centers for Disease Control and Prevention. *Guidelines for Prevention and Treatment of Opportunistic Infections in HIV-Infected Adults and Adolescents: Recommendations from CDC, the National Institutes of Health, and the HIV Medicine Association of the Infectious Diseases Society of America.* April 10, 2009. Available at www.aidsinfo.nih.gov/guidelines/.

- Centers for Disease Control and Prevention. *Updated guidelines for the use of nucleic acid amplification tests for the diagnosis of tuberculosis.* MMWR Morb Mortal Wkly Rep. 2009 Jan 16;58(1):7-10.

- Centers for Disease Control and Prevention. *Updated Guidelines for the Use of Rifamycins for the Treatment of Tuberculosis Among HIV-Infected Patients Taking Protease Inhibitors or Nonnucleoside Reverse Transcriptase Inhibitors.* Updated January 20, 2004. Available at www.aidsinfo.nih.gov/guidelines.

- Centers for Disease Control and Prevention. *Acquired rifamycin resistance in persons with advanced HIV disease being treated for active tuberculosis with intermittent rifamycin-based regimens.* MMWR Morb Mortal Wkly Rep. 2002 Mar 15;51(10):214-5. Available at www.aidsinfo.nih.gov/guidelines. Accessed June 30, 2010.

- Iseman MD. *A Clinician's Guide to Tuberculosis.* Philadelphia: Lippincott Williams & Wilkins; 2000.

- Mandell G, Bennett JE, Dolin R, et al. *Mandell, Douglas, and Bennett's Principles and Practice of Infectious Diseases, 7th Edition.* Philadelphia: Churchill Livingstone Elsevier; 2010.

- Manosuthi W, Sungkanuparph S, Tantanathip P, et al; N2R Study Team. *A randomized trial comparing plasma drug levels and efficacies between 2 nonnucleoside reverse transcriptase-inhibitor therapies in HIV-infected patients receiving rifampin: the N2R study.* Clin Infect Dis. 2009 Jun 15;48(12):1752-9.

- Reider HL. *Interventions for Tuberculosis Control and Elimination. Paris: International Union Against Tuberculosis and Lung Disease; 2002.* Available at www.tbrieder.org. Accessed June 30, 2010.

- U.S. Department of Health and Human Services. *Guidelines for the Use of Antiretroviral Agents in HIV-1-Infected Adults and Adolescents.* January 10, 2011. Available at www.aidsinfo.nih.gov/guidelines/.

Pelvic Inflammatory Disease

Background

Pelvic inflammatory disease (PID) is the syndrome resulting from the ascent of microorganisms from the vagina and cervix to the uterine endometrium, fallopian tubes, ovaries, or contiguous abdominal structures. Many episodes of PID go unrecognized, because of lack of symptoms or mild, nonspecific symptoms (e.g., dyspareunia, abnormal bleeding, and vaginal discharge). Infecting organisms may include *Neisseria gonorrhoeae* (GC) and *Chlamydia trachomatis* (CT), which are sexually transmitted, as well as anaerobic bacteria (*Gardnerella vaginalis* or *Haemophilus influenzae*), gram-negative rods (*Escherichia coli*), *Streptococcus agalactiae*, gastrointestinal flora, and mycoplasmas (*Mycoplasma hominis*). It is thought that PID generally is caused by sexually transmitted infections (STIs) and that additional organisms become involved after infection spreads and protective immunological barriers are disrupted.

Between 20% and 40% of women with cervical chlamydial infection and 10-20% of women with gonococcal infection eventually develop PID, but accurate estimates of the incidence of PID and infertility resulting from GC and CT are difficult to obtain. Hospitalizations for PID declined steadily throughout the 1980s and 1990s but remained relatively constant between 2000 and 2006, at approximately 80,000 annually.

PID is co-epidemic with HIV among some urban populations of reproductive age. Data on PID outcomes among HIV-infected women are limited. Many studies have documented no difference in length or severity of lower abdominal pain, vaginal discharge, fever, abnormal vaginal bleeding, or low back pain between HIV-infected and HIV-uninfected women with PID. However, there is a higher rate of tubo-ovarian abscesses and severe salpingitis and pyosalpinx among HIV-infected women.

Clinical presentation may include salpingitis, endometritis, tubal and ovarian abscess, and pelvic peritonitis, although PID may present with subtle or mild symptoms even in HIV-infected women. Long-term complications of PID may include infertility, ectopic pregnancy, pelvic adhesions, and chronic pain. After a single episode of PID, a woman's risk of ectopic pregnancy increases sevenfold. Approximately 13% of women are infertile after a single episode of PID, 25-35% after two episodes, and 50-75% after three or more episodes.

Diagnosis of PID usually is based on clinical findings, and providers should maintain a low threshold for diagnosing and promptly treating this disease, as it can wreak havoc on a woman's reproductive health. All women who are diagnosed with PID should be tested for GC and CT.

S: Subjective

The patient may complain of mild-to-moderate lower abdominal pain and tenderness, pain with intercourse, vaginal discharge, fever, chills, heavy menstrual bleeding, or other abnormal vaginal bleeding.

Inquire about the following during the history:

- Symptoms listed above, and duration
- Sexual history including new sex partner(s) and episodes of unprotected sex
- Last menstrual period
- Previous diagnosis of gonorrhea or chlamydia
- Previous abdominal or gynecologic surgery
- History of recent intrauterine device (IUD) placement (the risk of PID associated with IUD use is confined primarily to the first 3 weeks after insertion)

O: Objective

Check vital signs with special attention to temperature (may be elevated or normal).

Perform a focused physical examination. Check abdomen (bowel sounds, distention, rebound, guarding, masses, suprapubic and costovertebral angle [CVA] tenderness); perform complete pelvic examination looking for abnormal bleeding or discharge; uterine, adnexal, or cervical motion tenderness; pelvic masses or adnexal enlargement.

A: Assessment

A partial differential diagnosis includes the following:

- Pregnancy, uterine or ectopic
- Ruptured or hemorrhagic ovarian cyst
- Dysmenorrhea
- Appendicitis
- Pyelonephritis
- Diverticulitis
- Irritable bowel syndrome
- Cystitis
- Uterine fibroids/leiomyomas
- Ovarian torsion
- Mittelschmerz
- Kidney stones
- Pyelonephritis

P: Plan

Diagnostic Evaluation

A diagnosis of PID usually is based on clinical findings; however, the following can support a diagnosis and help rule out other causes of abdominal pain:

- Pregnancy test
- Nucleic acid amplification tests (NAAT) or culture for GC and CT
- Gram stain of endocervical discharge
- Microscopic examination of saline preparation of vaginal secretions

Often, diagnosis must be made and treatment initiated on the basis of clinical criteria. Current guidelines identify three "minimal criteria" found on pelvic examination in patients with PID:

- Cervical motion tenderness
- Uterine tenderness
- Adnexal tenderness

The following signs support a diagnosis of PID:

- Oral temperature >101°F (>38.3°C)

- Abnormal cervical or vaginal mucopurulent discharge

- Presence of abundant numbers of white blood cells on saline microscopy of vaginal secretions (this also can detect concomitant infections such as bacterial vaginosis and trichomoniasis)

- Elevated erythrocyte sedimentation rate (ESR)

- Elevated C-reactive protein (CRP)

- Laboratory documentation of cervical infection with GC or CT (the absence of infection from the lower genital tract, where samples are usually obtained, does not exclude PID and should not influence the decision to treat)

Definitive diagnosis may be made on the basis of:

- Endometrial biopsy with histopathologic evidence of endometritis

- Transvaginal sonogram or other imaging showing thickened, fluid-filled tubes with or without free pelvic fluid or tubo-ovarian complex

- Laparoscopic abnormalities consistent with PID

Treatment

Because clinical diagnostic criteria for PID are not always conclusive, presumptive diagnosis and early empiric treatment is common. The positive predictive value of a clinical diagnosis is 65-90%.

Empiric therapy for PID should be started in women who have one or more of the minimal criteria, plus pelvic or lower abdominal pain and risk factors for PID (sexually active young women, women at risk of STIs), unless another cause for the symptoms is identified.

Treatment considerations

Antimicrobial regimens must be broadly effective against likely pathogens (see below). HIV-infected women appear to respond as well to standard antibiotic regimens as do HIV-uninfected women. It is not known whether HIV-infected women with advanced immunosuppression should be treated more aggressively; decisions about whether to use oral or parenteral therapy must be individualized.

Resistance to fluoroquinolone by GC is widespread in the United States and elsewhere; thus, this class of antibiotics is no longer recommended for treatment of PID.

No evidence suggests that IUDs should be removed in women diagnosed with PID. However, caution should be used if the IUD remains in place, and close clinical follow-up is recommended.

The goals of treatment include the following:

- Alleviate the pain and systemic malaise associated with infection

- Achieve microbiological cure

- Prevent development of permanent tubal damage with associated problems, such as chronic pelvic pain, ectopic pregnancy, and infertility

- Prevent the transmission of infection to others

Indications for hospitalization of patients with PID include the following:

- Unsure diagnosis; surgical emergency cannot be excluded

- Pregnancy

- Patient does not respond clinically (within 72 hours) to oral antimicrobial therapy

- Tubo-ovarian abscess

- Severe illness with nausea and vomiting or high fever

- Inability to follow or tolerate outpatient regimen

Pregnancy

If the patient is pregnant, aggressive treatment is essential to prevent preterm delivery, fetal loss, and maternal morbidity. Some medications should be avoided to reduce the risk of fetal toxicity; these include doxycycline and gentamicin. Hospitalization for parenteral antibiotic therapy is recommended.

Antibiotic Regimens

Recommended Oral/Outpatient Regimens

- Ceftriaxone 250 mg IM in a single dose + doxycycline 100 mg PO BID for 14 days, with or without metronidazole 500 mg PO BID for 14 days

- Cefoxitin 2 g IM in a single dose and probenecid 1 g PO concurrently in a single dose + doxycycline 100 mg PO BID for 14 days, with or without metronidazole 500 mg PO BID for 14 days

- Other parenteral third-generation cephalosporin (e.g., ceftizoxime or cefotaxime) + doxycycline 100 mg PO BID for 14 days, with or without metronidazole 500 mg PO BID for 14 days

Alternative Oral Regimens

If parenteral cephalosporin therapy is not feasible, consult with an expert. Some evidence supports the use of amoxicillin/clavulanic acid with doxycycline, and azithromycin with or without metronidazole or ceftriaxone. Because of the prevalence of fluoroquinolone-resistant GC, use of fluoroquinolones is no longer recommended but may be considered, with or without metronidazole, if the community prevalence and patient's risk of gonorrhea is low. For more information, see the CDC STD Treatment Guidelines (see "References," below).

Recommended Parenteral Regimens

- Cefotetan 2 g IV Q12H + doxycycline 100 mg PO BID

- Cefoxitin 2 g IV Q6H + doxycycline 100 mg PO BID

- Clindamycin 900 mg IV Q8H + gentamicin loading dose IV or IM (2 mg/kg of body weight), followed by a maintenance dose (1.5 mg/kg) Q8H; single daily dosing (3-5 mg/kg) may be substituted

Alternative Parental Regimen

- Ampicillin/sulbactam 3 g IV Q6H + doxycycline 100 mg PO BID

Women who are started on oral antibiotics but do not respond within 72 hours should be reevaluated to confirm the diagnosis of PID and should be administered parenteral therapy on either an outpatient or inpatient basis. Patients who are treated with parenteral antibiotics usually can be transitioned to oral antibiotics within 24 hours of clinical improvement.

Follow-Up

- Patients should show significant clinical improvement within 3 days of initiation of therapy (e.g., improvement in fever, abdominal tenderness, and uterine, adnexal, and cervical motion tenderness). If the patient has not improved, consider hospitalization, additional diagnostic testing, or surgical intervention. Patients who are hospitalized for treatment initially may be switched to an oral regimen and be discharged on oral therapy after they have improved clinically.

- Evaluate sex partners and offer them treatment if they had sexual contact with the patient during the 60 days preceding the patient's onset of symptoms. Treat empirically for both chlamydia and gonorrhea.

- Some specialists recommend rescreening for GC and CT after therapy is completed in women with documented infection with these pathogens.

- Provide education about sexual risk reduction. Instruct patients to use condoms with every sexual contact to prevent reinfection with GC and CT, to prevent other STIs, and to prevent passing HIV to sex partners.

- Studies of patients treated for CT infection show reinfection rates as high as 13% within 4 months of treatment, highlighting the need for follow-up and partner treatment.

Patient Education

- Instruct patients to take all of their medications. Advise patients to take medications with food if they feel nauseated, and to contact the clinic promptly if they experience vomiting or are unable to take their medications.

- Sex partners from the previous 60 days need to be tested for sexually transmitted pathogens and treated as soon as possible with a regimen effective against GC and CT, even if they have no symptoms. Advise patients to inform their partners that they need to be tested and treated. Otherwise, they may be reinfected.

- Advise patients to avoid sexual contact until the infection has been cured.

- Provide education about sexual risk reduction. Instruct patients to use condoms with every sexual contact to prevent becoming reinfected, to prevent other STIs, and to prevent passing HIV to sex partners.

- Advise patients that PID can recur, and that they should contact the clinic if symptoms such as pain or fever develop.

- Patients must not drink beer, wine, or any other alcoholic beverage while taking metronidazole, and for at least 24-48 hours after the last dose. Metronidazole may cause a disulfiram-like reaction, resulting in severe nausea and vomiting. Note that patients taking ritonavir capsules may experience symptoms caused by the small amount of alcohol in the capsules; advise patients to contact the clinic if nausea and vomiting occur.

Section 6: Comorbidities, Coinfections, and Complications

References

- Abularach S, Anderson J. *Gynecologic Problems*. In: Anderson JR, ed. *A Guide to the Clinical Management of Women with HIV*. Rockville, MD: Health Resources and Services Administration, HIV/AIDS Bureau; 2005. Available at hab.hrsa.gov/publications/womencare05/WG05chap6.htm. Accessed June 30, 2010.

- Centers for Disease Control and Prevention. *Sexually Transmitted Diseases Treatment Guidelines*, 2010. MMWR 2010 Dec 17; 59 (No. RR- 12):1-110. Available at www.cdc.gov/STD/treatment/2010.

- Cohn SE, Clark RA. *Sexually transmitted diseases, HIV, and AIDS in women*. In: *The Medical Clinics of North America*, vol. 87; 2003:971-995.

- Handsfield HH, Sparling PF. *Gonococcal Infections*. In: Goldman L, Ausiello D, eds. *Cecil Medicine*; 23rd edition. Philadelphia: Saunders Elsevier; 2007.

- Handsfield HH, Sparling FP. *Neisseria Gonorrhoeae*. In: Mandell GL, Bennett JE, Dolin R, eds. *Mandell, Douglas, and Bennett's Principles and Practice of Infectious Diseases*. Vol. 7. New York: Churchill Livingstone; 2010.

- Trussell J. *Contraceptive Efficacy*. In: Hatcher RA, Trussell J, Nelson AL, et al. *Contraceptive Technology: 19th Revised Edition*. New York: Ardent Media; 2007.

- Trigg BG, Kerndt PR, Aynalem G. *Sexually transmitted infections and pelvic inflammatory disease in women*. Med Clin North Am. 2008 Sep;92(5):1083-113, x.

Pneumocystis Pneumonia

Background

Pneumocystis jiroveci pneumonia (previously called *Pneumocystis carinii* pneumonia, and still abbreviated PCP), is caused by an unusual fungus, *P. jiroveci*. Many humans appear to be infected in childhood, but clinical illness occurs only in people with advanced immunosuppression, either through new infection or reactivation of latent infection. More than 90% of PCP cases occur in patients with CD4 counts of <200 cells/μL. Cases of PCP in otherwise healthy young homosexual men were among the first recognized manifestations of AIDS, in 1981. The organism can affect many organ sites, but pneumonia is by far the most common form of disease. In the United States, the incidence of PCP has declined sharply since the use of prophylaxis and effective antiretroviral therapy (ART) became widespread, but PCP is still many patients' initial presenting opportunistic infection, and it is a significant cause of morbidity and mortality among HIV-infected patients.

S: Subjective

The patient reports fever, shortness of breath, particularly with exertion, nonproductive cough, night sweats, weight loss, or fatigue. Typically, the symptoms worsen over the course of days to weeks. Pleuritic pain and retrosternal pain or burning also may be present. There may be minimal symptoms early in the disease course of PCP.

Ask the patient about fever, fatigue, and weight loss, which may be present for weeks, with gradual worsening of shortness of breath. PCP may present less commonly with acute onset symptoms of fevers, chills, sweats, dyspnea, and cough.

Note: Given the possibility of HIV-associated tuberculosis (TB), patients with cough should be kept in respiratory isolation until TB is ruled out.

O: Objective

Perform a full physical examination, with particular attention to the following:

- Vital signs, including temperature, heart rate, blood pressure, respiratory rate, oxygen saturation at rest and after exertion (there is often a sharp drop in oxygen saturation with exertion)

- Appearance

- Lung examination

Patients may appear relatively well, or acutely ill. Tachypnea may be pronounced, and patients may exhibit such a high respiratory rate (e.g., >30 breaths per minute) that they are unable to speak without stopping frequently to breathe. Chest examination may be normal, or reveal only minimal rales, although coughing is common on deep inspiration. Cyanosis may be present around the mouth, in the nail beds, and on mucous membranes. Cough is either unproductive, or productive of a thin layer of clear or whitish mucus.

A: Assessment

A partial differential diagnosis includes the following:

- Pneumococcal pneumonia

- Other bacterial pneumonias

- TB

- Influenza

- *Mycobacterium avium* complex

- Lymphocytic interstitial pneumonitis

- Bronchitis

- Cytomegalovirus (CMV) pneumonitis

- Histoplasmosis
- Other fungal pneumonia, especially cryptococcosis
- Pulmonary Kaposi sarcoma
- Asthma, chronic obstructive pulmonary disease
- Congestive heart failure
- Pulmonary hypertension

P: Plan

Diagnostic Evaluation

- **CD4 cell count:** Check records for a recent CD4 count (CD4 is <200 cells/µL in >90% of PCP cases). Note that a CD4 count obtained in the setting of acute illness (e.g., when the patient presents with pneumonia) may be substantially lower than the usual baseline, and may be difficult to interpret.

- **Pulse oximetry at rest and after exercise:** Oxygen desaturation with exercise suggests an abnormal alveolar-arterial O2 gradient (A-a gradient).

- **Arterial blood gas (ABG):** Hypoxemia is common, as is elevation in A-a gradient. Generally, PO2 levels and A-a gradient are associated with disease severity. Poorer outcomes are seen with PO2 <70 mm Hg and A-a gradient >35 mm Hg.

- **Lactate dehydrogenase (LDH):** Elevated serum LDH (>300-500 IU/L) is common.

- **Chest X ray:** Typically shows bilateral interstitial infiltrates, but atypical patterns with cavitation, lobar infiltrates, nodules, or pneumothorax may occur, and chest X-ray findings may be normal in some cases. Upper-lobe predominance is common if the patient is receiving aerosolized pentamidine for PCP prophylaxis.

- **Thin-section chest computed tomography (CT) scan:** May show ground glass opacities; in a patient with clinical signs or symptoms of PCP, these are suggestive but not diagnostic of PCP.

- **Sputum induction:** The patient inhales saline mist to mobilize sputum from the lungs. The respiratory therapist collects expectorated sputum, which is stained with Giemsa and examined for *P. jiroveci* organisms. This technique is useful because of its noninvasive approach, but it requires an experienced technician, and therefore may not be available at all centers. Sensitivity varies widely (10-95%), depending on the expertise level of the staff at a particular center. (If there is any chance that the patient has TB, sputum induction should be performed in a confined space in a negative pressure area or near an exhaust fan vented safely outside, and samples should be sent for acid-fast bacilli [AFB] smear and culture.)

- **Bronchoscopy with bronchoalveolar lavage (BAL):** If induced sputum tests negative for PCP organisms, definitive diagnosis is made through detection of organisms in BAL fluid obtained during bronchoscopy. Sensitivity is >95% at centers with an experienced staff. BAL fluid can be evaluated for bacteria, mycobacteria, and fungi, as well as for *P. jiroveci*.

- Transbronchial biopsy may be performed if lung disease is progressive despite treatment, to look for diagnoses other than PCP. Open lung biopsy rarely is performed.

Treatment

Presumptive treatment often is initiated on the basis of clinical presentation, chest X-ray findings, and ABG results, while definitive diagnostic tests are pending. The standard and alternative treatment regimens are shown in Table 1.

Standard Therapy

Trimethoprim-sulfamethoxazole

Trimethoprim-sulfamethoxazole (TMP-SMX, Bactrim, Septra, cotrimoxazole) is the drug of choice: 15-20 mg/kg of the TMP component plus 75-100 mg/kg of the SMX component, divided into three or four doses daily and administered IV or PO for 21 days (a typical PO dose is two double-strength tablets TID). Adverse effects of TMP-SMX (e.g., rash, fever, leukopenia, anemia, gastrointestinal intolerance, hepatotoxicity, hyperkalemia) are common, mostly mild, and usually "treated through" successfully. Patients who have had previous reactions to sulfa drugs also may be desensitized successfully (see chapter *Sulfa Desensitization*). TMP-SMX requires dosage adjustment for patients with renal insufficiency.

Adjunctive corticosteroids

Adjunctive corticosteroids should be given if the patient's PO2 is <70 mm Hg (breathing room air) or the A-a gradient is >35 mm Hg. Corticosteroids should be given as early as possible (preferably before or with the first dose of antibiotic therapy) and within 36-72 hours of the start of anti-PCP therapy:

• Prednisone 40 mg BID days 1-5; 40 mg once daily on days 6-10; 20 mg once daily on days 11-21. IV methylprednisolone can be given, at 75% of the prednisone dosage.

Table 1. Preferred and Alternative PCP Therapy

Drugs	Dosages	Notes
Preferred Therapy		
TMP-SMX	TMP: 15-20 mg/kg plus SMX: 75-100 mg/kg in three or four divided doses daily, taken PO or IV for 21 days	Patients who have had previous reactions to sulfa drugs may be desensitized successfully. Adjust dosage for patients with renal insufficiency.
Alternative Therapies		
Pentamidine	4 mg/kg IV once daily for 21 days	Similar efficacy to TMP-SMX but greater toxicity (nephrotoxicity, pancreatitis, glucose dysregulation, cardiac arrhythmias). Usually reserved for patients with severe disease who require IV therapy.
Dapsone + trimethoprim	Dapsone* 100 mg PO once daily plus trimethoprim 15 mg/kg PO per day in 3 divided doses for 21 days	Appropriate for mild-to-moderate disease.
Clindamycin + primaquine	Clindamycin 600-900 mg IV Q6-8H (or 300-450 mg PO Q6-8H) plus primaquine* base 15-30 mg PO once daily for 21 days	Appropriate for mild-to-severe disease.
Atovaquone	750 mg PO BID for 21 days	For mild-to-moderate PCP only; not as potent as TMP-SMX.

* Use with caution in G6PD deficiency (most common among patients of African or Mediterranean descent).

Other therapy notes

- Patients started on IV therapy can be switched to an oral treatment regimen to complete the 3-week course when they are afebrile, have improved oxygenation, and are able to take oral medications.

- Paradoxical worsening of PCP resulting from presumed immune reconstitution inflammatory syndrome (see chapter *Immune Reconstitution Inflammatory Syndrome*) has been reported in some patients who initiated ART close to the time of diagnosis and treatment for PCP. However, recent data suggest that unless other compelling contraindications are present, early initiation of ART (near the time of initiating OI treatment) should be considered for most patients with most acute OIs, including PCP.

- Consultation with HIV experts is advisable when considering initiation of ART in the setting of PCP.

Treatment failures

The average time to clinical improvement for hospitalized patients is 4-8 days, so premature change in therapy should be avoided. For patients who fail to improve on appropriate therapy, it is important to exclude other diagnoses, rule out fluid overload, and consult an infectious disease specialist. Some patients do not respond to any therapy, and the mortality rate of hospitalized patients is about 15%.

Secondary Prophylaxis

Anti-PCP prophylaxis (chronic maintenance therapy) should be given to all patients who have had an episode of PCP. Prophylaxis should be continued for life, unless immune reconstitution occurs as a result of ART and the CD4 count has been >200 cells/μL for more than 3 months.

In patients with stable CD4 count of >200 cells/μL on effective ART, it is recommended that PCP prophylaxis be discontinued because it offers little clinical benefit but may cause drug toxicity, drug interactions, and selection of drug-resistant pathogens, plus it adds to the cost of care and to the patient's pill burden.

If PCP occurred at a CD4 count of >200 cells/μL, it is recommended to continue prophylaxis for life despite immune reconstitution; however, data to support this approach are limited.

Prophylactic therapy

Preferred:

- TMP-SMX, one double-strength tablet PO once daily, or one single-strength tablet PO once daily

Alternative:

- TMP-SMX: one double-strength tablet PO TIW (e.g., Monday, Wednesday, Friday)

- Dapsone* 100 mg PO once daily, or 50 mg PO BID

- Dapsone* 50 mg PO once daily + pyrimethamine 50 mg PO once weekly + leucovorin 25 mg PO once weekly

- Dapsone* 200 mg PO + pyrimethamine 75 mg + leucovorin 25 mg, all once weekly

- Aerosolized pentamidine 300 mg once monthly, via Respirgard II nebulizer (note: does not prevent toxoplasmosis). Warning: May increase the risk of extrapulmonary pneumocystosis, pneumothorax, and bronchospasm.

- Atovaquone suspension 1,500 mg PO once daily (with or without pyrimethamine 25 mg PO once daily + leucovorin 10 mg PO once daily)

* Use with caution in G6PD deficiency.

Primary Prophylaxis

Primary prophylaxis against PCP should be given to all HIV-infected patients with CD4 counts of <200 cells/µL or CD4 percentages of <14%, or a history of oral candidiasis; see chapter *Opportunistic Infection Prophylaxis*.

Patient Education

- Patients should be instructed to take all medications exactly as prescribed.

- Patients should call their health care providers if symptoms worsen.

- Patients being treated with TMP-SMX or dapsone who develop rash, fever, or other new symptoms should call their providers to be evaluated for a drug reaction.

- Patients should understand that taking anti-PCP prophylaxis is extremely important for preventing repeat episodes of illness. Patients should not stop taking these medicines without talking with their health care providers, and should not let their supply of medications run out.

References

- Centers for Disease Control and Prevention. *Guidelines for Prevention and Treatment of Opportunistic Infections in HIV-Infected Adults and Adolescents: Recommendations from CDC, the National Institutes of Health, and the HIV Medicine Association of the Infectious Diseases Society of America.* April 10, 2009. Available at www.aidsinfo.nih.gov/guidelines/.

- Leoung GS. *Pneumocystosis and HIV.* In: Coffey S, Volberding PA, eds. *HIV InSite Knowledge Base* [textbook online]; San Francisco: UCSF Center for HIV Information; April 2005.

- Masur H. *Pneumocystosis.* In: Dolin R, Masur H, Saag MS, eds. *AIDS Therapy, 2nd Edition.* Philadelphia: Churchill Livingstone; 2003:403-418.

- Stringer J, Beard CB, Miller RF, et al. *A new name (Pneumocystis jiroveci) for Pneumocystis from humans.* Emerg Infect Dis. 2002 Sep;8(9):891-6.

- Zolopa A, Andersen J, Powderly W, et al. *Early antiretroviral therapy reduces AIDS progression/death in individuals with acute opportunistic infections: a multicenter randomized strategy trial.* PLoS One. 2009;4(5):e5575.

Progressive Multifocal Leukoencephalopathy

Background

Classic PML

Progressive multifocal leukoencephalopathy (PML) is a demyelinating disease of the central nervous system (CNS) caused by reactivation of latent infection with JC virus, a polyomavirus that infects and lyses oligodendrocytes. Demyelination can occur along any part of the white matter, and often does so at multiple sites (hence the term multifocal). The severity of symptoms increases as demyelination progresses.

Among HIV-infected patients, PML occurs classically and most frequently in those with CD4 counts of <100 cells/μL. They typically present with multiple focal deficits of the cerebrum and brainstem, such as cognitive decline, focal weakness, and cranial nerve palsies, with one focal deficit often predominating. Symptoms typically progress over the course of several weeks. Imaging studies show noninflammatory, nonenhancing white matter lesions, without mass effect, with an anatomical location that maps to deficits on the neurological examination. A presumptive diagnosis of PML often can be made on the basis of the patient's clinical presentation and results of neuroimaging studies. Cerebrospinal fluid (CSF) often tests positive for JC virus DNA by polymerase chain reaction (PCR), although brain biopsy is sometimes needed for definitive diagnosis.

Although PML classically occurs in patients not receiving antiretroviral therapy (ART), it can occur in patients on ART, with suppressed HIV RNA but low CD4 counts. Among untreated patients, the interval between the first manifestation of neurologic symptoms and death may be as short as 3-4 months. Although the prognosis for patients with PML has improved with the use of potent ART, there is no specific treatment for PML, and mortality rates remain high. Patients who survive PML are likely to have permanent neurologic deficits.

Inflammatory PML

Whereas PML in the absence of ART usually is not an inflammatory condition, initiation of ART may cause an immune reconstitution-like syndrome, involving new or worsening neurologic deficits and inflammatory changes seen on brain imaging and biopsy specimens. (See chapter *Immune Reconstitution Inflammatory Syndrome*.) The initiation of ART in a patient with late-stage HIV-related disease may even reveal previously undetected PML. Although many patients with inflammatory PML improve or at least stabilize, some suffer exacerbation of symptoms, rapid progression of disease, cerebral edema, herniation, and death.

S: Subjective

The patient or a caregiver may note symptoms such as weakness, gait abnormalities, difficulties with speech, visual changes, altered mental status, personality changes, and seizures. Hemianopia, ataxia, dysmetria, and hemiparesis or hemisensory deficits are often seen. The onset is likely to be subacute, with progression over the course of weeks, though neurologic disturbances may become profound. PML is not associated with headache or fever; this may help to distinguish it from other opportunistic illnesses of the CNS.

O: Objective

- Measure vital signs.

- Perform a full physical examination, including a thorough neurologic and mental status and evaluation. Look for focal or nonfocal neurologic deficits, particularly cranial nerve abnormalities, visual field defects, weakness, gait abnormalities, and abnormalities in cognitive function, speech, or affect; deficits are likely to be multiple. The patient typically is alert.

- Review previous laboratory values, particularly CD4 count (usually <100 cells/μL in patients with PML).

A: Assessment

Rule out other causes of the patient's neurologic changes. A partial differential diagnosis includes the following:

- CNS lymphoma
- Toxoplasmosis
- HIV encephalopathy
- HIV dementia
- Other (non-HIV) forms of dementia
- Cerebrovascular disease
- Neurosyphilis
- CNS opportunistic infection (e.g., tuberculosis, cryptococcosis, and cytomegalovirus)
- Multiple sclerosis

P: Plan

Diagnostic Evaluation

Definitive diagnosis requires a brain biopsy and identification of characteristic pathological changes, or detection of JC virus DNA in CSF of patients with radiographic and clinical findings consistent with PML.

Presumptive diagnosis of PML often is made on the basis of clinical presentation, brain imaging, and laboratory tests. A brain biopsy should be considered with patients for whom a diagnosis is unclear.

Radiographic Studies

CNS imaging may reveal changes typical of PML, but is nonspecific. Magnetic resonance imaging (MRI) is more sensitive than computed tomography (CT) for detecting PML. Classic PML presents as single or multiple hypodense lesions in the subcortical white matter, with no surrounding edema. On MRI, lesions show increased T2 signal and little or no enhancement with gadolinium. On CT, PML lesions typically are nonenhancing. In some patients, and particularly in patients taking ART, PML lesions may show inflammatory changes, such as enhancement, and there may be cerebral edema.

CSF Evaluation

- CSF cell count, protein level, and glucose level generally are normal or show mild pleocytosis and slightly elevated protein.

- JC virus PCR assays are approximately 75-85% sensitive; detection of JC virus in a patient whose clinical presentation and radiographic imaging results are consistent with PML is adequate to make a diagnosis. A negative result with JC virus PCR does not rule out PML.

Other Studies

- Other diagnostic tests should be performed as indicated to rule out other potential causes of the patient's symptoms.

- A brain biopsy should be considered if the diagnosis is unclear.

Treatment

- There is no specific treatment for JC virus. Potent ART with maximal virologic suppression and effective immune reconstitution is the only treatment that may be effective for patients with PML. Even with ART, however, mortality rates approach 50%, and neurologic deficits are unlikely to be reversible.

- Initiate ART for patients who are not already receiving treatment. It is not clear whether antiretroviral agents with good CNS penetration are more effective than those that are less likely to cross the blood-brain barrier.

- For patients who are on ART with incomplete virologic suppression, change the ART regimen appropriately to achieve virologic suppression, if possible. For patients on ART with poor immunologic response, consider changing or intensifying therapy with the goal of improved immunologic recovery. (See chapter *Antiretroviral Therapy*.)

- If symptoms are caused by immune reconstitution, consider adding corticosteroids (e.g., dexamethasone) to help decrease inflammation.

- The following agents have been proposed as specific therapy for PML, but have not been shown to be effective by prospective studies and are not recommended for treatment: cidofovir, cytarabine, topotecan, interferon-alpha, and inhibitors of the serotonergic 5-HT2a receptor.

- Depending on the patient's cognitive and physical status, he or she may need a care provider in the home to assure that medications are taken on schedule.

- The patient is likely to need supportive care for personal hygiene, nutrition, safety, and prevention of accidents or injury; refer as indicated.

Patient Education

- Most patients diagnosed with PML will need supportive treatment for an undetermined period of time, and hospice referral should be considered if the patient does not show clinical improvement in response to ART.

- If the patient is receiving ART, be sure that caregivers, family members, and friends are taught about the medications and are able to help the patient with adherence.

- When a diagnosis of PML has been established or suspected, initiate a discussion of plans for terminal care (including wills, advanced directives, and supportive care and services) with the patient and family members or caregivers.

References

- Aksamit AJ. *Review of progressive multifocal leukoencephalopathy and natalizumab.* Neurologist. 2006 Nov;12(6):293-8.

- Centers for Disease Control and Prevention. *Guidelines for Prevention and Treatment of Opportunistic Infections in HIV-Infected Adults and Adolescents: Recommendations from CDC, the National Institutes of Health, and the HIV Medicine Association of the Infectious Diseases Society of America.* April 10, 2009. Available at www.aidsinfo.nih.gov/guidelines/.

- Koralnik IJ. *New insights into progressive multifocal leukoencephalopathy.* Curr Opin Neurol. 2004 Jun;17(3):365-70.

- Wyen C, Lehmann C, Fatkenheuer G, et al. *AIDS-related progressive multifocal leukoencephalopathy in the era of HAART: report of two cases and review of the literature.* AIDS Patient Care STDS. 2005 Aug;19(8):486-94.

Seborrheic Dermatitis

Background

Seborrheic dermatitis is one of the most common skin manifestations of HIV infection. It occurs in 3-5% of the general HIV-uninfected population but in up to 85-95% of patients with advanced HIV infection. Among HIV-infected individuals, seborrheic dermatitis often begins when their CD4 counts drop to the 450-550 cells/μL range. The disease is more likely to occur among young adults (because they have oilier skin) and males, and is more common in areas with cold, dry winter air. It is rarely found in African blacks, unless the person is immunocompromised. It is more common during times of mental stress and severe illness.

Seborrheic dermatitis is a scaling, inflammatory skin disease that may flare and subside over time. It is characterized by itchy reddish or pink patches of skin, accompanied by greasy flakes or scales. It most commonly occurs in the scalp and on the face, especially at the nasolabial folds, eyebrows, and forehead, but also may develop on the ears, chest, upper back, axillae, and groin. Dandruff is considered to be a mild form of seborrheic dermatitis. Occasionally, seborrheic dermatitis may be severe, may involve large areas of the body, and may be resistant to treatment. Severe manifestations are more likely with advanced HIV infection.

The etiology of seborrheic dermatitis is not entirely clear. *Malassezia* yeast (formerly called *Pityrosporum ovale*), a fungus that inhabits the oily skin areas of 92% of humans, is the most likely culprit. This same yeast also is thought to cause tinea versicolor and *Pityrosporum* folliculitis. Overgrowth of the *Malassezia* yeast in the oily skin environment, failure of the immune system to regulate the fungus, and the skin's inflammatory reaction to the yeast overgrowth appear to be the chief factors that cause the dermatitis.

S: Subjective

The patient complains of a new rash, sometimes itchy, or of "dry skin" that will not go away despite the application of topical moisturizers.

O: Objective

Perform a thorough evaluation of the skin with special attention to the scalp, medial eyebrows, eyelashes and eyelids, beard and other facial hair areas, nasolabial folds, postauricular areas, the concha of the auricle, glabella, umbilicus, central chest, back, axillae, and groin. Seborrheic dermatitis appears as white to yellow greasy or waxy flakes over red or pink patches of skin; however, discrete fine scales may indicate a mild form of the disease. Around the eyes, seborrheic dermatitis can cause eyelid erythema and scaling. The distribution usually is symmetrical.

A: Assessment

The diagnosis of seborrheic dermatitis is based on the characteristic appearance. A partial differential diagnosis includes psoriasis, atopic dermatitis, contact dermatitis, erythrasma, tinea capitus (can be present on the scalp without hair loss), rosacea, and rarely, dermatomyositis.

P: Plan
Treatment

- Antiretroviral therapy, if otherwise indicated.

- Specific treatments are divided into three types: antimycotic (first choice), antiinflammatory (second choice), and keratolytic. Shampoos may be used on the entire body.

- Topical antifungal medications: The azoles and ciclopirox have been well studied and shown to have both antifungal and antiinflammatory activity. Various preparations are available; selection can be based on cost and availability. Antifungals may be used in combination with topical corticosteroid therapy (see below). Effective antifungals include but are not limited to the following:

  - Ketoconazole (Nizoral) 2% cream or shampoo; ketoconazole is one of the most widely studied of all topical treatments

  - Bifonazole ointment, miconazole cream (Monistat), terbinafine (Lamisil) 1% solution or cream, or clotrimazole (Lotrimin) 1% cream, lotion, or solution

  - Ciclopiroxolamine (Loprox) 1% shampoo, gel, or cream

  - Zinc pyrithione (keratolytic/antifungal) shampoo or cream

- Topical corticosteroids generally are effective and may be used in combination with topical antifungal therapy (see above). Low-potency agents (e.g., hydrocortisone 1%) rather than high-potency corticosteroids (e.g., betamethasone dipropionate, triamcinolone), are recommended, especially for the face, to reduce the risk of adverse effects associated with all corticosteroids (e.g., atrophy, telangiectasias, and perioral dermatitis). Clobetasol shampoo has antiinflammatory effects.

- Selenium sulfide/sulfur preparations (the most common is selenium sulfide shampoo).

- Whole coal tar, crude coal tar extract: shampoos, creams, and gels.

- Lithium succinate or lithium gluconate ointment, available in some countries as a combination of lithium succinate 8% and zinc sulfate 0.05% (may have antifungal or antiinflammatory effects). Not for use on the scalp.

- Honey, 90% diluted with warm water, may be used to treat seborrheic dermatitis and dandruff.

- Azelaic acid, 15% gel or 20% cream, has sebosuppressive, antimicrobial, antifungal, and antiinflammatory activity (also used for acne and rosacea).

- Noncorticosteroid topical immunomodulators (calcineurin inhibitors):

  - Tacrolimus

  - Pimecrolimus

- Oral therapy may be used for patients who are refractory to topical treatment (may interact with protease inhibitors and nonnucleoside reverse transcriptase inhibitors; check for possible drug-drug interactions with antiretroviral and other medications before prescribing). There are limited data regarding the efficacy of systemic medication.

  - Fluconazole 300 mg once weekly for 2 weeks

  - Itraconazole 200 mg once daily for 7 days

  - Ketoconazole 200 mg once daily for no more than 4 weeks

  - Terbinafine 250 mg once daily for 4 weeks

Potential adverse effects:

- With all topical products: skin burning, stinging, dryness; allergic or contact dermatitis. Tar shampoos may discolor light hair, leave an oily film on hair, and leave an odor. Coal tar may be carcinogenic; use shampoo no more than twice a week, leave on skin or hair for 5 minutes, and rinse well.

- Topical corticosteroids may cause skin atrophy, telangiectasias, folliculitis, striae, and excessive hair growth. Risk of adverse effects is low and can be mediated by using product infrequently, diluting the product, or limiting the amount of time the product is on the skin (shampoos are ideal).

- With oral therapy, monitor for hepatotoxicity.

Patient Education

- Although topical and oral medicines can relieve symptoms, recurrence is common. Effective antiretroviral therapy should be considered to control the effects of HIV on the immune system and thereby treat the underlying cause of seborrheic dermatitis.

References

- Bikowski J. *Facial seborrheic dermatitis: A report on current status and therapeutic horizons.* J Drugs Dermatol. 2009 Feb;8(2):125-33.

- Dunic I, Vesic S, Jevtovic DJ. *Oral candidiasis and seborrheic dermatitis in HIV-infected patients on highly active antiretroviral therapy.* HIV Med. 2004 Jan;5(1):50-4.

- Faergemann J, Bergbrant IM, Dohse M, et al. *Seborrhoeic dermatitis and Pityrosporum (Malassezia) folliculitis: characterization of inflammatory cells and mediators in the skin by immunohistochemistry.* Br J Dermatol. 2001 Mar;144(3):549-56.

- Gupta AK, Bluhm R. *Seborrheic dermatitis.* J Eur Acad Dermatol Venereol. 2004 Jan;18(1):13-26; quiz 19-20.

- Gupta AK, Ryder JE, Nicol K, et al. *Superficial fungal infections: an update on pityriasis versicolor, seborrheic dermatitis, tinea capitis, and onychomycosis.* Clin Dermatol. 2003 Sep-Oct;21(5):417-25.

- Levin NA. *Beyond spaghetti and meatballs: skin diseases associated with the Malassezia yeasts.* Dermatol Nurs. 2009 Jan-Feb;21(1):7-13, 51; quiz 14.

- Naldi L, Rebora A. *Clinical practice: seborrheic dermatitis.* N Engl J Med. 2009 Jan 22;360(4):387-96.

- Rigopoulos D, Paparizos V, Katsambas A. *Cutaneous markers of HIV infection.* Clin Dermatol. 2004 Nov-Dec; 22(6):487-98.

- Waldroup W, Scheinfeld N. *Medicated shampoos for the treatment of seborrheic dermatitis.* J Drugs Dermatol. 2008 Jul;7(7):699-703.

Sinusitis

Background

Sinusitis is defined as an inflammation involving the membrane lining of any sinus, and is a frequent finding in people with HIV infection. It occurs very commonly as part of a viral upper respiratory infection (URI), and usually is self-limited. Bacterial sinusitis usually occurs as a secondary complication of a viral URI, which causes decreased patency of the nasal ostia, decreased nasal ciliary action, and increased mucus production. Acute sinusitis is defined as lasting up to 4 weeks, whereas chronic sinusitis persists for at least 12 weeks.

HIV-infected patients are susceptible to sinusitis for a number of reasons related to their immunosuppression. Pathophysiologic mechanisms for this susceptibility may include proliferation of lymphatic tissue contributing to nasal obstruction, defects in B-cell and T-cell immunity owing to HIV, and defects in production of immunoglobulins, specifically IgE, resulting in an exaggerated allergic response in the nasal mucosa. As in the general population, the most common pathogens causing acute bacterial sinusitis are *Streptococcus pneumoniae*, *Moraxella catarrhalis*, and *Haemophilus influenzae*. However, HIV-infected patients have a greater incidence of sinusitis caused by *Staphylococcus aureus* and *Pseudomonas aeruginosa*. The bacterial causes of chronic sinusitis are not well defined, but may involve more polymicrobial and anaerobic infections. In patients with severe immunosuppression, particularly those with CD4 counts of ≤50 cells/µL, sinusitis may be caused by *Aspergillus* and other fungal pathogens.

S: Subjective

The patient may complain of facial pain, frontal or maxillary headache, postnasal drip, or fever.

Ask the patient about specific symptoms, the duration and progression of symptoms, and treatments attempted.

- Fever
- Facial pain or pressure, headache; positional pain (worse when patient bends forward)
- Purulent or bloody nasal discharge
- Postnasal drip
- Nasal congestion
- Recent URI
- Malaise
- Chronic cough
- Maxillary tooth pain
- Ear pressure
- History of chronic sinusitis, seasonal allergies, antibiotic allergies, atopy
- Tobacco use, inhaled recreational drugs

O: Objective

- Document vital signs.
- Perform a careful physical examination focusing on the head and face, neck, and lungs. Examine the nose, mouth, ears, and sinuses.
  - Look for nares inflammation and drainage from sinus ostia.
  - Examine the tympanic membranes and external auditory canals.

- Evaluate the oropharynx for mucus drainage, lesions, and exudates.

- Check the teeth and gums for tenderness and erythema.

- Palpate for tenderness over frontal and maxillary sinus cavities.

- Examine the face and orbits for swelling or erythema.

- Perform cranial nerve examination.

- Auscultate the chest for abnormal lung sounds.

A: Assessment

A partial differential diagnosis includes the following:

- Allergic rhinitis

- Sinus blockage by other lesions such as Kaposi sarcoma or lymphoma (particularly if the CD4 count is <200 cells/µL) or fungal infections (if the CD4 count is <50 cells/µL)

- Dental abscess, caries

- Meningitis

- Vasculitis

- Trauma

P: Plan

Diagnostic Evaluation

Uncomplicated acute sinusitis usually is a clinical diagnosis. There are no symptoms, physical findings, or tests that reliably distinguish bacterial from viral sinusitis. Patients generally can be assumed to have bacterial sinusitis if symptoms do not resolve, or if they worsen, over the course of 7-10 days. Any patient with high fever or severe or unusual symptoms should be evaluated urgently for other causes of illness.

Imaging studies usually are not indicated for uncomplicated acute sinusitis. In patients with a poor response to empiric antibiotic therapy or worsening symptoms, and those with suspected chronic sinusitis, computed tomography (CT) scans of the paranasal sinuses are the best initial radiologic study. Standard X rays (sinus series) can detect cloudiness or air-fluid levels and will show mucosal thickening (a nonspecific finding in HIV-infected individuals).

Cultures of nasal aspirates are not useful for diagnosis, because nasal fluids do not accurately represent pathogens in the paranasal sinuses. Sinus aspirate cultures will give definitive diagnosis of a specific organism in the majority of cases; this may be considered in complicated cases. Definitive diagnosis of invasive fungal sinusitis requires tissue for culture.

Treatment

Treatment is multimodal. For viral sinusitis, treatment is based on symptom suppression; for bacterial sinusitis, an antibiotic is added to other therapies:

- Antihistamine: chlorpheniramine or other

- Decongestant: pseudoephedrine

- Nasal steroid (e.g., budesonide, fluticasone, mometasone, or triamcinolone) (see "Potential ARV Interactions," below)

- Nonsteroidal antiinflammatory drugs (NSAIDs): ibuprofen or other

- Cough suppressant as needed

- Mucolytic agent: guaifenesin

- Inhaled steam and saline nasal irrigation to promote sinus drainage

If acute bacterial sinusitis is suspected, treat as above and add an antibiotic for a 10-14 day course of therapy:

- Amoxicillin 500-1,000 mg TID

- Amoxicillin/clavulanate (Augmentin) 825/125 mg BID

- Cefpodoxime 200-400 mg BID
- Clindamycin 450 mg TID
- Levofloxacin 500 mg once daily or moxifloxacin 400 mg once daily

For chronic sinusitis, administer multimodal treatments as listed above for 3-4 weeks. The value of antibiotics in chronic sinusitis is unclear; consider especially if a trial of antibiotics has not been undertaken.

If symptoms persist or worsen, refer patients to an otolaryngologist for further evaluation and treatment.

Potential ARV Interactions

Protease inhibitors (PIs), particularly ritonavir-boosted PIs, may increase serum glucocorticoid levels if used concurrently with nasal steroids. Fluticasone (Flonase) nasal spray should not be used with ritonavir-boosted PIs unless expected benefits outweigh possible risks, and should be avoided, if possible, in patients taking unboosted PIs. Budesonide (Rhinocort Aqua) nasal spray should be avoided with ritonavir-boosted PIs. Interactions between PIs and other nasal steroids have not been well studied.

Patient Education

- Instruct patients in the correct use of medications used to treat sinusitis, including proper technique for nasal irrigation or steam inhalation, as required.
- Instruct patients to take antibiotics on schedule until the entire prescription is gone in order to prevent recurrence of the infection.
- Advise patients that drinking eight glasses (8-12 oz each) of fluid daily helps to keep the mucus thin enough to drain the sinus passages.
- Advise patients to call or return to clinic for swelling of the face or swelling around the eyes, increased facial tenderness, new or worsening fever, or other concerning symptoms.

References

- Gilbert DN, Moellering RC Jr., Eliopoulos GM, et al. *The Sanford Guide to Antimicrobial Therapy, 35th Edition.* Hyde Park, VT: Antimicrobial Therapy Inc.; 2005.
- Gurney TA, Lee KC, Murr AH. *Contemporary issues in rhinosinusitis and HIV infection.* Curr Opin Otolaryngol Head Neck Surg. 2003 Feb;11(1):45-8.
- Lee KC, Tami TA. *Otolaryngologic Manifestations of HIV.* In: Coffey S, Volberding PA, eds. *HIV InSite Knowledge Base* [textbook online]. San Francisco: UCSF Center for HIV Information; 1998. Available at hivinsite.ucsf.edu/InSite?page=kb-00&doc=kb-04-01-13. Accessed June 30, 2010.

Syphilis

Background

Syphilis is a sexually transmitted infection (STI) caused by the spirochete *Treponema pallidum*. It is a complex disease with protean variations that can mimic many common infections or illnesses. HIV infection may alter the natural history and management of syphilis, causing a more rapid course of illness, higher risk of neurologic complications, and potentially greater risk of treatment failure with standard regimens. Because many individuals with syphilis have no symptoms, or have symptoms that subside without treatment, sexually active individuals at risk of syphilis should receive regular screening for syphilis, as well as for other STIs. Many clinicians strongly recommend routine syphilis testing every 3-6 months for patients at risk of syphilis.

HRSA HAB Core Clinical Performance Measures

Percentage of adult clients with HIV infection who had a **test for syphilis** performed within the measurement year

(Group 2 measure)

There has been a resurgence of syphilis in metropolitan areas of the United States and western Europe. This trend is concerning, because syphilis can have major health consequences if it is undetected and untreated, and because it is associated with increased risk of new HIV infections. Risk assessment should be conducted at each patient visit for unprotected sex (including oral sex), multiple sex partners, and use of recreational drugs (methamphetamine and cocaine, in particular, are associated with high-risk sexual practices among men who have sex with men [MSM]). Asymptomatic persons at risk of acquiring syphilis should be screened at regular intervals (with rapid plasma reagin [RPR] or Venereal Disease Research Laboratory [VDRL] testing, as discussed below), depending on their risk factors. MSM with multiple partners should be tested every 3-6 months.

The natural history of untreated syphilis infection is divided into stages based on length of infection.

Primary Syphilis

Primary syphilis usually manifests after an incubation period of 1-3 weeks from exposure and is characterized by a painless self-limiting ulcer (chancre) at the site of sexual contact. HIV-infected individuals may have multiple or atypical chancres that could be misidentified. Some patients have no primary lesion, or have a primary lesion that is not visible. Associated regional lymphadenopathy can occur. HIV-infected individuals sometimes have a chancre concurrently with rash typical of secondary syphilis.

Secondary Syphilis

Secondary syphilis usually develops 2-8 weeks after initial infection and is caused by ongoing replication of the spirochete, with disseminated infection that may involve multiple systems. Rash is the most common presenting symptom; skin lesions may be macular, maculopapular, papular, or pustular, or they may appear as condyloma lata (which may look like the condyloma of papillomavirus). The rash often appears on the trunk and extremities and may involve the palms and soles of feet. Constitutional symptoms, lymphadenopathy, arthralgias, and myalgias are common, and neurologic or other symptoms may occur. In the absence of treatment, the manifestations of secondary syphilis last days to weeks, then usually resolve to the latent stages.

Latent Syphilis

Latent syphilis follows resolution of secondary syphilis. As in HIV-uninfected individuals, latent syphilis is asymptomatic and the diagnosis is determined by positive serologic tests. Latent syphilis is further classified as "early latent" if the infection is known to be <1 year in duration, "late latent" if the infection is known to be >1 year in duration, or "latent syphilis of unknown duration" if the duration of infection is not known.

Late or Tertiary Syphilis

Late or tertiary syphilis is caused by chronic infection with progressive disease in any system causing serious illness and death in untreated patients. The most common manifestations include neurosyphilis, cardiovascular syphilis, and gummatous syphilis.

Neurosyphilis

Neurosyphilis can occur at any time after initial infection, owing to spread of the spirochete to the central nervous system (CNS). In HIV-infected individuals, neurosyphilis may occur more commonly early in the course of infection, during secondary or latent syphilis. It is associated with neurologic symptoms, including cranial nerve abnormalities (particularly extraocular or facial muscle palsies, tinnitus, and hearing loss) or symptoms of meningitis. Uveitis and other eye disease may occur in conjunction with neurosyphilis.

S: Subjective

Symptoms depend on the site of initial infection, the stage of disease, and whether neurosyphilis is present. Symptoms are not present in all patients.

If symptoms are present, the patient may experience the following:

- Painless sore(s) or ulcer(s) in the genital area, vagina, anus, or oral cavity
- New rash, usually on the trunk, often on extremities, soles of the feet, or palms; patchy hair loss
- Fever, malaise, swollen glands, arthralgias, myalgias
- Altered mental status, weakness, paralysis
- Neurosyphilis: vision changes, eye pain, tinnitus, hearing loss, headaches, dizziness, generalized weakness, seizures, confusion, changes in personality or affect

Conduct a targeted history, asking the patient about symptoms listed above, including duration; inquire about other or associated symptoms. Ascertain the following:

- Previous diagnosis of syphilis
- New sex partners in past 90 days (for primary or secondary syphilis)
- Unprotected sex (oral, vaginal, anal)
- Date of last syphilis test
- Possibility of pregnancy

O: Objective

Check for fever, document other vital signs.

Perform a complete examination including the following:

- Skin and mucosal areas (including the genitals, palm, and soles): rash, gummas, granulomas, patchy hair loss

- Oropharynx: chancres, mucous patches, condyloma lata

- Lymph nodes

- Heart: murmurs

- Ophthalmic examination

- Neurologic examination (mental status, cranial nerves [including visual acuity], sensory, motor, reflexes, coordination, gait): abnormal mental status, visual acuity changes, extraocular movement abnormalities, neurosensory hearing loss, facial palsy, paraesthesias, paralysis, hemiplegia, hyperactive reflexes, ataxia

A: Assessment

Because syphilis has a wide range of manifestations, the differential diagnosis is broad. It is important to consider syphilis as a possible cause of many presenting illnesses. A partial differential diagnosis includes the following:

- Other causes of maculopapular rashes: pityriasis, drug eruption, condyloma, folliculitis, psoriasis, acute HIV infection

- Other causes of genital ulcerative disease: herpes simplex virus (HSV), chancroid

- Other causes of ocular disease; glaucoma, cytomegalovirus (CMV) retinitis, CMV immune reconstitution uveitis, HSV keratitis

- Other causes of neurologic disease: stroke, Bell palsy, CNS lymphoma, toxoplasmosis, meningitis

- Other causes of cardiac murmurs: bacterial endocarditis, congenital abnormalities

- Other causes of systemic symptoms (e.g., fever, malaise, adenopathy): acute HIV infection, acute hepatitis, other infections or malignancies

P: Plan
Diagnostic Evaluation
Darkfield examination and direct fluorescent antibody

Darkfield examination and direct fluorescent antibody (DFA) testing of a sample from suspicious genital or anal chancres or moist dermatologic lesions (not oral lesions) are definitive tests for syphilis, although these are not available in most clinic settings.

Serologic tests

Nontreponemal tests (RPR or VDRL) are most sensitive in primary and secondary syphilis when titers are high, though the response may be delayed in HIV-infected patients (nontreponemal test results typically are positive within 3 months after infection). Because false-positive results may occur, particularly in the setting of HIV infection, positive nontreponemal test results must be confirmed with a treponemal test. Titers may be used to follow response to treatment; a fourfold change in titer is considered a significant change. Note that the same nontreponemal test should be used consistently for a single patient; RPR titers cannot be compared with VDRL titers.

Treponemal antibody tests (TP-PA [*T. pallidum* particle agglutination] or FTA-ABS [fluorescent treponemal antibody absorption]) confirm a positive nontreponemal test. As an alternative, many laboratories have begun to use a treponemal test, e.g., an enzyme immunoassay (EIA) as an initial screen for syphilis infection, followed by a nontreponemal test for confirmation, to reduce the workload from the titration required for nontreponemal titers.

A false-negative RPR or VDRL result may occur, usually when the test is performed in early infection, before a sufficient antibody response has developed. Another possible cause of a false-negative nontreponemal result is the prozone phenomenon, seen when antibody concentrations are very high (usually in secondary syphilis) and the specimen is not diluted sufficiently. If serologic test results are negative and suspicion of syphilis is high, perform other diagnostic tests (e.g., biopsy) or request that the laboratory perform additional dilutions on nontreponemal test specimens.

Cerebrospinal fluid evaluation

- HIV-infected patients with neurologic or ocular signs or symptoms of syphilis, late latent syphilis, syphilis of unknown duration, or tertiary syphilis should undergo lumbar puncture (LP) and cerebrospinal fluid (CSF) analysis. CSF evaluation also is indicated for patients in whom treatment for early syphilis fails (see below). Routine CSF evaluation is not indicated for HIV-infected patients who have early syphilis without neurologic or ophthalmic signs or symptoms. CSF analysis should include the following:

  - CSF-VDRL: This test is specific but not very sensitive; a positive result is diagnostic but a negative result does not rule out neurosyphilis.

  - Leukocytes: Elevated white blood cell count (>10 cells/μL) is suggestive but not specific. Note that mononuclear pleocytosis (up to 5-20 cells/μL) is not uncommon in patients with HIV infection, particularly those with higher CD4 cell counts.

  - Some recommend checking CSF FTA-ABS. This is very sensitive but not very specific; a negative result indicates that neurosyphilis is highly unlikely.

Other testing

All patients who test positive for syphilis should be tested for gonorrhea and chlamydia, with sampling sites based on sexual practices and exposures (oropharyngeal, urethral, vaginal, or anorectal testing). Patients not known to be HIV infected also should be tested for HIV.

Treatment

Treatment of syphilis in HIV-infected individuals essentially is the same as in HIV-uninfected individuals, and depends on stage and the presence or absence of neurosyphilis. It is important to follow patients closely to assure the success of treatment. For further information, see the Centers for Disease Control and Prevention (CDC) *Sexually Transmitted Diseases Treatment Guidelines* (see "References," below).

An RPR or VDRL test should be sent on the day of treatment; the titer will be the reference point for assessing treatment efficacy (see "Follow-Up," below).

Early syphilis *(<1 year in duration [i.e., primary, secondary, and early latent]); nonneurologic*

- Recommended: benzathine penicillin G, 2.4 million units IM (single dose)

- Alternatives: note that penicillin is strongly preferred; consider allergy testing and desensitization to penicillin; in penicillin-allergic, nonpregnant patients, consider the following; note that these therapies are not as well proven in HIV-infected individuals; close monitoring for treatment response is recommended.

  - Doxycycline, 100 mg PO BID for 14 days

  - Tetracycline, 500 mg PO QID for 14 days

  - Ceftriaxone, 1 g IM or IV once daily for 10-14 days

  - High rates of treatment failure have been reported in patients treated with azithromycin (2 g, single dose); this regimen should be used only if other options are contraindicated and close follow-up is possible

Late latent syphilis *(>1 year in duration or of unknown duration; no evidence of neurologic disease)*

- CSF examination to rule out neurosyphilis should be done on all patients with a history of syphilis >1 year in duration or of unknown duration.

- If CSF examination result is negative, treat with benzathine penicillin G, 2.4 million units IM weekly for 3 consecutive weeks (7.2 million units in total).

- In penicillin-allergic clients, refer for desensitization to penicillin. As an alternative, some specialists consider doxycycline 100 mg PO BID for 28 days. Referral to infectious disease specialist and close clinical monitoring are required, as treatment efficacy is not proven in HIV-infected individuals.

Tertiary syphilis

Consult with specialists.

Neurosyphilis *(syphilis at any stage with neurologic or ocular symptoms or CSF findings of neurosyphilis)*

Ideally, patients should be hospitalized and given 2 weeks of penicillin IV under close observation. Penicillin-allergic patients should be referred for desensitization, if possible.

- Recommended: aqueous crystalline penicillin G, 18-24 million units IV per day (3-4 million units Q4H [or continuous infusion] for 10-14 days).

- Alternatives (require strict adherence with therapy):

  - Procaine penicillin 2.4 million units IM per day, plus probenecid 500 mg PO QID, both for 10-14 days

  - Some experts consider use of ceftriaxone 2 g IM or IV once daily for 10-14 days with close clinical monitoring

- Some experts recommend administration of benzathine penicillin, 2.4 million units IM weekly for 3 weeks, after completion of the standard 10- to 14-day course of therapy for neurosyphilis.

- Recheck CSF leukocyte count every 6 months until the cell count normalizes (if CSF pleocytosis was present at initial evaluation). If the leukocyte count is not lower at 6 months, consider retreatment (consult with a specialist).

Note that a **Jarisch-Herxheimer reaction** may occur after initial syphilis treatment, especially in primary, secondary, or even latent syphilis. This self-limited treatment effect should not be confused with an allergic reaction to penicillin. It usually begins 2-8 hours after the first dose of penicillin and consists of fever, chills, arthralgias, malaise, tender lymphadenopathy, and intensification of rash. It resolves within 24 hours and is best treated with rest and acetaminophen. Patients should be warned about the possibility of a Jarisch-Herxheimer reaction.

Pregnancy

Pregnant women should be treated with penicillin, if possible, using a regimen appropriate for the stage of infection (see above). Additional treatment may be indicated; consult with a specialist. Penicillin-allergic pregnant women should be referred for desensitization to penicillin. Doxycycline and tetracycline may cause fetal toxicity and should not be used during pregnancy; erythromycin is not sufficiently effective in treating syphilis in the fetus. Azithromycin and erythromycin do not have adequate efficacy in treating pregnant women or their fetuses and should not be used. The efficacy of ceftriaxone during pregnancy has not been studied adequately.

Women treated during the second half of pregnancy are at risk of contractions, early labor, and fetal distress if they develop a Jarisch-Herxheimer reaction; thus, they should be monitored carefully.

Sex partners

Syphilis is transmitted sexually only when mucocutaneous lesions of syphilis are present; this is uncommon after the first year of infection. Nevertheless, sex partners of a patient who has syphilis in any stage should be evaluated.

- Persons exposed within 90 days preceding the diagnosis of primary, secondary, or early latent syphilis should be treated presumptively, as they may be infected with syphilis even if they are seronegative.

- Persons exposed more than 90 days before the diagnosis of primary, secondary, or early latent syphilis should be treated presumptively if serologic test results are not available immediately and their follow-up is in doubt. Otherwise, they should receive serologic testing and be treated appropriately if the test result is positive. Note that some specialists recommend presumptive treatment of all persons potentially exposed to syphilis. For patients with primary syphilis, that means partners within the previous 3 months; for secondary, within 6 months; for early latent, within 1 year.

Follow-Up

All HIV-infected patients treated for syphilis should be evaluated clinically and serologically at 3, 6, 9, 12, and 24 months (at 6, 12, 18, and 24 months for latent syphilis) to rule out treatment failure. Treatment success is determined by a fourfold decrease in RPR or VDRL titer by 6-12 months (for primary and secondary syphilis) or 12-24 months (for latent syphilis) of treatment. Patients whose titers do not decrease appropriately probably either experienced treatment failure or were reinfected. Any patient with apparent treatment failure should undergo an LP for CSF analysis and be re-treated as appropriate. If at any time symptoms develop or nontreponemal test titers increase fourfold, CSF examination should be performed and appropriate treatment should be given.

Some patients retain reactive (low-titer) nontreponemal test results after successful treatment for syphilis. In these "serofast" individuals, reinfection with syphilis is indicated by a rise in test titer of at least fourfold.

Risk-reduction counseling

All patients with syphilis should receive risk evaluation and risk-reduction counseling. Evaluate each patient's sexual practices with regard to risk of acquiring STIs and of transmitting HIV. Work with the patient to reduce sexual risks.

Patient Education

- Instruct patients to go to clinic for treatment at the intervals recommended. If patients are given oral antibiotics (penicillin-allergic individuals), instruct them to take their medications exactly as prescribed.

- Warn patients about the possibility of a Jarisch-Herxheimer reaction and advise them about self-management of associated symptoms (e.g., acetaminophen or aspirin at usual doses, fluids, and rest).

- Instruct patients about the required follow-up laboratory and clinical evaluations necessary to document adequate treatment. Emphasize the need for regular evaluation of treatment efficacy.

- Sex partners from the previous 3-6 months (sometimes longer, depending on the stage of syphilis) need to be evaluated and treated as soon as possible, even if they have no symptoms. Advise patients to inform their partners that they need to be tested and treated.

- Syphilis is a reportable communicable disease in the United States. Patients will be contacted to assist with partner tracing and to ensure appropriate treatment.

- Provide education about sexual risk reduction. Review sexual practices and support patients in using condoms with every sexual contact to prevent becoming reinfected with syphilis or infected with other STIs, and to prevent passing HIV to sex partners.

References

- Centers for Disease Control and Prevention. *Guidelines for Prevention and Treatment of Opportunistic Infections in HIV-Infected Adults and Adolescents: Recommendations from CDC, the National Institutes of Health, and the HIV Medicine Association of the Infectious Diseases Society of America.* April 10, 2009. Available at www.aidsinfo.nih.gov/guidelines/.

- Centers for Disease Control and Prevention. *Sexually Transmitted Diseases Treatment Guidelines, 2010.* MMWR 2010 Dec 17; 59 (No. RR- 12):1-110. Available at www.cdc.gov/STD/treatment/2010.

- Golden MR, Marra CM, Holmes KK. *Update on syphilis: resurgence of an old problem.* JAMA. 2003 Sep 17;290(11):1510-4.

- Marra CM, Maxwell CL, Smith SL, et al. *Cerebrospinal fluid abnormalities in patients with syphilis: association with clinical and laboratory features.* J Infect Dis. 2004 Feb 1;189(3):369-76.

- Marra CM, Maxwell CL, Tantalo L, et al. *Normalization of cerebrospinal fluid abnormalities after neurosyphilis therapy: does HIV status matter?* Clin Infect Dis. 2004 Apr 1;38(7):1001-6.

- Mitchell SJ, Engelman J, Kent CK, et al. *Azithromycin-resistant syphilis infection: San Francisco, California, 2000-2004.* Clin Infect Dis. 2006 Feb 1;42(3):337-45.

- Paz-Bailey G, Meyers A, Blank S, et al. *A case-control study of syphilis among men who have sex with men in New York City: association with HIV infection.* Sex Transm Dis. 2004 Oct;31(10):581-7.

- Peterman TA, Heffelfinger JD, Swint EB, et al. *The changing epidemiology of syphilis.* Sex Transm Dis. 2005 Oct;32(10 Suppl):S4-10.

- Pope V. *Use of treponemal tests to screen for syphilis.* Infect Med. 2004 21(8); 399-404.

- Stolte IG, Dukers NH, de Wit JB, et al. *Increase in sexually transmitted infections among homosexual men in Amsterdam in relation to HAART.* Sex Transm Infect. 2001 Jun;77(3):184-6.

- Torian LV, Makki HA, Menzies IB, et al. *HIV infection in men who have sex with men, New York City Department of Health sexually transmitted disease clinics, 1990-1999: a decade of serosurveillance finds that racial disparities and associations between HIV and gonorrhea persist.* Sex Transm Dis. 2002 Feb;29(2):73-8.

Toxoplasmosis

Background

Toxoplasma gondii is a common intracellular protozoan that preferentially infects the central nervous system (CNS) of immunodeficient patients, causing severe neurologic disease. *T. gondii* also can cause local disease such as chorioretinitis and pneumonia. *Toxoplasma* has an infectious reservoir in almost all animals; humans acquire infection either through ingestion of tissue cysts contained in undercooked meat (usually pork, lamb, or beef) or oocysts on contaminated vegetables or through exposure to cat feces containing oocysts. There is no transmission by person-to-person contact.

HRSA HAB Core Clinical Performance Measures

Percentage of clients with HIV infection for whom *Toxoplasma* screening was performed at least once since the diagnosis of HIV infection

(Group 3 measure)

Clinical disease usually occurs through reactivation of latent infection in patients who have CD4 counts of <100 cells/μL. Seroprevalence varies widely, from 15% in the United States to 75% in some European countries, and even higher in certain resource-limited countries. In the absence of prophylaxis, toxoplasmic encephalitis occurs in more than 30% of patients with advanced HIV infection who are seropositive for *T. gondii*. There have been case reports of CNS toxoplasmosis in the setting of immune reconstitution on antiretroviral therapy (ART); see chapter *Immune Reconstitution Inflammatory Syndrome*.

CNS toxoplasmosis is an AIDS-defining condition that can be progressive and fatal. However, antimicrobial therapy, especially if given in conjunction with ART that results in immune reconstitution, can be successful in treating toxoplasmosis. Specific prophylaxis and effective ART also may be used to prevent toxoplasmosis in patients with advanced AIDS who have latent *T. gondii* infection (as demonstrated by the presence of anti-*Toxoplasma* immunoglobulin G [IgG] antibodies; see chapter *Preventing Exposure to Opportunistic and Other Infections*).

S: Subjective

The patient may complain of subacute onset of dull, constant headache, fever, visual changes or other focal neurologic symptoms, confusion, or disorientation. Seizures may occur. Caregivers may report subtle alterations in mental status or mood.

Take a careful history from the patient and caregivers about the symptoms listed above and their duration, progression, and severity. Inquire about other related symptoms. Ask whether the patient is taking *Toxoplasma* prophylaxis or ART.

O: Objective

- Measure vital signs (temperature, heart rate, blood pressure, respiratory rate).

- Perform a full physical examination including a thorough neurologic examination, looking for focal or nonfocal neurologic deficits, particularly weakness, cranial nerve abnormalities, visual field defects, gait disturbances, and abnormalities in speech, cognitive, or affective functions.

- Review previous laboratory values, particularly the following:

  - CD4 count (usually <50-100 cells/μL in patients with toxoplasmosis)

- *Toxoplasma* IgG (>95% of patients with toxoplasmosis have positive IgG)

A: Assessment

Rule out other infectious or neoplastic causes of headache, fever, and neurologic changes. A partial differential diagnosis includes the following:

- CNS lymphoma
- Cryptococcal meningitis
- Progressive multifocal leukoencephalopathy (PML)
- Tuberculous meningitis
- Brain abscesses of bacterial, fungal, or mycobacterial etiologies
- Herpes simplex virus or cytomegalovirus (CMV) encephalitis
- Primary HIV encephalopathy
- AIDS dementia complex
- Cerebrovascular accident secondary to hemorrhage, hypoxia, or emboli from vegetative endocarditis
- Neurosyphilis
- Other causes of chorioretinitis such as CMV, HIV, and cryptosporidiosis

P: Plan

Diagnostic Evaluation

Definitive diagnosis requires identification of *T. gondii* in tissue biopsy or body fluid samples from a patient with a compatible clinical presentation. Brain biopsy usually is not performed if toxoplasmosis is strongly suspected; instead, presumptive diagnosis is made on the basis of clinical presentation, laboratory and imaging tests, and response to therapy. Brain biopsy should be considered for patients who do not respond to therapy and for those whose diagnosis is unclear.

- Serum *Toxoplasma* IgG antibody test results are positive in nearly all patients with toxoplasmic encephalitis. A negative IgG test result makes the diagnosis very unlikely but does not rule it out. (Antibody titer changes are uncommon in reactivation disease and are not useful in making a diagnosis.)

- CNS imaging with computed tomography (CT) typically shows multiple contrast-enhancing mass lesions, but may show a single lesion or no lesions. Magnetic resonance imaging (MRI) is more sensitive than CT for CNS toxoplasmosis. Other imaging studies, such as single photon emission CT (SPECT), may be useful in distinguishing toxoplasmic lesions from CNS lymphoma.

- Polymerase chain reaction (PCR) tests for *T. gondii* in the cerebrospinal fluid have poor sensitivity.

- Other diagnostic tests should be performed as indicated to rule out other potential causes of the patient's symptoms.

- Patients with toxoplasmic encephalitis typically respond quickly to treatment. If clinical improvement is not seen after 10-14 days of appropriate treatment, or if clinical worsening is seen in the first week, consider brain biopsy for alternative diagnoses.

Treatment

Treatment consists of two phases: acute therapy and chronic maintenance therapy. If possible, consult with an expert on the management of toxoplasmosis.

Presumptive treatment often is begun on the basis of clinical presentation, positive *Toxoplasma* IgG, and results of brain imaging studies. If patients do not respond quickly to treatment, other diagnoses should be considered. The following recommendations are based on treatment guidelines published by the Centers for Disease Control and Prevention, National Institutes of Health, and HIV Medicine Association/Infectious Diseases Society of America (see "References," below).

Acute Therapy

Acute therapy should be given for at least 6 weeks, and until the patient has shown improvement by clinical and radiographic measures.

Preferred

- Pyrimethamine 200 mg PO as a single loading dose, then 50 mg (<60 kg body weight) to 75 mg (>60 kg body weight) once daily + sulfadiazine 1,000 mg (<60 kg body weight) to 1,500 mg PO Q6H (>60 kg body weight) + folinic acid (leucovorin) 10-25 mg once daily

Dosage adjustments to the lower end of therapeutic range of pyrimethamine and sulfadiazine may be considered for patients who have significant bone marrow suppression despite folinic acid supplementation. Monitor patients carefully for cytopenias, especially if they are taking other agents that cause bone marrow suppression, such as zidovudine, valganciclovir, and ganciclovir.

Note: Patients at risk of G6PD deficiency should be checked for G6PD deficiency before starting pyrimethamine.

Alternatives

- Pyrimethamine + folinic acid (administered as described above) + one of the following:

  - Clindamycin 600 mg PO or IV Q6H; recommended for patients with significant allergic reactions to sulfa medications

  - Atovaquone 1,500 mg PO Q12H

  - Azithromycin 1,200 mg PO once daily

- Trimethoprim-sulfamethoxazole (TMP-SMX) 5 mg/kg TMP and 25 mg/kg SMX PO or IV Q12H. TMP-SMX can be considered when the availability of other regimens is limited or when patients need IV therapy

- Atovaquone 1,500 mg PO BID + sulfadiazine 1,000-1,500 mg PO Q6H

Note: The regimens that contain sulfadiazine, TMP-SMX, or atovaquone also are effective in preventing *Pneumocystis jiroveci* pneumonia (PCP), so patients on these regimens do not need additional PCP prophylaxis.

Adjunctive corticosteroids (e.g., dexamethasone 4 mg PO or IV Q6H) may be indicated for patients with CNS mass effect or edema. Use is based on clinical judgment and should be discontinued as soon as it is feasible to do so.

Anticonvulsant therapy should be given to patients with seizures.

Ventilatory support may be necessary if severe CNS symptomatology is present.

Chronic Maintenance Therapy

After at least 6 weeks of initial therapy and significant clinical and radiologic improvement, chronic maintenance therapy can be considered.

Preferred

- Pyrimethamine 25-50 mg PO once daily + sulfadiazine 2,000-4,000 mg PO daily in 2-4 divided doses + folinic acid 10-25 mg PO once daily (also effective as PCP prophylaxis)

Alternatives

- Pyrimethamine 25-50 mg PO once daily + clindamycin 600 mg PO Q8H + folinic acid 10-25 mg PO once daily

- Atovaquone 750 mg PO Q6-12H +/- pyrimethamine 25 mg PO once daily (+ folinic acid 10 mg PO once daily) or sulfadiazine 2,000-4,000 mg PO daily in 2-4 divided doses (also effective as PCP prophylaxis)

- Limited data suggest that TMP-SMX also is effective

Chronic maintenance therapy generally should be continued for life. For patients who complete acute therapy successfully, have resolution of signs and symptoms of toxoplasmosis, and have immune reconstitution (with CD4 counts >200 cells/μL) for more than 6 months on ART, it is reasonable to consider discontinuing maintenance therapy. Some specialists would require resolution of CNS lesions on radiologic studies before discontinuation of therapy. Patients must be observed for recurrence of symptoms, and treatment should be restarted if the CD4 count decreases to <200 cells/μL.

Considerations During Pregnancy

All pregnant women should be tested for *T. gondii*. If the result is positive, evaluate the pregnant woman for signs or symptoms of toxoplasmosis and the neonate for evidence of congenital infection. Perinatal transmission usually occurs only with acute maternal infection, but in advanced HIV, it may occur with reactivation of chronic infection. If *T. gondii* infection occurs during pregnancy, consult with maternal-fetal and infectious disease specialists. Treatment for pregnant women is the same as for nonpregnant adults (see above). Note that sulfadiazine taken at the time of delivery may increase the risk of neonatal hyperbilirubinemia and kernicterus.

Patient Education

- Advise patients that antimicrobial therapy alone will not eradicate toxoplasmosis, but should decrease symptoms and improve quality of life. If medications are discontinued, the disease is likely to recur, unless the CD4 count increases to >100-200 cells/μL in response to ART.

- Inform patients that suppressive therapy must be continued to prevent recurrence. The duration of this therapy may be lifelong.

- It is essential for patients to take all medicines exactly as prescribed. If doses are missed, or if the medications are stopped and restarted, *Toxoplasma* can develop resistance to the medications. If patients are having trouble taking the medication on schedule, they should contact their health care provider immediately.

- Educate patients about the benefits of ART in strengthening the immune system and preventing opportunistic infections such as toxoplasmosis.

- Advise patients to contact the clinic promptly if symptoms worsen or if new symptoms develop.

- Toxoplasmosis is a late-stage HIV opportunistic infection that indicates profound immune suppression. Some patients may not respond to treatment or to ART. As with any patient who is at risk of a life-threatening HIV-related disease, clinicians should discuss advance directives and durable power of attorney with patients. Referral to a social worker, mental health clinician, or chaplain experienced in such issues may facilitate this discussion.

References

- Centers for Disease Control and Prevention. *Guidelines for Prevention and Treatment of Opportunistic Infections in HIV-Infected Adults and Adolescents: Recommendations from CDC, the National Institutes of Health, and the HIV Medicine Association of the Infectious Diseases Society of America.* April 10, 2009. Available at www.aidsinfo.nih.gov/guidelines/.

- Liesenfeld O, Wang SY, Remington JS. *Toxoplasmosis in the Setting of AIDS.* In: Merigan TC, Bartlett JG, Bolognesi D, eds. *Textbook of AIDS Medicine, 2nd Edition.* Baltimore: Williams and Wilkins; 1999:225-259.

- Subauste CS. *Toxoplasmosis and HIV.* In: Coffey S, Volberding PA, eds. *HIV InSite Knowledge Base* [textbook online]. San Francisco: UCSF Center for HIV Information; 2006. Available at hivinsite.ucsf.edu/InSite?page=kb-05-04-03. Accessed June 30, 2010.

Adverse Reactions to HIV Medications

Kirsten Balano, PharmD

Background

Clinicians and patients face many challenges associated with antiretroviral therapy (ART). These include making decisions about when to start therapy, what regimen to start with, when to change medications, and how to switch if a regimen is failing. Although clinical research guides the selection of antiretroviral (ARV) regimens, it is important to remember that the best regimen for any patient is the regimen that individual is willing and able to take. No regimen, no matter how potent, will be effective if the patient does not take it properly. Adherence to ART is one of the most important predictors of treatment efficacy. Although many factors may interfere with proper adherence to ART, adverse reactions to the medications are among the most important. In one trial, patients experiencing adverse events were 13 times less likely than those not experiencing adverse events to have the highest levels (95-100%) of adherence. Monitoring and managing adverse reactions to ARVs are crucial to establishing a successful HIV regimen.

Although adverse reactions are common and often predictable, their management must be individualized. Several factors will affect the management of adverse reactions, including comorbid conditions, the patient's other current medications, the availability of alternative medications, and the patient's history of medication intolerance. In some cases, the patient's report of the severity of adverse effects can be inconsistent with the clinical interpretation (i.e., some patients may overemphasize symptoms, whereas others underemphasize them), and this must be considered when determining the management of adverse reactions.

Using a case-based approach, this chapter suggests strategies for the evaluation and management of adverse effects, and it reviews several of the most commonly noted adverse effects in patients starting an ARV regimen. It is not intended as a comprehensive guide to adverse effects. For detailed information regarding assessment of symptoms, see the complaint-specific chapters found in section *Common Complaints* of this manual. For information on common adverse reactions to ARV agents and to medications used to prevent and treat opportunistic infections, see chapter *Antiretroviral Therapy* of this manual. In each case of suspected medication adverse effects, the patient should be evaluated for other possible causes of the symptoms. Consultation with an HIV expert can help in determining the best management strategy when symptoms may have multiple and overlapping causes.

S: Subjective

A patient presents 3 weeks after starting a new ARV regimen. She complains of fatigue, nausea, and rash. Her current ARV medications are nevirapine (NVP) plus a fixed-dose combination of zidovudine (ZDV), lamivudine (3TC), and abacavir (i.e., Trizivir). This was selected on the basis of her preferences and her past treatment history. She also is taking trimethoprim-sulfamethoxazole (TMP-SMX) as prophylaxis against PCP. Although she reports that she had not missed any doses of her medications and she likes the low pill burden of this regimen, she does not want to continue because she has been feeling so sick that she cannot adequately care for her children. She is asking to stop her ARV therapy because of "too many side effects."

The patient should be evaluated in the clinic for her complaints about adverse effects.

O: Objective

The following are suggestions for this evaluation; they are not intended to be a complete review of the workup and management of each symptom or objective finding. For more-detailed information, refer to the complaint-specific chapters of this manual, as noted above.

Vital signs: Fever may indicate a hypersensitivity reaction (HSR) or acute hepatitis attributable to medications, or an immune reconstitution inflammatory syndrome in relation to an opportunistic infection in the setting of early ART therapy. See chapter *Fever* for a more complete discussion about fever workup and considerations. Tachycardia or hypotension may suggest anemia, HSR, dehydration, infection, or another illness.

Physical examination: Pay special attention to the skin (rash, pallor), mucous membranes, and liver (enlargement or tenderness). Positive physical examination findings should be evaluated for severity and extent of involvement.

Laboratory tests: Check the complete blood count when monitoring drugs that may cause bone marrow toxicity (e.g., anemia, neutropenia). Perform a complete metabolic panel including electrolytes and liver function tests (LFTs). If the history suggests pancreatitis, evaluate amylase or lipase.

Other studies: Perform as indicated by symptoms and examination (e.g., chest X ray if respiratory symptoms are present).

A: Assessment

Step 1: Clarify the patient's reports of adverse reactions by requesting the following information for each symptom the patient describes:

- Characterize the symptoms by asking about severity, onset, timing, and frequency. It is helpful to have the patient describe whether the symptoms have been improving or worsening over time.

- Ask whether the patient has tried any remedies to alleviate the symptoms and whether they were helpful.

- Explore how the patient is currently taking the regimen. Open-end questions (e.g., "What are your current medications?" "How often do you take them?" "How many pills of each medicine do you take?" and "Do you take your medicines with or without food?") can be helpful in determining whether the patient has been taking medications correctly. Incorrect administration of medications (e.g., taking higher dosages than recommended) can lead to adverse effects and often is overlooked by providers.

Step 2: Assess the severity of the reaction against the need to continue the current regimen. For this assessment, it is important to have an understanding of the relative availability of alternative ARV regimens. Also try to determine the patient's risks for adverse reactions to specific medications. A review of the patient's clinical status, treatment history, resistance tests, and other testing is important.

- Most adverse effects are self-limited and mild-to-moderate in severity. With supportive care, patients often are able to continue their current medications. This is particularly true with regard to gastrointestinal symptoms (e.g., nausea, vomiting, bloating, diarrhea). Supportive care for gastrointestinal adverse effects includes reminding the patient to take medications with food (if appropriate), suggesting the use of symptomatic remedies (e.g., ginger-containing beverages or foods to relieve nausea [see "Nausea," below]), and prescribing medications such as antiemetics or antidiarrheals if needed. Other symptoms that can be monitored carefully with supportive care include fatigue, malaise, mild rashes, abdominal pain, and bloating.

- More severe reactions often require discontinuation of the offending medication. These include fever, liver function abnormalities, rash with mucous membrane involvement, or severe systemic symptoms.

- Determining which medication in a multidrug regimen is causing the reaction is often challenging because it is common for patients to concurrently take several medications with overlapping toxicities.

- Some patient factors affect the risk of particular adverse drug effects. For example, patients with higher CD4 cell counts at the time that nevirapine is initiated have a greater risk of hepatotoxicity (specifically, women with CD4 counts of >250 cells/μL or men with CD4 counts of >400 cells/μL), and patients with the HLA-B*5701 allele have higher rates of abacavir HSR (see "Abacavir Hypersensitivity Reaction," below).

- It is important to consider the possibility that non-ARV medications in the patient's regimen could be causing the adverse effects. Even with patients who have been on other non-ARV medications for months or years, initiation of a new ARV regimen (e.g., one with potent hepatic CYP 450 inhibition or induction effects) may alter serum levels of these other medications (see chapter *Drug-Drug Interactions with HIV-Related Medications*). For example, an increase in anxiety symptoms after starting a new ARV regimen could be attributable to altered drug concentrations of a chronic antidepressant or antianxiety medicine caused by an ARV, not to the new ARV medications themselves.

- The threshold for stopping a medication depends in part on the availability of alternative agents for the individual patient. Some patients have limited alternatives because their virus is resistant to other ARVs (e.g., patients on salvage ARV regimens) or because they have not tolerated certain ARVs in the past. For patients who develop significant adverse effects when starting their first ARV regimen, consider substituting alternative ARV medications (chosen with efficacy considerations in mind) that are better tolerated as early as possible to prevent nonadherence arising from a desire to avoid the adverse effects. For these situations, single-drug substitutions often improve tolerance and make it more likely that long-term viral suppression can be achieved.

- Some patients may refuse to attempt symptomatic treatment or to make substitutions in the ARV regimen. Although treatment interruptions generally should be avoided, in certain situations it may be best to discontinue all ARVs and return to an adherence-readiness assessment (see chapter *Adherence*) to determine when to restart ART and what medications to restart (see chapter *Antiretroviral Therapy*).

Gathering Additional Subjective and Objective Information

For the patient who reported nausea, fatigue, and rash 3 weeks after starting nevirapine and ZDV/3TC/abacavir (Trizivir) (see above), additional history, physical examination, and laboratory work yielded the following information:

- **Nausea:** This has been present since she started ART 3 weeks ago. She has had difficulty taking the ARVs with food, because of nausea. No actual vomiting or other abdominal pain has occurred. She has not tried any remedies. The nausea is not worsening and perhaps has improved slightly over the past few days.

- **Fatigue:** This has been present since she started ARVs 3 weeks ago. She is able to exercise and perform normal daily activities.

- **Vital signs:** Normal, with no fever or signs of hemodynamic changes.

- **Skin:** Skin and conjunctival pallor is noted, along with mild-to-moderate maculopapular rash on the trunk, back, and extremities.

Section 7: ARV Interactions and Adverse Events

These are associated with slight itching, but no pain. No mucous membrane involvement is noted. The rash has been present for 6 days, with slight improvement over the past day.

- **Abdomen:** Nontender, with normal liver size.
- **Complete blood count:** Normal, except for a slight increase in mean corpuscular volume (MCV), probably from ZDV therapy and not indicating macrocytic anemia.
- **LFTs:** Normal.
- **Pretreatment laboratory results:** CD4 count of 190 cells/µL, HLA-B*5701 negative.

Assessing Availability of Alternative Regimens

A clarified ARV history yielded the following information. The patient took ZDV for 5 months during one of her pregnancies a few years ago, and she recalls similar feelings of nausea and fatigue that caused her distress at the time. She was able to continue ZDV through the end of her pregnancy. She has taken several ritonavir-boosted protease inhibitors briefly in the past; she did not tolerate these and subsequently has refused treatment with protease inhibitors. Her virus is resistant to lamivudine and emtricitabine. She has no significant comorbidities. The patient has a number of treatment options, but these may be limited by tolerance issues (e.g., to protease inhibitors).

Summary Assessment

The patient's symptoms are mild and are most likely related to starting ARV therapy. The laboratory evaluation does not reveal significant abnormalities (e.g., anemia, transaminitis). In particular, the symptoms and signs and laboratory work are not consistent with HSR, hepatotoxicity, or other serious adverse effects. Thus, no additional workup is needed at this time. Careful monitoring is important because,

if symptoms do not improve over the next few days, the patient should have a more extensive workup for other possible causes of the various symptoms. If other causes of her symptoms are ruled out and she is unable to tolerate supportive care, alternative ARV medications (e.g., tenofovir, raltegravir, or perhaps unboosted protease inhibitors) could be substituted for medications in her current regimen (keeping in mind the need to maintain efficacy of the overall regimen).

P: Plan

A suggested treatment plan for the mild adverse effects exhibited by the patient described above is as follows:

Fatigue

Fatigue is a common adverse effect among patients who are starting ART. It is usually self-limited, and, with reassurance that symptoms should improve over a few weeks, most patients are able to continue their regimens without any changes. If fatigue does not resolve within the first weeks of treatment, it is important to rule out other causes of fatigue, including depression. For ZDV-containing regimens, clinicians should rule out ZDV-induced anemia, especially when patients are taking other medications that can cause bone marrow toxicity (e.g., TMP-SMX). Some patients experience fatigue from ZDV even without anemia. If fatigue persists for several weeks or becomes debilitating, and other causes are ruled out, consider replacing ZDV in this regimen. Patients taking regimens containing efavirenz also may complain of fatigue. With efavirenz, the fatigue often is related to sleep disturbances and other central nervous system (CNS) effects of this medication. Efavirenz-related CNS adverse effects, including fatigue, are likely to resolve over a period of days to weeks. Toxicities can be minimized by ensuring that patients take efavirenz on an empty stomach (1 hour before or 2 hours after eating). (See chapter *Fatigue*.)

Nausea

Nausea is another common adverse effect described by patients starting a new ARV regimen. As with fatigue, it usually is self-limited, and patients without other systemic symptoms, acute hepatitis, HSR, or pancreatitis usually can continue their regimens. Supportive care often helps patients to continue their regimens. For example, patients should take their medications with food, unless contraindicated for the ARV. Small, frequent snacks may be helpful for patients with significant nausea. Clinical trials have suggested that ginger extract may relieve nausea symptoms. Patients can take ginger (available in a variety of forms, including ginger ale, tea, cookies, and candies) or antiemetics.

Among the medications that the patient described above is taking, ZDV is the most likely culprit to cause persistent nausea. If nausea symptoms continue for several weeks despite taking the ARVs with food, using ginger, or taking other antiemetics, and if other underlying causes are ruled out, consider replacing ZDV in this regimen. (See chapter *Nausea and Vomiting*.)

Rash

Rash is a common adverse effect of certain ARVs and many other medications. It may present with a wide range of severity, as follows:

- Mild rash with no other related symptoms, resolving over the course of days or weeks

- Moderate rash, may be accompanied by systemic symptoms (e.g., fever, liver function abnormalities, myalgias)

- Life-threatening rashes (e.g., Stevens-Johnson syndrome, toxic epidermal necrolysis) associated with pain, mucous membrane involvement, fever, liver function changes, and myalgias

If a patient is taking two or more medications that have rash as a possible adverse effect, it may be difficult to determine which medicine is the most likely cause of the rash. In the case of the patient described above, rash may be related to one of three medications. Her rash currently is mild, but drug rash can range from mild to severe and life-threatening (including Stevens-Johnson syndrome).

- Abacavir

  - Mild abacavir rash: usually a self-limited reaction that can be treated symptomatically

  - Moderate to severe rash, with or without abacavir HSR (see "Abacavir Hypersensitivity Reaction," below): resolution of symptoms requires discontinuation of abacavir; in the case of HSR, repeat challenge with abacavir can be life-threatening (see below for more details)

- Nevirapine

  - Mild nevirapine rash: usually a self-limited reaction that can be treated symptomatically

  - Moderate to severe nevirapine rash, with or without hepatitis: requires discontinuation of nevirapine

- TMP-SMX reaction: may be mild or severe, and onset may be delayed

- Other reactions: can be caused by other medications, by immune reconstitution inflammatory effects, contact dermatitis, folliculitis, and other causes

If the clinician discontinues all of the suspect medications and the rash resolves, the patient will be relieved, but the clinician will not be able to determine which medication caused the rash. In cases of mild rash, it is reasonable to try to identify the offending agent by discontinuing one medication at a time (a substitution should be made for a discontinued ARV, to maintain regimen potency). This situation would require careful clinical judgment or consultation with an expert regarding the advantages or disadvantages of discontinuing each of the suspect medications.

Abacavir Hypersensitivity Reaction

Rash owing to abacavir may occur in isolation or as part of the abacavir HSR. Abacavir HSR should be suspected when two or more of the following symptoms are present: fever, rash, constitutional symptoms (malaise, fatigue, aches), respiratory symptoms (dyspnea, cough), or gastrointestinal symptoms (nausea/vomiting, abdominal pain, diarrhea). The initial symptoms of possible abacavir HSR are not life-threatening, and it is important to try distinguishing true abacavir HSR from isolated rash (without other hypersensitivity symptoms), self-limited adverse medication effects, or other illness (e.g., influenza).

The risk of abacavir HSR is closely linked to HLA-B*5701. The availability of genetic testing for this allele and avoidance of abacavir for use in patients with this allele has minimized the risk of abacavir HSR, but patients with symptoms that may be caused by abacavir HSR should be evaluated carefully to rule out a true abacavir HSR. Before starting an abacavir-containing regimen, patients should be tested for HLA-B*5701; patients who test positive for B*5701 should not be given abacavir.

Other Adverse Reactions

Patients may describe any number of adverse effects after starting new medications. Although some adverse effects are caused directly by the medications themselves, some symptoms may occur simply in the process of starting ART. The start of ART may precipitate a significant psychological shift in a patient's perception of self, in living with HIV infection, and in daily routine. In particular, patients who have kept their HIV infection distant from their "everyday" lives may notice significant psychological changes as they take

medications every day, go to the pharmacy to pick up medications, and make frequent visits to the clinic for evaluation and laboratory work. Some patients become depressed upon realizing that the severity of their illness now requires them to be on treatment. These psychological adjustments can cause significant symptoms that should be assessed and managed in a manner similar to the way in which pharmacologic adverse reactions are managed.

These psychological effects can be considered "process" effects from starting ART rather than adverse effects of the ARV medications themselves. As with the self-limited adverse effects of early-stage ARV therapy, process effects should become more tolerable over time as the medication regimen becomes routine for the patient. One of the most common process effects is fatigue. Many patients hope that their ARV regimen will give them increased energy and health, and they become frustrated when they notice increasing fatigue after starting the regimen. These patients must be evaluated to rule out common adverse effects that contribute to fatigue (e.g., anemia, hepatitis, lactic acidosis). Equally important, especially for patients beginning a new regimen, symptoms of fatigue could indicate depression or signal that the "process" of taking medications is emotionally difficult. Counseling, peer support, and antidepressant medications can be used to treat this type of fatigue. Often, once patients realize that some of the goals of treatment are being achieved (e.g., the CD4 cell count increases, the HIV viral load becomes undetectable, or symptoms of HIV infection resolve), they recognize the benefits of ARV medications, and their fatigue or other adverse symptoms associated with the process of starting the regimen This discussion has focused on the adverse reactions to ARV medications that patients are most likely to describe as they start a new regimen. Patients and providers also need to consider counseling about and management of long-term toxicities such as lipodystrophy, renal dysfunction, peripheral neuropathy, cardiac disease, diabetes, and dyslipidemia. As these long-term toxicities continue to challenge providers and patients alike, clinic trials and expert guidelines will provide support and information.

Clinicians are encouraged to report adverse reactions to medications to the U.S. Food and Drug Administration (FDA) MedWatch program by telephone at 800-FDA-1088, via fax at 800-FDA-0178, via the Internet at www.fda.gov/medwatch/report/, or by mail at MedWatch HF-2, FDA, 5600 Fishers Lane, Rockville, MD 20857.

Patient Education

- All medications have potential to cause adverse reactions, which are defined as negative, unintended effects of medication use.

- Advise patients to report any adverse reaction to their medical care provider as soon as possible.

- Before starting a new medication, medical care providers or pharmacists should counsel patients about the most common adverse effects and about any remedies that are available to minimize the severity of those effects.

- Advise patients to talk to their provider or pharmacist before starting any new medications (including over-the-counter medications and herbs) because some drugs may interact with ARVs or other medications and can increase side effects or cause unwanted reactions.

- Nausea is one of the most common adverse effects. Counsel patients that nausea can be minimized by taking medications with food (if indicated, as some medications should be taken on an empty stomach) or by using ginger-based food or beverages (e.g., ginger

ale, tea, cookies). If these measures do not work, patients should talk with their medical care provider; they may need medications to treat the symptoms.

- Counsel patients that they should not stop taking any medications unless instructed to do so by their medical care provider.

References

- Calmy A, Hirschel B, Cooper DA, et al. *A new era of antiretroviral drug toxicity.* Antivir Ther. 2009;14(2):165-79.

- Ickovics JR, Cameron A, Zackin R, et al. *Consequences and determinants of adherence to antiretroviral medication: results from Adult AIDS Clinical Trials Group protocol 370.* Antivir Ther. 2002 Sep;7(3):185-93.

- Montessori V, Press N, Harris M, et al. *Adverse effects of antiretroviral therapy for HIV infection.* CMAJ. 2004 Jan 20;170(2):229-38.

- Roca B. *Adverse drug reactions to antiretroviral medication.* Front Biosci. 2009 Jan;14:1785-92.

- U.S. Department of Health and Human Services. *Table 12: Antiretroviral Therapy-Associated Adverse Effects and Management Recommendations.* In: *Guidelines for the Use of Antiretroviral Agents in HIV-1-Infected Adults and Adolescents.* January 10, 2011. Available at aidsinfo.nih.gov/contentfiles/AA_Tables.pdf.

Section 7: ARV Interactions and Adverse Events

Drug-Drug Interactions with HIV-Related Medications

Kirsten Balano, PharmD

Background

Drug-drug interactions are common concerns of patients with HIV and their health care providers. The issues involved in evaluating drug interactions are complex. Although many questions can be articulated simply (e.g., "What antidepressant is least likely to have drug interactions with antiretroviral medications?"), the responses to these questions involve more complex concerns (e.g., "In choosing an antidepressant for my patient with HIV, I must consider efficacy, adverse effects, and tolerability as well as drug interactions.").

This complexity is increased because antiretroviral (ARV) agents, particularly protease inhibitors (PIs), nonnucleoside reverse transcriptase inhibitors (NNRTIs), and the CCR5 antagonist maraviroc, can cause or be affected by alterations in the activity of the cytochrome (CYP) P450 enzyme system in the liver, as well as by other mechanisms of drug metabolism. Interactions between an ARV and another drug (whether another ARV or a different type of medication) may result in an increase or a decrease in the serum levels of either the ARV or the interacting drug, potentially changing the effectiveness or the toxicity risk of substrate drugs. Understanding drug-drug interactions is challenging because of several factors, including the following:

- Different drugs affect different P450 enzymes.
- Some medications have dose-related responses that influence their effects on P450 enzymes.
- Formal pharmacokinetic studies on drug combinations are limited.
- Even when pharmacokinetic data exist for specific drug combinations, the clinical significance of any changes in pharmacokinetic parameters may not be clear.
- Patients taking ARVs often have complex drug regimens. Patients typically are taking three or more medications that could influence interactions. Pharmacokinetic studies that evaluate the clinical significance of drug interactions involving more than two medications are less likely to be available.
- Other metabolic pathways of medications such as P-glycoprotein (P-gp) and UDP-glucuronosyltransferase (UGT)-1A1, can be altered by drug interactions. The integrase inhibitor raltegravir, for example, is metabolized by UGT-1A1 and also is a substrate of P-gp.
- The P450 system is not the only influence on medication activity. Other influences include absorption, food-drug interactions, protein binding, altered activation of medications intracellularly, and altered efflux-pump activity.

Information on various drug-drug interactions is available in guidelines and via the Internet (see "Resources," below). Such resources can provide data regarding two-drug combinations, but rarely consider all the complexities outlined above. What follows, therefore, is a suggested approach to considering drug-drug interactions in managing HIV-infected patients and making patient-specific decisions.

S: Subjective

A new patient arrives for a clinic intake appointment. The patient receives medical care from a local infectious disease physician who treats only a handful of HIV-infected patients. The patient was recently released from hospital with a discharge diagnosis of pneumonia and *Mycobacterium avium* complex (MAC). The patient is not yet taking ARVs, but is likely to start in the next several weeks after the establishment of care and adherence support programs. Other problems include hyperlipidemia, erectile dysfunction, diabetes, depression, gastroesophageal reflux disease (GERD), and herpes. The clinician wants to review the patient's medication list to check for any potential drug-drug interactions.

O: Objective

Review the patient's pharmacy records for current medications, and ask about use of over-the-counter (OTC), herbal or natural products, and dietary supplements. As requested, the patient has brought in all medications from home for review. The current medication list includes the following:

- Clarithromycin 500 mg BID
- Ethambutol 1,000 mg once daily
- Rifabutin 300 mg once daily
- TMP-SMX (Septra, Bactrim) double strength, one tablet once daily
- Lovastatin 20 mg once daily
- Metformin 500 mg BID
- Bupropion 150 mg once daily
- Acyclovir 400 mg BID
- Omeprazole 20 mg once daily (patient buys OTC for heartburn)
- Milk thistle (silymarin) (patient takes as needed for energy and liver health)

A: Assessment

Step 1: Identify interactions and classify them as follows:

- Definite interactions
- Probable interactions
- Possible interactions

Definite Drug Interactions

A drug interaction is definite if a high level of evidence is available regarding the drug combination, the clinical significance of the interaction is well understood, and consensus exists regarding the management strategy (e.g., whether dosage adjustments are required, or concurrent use is contraindicated). Common definite interactions for HIV patients include the following:

- Certain combinations of HIV agents (e.g., certain PIs with NNRTIs, maraviroc with PIs or NNRTIs, tenofovir with atazanavir)
- Rifamycins and PIs, NNRTIs, or maraviroc
- Statins and PIs
- Erectile dysfunction agents and PIs
- Methadone and certain PIs or NNRTIs
- Fluticasone and PIs

Probable Drug Interactions

A drug interaction is probable if the limited available evidence suggests that an interaction may occur, even if the clinical outcome or significance may not be clearly established. Effective management of a probable interaction is based on assessment and clinical judgment about the risks and benefits of a particular combination for each patient. Examples of probable interactions with HIV-related medications include the following:

- Antidepressants and PIs or NNRTIs
- Oral contraceptives and PIs
- Warfarin and PIs or NNRTIs
- Proton pump inhibitors (PPIs) or H-2

blockers and atazanavir

- Certain antifungal agents and PIs or NNRTIs (except in the case of voriconazole, for which definite information on interactions is available)

- Certain antiepileptic medications and PIs or NNRTIs

Possible Drug Interactions

Possible drug interactions may be difficult to distinguish from probable drug interactions, but in these cases, only theoretical evidence is available. The proper management of such interactions requires weighing the risks and benefits of the combination and making sound clinical judgments. Examples of possible drug interactions with HIV medications include the following:

- Herbal products and PIs or NNRTIs (except in the case of St. John's wort, for which definite information on interactions is available)

- Antidiabetic medications and PIs or NNRTIs

- Antipsychotic agents and PIs or NNRTIs

Memorizing all the potential drug interactions is impossible. It is possible, however, to remember a few commonly encountered drug combinations that have the potential for clinically significant interactions. It is also important to recognize that PIs (particularly ritonavir) and NNRTIs very commonly interact with other medications. The above examples of definite, probable, and possible interactions are reasonable "red flag" drug combinations that can be recalled easily. In addition, certain Internet resources allow providers to submit all of a patient's current medications and planned additions (e.g., atazanavir/ritonavir as part of a new ARV regimen) and receive information on potential interactions (see "Resources," below). Finally, consultation with clinical pharmacists can aid in identifying and classifying potential

interactions.

P: Plan

Step 2: The patient described above will start an ARV regimen of atazanavir/ritonavir + tenofovir + emtricitabine. The PI may cause problematic drug-drug interactions with some of the patient's preexisting medications, and tenofovir interacts with atazanavir. Develop a plan for management when these ARVs are added. For this patient, the following definite interactions should be of concern:

- Rifabutin and atazanavir/ritonavir

- Lovastatin and atazanavir/ritonavir

- Tenofovir and atazanavir

- Clarithromycin and atazanavir/ritonavir

Refer to available references for management suggestions. Such references include the following:

- U.S. Department of Health and Human Services *Adult and Adolescent Antiretroviral Treatment Guidelines* (January 10, 2011), Tables 14, 15a-e, and 16 a-b

- *HIV InSite Database of Antiretroviral Drug Interactions* (www.hivinsite.ucsf.edu)

- University of Liverpool Drug Interactions Tables (www.hiv-druginteractions.org)

- Clinical Care Options (www. clinicaloptions.com)

Most of these resources include specific dosage adjustments or alternative agents to consider when managing these drug combinations. The suggestions for this patient are as follows:

- Rifabutin levels are increased by atazanavir/ritonavir. The rifabutin dosage should be decreased to 150 mg QOD with standard atazanavir/ritonavir dosing. Alternatively, discuss with the patient's primary care provider whether rifabutin is important to the current MAC regimen or whether the patient could be treated adequately with just clarithromycin + ethambutol to avoid the above interactions.

- Lovastatin levels are increased substantially by atazanavir/ritonavir; concurrent use with a PI can lead to potentially fatal rhabdomyolysis. Lovastatin should be discontinued when atazanavir/ritonavir is initiated. To manage hyperlipidemia, the patient should be switched to a statin whose metabolism is less affected by these PIs, such as pravastatin or low-dose atorvastatin (simvastatin, also is contraindicated for use by patients who take a PI).

- Tenofovir can decrease plasma concentrations of unboosted atazanavir, but can be safely administered with ritonavir-boosted atazanavir.

- Clarithromycin levels are increased by atazanavir/ritonavir; concurrent use can lead to QTc prolongation. If clarithromycin is co-administered with atazanavir/ritonavir, its dosage should be reduced by 50%.

Although this patient's current medication list does not contain an erectile dysfunction agent, the patient should be educated about the definite interactions and dosage adjustments recommended for patients using those agents with PIs. Some patients may obtain erectile dysfunction agents outside the care of their physician and, if unaware of the interactions and suggested dosage adjustments, may be at risk of life-threatening consequences.

The following probable or possible interactions should be considered if PIs are begun, including:

- Omeprazole with atazanavir/ritonavir
- Bupropion with atazanavir/ritonavir
- Milk thistle with atazanavir/ritonavir

The web-based resources and other references listed above include some information about these potential interactions. The following are suggestions:

- **Omeprazole**: PPIs and H2-blockers decrease serum levels of atazanavir, even when boosted with ritonavir, but the clinical significance of this interaction has not been demonstrated. In general, it may be best to avoid concomitant use of these acid-blocking medications with atazanavir by either discontinuing the GERD medication or switching to another ARV. Unboosted atazanavir should not be used with PPIs. For patients without evidence of ARV resistance in whom coadministration of these medications is judged unavoidable, atazanavir/ritonavir may be used, but doses of omeprazole should not exceed 20 mg and must be taken at least 12 hours prior to taking atazanavir/ritonavir. Note that tenofovir can also lower atazanavir levels, so increasing atazanavir to 400 mg/day with ritonavir 100 mg/day should be considered.

- **Bupropion and milk thistle:** Specific management or dosage adjustments based on data are not available. This patient should be monitored for increased or decreased effects of bupropion and educated about potential interactions with milk thistle. Clinical judgment and decision making with the primary care provider and other specialists (e.g., psychiatrists) may be required.

Consultation with clinical pharmacy services may assist in evaluating the potential significance of drug interactions and developing management strategies.

Patient Education

- Instruct patients that HIV medications, in particular PIs, NNRTIs, and maraviroc, have a high potential for significant drug interactions.

- Tell patients to bring all their medicines, including any herbal, nutritional, and dietary supplements and OTC remedies, with them to all medical appointments. If they cannot bring the actual containers with them, they should bring a list of current prescribed medications, supplements, and OTC medications.

- Patients should have their primary care provider or pharmacist review any newly prescribed medications along with their current list of medicines. This is especially important if another physician prescribes a new medication.

- Patients should not "borrow" medications from friends or family. Assure patients that if they have a problem that needs medical treatment, their primary care provider will discuss it and choose the safest treatments for them.

- Tell patients that, if they are considering buying a new nutritional or herbal supplement or an OTC product, they should consult their pharmacist or primary care provider about interactions with drugs on their current medication list.

- Not all drug interactions are cause for alarm. Some drug combinations are safe for certain people, but less safe for others. Warn patients not to stop taking any medicines without the advice of their primary care provider.

Resources

- *HIV InSite Database of Antiretroviral Drug Interactions* (hivinsite.ucsf.edu)

- University of Liverpool HIV Drug Interaction Charts (www.hiv-druginteractions.org)

- Clinical Care Options (www.clinicaloptions.com)

References

- Dickinson L, Khoo, S, Back D. *Pharmacokinetics and drug-drug interactions of antiretrovirals: an update.* Antiviral Res. 2010 Jan;85(1):176-89.

- Liedtke MD, Lockhart SM, Rathbun RC. *Anticonvulsant and antiretroviral interactions.* Ann Pharmacother. 2004 Mar;38(3):482-9.

- Piscitelli SC, Gallicano KD. *Interactions among drugs for HIV and opportunistic infections.* N Engl J Med. 2001 Mar 29;344(13):984-96.

- Rainey PM. *HIV drug interactions: the good, the bad, and the other.* Ther Drug Monit. 2002 Feb;24(1):26-31.

- Sheehan NL, Kelly DV, Tseng AL, et al. *Evaluation of HIV drug interaction web sites.* Ann Pharmacother. 2003 Nov;37(11):1577-86.

- Soodalter J, Sousa M, Boffito M. *Drug-drug interactions involving new antiretroviral drugs and drug classes.* Curr Opin Infect Dis. 2009 Feb;22(1):18-27.

- U.S. Department of Health and Human Services. *Guidelines for the Use of Antiretroviral Agents in HIV-1-Infected Adults and Adolescents.* January 10, 2011. Available at www.aidsinfo.nih.gov/guidelines/.

Antiretroviral Medications and Hormonal Contraceptive Agents

Background

Few pharmacokinetic or clinical studies have examined interactions between antiretroviral (ARV) medications and hormonal contraceptives, but it is known that certain protease inhibitors (PIs) and nonnucleoside reverse transcriptase inhibitors (NNRTIs) do interact with hormonal contraceptives. These interactions may increase the risk of medication failure or medication adverse effects — of either the ARV or the contraceptive. There are no known interactions between hormonal contraceptives and nucleoside analogues, integrase inhibitors, or CCR5 antagonists.

Oral Contraceptives

All oral contraceptives currently marketed in the United States, with the exception of progestin-only pills (which contain norethindrone), contain both ethinyl estradiol and a progestin (desogestrel, drospirenone, ethynodiol diacetate, levonorgestrel, norethindrone, norethindrone acetate, norgestimate, or norgestrel). The oral contraceptives ethinyl estradiol and norethindrone may interact in complex ways with PIs and NNRTIs. The mechanism of these interactions may be multifactorial and includes the activity of these agents on cytochrome P450 enzymes. Pharmacokinetic studies have shown changes (either increases or decreases) in levels of ethinyl estradiol and norethindrone in women who are taking certain PIs or NNRTIs. Other studies have shown decreases in levels of amprenavir in women taking oral contraceptives.

The clinical significance of these drug interactions has not been evaluated thoroughly, but may cause oral contraceptive failure, ARV failure, or medication toxicity, depending on whether drug levels are lowered or raised by the interacting drug. The consequences of decreased hormone levels may include an increased risk of pregnancy, so an alternative or additional method of contraception commonly is recommended. The consequences of decreased ARV levels may include virologic failure and development of resistance mutations. The consequences of a higher level of hormones may include risk of thromboembolism, breast tenderness, headache, nausea, and acne.

The available pharmacokinetic data are summarized in Table 1. For further discussion of oral and non-oral contraceptives for HIV-infected women, see chapter *Health Care of HIV-Infected Women Through the Life Cycle*.

Table 1. Interactions Between Antiretroviral Agents and Oral Contraceptives

☒ Use alternative/additional method or do not administer together　　❢ Use with caution　　✓ Safe to use in combination or no dosage adjustment necessary

Antiretroviral Agent	Pharmacokinetic Changes with Oral Contraceptives		Comments
Protease Inhibitors			
Atazanavir (ATV, Reyataz)	• EE AUC ↑ 48% • NE AUC ↑ 110%	❢	• OC should contain ≤30 mcg EE. Monitor for side effects, or use alternative method. • OCs containing <25 mcg EE or progestins other than norethindrone or norgestimate have not been studied.
ATV/r	• EE AUC ↓ 19% • 17-deacetyl norgestimate (active metabolite of NG) AUC ↑ 85%	❢	• OC should contain ≥35 mcg EE. • OCs containing progestins other than norethindrone or norgestimate have not been studied.
Darunavir (DRV, Prezista) DRV/r	• EE AUC ↓ 44% • NE AUC ↓ 14%	☒	• Use alternative or additional method of contraception.
Fosamprenavir (FPV, Lexiva)	• EE C_{min} ↑ 32% • NE C_{min} ↑ 45%; AUC ↑ 18% • Amprenavir AUC ↓ 22% • Amprenavir C_{min} ↓ 20%	☒	• Data are derived from studies with amprenavir (the active metabolite of FPV). • Risk of ARV failure and of EE or NE adverse effects: do not coadminister fosamprenavir with OCs. • Use alternative method of contraception.
FPV/r	• EE AUC ↓ 37% • NE AUC ↓ 34%	☒	• Risk of contraceptive failure and of ritonavir adverse effects. • Use alternative method of contraception.
Indinavir (IDV, Crixivan)	• EE AUC ↑ 24% • NE AUC ↑ 26%	✓	• No dosage adjustment is recommended. • Monitor for EE or NE adverse effects.
IDV/r	• No data	☒	• Risk of contraceptive failure; use alternative or additional method of contraception.
Lopinavir/r (LPV/r, Kaletra)	• EE AUC ↓ 42% • NE AUC ↓ 17%	☒	• Risk of contraceptive failure; use alternative or additional method of contraception.
Nelfinavir (NFV, Viracept)	• EE AUC ↓ 47% • NE AUC ↓ 18%	☒	• Risk of contraceptive failure; use alternative or additional method of contraception.
Ritonavir (RTV, Norvir)	• EE AUC ↓ 40%	☒	• Risk of contraceptive failure; use alternative method of contraception.
Saquinavir (SQV, Invirase)/r	• No data; theoretic EE ↓ • SQV kinetics not affected by OC	☒	• Risk of contraceptive failure; use alternative or additional method of contraception.
Tipranavir (TPV, Aptivus)/r	• EE AUC ↓ 48% • NE no significant change	☒	• Risk of contraceptive failure; use alternative or additional method of contraception.

Antiretroviral Agent	Pharmacokinetic Changes with Oral Contraceptives		Comments
Nonnucleoside Reverse Transcriptase Inhibitors			
Efavirenz (EFV, Sustiva)	• EE AUC ↑ 37% • No data available on NE component • NG AUC ↓ 64% • LN AUC ↓ 58-83%	☒	• Decrease in progestin levels: risk of contraceptive failure [including failure of emergency contraception (Plan B)]; use alternative or additional method of contraception.
Etravirine (ETR, Intelence)	• EE AUC ↑ 22% • NE AUC ↓ 5%	✓	• No dosage adjustment is necessary.
Nevirapine (NVP, Viramune)	• EE AUC ↓ 20% • NE AUC ↓ 19%	☒	• Risk of contraceptive failure; use alternative or additional method of contraception.
CCR5 Antagonist			
Maraviroc (MVC, Selzentry)	• No significant effect on EE or LN	✓	• Safe to use in combination.
Integrase Inhibitor			
Raltegravir (RAL, Isentress)	• No significant change in EE AUC or NG AUC	✓	• Safe to use in combination.

Adapted from U.S. Department of Health and Human Services. *Guidelines for the Use of Antiretroviral Agents in HIV-1-Infected Adults and Adolescents,* Table 15a. January 10, 2011. Available at www.aidsinfo.nih.gov/guidelines/.

Abbreviations: AUC = area under the time-concentration curve (drug exposure); C_{max} = maximum concentration; C_{min} = minimum concentration; EE = ethinyl estradiol; LN = levonorgestrel; NE = norethindrone; NG = norgestimate; OC = oral contraceptive; RTV = ritonavir; /r = low-dose ritonavir

Non-Oral Hormonal Contraceptives

Hormonal contraceptives using delivery methods other than oral include the following:

• Products containing both progestin and estrogen components: transdermal patch, vaginal ring

• Products containing a progestin alone (medroxyprogesterone acetate, levonorgestrel, norelgestromin, or etonogestrel): subcutaneous or IM injection, intrauterine system, implantable device

There has been little research on the interactions between ARVs and most of these agents. Theoretically, interactions with ARVs would be less likely with contraceptive methods that have primarily local action and minimal systemic absorption, and for injection or transdermal delivery systems, since first-pass metabolism is avoided. However, caution is still warranted, as this assumption has not been proven.

Because the transdermal patch and vaginal ring contain ethinyl estradiol, women who take ARVs that increase or decrease serum estradiol levels (see Table 1) are advised to use an alternative (or additional) contraceptive method. Small studies of depo-medroxyprogesterone acetate (DMPA, or Depo-Provera) have shown no significant interactions between DMPA and nelfinavir, efavirenz, or nevirapine. Interactions between DMPA and other ARVs have not been studied, but DMPA's interactions with PIs and NNRTIs would be expected to be similar to those of norethindrone (see Table 1). For other non-oral hormones, pending further study, an alternative (or additional) method of contraception should be considered.

References

- Abel S, Russell D, Ridgway C, et al. *Overview of the drug-drug interaction data for maraviroc (UK-427, 857)*. In: Program and abstracts of the 6th International Workshop on Clinical Pharmacology of HIV Therapy; April 28-30, 2005; Quebec. Abstract 76.

- Anderson MS, Wenning L, Moreau A, et al. *Effect of raltegravir on the pharmacokinetics of oral contraceptives*. In: Program and abstracts of the 47th Interscience Conference on Antimicrobial Agents and Chemotherapy; September 17-20, 2007; Chicago. Abstract A-1425.

- Bounds W, Guillebaud J. *Observational series on women using the contraceptive Mirena concurrently with anti-epileptic and other enzyme-inducing drugs*. J Fam Plann Reprod Health Care. 2002 Apr;28(2):78-80.

- Carten M, Kiser J, Kwara A, et al. *Pharmacokinetic interactions between the hormonal emergency contraception, levonorgestrel, and efavirenz*. In: Program and abstracts of the 17th Conference on Retroviruses and Opportunistic Infections. February 16-19, 2010; San Francisco. Abstract 934.

- Chu JH, Gange SJ, Anastos K et al. *Hormonal contraceptive use and the effectiveness of highly active antiretroviral therapy*. Am J Epidemiol. 2005 May 1;161(9):881-90.

- Cohn SE, Park JG, Watts DH, et al.; ACTG A5093 Protocol Team. *Depo-medroxyprogesterone in women on antiretroviral therapy: effective contraception and lack of clinically significant interactions*. Clin Pharmacol Ther. 2007 Feb;81(2):222-7.

- Gupta S. *Non-oral hormonal contraception*. Curr Ob Gyn. 2006 Feb;16(1):30-8.

- Heikinheimo O, Lehtovirta P, Suni J, et al. *The levonorgestrel-releasing intrauterine system (LNG-IUS) in HIV-infected women –* effects on bleeding patterns, ovarian function and genital shedding of HIV. Hum Reprod. 2006 Nov;21(11):2857-61.

- Implanon [package insert]. Kenilworth, NJ: Schering-Plough; 2009.

- Joshi AS, Fiske WD, Benedek IH, et al. *Lack of a pharmacokinetic interaction between efavirenz (DMP 266) and ethinylestradiol in healthy female volunteers*. In: Program and abstracts of the 5th Conference on Retroviruses and Opportunistic Infections; February 1-5, 1998; Chicago. Abstract 348.

- Kearney BP, Mathias A. *Lack of effect of tenofovir disoproxil fumarate on pharmacokinetics of hormonal contraceptives*. Pharmacotherapy. 2009 Aug;29(8):924-9.

- Liverpool HIV Pharmacology Group. *Drug Interactions Charts*. Available at www.hiv-druginteractions.org. Accessed June 30, 2010.

- Mayer K, Poblete R, Hathaway B, et al. *Efficacy, effect of oral contraceptive, and adherence in HIV infected women receiving Fortovase (saquinavir) soft gel capsule thrice and twice daily regimens*. In: Program and abstracts of the XIII International AIDS Conference; July 9-14, 2000; Durban, South Africa. Abstract TuPeB3226.

- McNicholl I. *Database of Antiretroviral Drug Interactions*. HIV InSite. San Francisco: UCSF Center for HIV Information. Available at hivinsite.ucsf.edu/insite?page=ar-00-02. Accessed June 30, 2010.

- Mitchell HS, Stephens E. *Contraception choice for HIV positive women*. Sex Transm Infect. 2004 Jun;80(3):167-73.

- Nanda K, Amaral E, Hays M, et al. *Pharmacokinetic interactions between depot medroxyprogesterone acetate and combination antiretroviral therapy*. Fertil Steril. 2008 Oct;90(4):965-71.

- Ouellet D, Hsu A, Qian J, et al. *Effect of ritonavir on the pharmacokinetics of ethinyloestradiol in healthy female volunteers.* Br J Clin Pharmacol. 1998 Aug;46(2):111-6.

- Scholler-Gyure M, Debroye C, Aharchi F, et al. *No effect of TMC125 on the pharmacokinetics of oral contraceptives.* In: Program and abstracts of the 8th International Congress on Drug Therapy in HIV Infection; November 12-16, 2006; Glasgow. Abstract P277.

- Sekar VJ, Lefebvre E, Guzman SS, et al. *Pharmacokinetic interaction between ethinyl estradiol, norethindrone and darunavir with low-dose ritonavir in healthy women.* Antivir Ther. 2008;13(4):563-9.

- Sevinsky H, Eley T, He B, et al. *Effect of efavirenz on the pharmacokinetics of ethinylestradiol and norgestimate in healthy female subjects.* In: Program and abstracts of the 48th Interscience Conference on Antimicrobial Agents and Chemotherapy; October 25-28, 2008; Washington. Abstract A-958.

- Tackett D, Child M, Agarwala S, et al. *Atazanavir: a summary of two pharmacokinetic drug interaction studies in healthy subjects.* In: Program and abstracts of the 10th Conference on Retroviruses and Opportunistic Infections; February 10-13, 2003; Boston. Abstract 543.

- Toronto General Hospital, Immunodeficiency Clinic. *Drug Interaction Tables.* Available at www.hivclinic.ca/main/drugs_interact. html. Accessed June 30, 2010.

- U.S. Department of Health and Human Services. *Guidelines for the Use of Antiretroviral Agents in HIV-1-Infected Adults and Adolescents.* January 10, 2011. Available at www.aidsinfo.nih.gov/guidelines/.

- Watts DH, Park JG, Cohn SE, et al. *Safety and tolerability of depot medroxyprogesterone acetate among HIV-infected women on antiretroviral therapy: ACTG A5093.* Contraception. 2008 Feb;77(2):84-90.

- Zieman M. *Overview of contraception.* Up to Date Online. June 1, 2009. Available at www.utdol.com/home/index.html. Accessed June 30, 2010.

Section 7: ARV Interactions and Adverse Events

Pain Syndrome and Peripheral Neuropathy

Background

The International Association for the Study of Pain defines pain as "an unpleasant sensory and emotional experience associated with actual or potential tissue damage or described in terms of such damage." Pain is subjective, it is whatever patient says it is, and it exists whenever the patient says it does. Pain is a common symptom in people with HIV infection, especially those with advanced disease. It occurs in 30-60% of HIV/AIDS patients and can diminish their quality of life significantly. Like cancer patients, HIV patients experience an average of 2.5 to 3 types of pain at once. Pain in HIV-infected patients may have many causes (as discussed below).

Peripheral Neuropathy

Pain from HIV-associated peripheral neuropathy is particularly common, and may be debilitating. Peripheral neuropathy is clinically present in approximately 30% of HIV-infected individuals and typically presents as distal sensory polyneuropathy (DSP). It may be related to HIV itself (especially at CD4 counts of <200 cells/μL), to medication toxicity (e.g., from certain nucleoside analogues such as stavudine or didanosine), or to the effects of chronic illnesses (e.g., diabetes mellitus). Patients with peripheral neuropathy may complain of numbness or burning, a pins-and-needles sensation, shooting or lancinating pain, and a sensation that their shoes are too tight or their feet are swollen. These symptoms typically begin in the feet and progress upward; the hands may be affected. Patients may develop difficulty walking because of discomfort, or because they have difficulty feeling their feet on the ground. Factors associated with increased risk of peripheral neuropathy include the following:

- Previous peripheral neuropathy
- Low CD4 count (<200 cells/μL)
- Previous AIDS-defining opportunistic infection or neoplasm
- Vitamin B12 deficiency
- Exposure to stavudine or didanosine
- Use of other drugs associated with peripheral neuropathy (e.g., isoniazid, dapsone, metronidazole, hydroxyurea, thalidomide, linezolid, ribavirin, vincristine)
- Use of other neurotoxic agents (e.g., alcohol)
- Diabetes mellitus

Section 8: Neuropsychiatric Disorders

Patients should be assessed carefully before the introduction of a potentially neurotoxic medication (including stavudine or didanosine), and the use of these medications for patients at high risk of developing peripheral neuropathy should be avoided.

Pain is significantly undertreated, especially among HIV-infected women, because of factors ranging from providers' lack of knowledge about the diagnosis and treatment of pain to patients' fear of addiction to analgesic medications. Pain, as the so-called fifth vital sign, should be assessed at every patient visit.

S: Subjective

Self-report is the most reliable method to assess pain.

The patient complains of pain. The site and character of the pain will vary with the underlying cause. Ascertain the following from the patient:

- Duration, onset, progression
- Distribution, symmetry
- Character or quality (e.g., burning, sharp, dull)
- Intensity
- Severity (using the 0-10 scale; see below)
- Neurologic symptoms (e.g., weakness, cranial nerve abnormalities, bowel or bladder abnormalities)
- Exacerbating or relieving factors
- Response to current or past pain management strategies
- Past medical history (e.g., AIDS, diabetes mellitus)
- Psychosocial history
- Substance abuse and alcohol use history (amount, duration)
- Medications, current and recent (particularly zalcitabine, didanosine, stavudine, and isoniazid)
- Nutrition (vitamin deficiencies)
- Meaning of the pain to the patient

Measuring the severity of the pain: Have the patient rate the pain severity on a numeric scale of 0-10 (0 = no pain; 10 = worst imaginable pain), a verbal scale (none, small, mild, moderate, or severe), or a pediatric faces pain scale (when verbal or language abilities are absent). Note that pain ratings >3 usually indicate pain that interferes with daily activities. Use the same scale for evaluation of treatment response.

Figure 1. Faces Pain Rating Scale (0-10)

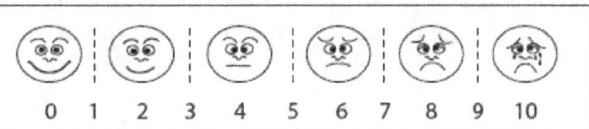

Quick screen for peripheral neuropathy: Ask about distal numbness and check Achilles tendon reflexes. Screening for numbness and delayed or absent ankle reflexes has the highest sensitivity and specificity among the clinical evaluation tools for primary care providers. For a validated screening tool, use the ACTG Brief Peripheral Neuropathy Scale (BPNS) to scale and track the degree of peripheral neuropathy (see www.hiv.va.gov/vahiv?page=pcm-403_peripheral#S4.2X).

O: Objective

Measure vital signs (increases in blood pressure, respiratory rate, and heart rate can correlate with pain). Perform a symptom-directed physical examination, including a thorough neurologic and musculoskeletal examination. Look for masses, lesions, and localizing signs. Pay special attention to sensory deficits (check for focality, symmetry, and distribution [such as "stocking-glove"]), muscular weakness, reflexes, and gait. Patients with significant motor weakness or paralysis, especially if progressive over days to weeks, should be evaluated emergently.

To evaluate peripheral neuropathy: Check ankle Achilles tendon reflexes and look for delayed or absent reflexes as signs of peripheral neuropathy. Distal sensory loss often starts with loss of vibratory sensation, followed by loss of temperature sensation, followed by onset of pain. Findings are usually bilateral and symmetric.

A: Assessment

Pain assessment includes determining the type of pain, for example, nociceptive, neuropathic, or muscle spasm pain.

Nociceptive pain occurs as a result of tissue injury (somatic) or activation of nociceptors resulting from stretching, distention, or inflammation of the internal organs of the body. It usually is well localized; may be described as sharp, dull, aching, throbbing, or gnawing in nature; and typically involves bones, joints, and soft tissue.

Neuropathic pain occurs from injury to peripheral nerves or central nervous system structures. Neuropathic pain may be described as burning, shooting, tingling, stabbing, or like a vise or electric shock; it involves the brain, central nervous system, nerve plexuses, nerve roots, or peripheral nerves. It is associated with decreased sensation and hypersensitivity.

Muscle spasm pain can accompany spinal

or joint injuries, surgeries, and bedbound patients. It is described as tight, cramping, pulling, and squeezing sensations.

Although pain in HIV-infected patients often results from opportunistic infections, neoplasms, or medication-related neuropathy, it is important to include non-HIV-related causes of pain in a differential diagnosis. Some of these other causes may be more frequent in HIV-infected individuals. A partial list for the differential diagnosis includes:

- Anorectal carcinoma
- Aphthous ulcers
- Appendicitis
- Arthritis, myalgias
- Candidiasis, oral or esophageal
- Cholecystitis
- Cryptococcal disease
- Cytomegalovirus colitis
- Dental abscesses
- Gastroesophageal reflux disease (GERD)
- Ectopic pregnancy
- Herpes simplex
- Herpes zoster
- Kaposi sarcoma
- Lymphoma
- Medication-induced pain syndromes (e.g., owing to growth hormone, granulocyte colony-stimulating factor)
- Medication-induced peripheral neuropathy (e.g., owing to didanosine, stavudine, isoniazid, vincristine)
- Other causes of peripheral neuropathy: diabetes, hypothyroidism, B12 deficiency, syphilis, cryoglobulinemia (especially in patients with hepatitis C coinfection)
- *Mycobacterium avium* complex
- Myopathy

- Pancreatitis
- Pelvic inflammatory disease
- Toxoplasmosis

P: Plan

Perform a diagnostic evaluation based on the suspected causes of pain.

Treatment

Treatment should be aimed at eliminating the source of pain, if possible. If symptomatic treatment of pain is needed, begin treatment based on the patient's pain rating scale, using the least invasive route. The goal is to achieve optimal patient comfort and functioning (not necessarily zero pain) with minimal medication adverse effects, negotiated with the patient. Use the three-step pain analgesic ladder originally devised by the World Health Organization (WHO); see Figure 2, below.

Nonpharmacologic interventions

The following interventions can be used at any step in the treatment plan:

- A therapeutic provider-patient relationship
- Physical therapy
- Exercise
- Relaxation techniques
- Guided imagery
- Massage
- Biofeedback
- Reflexology
- Acupuncture
- Thermal modalities (hot and cold compresses or baths)
- Transcutaneous electrical nerve stimulation (TENS)
- Spiritual exploration
- Prayer
- Deep breathing
- Meditation

- Enhancement of coping skills
- Self-hypnosis
- Humor
- Distraction
- Hobbies

Pharmacologic interventions
Principles of pharmacologic pain treatment

- The dosage of the analgesic is adjusted to give the patient adequate pain control.

- The interval between doses is adjusted so that the pain control is uninterrupted. It can take 4-5 half-lives before the maximum effect of an analgesic is realized.

- Chronic pain is more likely to be controlled when analgesics are dosed on a continuous schedule rather than "as needed." Sustained-release formulations of opioids should be used whenever possible.

- For breakthrough pain, use "as needed" medications in addition to scheduled-dosage analgesics. When using opiates both for scheduled analgesia for breakthrough pain, a good rule of thumb is to use 10% of the total daily dosage of opiates as the "as needed" opiate dose for breakthrough pain.

- Oral administration has an onset of analgesia of about 20-60 minutes, tends to produce more stable blood levels, and is cheaper.

- Beware of the risk of prolonged analgesic half-lives in patients with renal or hepatic dysfunction.

- Caution when using combination analgesics that are coformulated with ingredients such as acetaminophen, aspirin, or ibuprofen. Determine the maximum daily dosage of all agents.

The following three steps are adapted from the WHO analgesic ladder. Agents on higher steps are progressively stronger pain relievers but tend to have more adverse effects.

Figure 2. Pharmacologic Approaches to Pain Management: WHO Three-Step Ladder

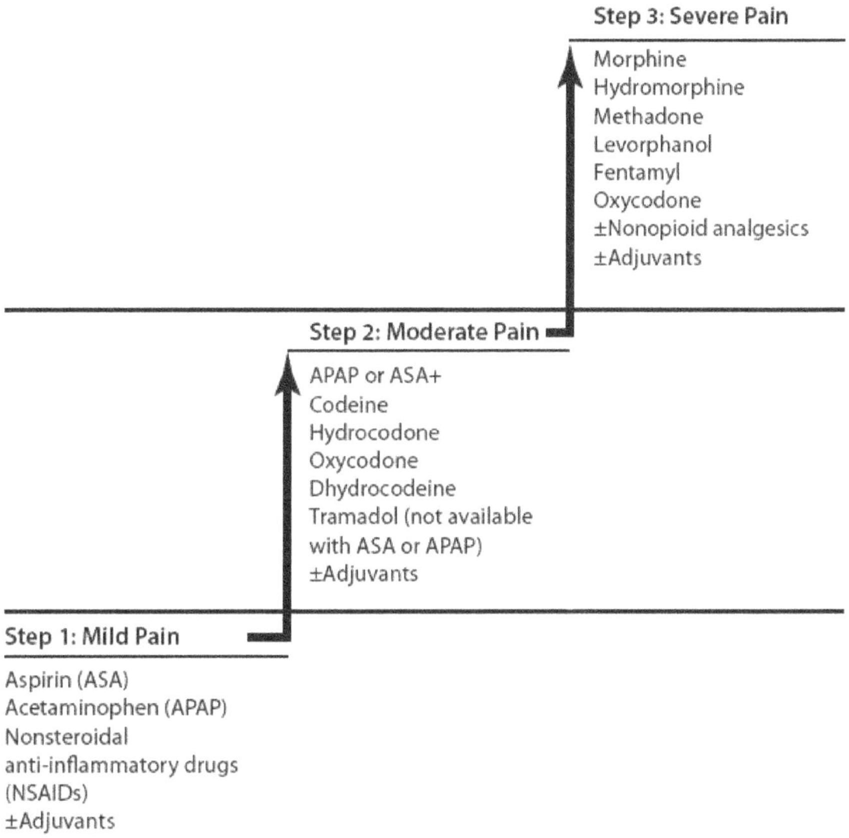

Step 3: Severe Pain

Morphine
Hydromorphine
Methadone
Levorphanol
Fentamyl
Oxycodone
±Nonopioid analgesics
±Adjuvants

Step 2: Moderate Pain

APAP or ASA+
Codeine
Hydrocodone
Oxycodone
Dhydrocodeine
Tramadol (not available
with ASA or APAP)
±Adjuvants

Step 1: Mild Pain

Aspirin (ASA)
Acetaminophen (APAP)
Nonsteroidal
anti-inflammatory drugs
(NSAIDs)
±Adjuvants

Adapted from World Health Organization. *Cancer Pain Relief and Palliative Care, Report of a WHO Expert Committee.* Geneva: World Health Organization; 1990.
Note: "Adjuvants" refers either to medications that are coadministered to manage an adverse effect of an opioid or to so-called adjuvant analgesics that are added to enhance analgesia.

Step 1: Nonopiates for mild pain (pain scale 1-3)

- The most common agents in this step include acetaminophen (650-1,000 mg PO Q6H as needed) and nonsteroidal antiinflammatory drugs (NSAIDs) such as ibuprofen 600-800 mg PO TID with food, and cyclooxygenase-2 (COX-2) inhibitors such as celecoxib and rofecoxib.

- A proton-pump inhibitor (such as omeprazole) can decrease the risk of gastrointestinal bleeding when using NSAIDs.

- Acetaminophen has no effect on platelets and no antiinflammatory properties; avoid use in patients with hepatic insufficiency, and in general limit to 4 g per day in acute use (or 2 g per day for patients with liver disease). Monitor liver function tests in chronic use.

- NSAIDs and acetaminophen can be used together for synergism.

- Note that COX-2 inhibitors have been associated with an increased risk of cardiovascular events and should be used with caution.

Section 8: Neuropsychiatric Disorders

Step 2: Mild opiates with or without nonopiates for moderate pain (pain scale 4-6)

- Most agents used to treat moderate pain are combinations of opioids and Step 1 agents. The most common agents are acetaminophen combined with codeine, oxycodone, or hydrocodone. Codeine can be dosed as codeine sulfate, separately from acetaminophen. Beware of acetaminophen toxicity in these combination drugs.

- Other agents include buprenorphine (partial opiate agonist).

- Tramadol (Ultram) is a centrally acting nonopiate that can be combined with NSAIDs. As with opiates, it is prone to abuse. Tramadol lowers the seizure threshold; avoid use for patients with a seizure history. Avoid coadministration with selective serotonin reuptake inhibitors (SSRIs) and monoamine oxidase inhibitors (MAOIs) because of the risk of serotonin syndrome.

Step 3: Opioid agonist drugs for severe pain (pain scale 7-10)

- Morphine is the drug of choice in this step. Start with short-acting morphine and titrate the dosage to adequate pain control, then divide the 24-hour total in half to determine the dosing for the sustained-release morphine, given Q12H. When converting from IV to PO morphine, PO dosage is about two to three times the parenteral dose.

- Other agents used are oxycodone, hydromorphone, fentanyl, levorphanol, methadone, codeine, hydrocodone, oxymorphone, and buprenorphine.

- Avoid meperidine because of the increased risk of delirium and seizures.

- Around-the-clock, sustained-release PO dosing will achieve optimum pain relief.

- Patients unable to take PO therapy may use transdermal fentanyl patches or do rectal administration of sustained-release tablets such as long-acting morphine. Note that the onset of analgesia with fentanyl patches can take more than 12 hours, and the analgesic effect can last more than 18 hours after the patch is removed.

- Anticipate and treat complications and adverse effects of opioid therapy, such as nausea, vomiting, and constipation. Constipation often leads to nausea and can be prevented with prophylactic stool softeners (such as docusate) and stimulant laxatives (such as senna).

Adjunctive treatments

The addition of antidepressant medications can improve pain management, especially for chronic pain syndromes. These agents, and anticonvulsants, usually are used to treat neuropathic pain (discussed in more detail below), but should be considered for treatment of other chronic pain syndromes as well.

Treatment of neuropathic pain

Assess the underlying etiology, as discussed above, and treat the cause as appropriate. Review the patient's medication list for medications that can cause neuropathic pain. Discontinue the offending agents, if possible. For patients on stavudine or didanosine, in particular, switch to another nucleoside analogue if suitable alternatives exist, or at least consider dosage reduction of stavudine to 30 mg BID (consult with an HIV expert). For patient on isoniazid, ensure that they are taking vitamin B6 (pyridoxine) regularly to avoid isoniazid-related neuropathy.

Nonpharmacologic interventions for neuropathic pain

The nonpharmacologic interventions described above can be useful in treating neuropathic pain.

Pharmacologic interventions for neuropathic pain

Follow the WHO ladder of pain management described above. If Step 1 medications are ineffective, consider adding antidepressants, anticonvulsants, or both before moving on to opioid treatments.

Antidepressants

Antidepressant medications often exert analgesic effects at dosages that are lower than those required for antidepressant effects. As with antidepressant effects, optimum analgesic effects may not be achieved until several weeks after starting therapy.

- **Tricyclic antidepressants (TCAs):** Note that ritonavir and other protease inhibitors may increase the level of TCAs, so start at the lowest dosage and titrate up slowly. Dosages may be titrated upward every 3-5 days, as tolerated. In general, use lower dosages for elderly patients, up to 100 mg QHS.

  - **Nortriptyline (Pamelor):** Starting dosage is 10-25 mg QHS. Usual maintenance dosage is 20-150 mg QHS.

  - **Desipramine (Norpramin):** Starting dosage is 25 mg QHS. Usual maintenance dosage is 25-250 mg QHS.

  - **Imipramine:** Starting dosage is 25 mg QHS. Usual maintenance dosage is 25-300 mg QHS.

  - **Amitriptyline (Elavil):** Starting dosage is 10-25 mg QHS. Usual maintenance dosage is 25-150 mg QHS. Amitriptyline has the highest rate of adverse effects among the TCAs, so other agents typically are preferred.

  Adverse effects include sedation, anticholinergic effects (e.g., dry mouth, urinary retention), QT prolongation, arrhythmias, and orthostatic hypotension. Monitor TCA levels and EKG at higher dosage levels. There is a risk of overdose if taken in excess.

- **SSRIs:** See chapter *Depression* for dosing, side effects, and drug interactions associated with this class of agents. SSRIs are less effective than TCAs in treating chronic pain.

- **Venlafaxine (Effexor):** Starting dosage is 37.5 mg daily. Usual maintenance dosage is 75-300 mg daily in divided doses or by extended-release formulation (Effexor XR). Note that there are limited data on using venlafaxine for patients with HIV infection.

- **Duloxetine (Cymbalta):** Starting dosage is 30-60 mg daily. Dosages of >60 mg per day are rarely more effective for either depression or pain treatment. Note that there are limited data on using duloxetine for patients with HIV infection.

Anticonvulsants

The following agents may be effective for neuropathic pain:

- **Gabapentin (Neurontin):** Considered first-line for HIV sensory neuropathy for its tolerability. Starting dosage is 100-300 mg QHS; may be increased every 3-5 days to BID or TID to achieve symptom relief. Monitor response and increase the dosage every 1-2 weeks by 300-600 mg/day. Usual maintenance dosage is 1,200-3,600 mg/day in divided doses. Adverse effects include somnolence, dizziness, fatigue, weight gain, and nausea. To discontinue, taper over the course of 7 or more days.

- **Pregabalin (Lyrica):** Starting dosage is 25-50 mg TID; may be increased by 25-50 mg per dose every 3-5 days as tolerated to achieve symptom relief. Maximum dosage is 200 mg TID. Adverse effects are similar to those of gabapentin. To discontinue, taper over the course of 7 or more days.

- **Lamotrigine (Lamictal):** Starting dosage is 25 mg QOD; titrate slowly to 200 mg BID over the course of 6-8 weeks to reduce the risk of rash (including Stevens-Johnson syndrome). Adverse effects include sedation, dizziness, ataxia, confusion, nausea, blurred vision, and rash. Note that lopinavir/ritonavir (Kaletra) may decrease lamotrigine levels; higher dosages may be needed. To discontinue, taper over the course of 7 or more days.

- Although phenytoin and carbamazepine have some effectiveness in treating neuropathy, they have significant drug interactions with protease inhibitors and nonnucleoside reverse transcriptase inhibitors, and their use with HIV-infected patients is limited. Topiramate and valproic acid have been used for migraine prophylaxis and anecdotally may be useful for treating peripheral neuropathy, but have not been well-studied in HIV-related neuropathies.

Treatment of Muscle Spasm Pain

Stretching, heat, and massage may help the pain of muscle spasm. This pain also can respond to muscle relaxants such as baclofen, cyclobenzaprine, tizanidine, benzodiazepines, as well as intraspinal infusion of local anesthetics for spinal injuries.

Substance Abuse, HIV, and Pain

- Some health care providers hesitate to treat pain in patients with current or past substance abuse because of concern about worsening these patients' dependence on opioids or suspicion that such patients are seeking pain medications for illicit purposes. However, the following points should be considered:

- Many patients with current or past substance abuse do experience pain, and this pain should be evaluated by care providers and treated appropriately.

- Failure to distinguish among addiction, tolerance, and dependence can lead to undertreatment of chronic pain by health care providers.

- Addiction (substance abuse) is a complex behavioral syndrome characterized by compulsive drug use for the secondary gain of euphoria.

- Pharmacologic tolerance refers to the reduction of effectiveness, over time, of a given dosage of medication.

- Physical dependence is the consequence of neurophysiologic changes that take place in the presence of exogenous opioids.

- Aberrant use of pain medications, if it develops, is best managed by an interdisciplinary team of providers from HIV clinical care, psychiatry, psychology, pharmacy, social services, and drug addiction management.

- Drug-drug interactions between certain antiretroviral medications and methadone can decrease methadone serum concentrations (see chapter *Drug-Drug Interactions with HIV-Related Medications*). If this occurs, methadone dosages may need to be increased to prevent opiate withdrawal.

- As part of chronic pain management in patients with substance abuse, consider establishing a written pain-management contract to be signed by the clinician and the patient. The contract should:

  - Clearly state limits and expectations for both the patient and provider.

  - Identify a single clinician responsible for managing the pain regimen.

  - Tell the patient what to do if the pain regimen is not working.

  - Describe the procedure for providing prescriptions (e.g., one prescription given to the patient, in person, for a limited period of time, such as 1 month).

  - List the rules for dealing with lost medications or prescriptions.

Patient Education

- Pain management is part of HIV treatment, and patients should give feedback to allow the best treatment decisions. If pain persists for more than 24 hours at a level that interferes with daily life, patients should inform their health care provider so that the plan can be changed and additional measures, if needed, can be tried.

- Patients should not expect full pain relief in most cases, but enough relief that they can perform their daily activities.

- "Mild" pain medications (e.g., NSAIDs, aspirin, acetaminophen) usually are continued even after "stronger" medications are started because their mechanism of action is different than that of opiates. This combination of pain medication has additive effects, so that pain may be controllable with a lower narcotic dosage.

- Patients taking "around-the-clock" medications, should take them on schedule. Those taking "as needed" medications should take them between doses only if they have breakthrough pain.

- Opiates may cause severe constipation. Patients must remain hydrated and will likely need stool softeners, laxatives, or other measures. They should contact their health care provider promptly if constipation occurs.

- Patients should avoid use of recreational drugs and alcohol when taking opiates because opiates can interact with them or cause additive adverse effects, possibly resulting in central nervous system depression, coma, or death.

- Patients taking opiates should avoid driving and operating machinery.

References

- Alexander C. *Palliative and End-of-Life Care.* In: Anderson JR, ed. *A Guide to the Clinical Care of Women with HIV.* Rockville, MD: Health Services and Resources Administration; 2005. Available at hab.hrsa.gov/publications/womencare05/. Accessed June 30, 2010.

- American Academy of HIV Medicine. *Pain Management.* In: AAHIVM *Fundamentals of HIV Medicine* (2007 ed.). Washington, DC: American Academy of HIV Medicine; 2007.

- Association of Nurses in AIDS Care. *Pain.* In: Kirton C, ed. *Core Curriculum for HIV/AIDS Nursing, 2nd Edition.* Thousand Oaks, CA: Sage Publications; 2003;143-155.

- Breitbart W. *Suicide Risk and Pain in Cancer and AIDS.* In: Chapman CR, Foley KM, eds. *Current and Emerging Issues in Cancer Pain: Research and Practice.* New York: Raven Press; 1993;49-66.

- Cherry CL, Wesselingh SL, Lal L, et al. *Evaluation of a clinical screening tool for HIV-associated sensory neuropathies.* Neurology. 2005 Dec 13;65(11):1778-81.

- Gonzalez-Duarte A. Robinson-Papp J, Simpson DM. *Diagnosis and management of HIV-associated neuropathy.* Neurol Clin. 2008 Aug;26(3):821-32, x.

- Hahn K, Arendt G, Braun JS, et al. *A placebo-controlled trial of gabapentin for painful HIV-associated sensory neuropathies.* J Neurol. 2004 Oct;251(10):1260-6.

- McArthur J, Brew B, Nath A. *Neurological complications of HIV infection.* Lancet Neurol. 2005 Sep;4(9):543-55.

- O'Neill WM, Sherrard JS. *Pain in human immunodeficiency virus disease: a review.* Pain. 1993 Jul;54(1):3-14.

- Singer EJ, Zorilla C, Fahy-Chandon B, et al. *Painful symptoms reported by ambulatory HIV-infected men in a longitudinal study.* Pain. 1993 Jul;54(1):15-9.

- Slaughter A, Pasero C, Manworren R. *Unacceptable pain levels.* Am J Nurs. 2002 May;102(5):75, 77.

- Swica Y, Breitbart W. *Treating pain in patients with AIDS and a history of substance use.* West J Med. 2002 Jan;176(1):33-9.

- Weinreb NJ, Kinzbrunner BM, Clark M. *Pain Management.* In: Kinzbrunner BM, Weinreb NJ, Policzer JS, eds. *20 Common Problems: End-of-life Care.* New York: McGraw Hill Medical Publishing Division; 2002:91-145.

- U.S. Department of Health and Human Services. *Management of Cancer Pain.* Rockville, MD: Department of Health and Human Services; 1994.

- U.S. Department of Health and Human Services. *Guidelines for the Use of Antiretroviral Agents in HIV-1-Infected Adults and Adolescents.* January 10, 2011. Available at www.aidsinfo.nih.gov/guidelines/.

- World Health Organization. *Cancer Pain Relief and Palliative Care, Report of a WHO Expert Committee.* Geneva: World Health Organization; 1990.

Section 8: Neuropsychiatric Disorders

HIV-Associated Dementia and Other Neurocognitive Disorders

Background

HIV is a neurotropic virus that directly invades the brain shortly after infection. HIV replicates in brain macrophages and microglia, causing inflammatory and neurotoxic host responses. HIV may cause cognitive, behavioral, and motor difficulties. These difficulties may range in severity from very mild to severe and disabling; if moderate or severe, they constitute minor cognitive motor disorder (MCMD) or HIV-associated dementia (HAD), respectively. These conditions are distinguished from the milder cognitive changes seen in some people with HIV infection by the greater impact and duration of the functional deficits. MCMD is thought to involve neuronal cell dysfunction, whereas HAD often involves actual cell death.

> **A note on nomenclature:** There have been multiple shifts in the nomenclature used to describe HIV-associated neurocognitive disorders. The most recent proposed system, published in the journal *Neurology* in 2007, suggests three categories: asymptomatic neurocognitive impairment (ANI), mild neurocognitive disorder (MND), and HAD. However, the diagnoses of ANI and MND require neuropsychological testing that is more likely to be available in research settings as opposed to clinical settings. This chapter will therefore address the clinical diagnoses of MCMD and HAD.

Both MCMD and HAD are AIDS-defining conditions (listed as "Encephalopathy, HIV related" in the classification system used by the U.S. Centers for Disease Control and Prevention), and are risk factors for death. Neurocognitive disorders associated with HIV are among the most common and clinically important complications of HIV infection. However, they are diagnoses of exclusion, and other medical causes must be ruled out.

Risk factors for developing an HIV-associated neurocognitive disorder include the following:

- Older age
- Female gender
- More advanced HIV disease (including CD4 count <100 cells/μL, wasting)
- High plasma HIV RNA (viral load)
- Comorbid conditions (especially anemia and infection with cytomegalovirus, human herpesvirus 6, and JC virus)
- History of injection drug use (especially with cocaine)
- History of delirium

The use of effective antiretroviral therapy (ART) that maintains the plasma HIV RNA at undetectable or low values is the best way to prevent and treat HIV-related neurocognitive disorders. Thus, it is essential to choose an ART regimen that takes into consideration resistance testing and adherence issues.

Minor Cognitive Motor Disorder

MCMD is characterized by mild impairment in functioning and may escape diagnosis by the clinician. The course and onset of MCMD can vary dramatically. The more demanding the activities of a particular individual, the more likely that person would be to notice the difficulties. MCMD does not necessarily progress to dementia.

HIV-Associated Dementia

HAD is characterized by symptoms of cognitive, motor, and behavioral disturbances. There is often a progressive slowing of cognitive functions, including concentration and attention, memory, new learning, sequencing and problem solving, and executive control. HAD also can present with behavioral changes, which mainly take the form of apathy, loss of motivation, poor energy, fatigue, and social withdrawal. Motor changes, including slowing, clumsiness, unsteadiness, increased tendon reflexes, and deterioration of handwriting may occur.

S: Subjective

If a neurocognitive disorder is suspected, obtain a history of the patient's symptoms (see below). Whenever possible, obtain a parallel history of the patient's past history and recent mental status changes from significant others or caretakers.

Patient self-reports of cognitive problems and bedside cognitive status tests may be insensitive, particularly to subtler forms of impairment.

To help clarify factors that may be causing the changes in mental status, inquire about the following:

- Acuity of onset
- Recent changes or events
- Medications, particularly new medications
- Drug and alcohol use
- Symptoms of opportunistic illnesses, other infections
- HIV history, including duration, CD4 cell count, HIV viral load, history of ART
- History of other medical and psychiatric disorders

Section 8: Neuropsychiatric Disorders

Ask about the following symptoms:

MCMD	HAD
Patients may complain of: • Difficulty with complex tasks • Mild memory problems • Distractibility/confusion • A need to make lists • Problems with adherence to medications **Diagnostic Criteria*** The patient displays at least two of the following symptoms for >1 month: • Impaired attention/ concentration • Mental slowing • Impaired memory • Slowed movements • Impaired coordination • Personality change, irritability, or emotional lability	Patients may present with: • Memory problems • Distractibility • Anger, irritability, or emotional lability • Fatigue, psychomotor slowness • Sadness • Poor balance, clumsiness • Decreased attention or concentration • Social withdrawal • Reduced speed of information processing • Executive dysfunction (e.g., in realms of abstraction, divided attention, shifting cognitive sets) • Language problems • Visuospatial difficulties • Apraxias • Psychotic symptoms (in late stage) • Severe verbal memory loss (in late stage) • Seizures (in late stage) • Mutism (in late stage) **Diagnostic Criteria*** The patient displays at least two of the following cognitive symptoms for >1 month: • Impaired attention/concentration • Slowing in processing information • Difficulty with abstraction/reasoning • Difficulty with visuospatial skills • Impaired memory/learning • Impaired speech/language AND At least one of the following: • Acquired abnormality in motor function by clinical examination or neuropsychological testing • Decline in motivation, emotional control, or social behavior

* American Academy of Neurology, AIDS Task Force (see "References," below)

O: Objective

• Check temperature and other vital signs (MCMD and HAD are not associated with fever).

• Perform a complete physical examination with special attention to signs of opportunistic illnesses.

• Perform a thorough neurological examination, including funduscopy. Rule out focal neurologic deficits.

• Perform Mini-Mental State Examination (note that this is not sensitive for HIV-associated neurocognitive disorders; negative results do not rule out these conditions).

• Consider a neuropsychological screening test such as the Modified HIV Dementia Scale (see Figure 1). Others are noted in "Laboratory and Diagnostic Evaluation," below.

Figure 1. Modified HIV Dementia Scale

Maximum Score	Score	Exercise
N/A	N/A	**Memory/Registration:** State four words for the patient to recall (dog, hat, green, peach), pausing 1 second between each each. Then ask the patient to restate all four.
6	(__)	**Psychomotor Speed:** Ask the patient to write the alphabet in upper case letters horizontally across the page; record time: ____ seconds. ≤21 sec = 6 21.1 - 24 sec = 5 24.1 - 27 sec = 4 27.1 - 30 sec = 3 30.1 - 33 sec = 2 33.1 - 36 sec = 1 >36 sec = 0
4	(__)	**Memory Recall:** Ask the patient to restate the four words from Memory/Registration above. Give one point for each correct response. For words not recalled, prompt with a "semantic" clue, as follows: animal (dog); piece of clothing (hat), color (green), fruit (peach). Give 1/2 point for each correct after prompting.
2	(__)	**Construction:** Copy the cube below; record time:____ seconds. (<25 sec = 2; 25 - 35 sec = 1; >35 sec = 0)

Maximum score: 12 points; a score of <7.5 points suggests possible HAD (note, this test is not specific)
Adapted from McArthur JC. *Minor cognitive motor disorder: Does it really exist?* Hopkins HIV Rep. Nov 1996;8(4):8.

A: Assessment

A differential diagnosis includes the following medical conditions, which may present with cognitive changes or delirium:

- Substance use: intoxication or withdrawal from alcohol, opioids, stimulants, etc.
- Psychiatric disorders, especially major depression
- Metabolic or systemic disorders, including hepatic encephalopathy, vitamin B12 or folate deficiency, uremia, endocrine disorders (e.g., hypogonadism)
- Central nervous system (CNS) opportunistic infections, such as cytomegalovirus encephalitis, cryptococcal meningitis, tuberculous meningitis, CNS toxoplasmosis, and progressive multifocal leukoencephalopathy (PML)
- Systemic infections
- Brain tumors, including CNS lymphoma and metastatic disease
- Other causes of cognitive impairment and dementia (e.g., neurosyphilis, substance-induced dementia, vascular dementia, brain injury, Alzheimer disease, and hydrocephalus)
- Medication adverse effects: antiretroviral (ARV) medications (especially efavirenz), psychotropic medications, interferon, anticholinergics, and others
- Poisoning with toxic substances

P: Plan
Laboratory and Diagnostic Evaluation

A change in the mental status of an HIV-infected person should prompt a thorough search for underlying biological causes. As noted above, HIV-related neurocognitive disorders are diagnoses of exclusion, and other causes of the patient's symptoms should be ruled out.

Perform the following tests:

- Laboratory tests: Complete blood count, electrolytes and creatinine, liver function, thyroid function, vitamin B12, rapid plasma regain (RPR) or Venereal Disease Research Laboratory (VDRL).

- Toxicology tests if substance use is suspected (e.g., opioids, ethanol, amphetamines).

- Brain imaging studies (computed tomography [CT] scan or magnetic resonance imaging [MRI]); rule out space-occupying masses and other lesions; cortical atrophy may be seen in advanced HAD; this finding is not specific.

- Cerebral spinal fluid (CSF) tests if CNS infection is suspected.

- Consider tests for neurocognitive impairment as noted in the table below; most of these can be found on the website of the New York State Department of Health AIDS Institute (www.hivguidelines.org).

- Refer to an HIV-experienced neuropsychologist, neurologist, or psychiatrist, if available.

Tests for Identifying and Staging HIV-Related Neurocognitive Impairment	
HIV Dementia Scale	• Screens for the memory and attention deficits and psychomotor slowing that are typical of HAD • Requires training to administer and, therefore, may not be ideal for a clinic setting
Modified HIV Dementia Scale	• Designed specifically for use by non-neurologists and, therefore, may be more useful than the HIV Dementia Scale for a primary care setting • Requires approximately 5 minutes to administer • See Figure 1, above.
Mental Alternation Test	• Useful for assessing patients with early dementia, who will show impairments in timed trials
Memorial Sloan-Kettering (MSK) Scale	• Can be used for assessing severity • Combines the functional impact of both cerebral dysfunction (dementia) and spinal cord dysfunction (myelopathy); the two entities can be separated and staged independently
Trail Making Test, Parts A and B (from the Halstead-Reitan Neuropsychological Battery)	• May be used as a screening tool, but results require interpretation by a neuropsychologist • May be used at the bedside to track a patient's response to ART over time
Grooved Pegboard (dominant and nondominant hand)	• May be used as a screening tool and does not require literacy

Treatment

There are no specific treatments for HIV-associated neurocognitive disorders, but ART may reverse the disease process, and a number of therapies may be helpful. The treatment of MCMD and HAD ideally utilizes a multidisciplinary approach that may involve HIV specialists, neurologists, psychiatrists, psychologists, nurse practitioners, social workers, and substance-use counselors.

Neurocognitive impairment in patients with HIV infection often is multifactorial. In addition to treating HIV-associated neurocognitive disorders themselves, it is important to correct, as much as possible, all medical conditions that may adversely affect the brain (e.g., psychiatric comorbidities, endocrinologic abnormalities, adverse medication effects). For patients using alcohol or illicit or nonprescribed drugs, implement strategies to reduce their use; these agents can further impair cognition.

Pharmacologic Management of HIV-Associated Neurocognitive Disorders

- **ART:** Maximal suppression of HIV replication via ART may partially or fully reverse HIV-associated neurocognitive disorders, and ART is the treatment of choice for both treatment and prevention of HIV-associated neurocognitive disorders, including dementia. In general, ART regimens that effectively suppress HIV RNA in the serum also suppress HIV in the CNS. However, ARV medications vary in their ability to penetrate the blood-brain barrier and, therefore, in their ability to act directly on the HIV virus in the CNS. Limited data suggest that using ARVs with good CNS penetration may be important in treating or preventing neurocognitive disorders, and some experts recommend the use of these ARVs, if otherwise appropriate, for patients with HIV dementia. ARVs with the best CNS penetration include the nucleoside reverse transcriptase inhibitors (NRTIs) abacavir, emtricitabine, and zidovudine (AZT, ZDV); the nonnucleoside reverse transcriptase inhibitor (NNRTI) nevirapine; the protease inhibitors (PIs) indinavir/ritonavir and lopinavir/ritonavir; and the CCR5 antagonist maraviroc. There currently is no role for testing levels of HIV RNA in the CSF outside research settings.

- **Stimulants:** Stimulant medications (e.g., methylphenidate, dextroamphetamine) have been used as palliative agents to help manage symptoms of fatigue, decreased concentration, and memory deficits among patients with MCMD and HAD. Starting dosages of both is 5 mg/day; maximum dosage is 60 mg/day. The response to stimulants is idiosyncratic and varies from patient to patient; begin with the lowest dose of 5 mg QAM and titrate upward as needed. If BID dosing is required as a result of afternoon fatigue, the afternoon dose should be taken before 2 PM to prevent interference with sleep. Consider referral to a psychiatrist or neurologist for evaluation and initiation of treatment; after a stable dosage is achieved, treatment may be continued. These medications should be used with caution for patients who have a history of stimulant abuse.

- For comorbid depression, consider prescribing antidepressant medications as for other medically ill HIV-infected patients (see chapter *Depression*).

- Antipsychotic medications may be useful in treating agitation and hallucinations but should be used for patients with dementia only when nonpharmacologic measures are insufficient for patient management; consult with a psychiatrist. All antipsychotic medications increase the risk of death in elderly patients with dementia. Start antipsychotic medications at the lowest possible dosage and increase slowly as needed.

- Many agents are being studied for either their neuroprotective effects or their therapeutic effects on HIV-associated neurocognitive disorders. The data are not sufficient at present to make specific recommendations. Patients with dementia often are sensitive to medication side effects; follow closely.

- Benzodiazepines have been shown to increase confusion and decrease concentration, and generally should be avoided.

Nonpharmacologic Management of MCMD and Mild HAD

- Encourage patients to remain appropriately active

- Explain the benefits of structured routines

- Encourage good nutrition

- Use strategies to minimize use of alcohol and illicit drugs

- Use memory aids such as lists

- Simplify complex tasks, especially drug regimens

- When giving instructions, do the following:

  - Repeat information

  - Write instructions to provide structure for patients and caregivers

  - Ask patients to express the information and instructions in their own words

- Adherence to medical regimens, including ART, often is particularly difficult for patients with neurocognitive disorders. Encourage use of medication adherence tools such as pill boxes, alarms, and, if available, packaged medications (e.g., blister packs) or prefilled medi-sets. Encourage patients to enlist adherence support from family members and friends.

- Cognitive skills building can be helpful (e.g., reading, solving puzzles, intellectual conversation).

Nonpharmacologic Management of Moderate to Severe HAD

The strategies noted above should be utilized, but additional measures are needed.

Management of patients with severe or late-stage HAD requires an evaluation of their safety and a determination of the environment and level of supervision that are needed. The clinician should attend to the following:

- Help determine whether patients can be left alone at home or whether doing so would present the risk of them wandering away or sustaining an injury in the home (e.g., from the use of an appliance such as the oven).

- For patients who cannot be left alone at home, assess options for support (e.g., help from family members or paid home attendants).

- Utilize fall prevention strategies.

- For patients who smoke, decide whether smoking can be done safely; if smoking is deemed unsafe, consider smoking cessation programs or supervision.

- If lesser measures fail, explore options for placement in a skilled nursing facility.

Additional helpful strategies for managing patients who are confused, agitated, or challenged by their experience include the following:

- Keep their environments familiar to the extent possible (e.g., in terms of objects, people, locations).

- Redirect or distract patients from inappropriate behavior.

- Remain calm when patients become confused or agitated; refrain from confronting an agitated patient; reorient confused or agitated patients.

- Provide a clock and calendar in the room to help keep patients oriented to time and to day of the week.

Section 8: Neuropsychiatric Disorders

- Provide lighting that corresponds with day and night.
- Emphasize routines.
- Ensure that patients who require eyeglasses or hearing aids wear them to help lessen confusion and disorientation.
- Prepare patients for any planned changes.
- Ensure that patients are receiving their prescribed medications.
- Protect wandering patients.
- Supervise any cigarette smoking.
- Offer activities that keep their minds alert.
- Educate family members about the nature of dementia and methods for helping patients maintain activities of daily living.
- Suggest that patients or their family members make arrangements for financial, health, and other matters in the event they become unable to make decisions about their affairs (e.g., advance health care directives, durable powers of attorney, wills).

Patient Education

- Advise patients that ART can be effective in preventing and treating HIV-related neurocognitive impairment.
- Inform patients and family members of the many other strategies may aid in managing neurocognitive impairment. Such strategies may help patients maintain the highest possible level of skills and independence.
- Family members and significant others can be important sources of support (e.g., by providing assistance with medication adherence).
- Advise patients with advanced HAD that placement in a residential facility may be the best option for ensuring their safety.

References

- American Academy of Neurology. *Nomenclature and research case definitions for neurologic manifestations of human immunodeficiency virus-type 1 (HIV-1) infection. Report of a Working Group of the American Academy of Neurology AIDS Task Force.* Neurology. 1991 Jun;41(6):778-85.

- Antinori A, Arendt G, Becker JT, et al. *Updated research nosology for HIV-associated neurocognitive disorders.* Neurology. 2007 Oct 30;69(18):1789-99.

- Brew B, Pemberton L, Cunningham P, et al. *Levels of human immunodeficiency virus type 1 RNA in cerebrospinal fluid correlate with AIDS dementia stage.* J Infect Dis. 1997 Apr;175(4):963-6.

- Cherner M, Cysique L, Heaton RK, et al.; HNRC Group. *Neuropathologic confirmation of definitional criteria for human immunodeficiency virus-associated neurocognitive disorders.* J Neurovirol. 2007;13(1):23-8.

- Cohen MA, Gorman JM. *Comprehensive Textbook of AIDS Psychiatry.* New York: Oxford University Press; 2008.

- Evers S, Rahmann A, Schwaag S, et al. *Prevention of AIDS dementia by HAART does not depend on cerebrospinal fluid drug penetrance.* AIDS Res Hum Retroviruses. 2004 May;20(5):483-91.

- McArthur JC, McClernon DR, Cronin MF, et al. *Relationship between human immunodeficiency virus-associated dementia and viral load in cerebrospinal fluid and brain.* Ann Neurol. 1997 Nov;42(5):689-98.

- New York State Department of Health AIDS Institute. *Mental Health Care for People with HIV Infection: Clinical Guidelines for the Primary Care Practitioner.* Available at www.hivguidelines.org. Accessed June 30, 2010.

- Power C, Selnes OA, Grim JA, et al. *HIV dementia scale: a rapid screening test.* J Acquir Immune Defic Syndr Hum Retrovirol. 1995 Mar 1;8(3):273-8.

- Price RW, Epstein LG, Becker JT, et al. *Biomarkers of HIV-1 CNS infection and injury.* Neurology. 2007 Oct 30;69(18):1781-8.

- Rippeth JD, Heaton RK, Carey CL, et al.; HNRC Group. *Methamphetamine dependence increases risk of neuropsychological impairment in HIV infected persons.* J Int Neuropsychol Soc. 2004 Jan;10(1):1-14.

- Schifitto G, Navia BA, Yiannoutsos CT, et al.; Adult AIDS Clinical Trial Group (ACTG) 301; 700 Teams; HIV MRS Consortium. *Memantine and HIV-associated cognitive impairment: a neuropsychological and proton magnetic resonance spectroscopy study.* AIDS. 2007 Sep 12;21(14):1877-86.

- Shiu C, Barbier E, Di Cello F, et al. *HIV-1 gp120 as well as alcohol affect blood-brain barrier permeability and stress fiber formation: involvement of reactive oxygen species.* Alcohol Clin Exp Res. 2007 Jan;31(1):130-7.

- U.S. Department of Health and Human Services. *Guidelines for the Use of Antiretroviral Agents in HIV-1-Infected Adults and Adolescents.* January 10, 2011. Available at www.aidsinfo.nih.gov/guidelines/.

Major Depression and Other Depressive Disorders

Background

Major depression is the most prevalent psychiatric comorbidity and a common cause of significant morbidity among people with HIV infection. The etiology may be multifactorial, as with depression in HIV-uninfected persons, but HIV infection may bring additional complexity. A diagnosis of HIV may cause a psychological crisis, but also may complicate underlying psychological or psychiatric problems (e.g., preexisting depression, anxiety, or substance abuse). Direct viral infection of the central nervous system (CNS) can cause several neuropsychiatric syndromes. In addition, both HIV-related medical conditions and HIV medications can cause or contribute to depression.

HRSA HAB Core Clinical Performance Measures

Percentage of new clients with HIV infection who have had a **mental health screening**

(Group 3 measure)

Patients with untreated depression experience substantial morbidity and may become self-destructive or suicidal. They are at continuing risk of engaging in unsafe behaviors that may lead to HIV transmission and poor adherence to care and treatment.

Major depression in persons with comorbid medical illness, including HIV infection, has been associated with the following:

- Decreased survival
- Impaired quality of life
- Decreased adherence to antiretroviral therapy (ART)
- Increased risk behaviors
- Suicide
- Longer hospital stays and more frequent medical visits (e.g., emergency room, medical clinics)
- Higher treatment costs

Stress and depressive symptoms, especially when they occur jointly, are associated with diminished immune defenses in HIV-infected individuals, and severe depression is associated with higher mortality rates. Anxiety symptoms are common among people with major depression (see chapter *Anxiety*). Psychotic symptoms may occur as a component of major depression and are associated with an increased risk of suicide. Even one or two symptoms of depression increase the risk of an

episode of major depression.

All clinicians should do the following:

- Maintain a high index of suspicion for depression and screen frequently for mood disorders.
- Elicit any history of psychiatric diagnoses or treatment.

Rule out medical conditions that may cause mood or functional alterations.

Refer for psychiatric evaluation and psychosocial support, including, as appropriate, to substance abuse counselors and domestic violence service providers.

A screening test for depression such as the Patient Health Questionnaire-2 (PHQ-2) should be administered yearly or whenever a patient's complaints or symptoms suggest depressive disorders.

PHQ-2

Over the past 2 weeks, how often have you been having little interest or pleasure in doing things?

0 = Not at all
1 = Several days
2 = More than half the days
3 = Nearly every day

Over the past 2 weeks, how often have you been feeling down, depressed, or hopeless?

0 = Not at all
1 = Several days
2 = More than half the days
3 = Nearly every day

Calculate the total point score:_____

Score interpretation:

Score	Probability of major depressive disorder (%)	Probability of any depressive disorder (%)
1	15.4	36.9
2	21.1	48.3
3	38.4	75.0
4	45.5	81.2
5	56.4	84.6
6	78.6	92.9

Depression is diagnosed, as in HIV-uninfected individuals, according to the criteria of the *Diagnostic and Statistical Manual of Mental Disorders* (DSM)-IV.

Major Depression

The patient may complain of either or both of two cardinal symptoms:

- Diminished interest or pleasure in activities
- Depressed mood, sadness

If either or both of these are present, other complaints may be used to diagnose major depression, including the following:

- Decreased ability to concentrate
- Appetite changes with weight changes (increase or decrease)
- Fatigue or loss of energy
- Feelings of worthlessness or guilt
- Insomnia or hypersomnia
- Psychomotor agitation or retardation
- Recurrent thoughts of death or suicide

The diagnosis of major depression is made if five of the above symptoms occur on most days for at least 2 weeks. Depressed mood or diminished interest or pleasure must be one of the five symptoms present.

Other subjective symptoms of depression may include:

- Hopelessness
- Helplessness
- Irritability or anger
- Somatic complaints in addition to those noted above

Other Depressive Disorders

- **Dysthymia** is another very common depressive disorder found among HIV-infected patients. It is not uncommon for dysthymia to coexist with major depression, and the treatments for the two conditions are similar.

Dysthymia is characterized by more chronic but less severe symptoms than those found in major depression. The diagnosis is made when a person has had a depressed mood for most of the day, for more days than not, for at least two years. While depressed, the patient exhibits two or more of the following symptoms:

- Poor appetite or overeating
- Insomnia or hypersomnia
- Low energy or fatigue
- Low self-esteem
- Poor concentration or difficulty making decisions
- Feelings of hopelessness

In addition, the symptoms must cause clinically significant distress or impairment in functioning, and there can have been no major depressive episode during the first two years of the disturbance.

- **Bipolar disorder:** Major depression may be a manifestation of bipolar disorder. Bipolar disorder should be ruled out before giving an antidepressant to a patient with major depression, as bipolar disorder usually requires the use of mood stabilizers before, or instead of, beginning antidepressant medications (antidepressant therapy may precipitate a manic episode). Bipolar disorder should be suspected if a patient has a history of episodes of high energy and activity with little need for sleep, has engaged in risky activities such as buying sprees and increased levels of risky sexual behavior, or has a history of taking mood stabilizers (lithium and others) in the past. If bipolar disorder is suspected, refer the patient to a psychiatrist for further evaluation and treatment.
- **Other forms of depression** include adjustment disorder with depressed mood (acute reaction to a life crisis, such as the loss of a job) and depressive disorder not otherwise specified.

- **Bereavement** is not a disorder but may be accompanied by symptoms that look similar to those of major depression. The diagnosis of major depression generally is not given unless depressive symptoms persist for 2 months after the loss.

S: Subjective

- Inquire about the symptoms listed above, and about associated symptoms.
- Take a careful history of the timing and duration of symptoms, their relationship to life events (e.g., HIV testing, loss of a friend, onset of physical symptoms), and any other physical changes noted along with the mood changes.
- Elicit personal and family histories of depression, bipolar disorder, or suicidal behavior.
- Probe for suicidal thoughts, plans, and materials to execute the plans (see chapter *Suicide Risk*).
- Inquire about hallucinations, paranoia, and other symptoms.
- Ask about current and past medication use and substance abuse.

O: Objective

Perform mental status examination, including evaluation of affect, mood, orientation, appearance, agitation, or psychomotor slowing; perform thyroid examination, inspection for signs of self-injury, and neurologic examination if appropriate.

A: Assessment
Partial Differential Diagnosis

Rule out nonpsychiatric causes of symptoms, which may include the following:

- Hypothyroidism or hyperthyroidism
- Hypotestosteronism (hypogonadism) —

very common with HIV disease in both men and women

- Other endocrine disorders such as Addison disease

- Substance-induced mood disorder (intoxication or withdrawal)

- Medication adverse effects (e.g., from steroids, efavirenz, isoniazid, or interferon-alfa)

- HIV dementia or minor cognitive motor disorder

- HIV encephalopathy

- Neurosyphilis

- Opportunistic illnesses affecting the CNS (e.g., toxoplasmosis, cryptococcal disease, CNS cytomegalovirus, progressive multifocal leukoencephalopathy)

- Vitamin B12, folate (B6), zinc, vitamin A, or vitamin D deficiency

P: Plan

Evaluation

The diagnosis is based on clinical criteria as indicated above. Rule out medical and other causes. An initial screening includes the following:

- Complete blood count, electrolytes, creatinine, blood urea nitrogen (BUN), glucose

- Thyroid function tests (thyroid stimulating hormone [TSH], T4)

- Vitamin B12, vitamin D, and folate levels

- Testosterone (both in men and women)

- Other tests as suggested by history and physical examination

Treatment

Refer immediately for psychiatric evaluation or treatment if the patient is:

- Hopeless

- Suicidal (see chapter *Suicide Risk*)

- Displaying psychotic symptoms

- Debilitated or functionally impaired by severe symptoms

- Not responding to treatment

The combination of psychotherapy and antidepressant medication is more effective than either treatment modality alone. Social support interventions (e.g., community-based HIV support groups) also can help; refer to available resources. Patients should be encouraged to discontinue alcohol or substance use, and should be referred for treatment as indicated.

Psychotherapy

Individual psychotherapy with a skilled, HIV-experienced mental health professional can be very effective in treating depression. Several specific types of individual and group psychotherapies for depression (e.g., interpersonal therapy, cognitive-behavioral therapy, behavioral activation, supportive psychotherapy, coping effectiveness) have been shown to be effective for HIV-infected individuals.

Pharmacotherapy

For most patients, a selective serotonin reuptake inhibitor (SSRI) or a selective norepinephrine reuptake inhibitor (SNRI) is the most appropriate initial treatment for depression. For patients who experience treatment failure with these agents (or have an incomplete response) at a customary therapeutic dosage, consultation with a psychiatrist is recommended.

When selecting antidepressant medications, consider their side effect profiles as a means to manage other symptoms the patient may be experiencing. For example, activating antidepressants (taken in the morning) may help patients who complain of low energy; antidepressants that increase appetite may be useful for patients with wasting syndrome; sedating antidepressants (taken at bedtime) may help patients with insomnia. Medications that may be lethal if overdosed (e.g., tricyclic antidepressants) should not be prescribed to patients for whom suicidality may be a concern.

The information below describes specific antidepressant medications, with information on dosage and possible adverse effects. Most antidepressants should be started at low dosages and gradually titrated upward to avoid unpleasant side effects that might lead to nonadherence. Antidepressant effect usually is not noticed until 2-4 weeks after starting a medication. If there is no improvement in symptoms in 2-4 weeks, and there are no significant adverse effects, the dosage may be increased.

A therapeutic trial consists of treatment for 4-6 weeks at a therapeutic dosage. If the patient's symptoms have not improved, an increase in dosage or a switch to another medication should be considered. Patients who remain depressed should be referred to a psychiatrist.

Monitor all patients closely after starting them on antidepressant medications. Some patients may be at risk of worsening depression, including suicidality, after initiation of therapy; improved energy is the initial effect of antidepressants, whereas hopelessness and sadness improve later. In addition, some young persons are at risk of worsening depression caused by antidepressants. Black-box warnings advise that antidepressants may cause increased risk of suicidality in children, adolescents, and young adults (<24 years of age) with major depressive or other psychiatric disorders, especially during the first month of treatment.

Medications should be continued for 6-9 months beyond the resolution of symptoms to reduce the risk of recurrence. After this time, treatment may be tapered down gradually if the patient wishes, with careful monitoring for recurrence of symptoms. The risk of recurrence is higher if the first depressive episode is inadequately treated or if the patient has had multiple depressive episodes. For patients with recurrent depression, consider long-term maintenance antidepressant treatment. See "Discontinuing antidepressant medication," below.

Potential ARV Interactions

Interactions may occur between certain ARVs and agents used to treat depression. Some combinations may be contraindicated and others may require dosage adjustment. Refer to medication interaction resources or consult with an HIV expert, psychiatrist, or pharmacist before prescribing.

Some ARV medications (particularly protease inhibitors [PIs]) may affect the metabolism of some antidepressants via cytochrome P450 interactions. For example, ritonavir can significantly increase serum levels of tricyclic antidepressants, increasing the risk of tricyclic toxicity. In the case of most other antidepressants, interactions with ARVs generally are not clinically significant, but most antidepressants used concomitantly with PIs should be started at low dosages and titrated cautiously to prevent antidepressant adverse effects and toxicity. On the other hand, some PIs may decrease levels of paroxetine, sertraline, and bupropion, and efavirenz also lowers sertraline and bupropion levels; these antidepressants may require upward titration if used concurrently with interacting ARVs. Further information is presented under individual agents and classes, below.

For patients who are starting ARV medications (particularly PIs) and are on a stable antidepressant regimen, monitor carefully for adverse effects and for efficacy of the antidepressant; dosage adjustments may be required.

Section 8: Neuropsychiatric Disorders

The available antidepressant medications (SSRIs and SNRIs), including therapeutic dosages and possible positive and negative effects, are listed in Table 1.

Table 1. SSRI and SNRI Antidepressant Medications and Possible Positive and Negative Effects

Medication/Usual Dosage	Possible Positive Effects	Possible Negative Effects
SSRIs	No anticholinergic or cardiovascular effects, nonfatal in overdose; may help treat anxiety	Sexual dysfunction (men and women) Serotonin withdrawal syndrome if discontinued abruptly
Citalopram (Celexa): 10-60 mg once daily	May have lower risk of significant drug-drug interactions than other SSRIs	Mild nausea, possible sedation
Escitalopram (Lexapro): 10-20 mg once daily	May have lower risk of significant drug-drug interactions than other SSRIs	Mild nausea, possible sedation
Fluoxetine (Prozac): 10-40 mg once daily	Rarely sedating, often energizing, lower risk of SSRI withdrawal syndrome if discontinued abruptly	Insomnia, agitation, nausea, headache, sexual dysfunction in men and women, long half-life
Paroxetine (Paxil): 10-40 mg once daily	May be sedating (for patients experiencing sedation with paroxetine, dose at bedtime; can be useful with depression-associated insomnia)	Insomnia, agitation (for patients experiencing these effects, administer dose in mornings), nausea, headache, higher risk of SSRI withdrawal syndrome, weight gain
Sertraline (Zoloft): 50-200 mg once daily	May have lower incidence of significant drug-drug interactions compared with fluoxetine and paroxetine	Insomnia, agitation, nausea, headache
SNRIs		Nausea, headache, nervousness, sexual dysfunction (men and women) Serotonin withdrawal syndrome if discontinued abruptly
Duloxetine (Cymbalta): 30-60 mg once daily	May be used also for pain management and neuropathy; may have lower risk of significant drug-drug interactions compared with SSRIs	Nausea, somnolence
Venlafaxine (Effexor): 37.5-75 mg BID or TID OR Venlafaxine XR (Effexor XR): 75-375 mg once daily	May have lower risk of significant drug-drug interactions compared with SSRIs	Hypertension (monitor blood pressure at higher dosages) Higher risk of SSRI/SNRI withdrawal syndrome
Desvenlafaxine (Pristiq): 50 mg once daily	May have lower risk of significant drug-drug interactions compared with SSRIs	Higher risk of SSRI/SNRI withdrawal syndrome

Section 8: Neuropsychiatric Disorders

Other agents

- **Bupropion (Wellbutrin and others):** Bupropion is available in immediate-release form (requires TID dosing), sustained-release (SR) (requires BID dosing), or extended-release (XL) (once-daily dosing) formulations. At higher bupropion dosages, there is an increased risk of seizures, and this drug is contraindicated in patients who have risk factors for seizures. For patients taking PIs, caution should be used as the dosage approaches 300-400 mg per day because of possible increases in levels of bupropion (however, tipranavir and efavirenz may decrease bupropion levels). Bupropion may have an activating effect, which some patients may experience as agitation, insomnia, or both, and also may have an appetite suppressant effect. It usually does not cause sexual dysfunction, and therefore may be helpful for individuals with depression who experience adverse sexual effects with other antidepressant agents.

- **Mirtazapine (Remeron):** (15-45 mg QPM) May have lower risk of significant drug-drug interactions compared with SSRIs; can be useful when weight gain and sleep induction are needed. Potential adverse effects include sedation, increased appetite, weight gain, constipation, and dry mouth. Note that the higher dosages may result in increased activation owing to increased NE receptor antagonism.

- **Tricyclics:** Tricyclic antidepressants may be effective, but in general have a higher risk of adverse effects than do SSRIs and SNRIs. They also are more dangerous (potentially fatal) in overdose. Adverse effects include anticholinergic effects, sedation, and cardiac conduction abnormalities. Levels of tricyclics are increased by ritonavir, so lower dosages may be needed for patients taking ritonavir or ritonavir-boosted PIs.

Routine monitoring of blood levels of tricyclics should be performed on patients receiving higher doses *(e.g., 100 mg per day; 50 mg for nortriptyline)*, those on concurrently on ritonavir, and those with risk factors for cardiac conduction abnormalities. A routine electrocardiogram should be performed before prescribing tricyclics, and this class of drugs should not be prescribed to patients with cardiac conduction problems.

The adverse effects of tricyclics can be used to treat insomnia or diarrhea, for example, and tricyclics can be effective for neuropathic pain.

- **Imipramine (Tofranil):** FDA indications for depression and chronic pain. The full recommended dosage for either problem is 150-300 mg QHS. Starting dosage: 25-75 mg PO QHS.

- **Doxepin (Sinequan):** FDA indications for depression and anxiety at adult dosages of 150-300 mg QHS. Starting dosage: 25-75 mg PO QHS.

- Three other available tricyclics have an FDA indication for depression only: **nortriptyline (Pamelor)** at dosages of 50-150 mg QHS; **desipramine (Norpramin)** at dosages of 50-200 mg a day; and **protriptyline (Vivactil)** at dosages of 5-10 mg, either TID or QID.

- **Tricyclics need to be started at low dosages and titrated gradually.** Lower dosages often are more appropriate for patients who are elderly, medically ill, or taking ritonavir or a ritonavir-boosted PI.

- Trazodone (Desyrel): a highly sedating antidepressant that is rarely used at an antidepressant dosage. Rather, it is often given at lower dosage for insomnia associated with depression, at a dosage of 25-50 mg 1-2 hours before bedtime. Ritonavir and other PIs can increase trazodone levels significantly; start at low dosage and use the lowest effective dosage; monitor for adverse effects; do not use with saquinavir/ritonavir.

- Nefazodone (Serzone): an antidepressant that usually should be avoided in people with HIV infection. Little information on interactions with ARVs is available, but it appears that nefazodone may increase levels of maraviroc and saquinavir, and that ritonavir may increase nefazodone levels. It has a black-box warning for severe liver toxicity. If the patient has ever had liver toxicity from the drug, restarting it is contraindicated.

- St. John's wort: an herbal antidepressant that can significantly decrease serum concentrations of PIs, NNRTIs, and maraviroc; it is contraindicated for use by patients taking those ARVs.

- Treatment may involve antidepressant combinations, including psychostimulants; consult with a psychiatrist.

Discontinuing antidepressant medication

Antidepressant medication generally should be continued for at least 6 months following improvement from a first episode of major depression. Longer term, and even indefinite, maintenance treatment may be necessary for people with recurrent major depression. When discontinuing antidepressants, except for the few mentioned above (e.g., fluoxetine), they need to be tapered gradually to avoid withdrawal symptoms (as below) or rebound depression.

Abrupt discontinuation of SSRI and SNRI antidepressants often precipitates the emergence of unpleasant withdrawal symptoms. This is particularly true for paroxetine and venlafaxine. Withdrawal symptoms may include confusion, agitation, irritability, sensory disturbances, and insomnia. The abrupt discontinuation of SSRIs is associated with a return or worsening of depressive symptoms.

Brain stimulation treatments

There are a variety of brain stimulation treatments that usually are reserved for patients who have inadequate responses to medication. Electroconvulsive therapy (ECT) is the best known of these treatments and, despite the stigma associated with it, is more effective than antidepressant medication. Newer brain stimulation treatments also are available. These treatments require referral to the specialty care locations that offer them. Antidepressant medication often is used for maintenance after stabilization with ECT, but for some people, maintenance ECT is needed to prevent the relapse of depression.

Patient Education

- Providers should explain to patients that illness (physical or emotional) is not a character flaw or a moral or spiritual weakness. It is a common aspect of HIV infection. Sadness is a normal part of life, but major depression always is abnormal and often can be alleviated with medication, psychotherapy, or both.

- Providers should help patients identify the symptoms of depression and the factors that led them to seek treatment. Patients will need to monitor themselves for recurrences or exacerbations and get help if the symptoms recur. Patients should be told to contact providers if they notice changes in their sleep, appetite, mood, activity level, or concentration, or if they notice fatigue, isolation, sadness, or feelings of helplessness.

- When starting an antidepressant medication, patients should expect that it will take 2-4 weeks for them to notice any improvement. Their symptoms should continue to decrease over the following weeks. If they do not have much improvement in symptoms, providers may choose to adjust the dosage of the medication or to change medications. Patients must continue taking their medications so that the symptoms of depression do not return.

- Providers should let patients know that St. John's wort can lower levels of ARVs and cannot be taken if they are on ART.

- Antidepressants typically are given for a long time, usually for a year or longer, to help patients with the chemical imbalances associated with major depression. Patients should be told that they should not suddenly stop antidepressants they have been taking for a long time, and that these medications need to be discontinued gradually.

- Some patients develop problems with sexual function while they are taking antidepressants. They should report any problems to their prescribers. (Note: Providers should let patients know that sexual well-being is fundamental to quality of life and can be talked about and addressed in the clinical setting.)

References

- American Psychiatric Association. *Diagnostic and Statistical Manual of Mental Disorders.* Washington: American Psychiatric Association; 1994.

- Himelhoch S, Medoff DR, Oyeniyi G. *Efficacy of group psychotherapy to reduce depressive symptoms among HIV-infected individuals: a systematic review and meta-analysis.* AIDS Patient Care STDS. 2007 Oct;21(10):732-9

- Ickovics JR, Hamburger ME, Vlahov D, et al.; HIV Epidemiology Research Study Group. *Mortality, CD4 cell count decline, and depressive symptoms among HIV-seropositive women: longitudinal analysis from the HIV Epidemiology Research Study.* JAMA. 2001 Mar 21;285(11):1466-74.

- Kroenke K, Spitzer RL, Williams JB. *The Patient Health Questionnaire-2: validity of a two-item depression screener.* Med Care. 2003 Nov;41(11):1284-92.

- Leserman J, Petitto JM, Perkins DO, et al. *Severe stress, depressive symptoms, and changes in lymphocyte subsets in human immunodeficiency virus-infected men.* A 2-year follow-up study. Arch Gen Psychiatry. 1997 Mar;54(3):279-85.

- Maye TJ, Vittinghoff E, Chesney MA, et al. *Depressive affect and survival among gay and bisexual men infected with HIV.* Arch Intern Med. 1996 Oct 28;156(19):2233-8.

- New York State Department of Health AIDS Institute. *Mental Health Care for People with HIV Infection: Clinical Guidelines for the Primary Care Practitioner.* Available at www.hivguidelines.org. Accessed June 30, 2010.

- Schatzberg AF, Nemeroff CB, eds. *Essentials of Clinical Psychopharmacology.* Washington: American Psychiatric Press; 2006.

- Sikkema KJ, Hansen NB, Ghebremichael M, et al. *A randomized controlled trial of a coping group intervention for adults with HIV who are AIDS bereaved: longitudinal effects on grief.* Health Psychol. 2006 Sep;25(5):563-70.

- Stober DR, Schwartz JAJ, McDaniel JS, et al. *Depression and HIV disease: prevalence, correlates and treatment.* Psych Annals. 1997;27(5):372-377.

- U.S. Department of Health and Human Services. *Guidelines for the Use of Antiretroviral Agents in HIV-1-Infected Adults and Adolescents.* January 10, 2011. Available at www.aidsinfo.nih.gov/guidelines/.

- Wainberg ML, Faragon J, Cournos F, et al. *Psychiatric Medications and HIV Antiretrovirals: A Guide to Interactions for Clinicians, 2nd Edition.* Laminated booklet produced by the New York/New Jersey AIDS Education & Training Center, U.S. Health Resources and Services Administration; 2008.

Section 8: Neuropsychiatric Disorders

Suicide Risk

Background

Transient suicidal thoughts are common for some people throughout the course of HIV disease and often do not indicate significant risk of suicide. However, persistent suicidal thoughts with associated feelings of hopelessness and intent to die are very serious and must be assessed promptly and carefully. Compared with people at high risk of suicide who are not HIV infected, people living with HIV have significantly increased frequency and severity of both suicidal ideation and thoughts of death. The risk of suicide is especially high for patients who are depressed and for those at pivotal points in the course of HIV infection. Stigma, quality of life concerns, and issues regarding disclosure may be contributing factors.

HRSA HAB Core Clinical Performance Measures

Percentage of new clients with HIV infection who have had a **mental health screening**

(Group 3 measure)

Suicidality may be the direct physiological result of HIV (e.g., owing to the impact of HIV in the brain), a reaction to chronic pain, an emotional reaction to having a chronic and life-threatening illness (e.g., major depression as a result of physical illness or psychiatric side effects caused by medications used to treat HIV infection and associated comorbidities). Many events may trigger suicidal thoughts among people with HIV. Such events include learning of their positive HIV status, disclosing to family and friends, starting antiretroviral therapy (ART), noticing the first symptoms of infection, having a decrease in CD4 cell count, undergoing a major illness or hospitalization, receiving an AIDS diagnosis, losing a job, experiencing major changes in lifestyle, requiring evaluation for dementia, and losing a significant relationship.

Evaluation of suicide risk must be included as part of a comprehensive mental health evaluation for HIV-infected patients. Note that asking patients about suicidal thoughts does not increase their risk of suicide.

Risk factors for suicide attempts include the following:

- Previous suicide attempts
- Abandonment by or isolation from, family, friends, or significant others
- Age >45 for men, >55 for women; or teen years
- Male gender
- Gay sexual orientation
- Transgender
- Any acute change in health status; worsening of HIV-related illness or other physical illnesses
- Family history of completed suicide
- Alcohol and other substance misuse, abuse, or dependence
- Relapse into drug use after significant recovery
- Severe anxiety, depression, psychotic disorder, or other mental health disorder
- Domestic violence
- Social isolation (e.g., being single, divorced, or alone, or experiencing the death of a spouse)
- Multiple losses or recent stressors
- Financial difficulty, unemployment

- Hopelessness and lack of pleasure
- Impulsivity
- Pain
- Perception of poor prognosis
- Perception of poor social support
- Planning for death
- Stigmatization associated with illness, sexual orientation, substance use history, or other factors
- Fear of HIV-associated dementia

Protective factors include the following:

- Strong psychosocial support
- Evidence of good coping mechanisms
- Cultural and religious beliefs against suicide
- Reasons for living
- No specific plan for suicide

S: Subjective

The patient expresses or exhibits, or a personal care giver discloses, the following:

- Active suicidal ideation with intent and plan, such as giving away significant personal belongings, saying goodbye, acquiring the means (e.g., gun, pills), writing a suicide note
- Depressed mood, hopelessness, agitation, intoxication with alcohol or other drugs
- Passive withdrawal from therapy or medical care or decreased adherence (e.g., stopping medications, missing appointments)
- A desire for HIV disease to progress more rapidly

Inquire about the following during the history (again, note that asking patients about suicidal thoughts does not increase their risk of suicide):

- Previous suicide attempt(s) — one of the best predictors of eventual death by suicide
- Friend or family member who has committed suicide
- Personal or family history of depression
- Previous episode of psychosis
- Presence of risk factors described above

Probe for other depressive symptoms and the immediacy of potential suicidal intent. Sample questions may include the following:

- "It sounds as if you're in great pain. Have you ever thought that life is not worth living?"
- "Do you often think of death?"
- "Do you think about hurting yourself?"
- "How might you do that?"
- "Do you have a plan?" Ask whether the patient has access to the components of the plan (e.g., gun, pills)
- "Is this something you feel you might do?"
- "What would prevent you from doing this?"
- "Have you ever attempted suicide? What did you do?"

O: Objective

- Perform a mental status examination and suicide assessment.
- Look for signs of self-inflicted injuries such as wrist lacerations or neck burns.
- Look for signs of depression, agitation, or intoxication.

A: Assessment

See chapter *Depression* for differential diagnosis of possible causes of depression and suicidality.

P: Plan

Evaluation

Evaluate the patient for depression, risk factors for suicide, and contributing psychiatric illnesses or situational stressors. Determine the immediacy of potential suicidal intent. If a mental health professional is available on site or can be summoned, an urgent consultation often is helpful in making these determinations.

Treatment

- If the patient exhibits active suicidal ideation with a plan, hospitalize the patient immediately, preferably in a psychiatric facility.

- If suicidal thoughts are passive, refer for evaluation for specific psychiatric disorders and refer for psychotherapy with an HIV-experienced mental health provider.

- Encourage the patient to contact you or another specified clinician for help, or to go to a hospital if suicidal ideation worsens or patient worries about acting upon suicidal thoughts.

- Note that making a contract with a patient against suicide is not recommended; research shows is not effective, and it can provide a false sense of security.

- Inform patients about local suicide prevention resources, including suicide hotlines, emergency response (e.g., 911), and local emergency departments.

- Contact the patient between appointments. Enlist the help of significant others (if the patient agrees); invite them to accompany the patient on the next visit and see all of them together. Consider a support group or peer referral, if available.

- Consider dispensing medications on a weekly basis for the following purposes:
  - Monitoring emotional status and treatment adherence
  - Preventing the availability of lethal doses of medications

- Perform appropriate follow-up. In consultation with a skilled mental health provider, be sure that the patient is receiving appropriate ongoing treatment for underlying or persisting psychiatric illness. Assess at each visit for adherence to mental health care and for recurrence of symptoms.

Patient Education

- Suicidal ideation and severe depression are not normal aspects of HIV infection, and usually can be treated effectively.

- Patients should report suicidal thoughts to their health care providers.

- Inform patients about local suicide prevention resources, including suicide hotlines, emergency response (e.g., 911), and local emergency departments.

References

- Cournos F, Lowenthal D, Cabaniss D. *Clinical Evaluation and Treatment Planning: A Multimodal Approach.* In: Tasman A, Kay J, Lieberman JA, et al., eds. *Psychiatry, Third Edition.* Hoboken, NJ: John Wiley & Sons; 2008;525-45.

- Gielen AC, McDonnell KA, O'Campo PJ, et al. *Suicide risk and mental health indicators: Do they differ by abuse and HIV status?* Women's Health Issues. 2005 Mar-Apr;15(2):89-95.

- Goldstein RB, Black DW, Nasrallah A., et al. *The prediction of suicide: Sensitivity, specificity and predictive value of a multivariate model applied to suicide among 1906 patients with affective disorders.* Arch Gen Psychiatry. 1991 May;48(5):418-22.

- Kelly B, Raphael B, Judd F, et al. *Suicidal ideation, suicide attempts, and HIV infection.* Psychosomatics. 1998 Sep-Oct;39(5):405-15.

- Kessler RC, Borges G, Walters EE. *Prevalence of and risk factors for lifetime suicide attempts in national comorbidity survey.* Arch Gen Psychiatry. 1999 Jul;56(7):617-26.

- Komiti A, Judd F, Grech P, et al. *Suicidal behaviour in people with HIV/AIDS: a review.* Aust N Z J Psychiatry. 2001 35(6):747-57.

- Mountain Plains AIDS Education and Training Center. *HIV and Suicide: Risk Assessment and Intervention.* 2007.

- New York State Department of Health AIDS Institute. *Mental Health Care for People with HIV Infection: Clinical Guidelines for the Primary Care Practitioner.* Available at www.hivguidelines.org. Accessed June 30, 2010.

- Robertson K, Parsons TD, Van Der Horst C, et al. *Thoughts of death and suicidal ideation in nonpsychiatric human immunodeficiency virus seropositive individuals.* Death Stud. 2006 Jun;30(5):455-69.

- Roy A. *Characteristics of HIV patients who attempt suicide.* Acta Psychiatr Scand. 2003 Jan;107(1):41-4.

- Wainberg ML. *Mental Health Issues in HIV-Positive Patients.* Presentation at the 3rd annual Mountain-Plains AIDS Education and Training Center Faculty Development Conference, Keystone, CO. Mountain Plains AIDS Education and Training Center; 2005.

Anxiety Disorders

Background

Anxiety symptoms are common and can develop or recur for many reasons, including a patient's worries about HIV infection and treatment, or issues unrelated to HIV. Symptoms can range from mild distress to full-blown anxiety disorders. Symptoms of anxiety can mimic symptoms of physical illness, and an appropriate workup should be performed to rule out other illnesses. Use of illicit drugs (e.g., amphetamines, cocaine) or alcohol can cause or substantially worsen anxiety symptoms; all patients should be screened for substance use.

HRSA HAB Core Clinical Performance Measures

Percentage of new clients with HIV infection who have had a **mental health screening**

(Group 3 measure)

Anxiety disorders include generalized anxiety disorder, obsessive-compulsive disorder, specific phobia, social phobia, acute stress disorder, posttraumatic stress disorder (PTSD), and panic disorder. This chapter focuses primarily on anxiety symptoms and generalized anxiety disorder. See chapters *Panic Disorder* and *Posttraumatic Stress Disorder* for further information about these conditions.

S: Subjective

The criteria for a diagnosis of generalized anxiety disorder include unrealistic or excessive worry about two or more life circumstances for >6 months, and at least three of the following subjective complaints:

- Restlessness or feeling keyed-up or on edge
- Difficulty concentrating or mind going blank
- Irritability
- Muscle tension
- Being easily fatigued
- Sleep disturbance (difficulty falling or staying asleep, or restless, unsatisfying sleep)

Other subjective complaints may include the following:

- Shortness of breath or smothering sensations
- Palpitations or accelerated heart rate
- Dizziness or lightheadedness
- Exaggerated startle response
- Trembling, twitching, or feeling shaky
- Dry mouth

- Flushes or chills
- Frequent urination
- Muscle aches or soreness
- Nausea, diarrhea, or other abdominal distress
- Skin rashes
- Sweating or cold, clammy hands
- Trouble swallowing or "lump in the throat"

Ask about the symptoms indicated above, and about the following:

- Anxiety patterns (e.g., constant or intermittent; timing, duration, precipitants)
- Onset: sudden or gradual
- Caffeine intake
- Recreational drug or alcohol use (current or recent)
- Concomitant illnesses (e.g., cardiac, pulmonary, endocrine)
- Family history of similar problems
- Medications, supplements, and herbal preparations
- History of previous episodes

- Recent stressors
- Sleep disturbances
- Other physical symptoms

O: Objective

Measure vital signs, with particular attention to heart rate (tachycardia) and respiratory rate (shortness of breath, hyperventilation).

Perform a physical examination, including mental status and neurologic, cardiopulmonary, and thyroid examinations.

A: Assessment

A differential diagnosis may include the following medical conditions:

- Substance use (e.g., amphetamines, cocaine)
- Substance or medication withdrawal (e.g., alcohol, benzodiazepines)
- Excessive caffeine intake
- Electrolyte imbalances
- Heart disease, arrhythmias
- Hyperthyroidism
- Hypoglycemia
- Immune disorders
- Respiratory disease, hypoxia
- Medication adverse effects (e.g., with efavirenz, isoniazid, steroids, theophylline, or stimulants)
- Sleep disturbances or sleep deprivation
- Allergic reactions
- Anemia
- Central nervous system (CNS) or opportunistic infections or malignancies
- Systemic or other infections
- Vitamin B12 deficiency

P: Plan

Diagnostic Evaluation

Perform the following tests:

- Blood glucose, electrolytes
- Thyroid function tests (TSH, T4)
- Electrocardiogram (EKG) if patient has shortness of breath or palpitations
- Arterial blood gases (if frank difficulty breathing is not self-limited)
- Other tests as indicated by symptoms and physical examination

Treatment

Once medical disorders have been ruled out, and the diagnosis of an anxiety disorder is established, several options are available:

Psychotherapy

Options include cognitive-behavioral therapy, interpersonal therapy, exposure therapy, a stress-management group, relaxation therapy, visualization, guided imagery, supportive psychotherapy, and psychodynamic psychotherapy. Long-term psychotherapy may be indicated if experienced professionals are available and the patient is capable of forming an ongoing relationship. If possible, refer to an HIV-experienced therapist. The type of psychotherapy available to the patient often depends on the skills and training of the practitioners in a given health care system or region. In addition, the patient may be referred to available community-based support.

Pharmacotherapy

Medications, with or without psychotherapy, may alleviate symptoms of anxiety. Patients with advanced HIV disease, like geriatric patients, may be more vulnerable to the CNS effects of certain medications. Medications that affect the CNS should be started at low dosage and titrated slowly. Similar precautions should apply to patients with liver dysfunction.

- **Antidepressants:** Selective serotonin reuptake inhibitors (SSRIs) and selective norepinephrine reuptake inhibitors (SNRI) are effective in treating patients with anxiety. They are favored for long-term use when a specific anxiety disorder is present and persistent. These medications do not cause tolerance or pose a risk of addiction. Below is a list of antidepressants that includes their U.S. Food and Drug Administration (FDA) approvals for specific anxiety disorders and the usual recommended dosages. FDA recommendations are based on availability of specific study data, but all SSRIs (regardless of whether they have an FDA indication for anxiety) may be helpful for a broad range of anxiety disorders.

  Common adverse effects of SSRIs and SNRIs include sexual dysfunction, sleep disturbance, and nausea. For patients who are medically ill, these medications should be started at low dosage and titrated up slowly; a low dosage may be effective. These medications also should be down-tapered slowly; SSRI/SNRI discontinuation syndrome may occur if they are discontinued abruptly.

  See chapter *Depression* for further information about antidepressant medications, including adverse effects.

- **SSRI antidepressants:**

  - Fluoxetine (Prozac): FDA indication for panic disorder with a recommended dosage of 20 mg once daily. Also recommended for obsessive-compulsive disorder, but higher dosages are needed, sometimes up to 80 mg daily.

  - Escitalopram (Lexapro): FDA indication for generalized anxiety disorder at a dosage of 10 mg once daily.

  - Citalopram (Celexa): Does not have specific FDA indications for anxiety disorders. Suggested dosage: start at 10 mg once daily and titrate as needed; maximum dosage: 60 mg daily.

  - Paroxetine (Paxil): FDA indications for obsessive-compulsive disorder and panic disorder both at a recommended dosage of 40 mg once daily. Also indicated for social anxiety disorder at a dosage of 20-40 mg daily. Usual starting dosage: 10 mg daily.

  - Sertraline (Zoloft): FDA indications for panic disorder and PTSD at dosages of 50-200 mg once daily. Usual starting dosage: 25 mg daily.

- **SNRI antidepressants:**

  - Venlafaxine timed-release formulation (Effexor XR): FDA indication for generalized anxiety disorder, at recommended dosages of 75-225 mg per day. **Note:** There is a risk of hypertension at the higher dosages of venlafaxine; monitor blood pressure.

  - Duloxetine (Cymbalta): FDA indication for generalized anxiety disorder at a recommended dosage of 60 mg once daily.

- **Other antidepressants:**

  - Some sedating antidepressants are effective, nonaddictive agents that are helpful when taken at bedtime for both insomnia and anxiety symptoms. These include trazodone (Desyrel) 25-100 mg QHS or imipramine (Tofranil) 25 mg QHS. Note that imipramine and other tricyclics must be used with caution but are not contraindicated for use by patients taking ritonavir (including ritonavir-boosted protease inhibitors [PIs]).

  - Gabapentin (Neurontin), a mood stabilizer, may be given at dosages of 200-400 mg BID to QID and may sometimes help to diminish anxiety.

Section 8: Neuropsychiatric Disorders

- **Anxiolytics:** Short-term use of benzodiazepines sometimes is appropriate for mild and brief situational anxiety symptoms, even without the presence of a specific anxiety disorder. For longer-term use, non-benzodiazepines (e.g., buspirone [see below], SSRIs, or SNRIs) are preferred.

  - Buspirone (BuSpar) is a nonaddictive anxiolytic. Start at 5 mg PO TID. If symptoms persist, the dosage can be increased by 5 mg per dose each week to a maximum of 10-15 mg TID (for a total daily dosage of 30-45 mg). It will take several weeks for patients to notice a decrease in anxiety; low-dose benzodiazepines may be used during this interval. The major potential adverse effects of buspirone are dizziness and lightheadedness.

  - Consider intermediate half-life benzodiazepines such as lorazepam (Ativan) 0.5 mg PO Q8H or oxazepam (Serax) 10 mg PO Q6H if buspirone is not tolerated or to alleviate anxiety symptoms until buspirone takes effect. Longer-acting benzodiazepines such as clonazepam (Klonopin) also may be useful at dosages of 0.25-0.5 mg PO BID.

  - Benzodiazepines generally should be used only for acute, short-term management because of the risk of tolerance and physiologic dependence. These risks are even more problematic for patients with a history of addiction.

Potential ARV Interactions

Interactions may occur between certain ARVs and agents used to treat anxiety. Some combinations may be contraindicated and others may require dosage adjustment. Refer to medication interaction resources or consult with an HIV expert, psychiatrist, or pharmacist before prescribing.

Antidepressants

- Some ARV medications (particularly PIs) may affect the metabolism of some antidepressants via cytochrome P450 interactions. For most SSRIs and SNRIs, interactions with ARVs generally are not clinically significant; in the case of tricyclics, their levels may be significantly increased by ritonavir. On the other hand, some PIs may decrease levels of paroxetine and sertraline, and efavirenz also lowers sertraline levels. See chapter *Depression* for further information.

Anxiolytics

- PIs and nonnucleoside reverse transcriptase inhibitors (NNRTIs) may raise blood concentrations of many benzodiazepines. Consider using a benzodiazepine metabolized by glucuronidation (e.g., lorazepam, oxazepam), particularly in patients with liver disease. For benzodiazepines metabolized by the CYP system, start at low dosages and titrate slowly. Other CNS depressants and alcohol should be avoided in patients taking these benzodiazepines.
  - Midazolam (Versed) and triazolam (Halcion) are contraindicated for use with all PIs and with delavirdine and efavirenz.
- Buspirone levels may be increased by ritonavir-boosted PIs, and may be decreased by CYP inducers. Monitor patients for adverse effects and for efficacy.

Patient Education

- Behavioral interventions can help to reduce anxiety, but may take practice. Patients should seek help from a therapist or another experienced source.

- Advise patients that misuse of alcohol or illicit drugs can cause or substantially worsen anxiety symptoms; advise patients to decrease or eliminate use. Refer for substance abuse treatment if indicated.

- Inform patients that they may develop problems with sexual function because of antianxiety medications. Patients should report any problems to their prescribers. (Note: Providers should let patients know that sexual well-being is fundamental to quality of life and can be talked about and addressed in the clinical setting.)

References

- American Psychiatric Association. *Diagnostic and Statistical Manual of Mental Disorders.* Washington: American Psychiatric Association; 1994.

- New York State Department of Health AIDS Institute. *Mental Health Care for People with HIV Infection: Clinical Guidelines for the Primary Care Practitioner.* Available at www. hivguidelines.org. Accessed June 30, 2010.

- U.S. Department of Health and Human Services. *Guidelines for the Use of Antiretroviral Agents in HIV-1-Infected Adults and Adolescents.* January 10, 2011. Available at www.aidsinfo.nih.gov/ guidelines/.

- Wainberg ML, Faragon J, Cournos F, et al. *Psychiatric Medications and HIV Antiretrovirals: A Guide to Interactions for Clinicians, 2nd Edition.* Laminated booklet produced by the New York/New Jersey AIDS Education & Training Center, U.S. Health Resources and Services Administration; 2008.

Panic Disorder

Background

Panic disorder is an anxiety disorder whose essential feature is the presence of recurrent, unexpected panic attacks. Panic attacks are discrete, sudden-onset episodes of intense fear or apprehension accompanied by specific somatic or psychiatric symptoms (e.g., palpitations, shortness of breath, fear of losing control). A patient is diagnosed as having panic disorder when he or she has experienced such attacks, and at least one of the attacks has been followed by ≥1 month of persistent concern about additional attacks, worry about the implications or consequences of the attack, or a significant change in behavior related to the attack.

Panic disorder is classified as being either with or without agoraphobia. Agoraphobia refers to anxiety about being in places or situations from which escape might be difficult or embarrassing, or in which help might not be available in the event of a panic attack or panic-like symptoms. These situations might include being alone outside one's home, being in a crowd, being on a bridge, driving, traveling in a bus or train, or even visiting health care providers for medical appointments. The patient avoids these situations or endures them with marked distress.

The symptoms of panic disorder usually begin in late adolescence to the mid-30s and may coincide with the presentation of major depressive disorder, social phobia, or generalized anxiety disorder. Panic disorder can interfere with the ability to conduct activities of daily living. Patients with panic disorder have an increased incidence of suicide.

Symptoms may mimic those of various physical illnesses or be caused by other medical conditions (e.g., hyperthyroidism, brain tumors, adrenal tumors, heart arrhythmias, hypoglycemia, anemia). Substance or alcohol intoxication or withdrawal also may cause panic symptoms. Patients with panic symptoms should be evaluated for other causative conditions

Major depressive disorder occurs in 50% to 65% of people with panic disorder. Major depression may precede or follow the onset of panic disorder. Patients with panic disorder therefore should be screened for depression initially and periodically thereafter (see chapter *Depression*). Anxiety also commonly is experienced by persons with panic disorder; see chapter *Anxiety* for further information about this condition.

S: Subjective

The patient complains of discrete periods of intense fear or discomfort in which four or more of the following symptoms developed abruptly and reached a peak within 10 minutes:

- Shortness of breath or smothering sensation
- Sweating
- Trembling or shaking
- Dizziness, lightheadedness, faintness, or feeling of unsteadiness

- Numbness or tingling sensations
- Chest pain or discomfort
- Palpitations or accelerated heart rate
- Hot flashes or chills
- Sensation of choking
- Depersonalization or derealization
- Fear of dying
- Fear of going crazy or losing control
- Nausea or abdominal distress

Other subjective complaints may include the following:

- Apprehension about the outcome of routine activities and experiences

- Anticipation of a catastrophic outcome from a mild physical symptom or from medication side effects

- Discouragement and demoralization

Panic attacks are, by definition, self-limited and they peak quickly. Symptoms that persist continuously for longer periods suggest other causes.

Ask about the symptoms indicated above and about the following:

- Frequency, duration, and onset of panic episodes

- Possible precipitants, (e.g., settings in which attacks occur), situations (e.g., being alone outdoors [agoraphobia]), relationship to food or hunger

- Current medications, herbal products, and supplements; recent medication changes

- Multiple visits to health care providers with complaints suggesting panic attacks

- Family history of mood and psychiatric illnesses, particularly anxiety and panic

- Use of recreational drugs (especially stimulants such as cocaine or amphetamines), alcohol (current and recent), and caffeine

- Sleep disturbances

- Concomitant illnesses (e.g., endocrine, cardiac, pulmonary)

- Any associated or concurrent symptoms that could suggest a medical etiology

- Screen for depression (see chapter *Depression*)

O: Objective

Measure vital signs, with particular attention to heart rate (tachycardia) and respiratory rate (shortness of breath, hyperventilation). Perform a complete physical examination, including thyroid, cardiac, pulmonary, and neurologic evaluation.

During actual panic attacks, patients may have increases in heart rate, respiratory rate, or systolic blood pressure.

A: Assessment

A differential diagnosis may include the following conditions:

- Congestive heart failure, myocardial ischemia, arrhythmias

- Hyperthyroidism

- Intoxication with or withdrawal from psychoactive substances (e.g., amphetamines, cocaine, hallucinogens, caffeine, medications)

- Hypoglycemia

- Hypoxia

- Hyperparathyroidism

- Medication side effects

- Pheochromocytoma

- Adrenal disorders, Cushing syndrome, electrolyte abnormalities

- Respiratory infection

- Seizure disorder

- Vestibular dysfunction

- Allergic reactions

- Posttraumatic stress disorder

- Social phobia or specific phobia (specific phobia is a response to a specific stimulus, whereas a patient with panic attacks is unsure when they will recur and what will trigger them)

- Obsessive compulsive disorder

- Separation anxiety disorder

P: Plan

Diagnostic Evaluation

Perform the following tests:

- Electrolytes, blood glucose

- Thyroid function tests (thyroid stimulating hormone [TSH], T4)

- Arterial blood gases if the patient has persistent shortness of breath

- Electrocardiogram if chest pain or other cardiac symptoms are present

- Other tests as indicated by symptoms and physical examination

Treatment

Once other diagnoses have been ruled out, consider the following treatments:

Psychotherapy

Options include cognitive-behavioral therapy, interpersonal therapy, exposure therapy, a stress-management group, relaxation therapy, visualization, guided imagery, supportive psychotherapy, and psychodynamic psychotherapy. Long-term psychotherapy may be indicated if experienced professionals are available and the patient is capable of forming an ongoing relationship. If possible, refer to an HIV-experienced therapist. The type of psychotherapy selected often will depend on the skills and training of the practitioners available in a given health care system or region. In addition, refer the patient to available community-based support. Emergency referrals may be needed for the most anxious patients and those with comorbid depression.

Pharmacotherapy

Patients with advanced HIV disease, like geriatric patients, may be more vulnerable to the central nervous system (CNS) effects of certain medications. Medications that affect the CNS should be started at low dosage and titrated slowly. Similar precautions should apply to patients with liver dysfunction.

Options

Five medications have an approved indication by the U.S. Food and Drug Administration (FDA) for panic disorder. These are the serotonin reuptake inhibitors (SSRIs) and benzodiazepines listed below. For most patients, SSRIs are preferable to benzodiazepines for the treatment of panic disorder because they do not have the potential for addiction and they do not pose the same level of risk if drug interactions cause an elevation of their levels. Other medications used to treat anxiety disorders, such as serotonin/norepinephrine reuptake inhibitor (SNRI) may be considered, and some of them are less likely to interact with ARV medications. See chapter *Anxiety* for descriptions of these medications.

SSRI antidepressants approved for panic disorder include the following:

- Fluoxetine (Prozac), recommended dosage 20 mg PO once daily (usual starting dosage 10 mg daily)

- Paroxetine (Paxil), recommended dosage 40 mg PO once daily (usual starting dosage 10 mg daily)

- Sertraline (Zoloft), recommended dosage 50-200 mg PO once daily (usual starting dosage 25 mg daily)

Benzodiazepines approved for panic disorder include the following:

- Clonazepam (Klonopin), recommended dosage 0.5-2 mg PO BID

- Alprazolam (Xanax), recommended dosage 0.5-3 mg PO TID or Xanax XR at a recommended dosage of 3-6 mg PO once daily. Start at low dosage, may increase every 3-4 days in increments of ≤1 mg/day if tolerated.

Potential ARV Interactions

Interactions may occur between certain ARVs and agents used to treat panic. Some combinations may be contraindicated and others may require dosage adjustment. Refer to medication interaction resources or consult with an HIV expert or pharmacist before prescribing.

Some ARV medications (particularly protease inhibitors [PIs]) may affect the metabolism of some SSRIs via cytochrome P450 interactions. These generally are not clinically significant, but SSRIs used concomitantly with PIs should be started at low dosages and titrated cautiously to prevent antidepressant adverse effects and toxicity. On the other hand, some PIs may decrease levels of paroxetine and sertraline, and efavirenz also lowers sertraline levels; these antidepressants may require upward titration if used concurrently with interacting ARVs.

PIs can significantly elevate the levels of clonazepam and alprazolam, resulting in the potential for severe sedation or respiratory depression. For patients receiving clonazepam or alprazolam, it is recommended that these medications be used at the lowest dosages for the shortest duration possible.

Patient Education

- Inform patients that behavioral interventions can help to reduce the frequency and severity of panic attacks.

- Some antidepressants and antianxiety medications can prevent or reduce the severity of panic attacks.

- Advise patients that they may develop problems with sexual function because of the medications. Patients should report any problems to their prescribers. (Note: Providers should let the patient know that sexual well-being is fundamental to quality of life and can be talked about and addressed in the clinical setting.)

References

- American Psychiatric Association. *Diagnostic and Statistical Manual of Mental Disorders.* Washington: American Psychiatric Association; 1994.

- New York State Department of Health AIDS Institute. *Mental Health Care for People with HIV Infection: Clinical Guidelines for the Primary Care Practitioner.* Available at www.hivguidelines.org/. Accessed June 30, 2010.

- U.S. Department of Health and Human Services. *Guidelines for the Use of Antiretroviral Agents in HIV-1-Infected Adults and Adolescents.* January 10, 2011. Available at www.aidsinfo.nih.gov/guidelines/.

- Wainberg ML, Faragon J, Cournos F, et al. *Psychiatric Medications and HIV Antiretrovirals: A Guide to Interactions for Clinicians, 2nd Edition.* Laminated booklet produced by the New York/New Jersey AIDS Education & Training Center, U.S. Health Resources and Services Administration; 2008.

Posttraumatic Stress Disorder

Francine Cournos, MD; Milton Wainberg, MD

Background

Symptoms of posttraumatic stress disorder (PTSD) can develop after exposure to a traumatic event. A traumatic event may be a single instance, such as a car accident or experience of a natural disaster, or an ongoing pattern of events, such as continuous neglect, physical or sexual abuse, or chronic exposure to war or violent conflict. PTSD causes intrusive memories, hyperarousal, and psychological numbing or avoidance, among other symptoms. It may impair an individual's psychological and physical functioning, decreasing immune system function and increasing susceptibility to illness. Untreated PTSD can increase the risk of HIV transmission or acquisition and worsen the course of HIV treatment.

Individuals with PTSD may experience depression, anxiety, social isolation, impairments in trust and attachments, and feelings of anger, and PTSD often coexists with depression, anxiety, or other psychiatric illnesses. PTSD may be associated with increased risk-taking behavior (e.g., substance abuse, unsafe sex).

The rate of PTSD among individuals with HIV infection (in whom the lifetime prevalence is possibly as high as 42%) is higher than that of the general population (1.3%-7.8%). Women experience PTSD at a higher rate than men. The likelihood of developing PTSD increases in relation to the severity of or proximity to the traumatic event. A history of traumatic experiences may increase an individual's risk of developing PTSD after a new trauma. Although a diagnosis of HIV may trigger PTSD symptoms, a history of trauma or abuse often is present as well. A personal or family psychiatric history may increase the likelihood of developing PTSD.

PTSD is diagnosed, as in HIV-uninfected individuals, according to the criteria of the *Diagnostic and Statistical Manual of Mental Disorders* (DSM)-IV (see "References," below). It is treatable through diverse therapies and psychopharmacology.

S: Subjective

The following reflect DSM-IV diagnostic criteria; include them in the history.

- The person experienced, witnessed, or was confronted with an event or events that involved actual or threatened death, serious injury, or a threat to the physical integrity of self or others.

- The person's response involved intense fear, helplessness, or horror.

- The patient complains of persistently reexperiencing the event in one or more of the following ways:

  - Recurrent and intrusive distressing recollections of the event, including images, thoughts or perceptions

  - Recurring distressing dreams of the event

  - Acting or feeling as if the traumatic event were recurring (includes a sense of reliving the experience, illusions, hallucinations and dissociative flashback episodes, including those that occur when awakening or intoxicated)

  - Intense psychological distress at exposure to internal or external cues that symbolize or resemble an aspect of the traumatic event

  - Physiological reactivity on exposure to internal or external cues that symbolize or resemble an aspect of the traumatic event

Other complaints may include the following:

- Overwhelming emotions caused by memories of the event
- Emotional numbness
- Disruptions in consciousness, memory, or identity
- Depersonalization (i.e., a feeling of watching oneself act, while having no control over a situation)
- Derealization (i.e., alteration in the perception or experience of the external world so that it seems strange or unreal)
- Feelings of estrangement from others
- Episodes of lost time

The patient may experience the following:

- Recurrent distressing recollections of the event
- Recurrent distressing dreams of the event
- Illusions/hallucinations of the event actually occurring
- Psychological distress triggered by cues reminiscent of the event
- Avoidance of thoughts, feelings, or conversation associated with the event
- Avoidance of activities, places, or people associated with the event
- Inability to recall important aspects of the event
- Diminished interest in significant activities
- Detachment
- Restricted range of affect
- Difficulty falling or staying asleep
- Irritability or outbursts of anger
- Difficulty concentrating
- Hypervigilance

Also screen for the following:

- Clinical depression
- Anxiety disorders
- Alcohol or other substance-use disorders

O: Objective

- Check vital signs, with particular attention to heart rate (tachycardia) and respiratory rate (shortness of breath, hyperventilation).
- Perform a physical examination, including mental status and neurologic examination (tremor, hyperreflexia, focal abnormalities).
- Look for signs of physical trauma or sexual assault.

A: Assessment

A differential diagnosis may include the following:

- Substance use (e.g., amphetamines, cocaine)
- Substance withdrawal (e.g., alcohol, benzodiazepines)
- Electrolyte imbalances
- Excessive caffeine intake
- Hyperthyroidism
- Medications effects (e.g., efavirenz, isoniazid, steroids, theophylline)
- Allergic reactions
- Head trauma
- Hypoglycemia
- Sleep disturbances or sleep deprivation
- Central nervous system (CNS) or opportunistic infections or malignancies
- Systemic or other infections
- Respiratory disease
- Heart disease, arrhythmias
- Anemia
- Vitamin B12 deficiency

P: Plan

Evaluation

Perform the following tests:

- Complete blood count, electrolytes, creatinine, blood urea nitrogen, glucose
- Thyroid function tests (thyroid stimulating hormone [TSH], T4)
- Vitamin B12 levels
- Other tests as suggested by history and physical examination

Treatment

Once other diagnoses have been ruled out and the diagnosis of PTSD is established, several treatment options are available.

Psychotherapy

Options include individual cognitive-behavioral therapy, dialectical-behavioral therapy, interpersonal therapy, exposure therapy, a stress-management group, relaxation therapy, visualization, guided imagery, supportive psychotherapy, and psychodynamic psychotherapy. Long-term psychotherapy may be indicated if experienced professionals are available and the patient is capable of forming an ongoing relationship. If possible, refer to an HIV-experienced therapist. The specific psychotherapy often depends on the skills and training of the practitioners available in a given health care system or region. In addition, refer the patient to available community-based support.

Pharmacotherapy

Antidepressants

Most antidepressants should be started at low dosages and gradually titrated upward to avoid unpleasant side effects. Therapeutic effects may not be noticed until 2-4 weeks after starting a medication. If there is no improvement in symptoms in 2-4 weeks, and there are no significant adverse effects, the dosage may be increased. Before prescribing a medication, always remember to check for drug-drug interactions, particularly with concurrent antiretrovirals (ARVs). See "Potential ARV Interactions," below, and chapter *Depression* for further information about antidepressants, including possible adverse effects and interactions with ARVs.

- **Selective serotonin reuptake inhibitors (SSRIs)** have the strongest evidence for efficacy and tolerability for PTSD and are first-line medication treatment. Two SSRI antidepressants have a specific indication for PTSD approved by the U.S. Food and Drug Administration (FDA): sertraline (Zoloft) at recommended dosages of 50-200 mg per day (usual starting dosage: 25 mg daily) and paroxetine (Paxil) at recommended dosages of 20-50 mg per day (usual starting dosage: 25 mg daily). Other SSRIs include fluoxetine (Prozac), citalopram (Celexa), and escitalopram (Lexapro).

- The **serotonin-norepinephrine reuptake inhibitor (SNRI)** antidepressants such as venlafaxine (Effexor) and duloxetine (Cymbalta), as well as the antidepressant mirtazapine (Remeron), are second-line treatments if SSRIs prove ineffective or are not well tolerated.

- **Tricyclic antidepressants (TCAs)** may be employed if the individual has had a good response to them in the past and they do not cause severe side effects, or if the individual has failed to respond to or cannot tolerate SSRIs or SNRIs. TCAs in low dosages also may be used for sleep; see chapter *Insomnia*.

Anxiolytics

Antianxiety medications have not been shown to be effective treatments for PTSD when used alone but may be effective, as adjunctive therapy, in reducing anxiety symptoms. Treatment may include intermediate half-life benzodiazepines such as oxazepam (Serax)

10 mg PO Q6H or lorazepam (Ativan) 0.5 mg PO Q8H. Longer-acting benzodiazepines such as clonazepam (Klonopin) may be useful at dosages of 0.25-0.5 mg PO BID. Levels of many benzodiazepines may be increased by certain protease inhibitors and nonnucleoside reverse transcriptase inhibitors; see "Potential ARV Interactions," below.

Benzodiazepines can reduce anxiety rapidly, often within hours, but may have counterbalancing side effects early in the course of their use that include sedation and incoordination. In addition, physical dependency may develop in patients who use them for more than a few weeks. Benzodiazepines are not recommended for people who have a history of alcohol abuse or dependence. Benzodiazepines ideally would be used only briefly and intermittently to quell acute and severe anxiety symptoms.

Buspirone (BuSpar) is a nonaddictive anxiolytic. It usually must be taken for at least 1-2 weeks before anxiety symptoms begin to lessen. Starting dosage is 5 mg PO TID. If symptoms persist, the dosage can be increased by 5 mg per dose each week to a maximum of 10-15 mg PO TID (for a total daily dosage of 30-45 mg). Low-dose benzodiazepines may be used during the initial weeks of buspirone therapy, until the effects of buspirone are felt. The major potential adverse effects of buspirone are dizziness and lightheadedness.

Anticonvulsants

Mood stabilizers such as valproate (Depakote), carbamazepine (Tegretol), lamotrigine (Lamictal), and topiramate (Topamax) may be added for patients with a partial response to an antidepressant. They may be particularly helpful for those who have considerable irritability, anger, or hostility, as well as those with reexperiencing symptoms (e.g., flashbacks, intrusive memories). Gabapentin (Neurontin) 200-400 mg BID or QID sometimes helps to diminish anxiety.

Treatment with these agents usually should be done by or in consultation with a psychiatrist.

Antipsychotics

Older and newer antipsychotics (aripiprazole, olanzapine, paliperidone, quetiapine, risperidone, and ziprasidone) may be suitable for individuals with psychotic features of PTSD or those who have a comorbid psychotic illness. These medications also may be helpful for some individuals who have not benefited from medications indicated for PTSD. Adverse effects may include dyslipidemia, hyperglycemia, weight gain, and sudden cardiac death. Consultation with a psychiatrist is recommended.

Other medications

A variety of other medications have been used as adjunctive treatment when insomnia and nightmares persist despite adequate use of psychotropic medications. Research is still quite limited, but suggests that the antihypertensive drugs clonidine (Catapres) and prazosin (Minipress) may help with the insomnia and nightmares of PTSD.

Patients with advanced HIV disease, as with geriatric patients, may be particularly vulnerable to the CNS effects of certain medications. Medications that affect the CNS should be started at low dosage and titrated slowly. Similar precautions should apply to patients with liver dysfunction.

Potential ARV Interactions

Interactions may occur between certain antiretrovirals and agents used to treat PTSD. Some combinations may be contraindicated and others may require dosage adjustment. Refer to medication interaction resources or consult with an HIV expert or pharmacist before prescribing.

Antidepressants

- Levels of many SSRIs and SNRIs may be increased or decreased by certain PIs or NNRTIs. These interactions generally are not clinically significant, but most agents should be started at low dosages and titrated cautiously while monitoring efficacy and adverse effects. See chapter *Depression*.

- Tricyclic levels can be increased substantially by ritonavir. If they are used for patients taking ritonavir or ritonavir-boosted PIs, they should be started at low dosage, patients should be followed closely, and tricyclic levels should be monitored.

Anxiolytics

- Protease inhibitors (PIs) and nonnucleoside reverse transcriptase inhibitors may raise blood concentrations of many benzodiazepines. If benzodiazepines are used, they should be started at low dosage, and other CNS depressants should be avoided. Consult with a clinical pharmacist before prescribing. See chapters *Anxiety* and *Insomnia* for additional information.

  - Midazolam (Versed) and triazolam (Halcion) are contraindicated for use with all PIs and with delavirdine and efavirenz.

- Buspirone levels may be increased by ritonavir-boosted PIs and may be decreased by CYP inducers. Monitor patients for adverse effects and for efficacy

Anticonvulsants

- Most anticonvulsants may have significant interactions with certain ARVs and other medications; check for drug-drug interactions before prescribing

Antipsychotics

- Potential interactions vary according to the specific medications used; consult with a pharmacist or psychiatrist.

Patient Education

- Explain to patients that illness (physical or emotional) is not a character flaw or a moral or spiritual weakness.

- Inform patients that both behavioral interventions and medication can be very helpful in treating PTSD. If one strategy is not successful, many others are available.

- Advise patients that psychiatric medications are often given for a long time, usually for a year or longer.

- Advise patients that, when they start taking an antidepressant medication for PTSD, they should expect that it will take 2-4 weeks for them to notice any improvement. Their symptoms should continue to decrease over the following weeks. If they do not have much improvement in symptoms, providers may choose to adjust the dosage of the medication or to change medications. Patients must continue taking their medications so that symptoms do not return.

- Advise patients that they may develop problems with sexual function because of psychiatric medications. They should report any problems to their prescribers.

References

- American Psychiatric Association. *Diagnostic and Statistical Manual of Mental Disorders.* Washington: American Psychiatric Association; 1994.

- Cohen M, Hoffman RG, Cromwell C, et al. *The prevalence of distress in persons with human immunodeficiency virus infection.* Psychosomatics. 2002 Jan-Feb;43(1):10-5.

- Essock SM, Dowden S, Constantine NT, et al.; Five-Site Health and Risk Study Research Committee. *Risk factors for HIV, hepatitis B, hepatitis C among persons with severe mental illness.* Psychiatr Serv. 2003 Jun;54(6):836-41.

- McNicholl I. HIV *InSite Database of Antiretroviral Drug Interactions.* San Francisco: UCSF Center for HIV Information. Available at hivinsite.ucsf.edu/insite?page=ar-00-02. Accessed June 30, 2010.

- New York State Department of Health AIDS Institute. *Mental Health Care for People with HIV Infection: Clinical Guidelines for the Primary Care Practitioner.* Available at www.hivguidelines.org. Accessed June 30, 2010.

- New York State Department of Health AIDS Institute. *Trauma and Post-Traumatic Stress Disorder in Patients with HIV/AIDS;* 2007. Available at www.hivguidelines.org. Accessed June 30, 2010.

- van Liempt S, Vermetten E, Geuze E, et al. *Pharmacotherapeutic treatment of nightmares and insomnia in posttraumatic stress disorder: an overview of the literature.* Ann N Y Acad Sci. 2006 Jul;1071:502-7.

Insomnia

Background

Insomnia is a common accompaniment to HIV infection, especially as the disease progresses and complications worsen. Once present, insomnia tends to be chronic, unlike the transient disturbances of sleep that are a normal part of life. Most insomnia related to HIV can be characterized by the amount, quality, or timing of sleep. Insomnia may cause progressive fatigue and diminished functioning.

S: Subjective

The patient may complain of the following:

- Difficulty initiating sleep
- Early-morning awakening
- Mind-racing thoughts (e.g., "I can't turn off my thoughts.")
- Difficulty maintaining sleep
- Nonrestorative sleep (i.e., although the amount of sleep is adequate, the patient does not feel rested upon awakening)
- Nighttime restlessness

Ask about the symptoms above, and about the following:

- Determine the patient's bedtime sleep habits; request additional history from a sleep partner, if possible.
- Try to quantify how long the patient actually sleeps each night.
- Ask about the following:
  - Alcohol and recreational drug use
  - Caffeine intake (quantity, times of day)
  - Nightmares, life stressors
  - Concurrent medications that may cause insomnia as an adverse effect (e.g., efavirenz, corticosteroids, pseudoephedrine, and decongestants)
  - Medications (prescription or over-the-counter) or supplements used to promote sleep

- Shift work, exercise, nighttime reflux or heartburn, snoring, and periods of apnea (not breathing)
- Collar size (size >16 more often associated with sleep apnea)
- Screen for depression and anxiety.

O: Objective

Perform a general symptom-directed physical examination, including evaluation of body habitus, neurologic status, and mental status.

A: Assessment

A partial differential diagnosis includes the following:

- Alcohol intake (interferes with sleep 2-4 hours after ingestion, may cause nocturnal awakening)
- Caffeine intake
- Recreational drug use
- Anxiety disorder
- Major depression (insomnia is a primary symptom)
- Transient insomnia related to acute stress
- Cognitive impairment
- Disturbance of the sleep/wake cycle because of excessive time in bed or inadequate sleep hygiene (e.g., noise in the bedroom)
- Medication adverse effects (e.g., from steroids, efavirenz)

- Other identifiable sleep disorders (e.g., obstructive sleep apnea, periodic leg movements)

Pain

Underlying systemic medical conditions that can interfere with sleep, such as delirium, lung disease, congestive heart failure, renal failure, diarrhea, and incontinence

P: Plan

Evaluation

The diagnosis usually is based on history. A sleep evaluation (including polysomnography) may be indicated when a physiologic cause (e.g., obstructive sleep apnea) is suspected or insomnia is severe.

Treatment

Treat underlying illnesses that may be causing or contributing to insomnia.

- Manage correctible medical conditions that may interfere with sleep.

- Treat depression and anxiety disorders. These are very common contributors to insomnia among people with HIV infection. See chapters *Depression, Anxiety,* and *Panic Disorder.*

- If the patient is suspected of having sleep apnea, periodic limb movements in sleep, or restless limb syndrome, refer to a specialist in sleep medicine for evaluation.

The following options are available for treatment:

Behavioral strategies

- To correct deleterious sleep habits, patients should do the following:

  - Establish a bedtime routine.

  - Avoid stimuli before bedtime.

  - Avoid vigorous exercise within 3-4 hours of bedtime.

  - Reduce or eliminate daytime napping.

  - Avoid eating, reading, watching TV, or working in bed.

  - Wake up at the same time each day regardless of total hours of sleep.

  - Have a dark, cool, quiet, comfortable environment conducive to sleep.

  - Place the bedroom clock out of sight.

- If unable to fall sleep after 15-20 minutes, the patient should get up, go into another room for nonstimulating activity in dim light (such as reading), and not go back to bed until sleepy.

- The patient should discontinue use of caffeine, central nervous system stimulants, alcohol, and tobacco, with tapering if necessary, to avoid withdrawal symptoms.

- Teach or refer the patient for relaxation techniques.

Pharmacotherapy

Choosing a pharmacologic agent for insomnia

A number of medications may be effective in treating insomnia. In selecting a medication for an individual patient, consider the following about a specific medication:

- Is it likely to improve symptoms that may be contributing to the patient's insomnia (e.g., depression, anxiety, psychosis, neuropathic pain)?

- Does it pose risks to the patient based on comorbid medical conditions (e.g., benzodiazepines should not be given to patients with sleep apnea, tricyclic antidepressants should not be given to patients with cardiac conduction problems)?

- Does it have adverse interactions with other medications, (e.g., zolpidem [Ambien], zaleplon [Sonata], and eszopiclone [Lunesta] should be used with caution in patients taking protease inhibitors [PIs])?

- Is it the optimal agent for a patient with a current or past history of alcohol or sedative abuse/dependence?

- Is it affordable (e.g., formulary or co-pay issues)?

Treatment considerations

There are limited data to guide the frequency (nightly, intermittently, as needed) and duration (brief, intermediate, long-term) of hypnotic medications. Hypnotics generally should be prescribed at the lowest effective dosage for the shortest possible period. The greater the degree of physical illness, the more likely the patient will need a low dosage of a hypnotic agent. When long-term treatment is necessary, benzodiazepines pose the greatest risk of tolerance, abuse, and dependence.

Possible adverse effects of all hypnotics include excess sedation, daytime grogginess, and disruption of the sleep architecture (e.g., causing sleepwalking).

Interactions may occur between certain antiretrovirals (ARVs) and agents used to treat insomnia. Some combinations may be contraindicated and others may require dosage adjustment. Refer to medication interaction resources or consult with an HIV expert, psychiatrist, or pharmacist before prescribing.

Agents with FDA-Approved Indications for Insomnia

Antihistamines

- The antihistamines diphenhydramine, doxylamine, and hydroxyzine, given at doses of 25-50 mg QHS, can be used for sleep. Adverse anticholinergic effects often interfere with long-term use.

Antidepressants

- Trazodone, 25 -50 mg; maximum dose: 200 mg QHS.
  - Trazodone, a triazolopyridine derivative antidepressant and sedative, is the only antidepressant with a U.S. Food and Drug Administration (FDA) indication for insomnia, and it is widely used for this purpose. However, levels are increased by ritonavir-boosted PIs. Do not use with saquinavir/ritonavir; use lower dosages for patients receiving other PIs. Trazodone may (rarely) cause priapism. Trazodone can be used for an indefinite period of time as it is not associated with tolerance or addiction.

Non-benzodiazepine hypnotics (agonists of the benzodiazepine receptor)

- Zolpidem (Ambien) 5-10 mg, zolpidem-CR (Ambien-CR) 6.25-12.5 mg, zaleplon (Sonata) 5-10 mg, and eszopiclone (Lunesta) 2-3 mg QHS.
  - These newer hypnotic agents are benzodiazepine receptor agonists with shorter half-lives than benzodiazepines and are not likely to result in day-after drowsiness. They may have decreased addiction potential compared with benzodiazepine hypnotics. Patients should be advised to use these hypnotics on an as-needed basis rather than nightly; it is easier for patients to discontinue a drug that they are not taking every day. The inhibition of CYP 3A4 enzyme activity by PIs may increase levels of these benzodiazepine receptor agonists, particularly eszopiclone; this may cause excessive sedation or respiratory depression.

Melatonin agonists

- Ramelteon (Rozerem), 8 mg QHS.
  - The first of a new class of melatonin agonists to receive FDA approval, ramelteon may have some advantages over sedative/hypnotic agents, such as reduced dependence and overuse. However, it may have severe adverse reactions, including hypersensitivity reactions such as anaphylaxis and angioedema. Long-term interactions with ARV agents are unknown.

Benzodiazepine hypnotics

- A number of benzodiazepines have FDA-approved indications for the short-term treatment of insomnia. They carry a risk of addiction and residual drowsiness the following day.
- Metabolized by glucuronidation; predicted to have few drug interactions with ARVs:
  - Temazepam (Restoril) 7.5-30 mg; intermediate half-life
  - Lorazepam (Ativan), 2-4 mg; intermediate half-life
- Metabolized by CYP 34A; PIs may prolong their duration, resulting in excessive daytime somnolence. These may be most beneficial for use with patients whose insomnia is associated with anxiety:
  - Flurazepam (Dalmane) 15-30 mg
  - Quazepam (Doral) 7.5-15 mg
  - Estazolam (ProSom) 1-2 mg
- Clonazepam (Klonopin) at a dose of 0.5-2 mg has been approved for treatment of periodic leg movements. PIs may prolong its duration and increase risk of adverse effects; start at low dosage and titrate slowly.
- Triazolam (Halcion), another approved agent for insomnia, is contraindicated for use with all PIs and some nonnucleoside reverse transcriptase inhibitors (NNRTIs) (delavirdine, efavirenz) because of potentially life-threatening reactions (e.g., respiratory depression).

Agents Used for Sedating Side Effects (no FDA Indication for Insomnia)

Antidepressants

- Tricyclic antidepressants at doses of 10-50 mg can be beneficial for sleep, but they have longer half-lives than short-acting hypnotic agents, and potential adverse effects include cardiac dysrhythmias and pulmonary complications. Also, levels of tricyclics are elevated by ritonavir and lower dosages may be needed for patients taking ritonavir or ritonavir-boosted PIs. Routine testing of tricyclic blood levels should be performed on patients receiving higher doses (eg, 100 mg per day; 50 mg for nortriptyline), those on concurrently on ritonavir, and those with risk factors for cardiac conduction abnormalities. A routine electrocardiogram should be performed before prescribing tricyclics, and this class of drugs should not be prescribed to patients with cardiac conduction problems. However, tricyclic antidepressants also have characteristics that may benefit some patients, including treatment of chronic pain, promotion of weight gain, and reduction of diarrhea. Amitriptyline (Elavil) and doxepin (Sinequan) are the most sedating of the tricyclic antidepressants and therefore are the drugs in this class most often used for sleep.

- The tetracyclic antidepressant mirtazapine (Remeron) is sedating and has been effective in treating insomnia at low dosages (7.5-15 mg). Higher dosages may result in increased activation owing to increased NE receptor antagonism.

- The selective serotonin reuptake inhibitor (SSRI) antidepressants are not sufficiently sedating to be used as sleeping agents, but when insomnia is caused by depression, sleep will improve as the depression lifts.

Anticonvulsants

- Gabapentin (Neurontin) can be useful for patients with insomnia and has been demonstrated to be particularly beneficial for patients with alcohol and other substance-use disorders; it is widely prescribed for neuropathic pain. Tiagabine (Gabitril) has demonstrated efficacy in adults with insomnia.

Patient Education

- Instruct patients in behavioral interventions that can help to reduce insomnia.

- Additional interventions are available when behavioral interventions are not sufficient.

- Patients should report new or worsening symptoms to their health care provider. These may be not only signs of worsening insomnia, but also symptoms of anxiety, depression, medications, or changes in medical conditions.

References

- Ford DE, Kamerow DB. *Epidemiologic study of sleep disturbances and psychiatric disorders. An opportunity for prevention?* JAMA. 1989 Sep 15;262(11):1479-84.

- Insomnia and HIV: A Biopsychosocial Approach. In: *Comprehensive Textbook of AIDS Psychiatry*; Cohen MA, Gorman JM, eds. New York: Oxford University Press; 2008;163-72.

- Kuppermann M, Lubeck DP, Mazonson PD, et al. *Sleep problems and their correlates in a working population.* J Gen Intern Med. 1995 Jan;10(1):25-32.

- McNicholl I. *HIV InSite Database of Antiretroviral Drug Interactions.* San Francisco: UCSF Center for HIV Information. Available at hivinsite.ucsf.edu/insite?page=ar-00-02. Accessed June 30, 2010.

- Ohayon MM, Roth T. *Place of chronic insomnia in the course of depressive and anxiety disorders.* J Psychiatr Res. 2003 Jan-Feb;37(1):9-15.

- Reid S, Dwyer J. *Insomnia and HIV infection: a systematic review of prevalence, correlates, and management.* Psychosom Med. 2005 Mar-Apr;67(2):260-9.

- Schutte-Rodin S, Broch L, Buysse D, et al. *Clinical guideline for the evaluation and management of chronic insomnia in adults.* J Clin Sleep Med. 2008 Oct 15;4(5):487-504.

- Sleep and Sleep-Wake Disorders. In: *Psychiatry, 3rd Edition*, Vol. 2008; Tasman A Kay J, Lieberman JA, et al., eds. London: J. Wiley & Sons, 2008:1626-57.

- Sleep and Wakefulness Disorders. In: *The Merck Manual of Diagnosis and Therapy, 18th ed.*; Beers MH, Porter RS, Jones TV, eds. Whitehouse Station, NJ: Merck & Co.; 2006:1834-40.

- Wainberg ML, Faragon J, Cournos F, et al. *Psychiatric Medications and HIV Antiretrovirals: A Guide to Interactions for Clinicians, 2nd ed.* Laminated booklet produced by the New York/New Jersey AIDS Education and Training Center, Health Resources and Services Administration; 2008.

Oral Health

Background

Examination of the oral cavity should be included in both the initial and interim physical examination of all HIV-infected patients. Patients with lesions suspected to be oral manifestations of HIV disease should be referred to a dental health expert with experience in treating oral lesions associated with HIV/AIDS. Other oral lesions may be a sign of a systemic disease, a side effect of medications, or a result of poor oral hygiene.

The following is an overview of conditions commonly seen in patients with HIV infection. See chapters *Oral Hairy Leukoplakia, Oral Warts, Oral Ulceration,* and *Necrotizing Ulcerative Periodontitis and Gingivitis* for more information about those conditions.

HRSA HAB Core Clinical Performance Measures

Percentage of clients with HIV infection who received an **oral examination by a dentist** at least once during the measurement year

(Group 2 measure)

Xerostomia (Dry Mouth)

S: Subjective

The chief complaint may be a dry, "sticky," or possibly a burning sensation in the mouth, or an inability to "taste" food. The patient may present with difficulty swallowing.

O: Objective

The oral mucosal tissues appear dry and sometimes "shiny" in appearance. The lips may be dry and cracked, and the tongue is dry. Dental decay may be present on the cervical portion of the teeth (near the gingival margin or "gumline"). Oral candidiasis (thrush) may or may not be present.

A: Assessment

The differential diagnosis for the cause of xerostomia includes medication side effects (e.g., from anticholinergics), systemic diseases (e.g., Sjögren syndrome), adverse effects of radiation therapy, and salivary gland diseases.

P: Plan

Identify the cause of xerostomia and modify, if possible. Treat with artificial saliva products or oral lubricant products (e.g., Salivart, Biotene Oral Balance Dry Mouth Relief Moisturizing Gel, or TheraSpray). Discourage sucking on hard candies with sugar that can promote caries (dental decay); encourage patients to use sugar-free gums and candies to help promote salivary function. Promote good oral hygiene with flossing and brushing with a fluoride toothpaste, and encourage regular (every 3-4 months) dental recall visits. Severe cases of xerostomia may be treated by prescribing cholinergic stimulants such as pilocarpine (Salagen).

Burning Mouth Syndrome; Atrophic Glossitis

S: Subjective

The patient may complain of a constant burning sensation in the mouth or a numbness or tingling feeling of the tongue. Eating certain foods or spices may trigger the burning sensation. The patient also may complain of dry mouth or a metallic taste in the mouth.

O: Objective

The tongue and oral mucosal tissues may be normal in appearance or there may be a slight redness on the tip and lateral margins of the tongue. In other cases, the tongue may appear "bald," owing to the loss of papillae on the dorsal surface, and it may be "beef red" in color.

A: Assessment

Possible systemic etiologies include nutritional and vitamin deficiencies (atrophic glossitis), chronic alcoholism, medication adverse effects, diabetes mellitus, and gastric reflux. Local etiologies include denture irritation, oral habits such as tongue or cheek biting, and excessive use of certain toothpastes or mouthwashes. Psychological factors and nerve damage also may cause burning mouth. Erythematous candidiasis also can present as a burning sensation.

P: Plan

Identify the cause of the burning sensation, if possible, by review of the medical history and by performing diagnostic tests as indicated (e.g., complete blood count, biopsy, or oral cytological smears). Once the underlying cause is identified, treatment may be as simple as changing a dentifrice or eliminating the identified irritant, or the condition may require systemic treatment.

Recurrent Aphthous Ulceration (RAU)

S: Subjective

The patient complains of a painful ulcer or ulcers in the mouth that recur.

O: Objective

The typical appearance of an aphthous ulcer is a "red raised border with a depressed, necrotic (white-to-yellow pseudomembrane) center." Aphthous ulcers tend to present on nonkeratinized or nonfixed tissues such as the buccal mucosa or posterior oropharynx and may be small or large, solitary or in clusters, and can resemble intraoral herpetic lesions (although herpetic lesions tend to present on keratinized tissues such as the roof of the mouth and gingival tissues).

A: Assessment

The differential diagnosis includes traumatic ulcers and herpes simplex virus ulcers.

P: Plan

The diagnosis usually is based on appearance. For further information, see chapter *Oral Ulceration*.

Recurrent Herpes Simplex

S: Subjective

The patient complains of a locally painful ulcer or ulcers on the lips or intraoral areas.

O: Objective

Herpes lesions are located on the lips, gingival tissues, or the hard palate. They may appear as small vesicular lesions that rupture, forming small ulcers. They may rupture and coalesce into larger lesions.

A: Assessment

The differential diagnosis includes aphthous ulcer and traumatic ulcer.

P: Plan

The diagnosis usually is based on appearance. For further information, see chapters *Oral Ulceration* and *Herpes Simplex, Mucocutaneous*.

Periodontal Disease

The medical evaluation of patients with HIV infection should include assessment of periodontal health. Whereas the same type of plaque-induced periodontal diseases can be seen in both immunocompetent and immunosuppressed individuals, periodontal disease in HIV-infected patients can be a marker of HIV disease progression. In the HIV-infected patient with periodontal disease, it is important to distinguish whether the periodontitis represents an aggressive or chronic presentation unique to those with HIV disease. In addition, it is important to determine whether the patient has an inflammatory oral disease process that may further compromise his or her health.

Various illnesses and systemic factors (e.g., diabetes mellitus, hormonal abnormalities, medications, and malnutrition) can complicate the clinical presentation of periodontal disease. If significant periodontal disease is suspected, refer to an experienced dentist for diagnosis and treatment. Gingivitis, a milder form of periodontal disease, usually is reversible with proper professional and home oral health care. For further information on necrotizing ulcerative periodontitis or necrotizing ulcerative gingivitis, see chapter *Necrotizing Ulcerative Periodontitis and Gingivitis.*

S: Subjective

The patient may complain of red, swollen, or painful gums, which may bleed spontaneously or with brushing; chronic bad breath or bad taste in the mouth; loose teeth or teeth that are separating; or a "bite" that feels abnormal.

O: Objective

Examine the gingival tissues. Periodontitis appears as localized or generalized gingival inflammation. The gingivae appear bright red or reddish-purple, ulcerated, or necrotic. Spontaneous gingival hemorrhage and purulent discharge may be evident around the teeth, especially if pressure is applied to the gingivae. Fetor oris may be present.

A: Assessment

The differential diagnosis includes gingivitis, periodontitis, trench mouth, and oral abscesses. Diagnosis usually is based on appearance. Patients with severe or recalcitrant disease should be referred to a dental care provider for definitive diagnosis and treatment.

P: Plan

Treatment may include:

- Warm saline rinses
- Daily brushing and flossing
- Antimicrobial mouth rinse (e.g., Listerine, chlorhexidine)
- Antibiotic therapy

For further information, see chapter *Necrotizing Ulcerative Periodontitis and Gingivitis.*

Dental Caries Caused by Methamphetamine and Cocaine Use

Dental decay seen in individuals who smoke methamphetamine or crack cocaine, or use cocaine orally, often is referred to as "meth mouth."

S: Subjective

The chief complaint may be pain in one or more teeth. However, if the condition is chronic, the patient may not complain of pain.

O: Objective

In meth mouth, the enamel on all teeth or multiple teeth is grayish-brown to black in color (owing to decay), and appears "soft" (this has been described as a "texture less like that of hard enamel and more like that of a piece of ripened fruit"). Oral mucosal tissues appear dry as a result of decreased salivary flow. The gingiva appears red or inflamed, and there may be spontaneous bleeding of the gingiva around the teeth.

Another pattern of dental decay can be seen in cocaine users who rub the drug along the gingiva in order to test its strength or purity. This can lead to localized dryness of the gingival tissues. Consequently, plaque sticks to the cervical portion of the teeth in the area where the cocaine is rubbed, resulting in dental caries along the cervical portion of the teeth.

A: Assessment

The differential diagnosis includes other causes of caries.

P: Plan

Refer to a dentist for appropriate care, which may involve restorative, endodontic therapy, periodontal care, and oral surgery. In severe cases, extraction of the involved teeth and replacement with a partial or complete denture may be necessary. Encourage proper oral hygiene; evaluate sucrose intake.

Oral Cancer

S: Subjective

Oral malignancies may be symptomatic or asymptomatic. Data suggest two distinct pathways for the development of oropharyngeal cancer: one driven predominantly by the carcinogenic effects of tobacco or alcohol (or both), another by genomic instability induced by human papillomavirus.

The patient may complain of a mouth sore that fails to heal or that bleeds easily, or a persistent white or red (or mixed) patch. The patient may note a lump, thickening, or soreness in the mouth, throat, or tongue; difficulty chewing or swallowing food; difficulty moving the jaw or tongue; chronic hoarseness; numbness of the tongue or other areas of the mouth; or a swelling of the jaw, causing dentures to fit poorly or become uncomfortable.

O: Objective

Perform a thorough evaluation of the oropharynx, as well as lymph nodes in the head and neck. Suspicious lesions may occur on the lips, tongue, floor of the mouth, palate, gingiva, or oral mucosa, and may appear as an ulcer or a soft-tissue mass or masses that can be pink, reddish, purple, white, or mixed red and white. The lesion typically is indurated and

may be painful. It may enlarge rapidly between examinations.

A: Assessment

The differential diagnosis includes oral squamous cell carcinoma, lymphoma, Kaposi sarcoma, traumatic ulcer, hyperplasia, and hyperkeratosis.

P: Plan

An ulcerated lesion or symptom described above that is present for 2 weeks or longer should be evaluated promptly by a dentist or physician. If cancer is suspected, a biopsy should be obtained to make a definitive diagnosis. Treatment will be based on the specific diagnosis.

Bruxism

S: Subjective

The patient may complain of chronic facial or jaw pain, sensitive teeth, earache, or waking up with a headache or facial pain. Often, the patient is not aware that he or she is clenching or grinding the teeth. Bruxism very often is a result of increased stress or anxiety, causing the patient consciously or unconsciously to clench or grind the teeth. However, some people may be "nighttime bruxers" and grind their teeth while sleeping, often loudly enough to wake others sleeping in the same room.

O: Objective

Perform a focused evaluation of the oropharynx, jaw, and facial muscles. The teeth may appear shortened, flattened, or worn down as a result of chronic grinding or clenching of the teeth. There may be hyperkeratotic lesions on the inside of cheeks as a result of chronic grinding or biting. There may be tenderness with palpation of facial muscles.

A: Assessment

The differential diagnosis includes other causes of facial or jaw pain, including caries, dental abscesses, and trauma.

P: Plan

Refer the patient to a dentist for treatment. Treatment may include wearing a bite guard or psychological or behavioral management therapy.

Oral Piercing

S/O/A: Subjective/Objective/Assessment

Jewelry worn in piercings in the tongue, lips, or cheeks can chip or fracture the teeth. Chronic rubbing of jewelry against the gingiva can cause the gingiva to recede, leading to periodontal problems. (These complications occur apart from procedure- or technique-associated complications associated with body piercing, such as inflammation and infection, bleeding, and transmission of bloodborne pathogens.)

P: Plan

Refer the patient to a dentist for treatment. Recommend plastic tongue jewelry as opposed to metal to prevent fracture of teeth. Removal of the jewelry may be warranted.

Maxillary Tori; Mandibular Tori

S: Subjective

The patient may complain of a "lump" in the roof or floor of the mouth, or behind the lower front teeth.

O: Objective

Exostosis of normal bone (covered by oral mucosal tissue) can appear as a nodular or lobulated protuberance centrally located on the hard palate (maxillary tori) or unilaterally or bilaterally located behind the mandibular incisors (mandibular tori). This develops slowly and the patient may become aware of exophytic growth only if the area is inadvertently traumatized.

A: Assessment

Differential diagnosis includes other benign or malignant lesions, including oral cancer.

P: Plan

No treatment is indicated unless the exostosis interferes with speech or swallowing, or removal is needed for fabrication of dentures or a partial denture. Tori are a variation of normal anatomy.

References

- Cherry-Peppers G, Daniels CO, Meeks V, et al. *Oral manifestations in the era of HAART.* J Natl Med Assoc. 2003 Feb;95(2 Suppl 2):21S-32S.

- Davey M. *Grisly effect of one drug: "meth mouth."* New York Times. June 11, 2005. Available online at www.nytimes.com.

- DePaola LG. *The Importance of Oral Health in HIV Disease.* NUMEDIX. 2003; 4(2):68-69.

- Ibsen O, Phelan J. *Oral Pathology for the Dental Hygienist;* 4th ed. Philadelphia: W.B. Saunders; 2004.

- Mayo Foundation for Medical Education and Research. *Canker Sore* (April 15, 2004); *Cold Sore* (April 28, 2004); *Bad Breath* (July 20, 2004); *Bruxism/Teeth Grinding* (May 19, 2005); *Burning Mouth Syndrome* (September 23, 2004); *Trench Mouth* (October 24, 2004); and *Behind Your Smile: What's Your Mouth Made Of?* (February 18, 2005). Available online at www.mayoclinic.com. Accessed June 1, 2010.

- National Institutes of Health, National Institute of Dental and Craniofacial Research. *Dry Mouth.* Bethesda, MD: National Oral Health Information Clearinghouse; June 1999. NIH Publication #99-3174. Available online at www. nidcr.nih.gov/HealthInformation/ DiseasesAndConditions/ DryMouthXerostomia/DryMouth.htm.

- National Institutes of Health, National Institute of Dental and Craniofacial Research. *TMD/TMJ: Temporomandibular Disorders.* Bethesda, MD: National Oral Health Information Clearinghouse; May 2005. NIH Publication #94-3487. Available online at www.nidcr.nih.gov/ HealthInformation/DiseasesAndConditions/ TMDTMJ/default.htm.

- Newland JR, Meiller TF, Wynn R, et al. *Oral Soft Tissue Diseases: A Reference Manual for Diagnosis and Management*; 2nd ed. Hudson, OH: Lexi-Comp; 2002.

- Nittayananta W, ed. *Oral Manifestations of HIV Infection: Current Update with Asian Focus.* Bangkok; 2004. Available online at www.hivdent.org/oralm/ oralmOMHI082004.htm [purchase information].

Oral Ulceration

Background

Oral ulcerations appear as necrotic or eroded areas on the oral mucosa, including the tongue. Most such lesions are idiopathic (aphthous) or of viral etiology (e.g., herpes simplex virus [HSV]; rarely herpes zoster [VZV]). Oral ulcerations may be caused by fungal, parasitic, or bacteriologic pathogens; malignancy; or other systemic processes. This chapter will focus on herpetic and aphthous ulcers.

Herpetic ulcerations tend to appear on keratinized tissues such as the hard palate or gingiva. Recurrent aphthous ulcers tend to manifest on nonkeratinized tissues such as buccal mucosa, soft palate, and lingual (bottom) surface of the tongue, and, by definition, recur.

S: Subjective

The patient complains of painful ulcerated areas in mouth. He or she may have difficulty eating, drinking, swallowing, or opening the mouth, and may complain of sore throat.

Inquire about previous occurrences of oral ulcerative disease as well as ulcerative gastrointestinal diseases, including HSV, cytomegalovirus (CMV), or histoplasmosis. Ask about recent sexual exposures. Inquire about recent trauma or burns. Note current medications and any recent changes in medications; obtain history of tobacco (smoked and chewed) and alcohol use.

O: Objective

Look for red or white-bordered erosions or ulcerations varying in size from 1 mm to 2 cm on the buccal mucosa, oropharynx, tongue, lips, gingiva, and hard or soft palate. Lesions caused by HSV tend to be shallow and occur on keratinized tissues. HSV lesions may appear as clusters of vesicles that may coalesce into ulcerations with scalloped borders. Aphthous ulcers present with a white or gray pseudomembrane surrounded by a halo of inflammation.

A: Assessment

Rule out syphilis and other suspected pathogens as well as trauma, seizure, and other physical injury.

P: Plan

Diagnostic Evaluation

The diagnosis of HSV and aphthous ulcers usually is made on the basis of characteristic lesions. Location, duration, and recurrence are key elements in determining the nature of the oral ulcer. As mentioned previously, HSV-related ulcers most often present on keratinized fixed tissues; aphthous ulcers appear on nonfixed tissues such as buccal mucosa, and have a tendency to recur. Check the absolute neutrophil count (ANC), as a low count (<500 cells/µL) may be associated with nonresponsive ulcerative disease. If diagnosis is uncertain, it is possible to perform HSV culture or HSV antigen detection using direct florescent antibody (DFA) testing on oral ulcerations that appear on keratinized tissues or the dorsal and lateral surfaces of the tongue, scraping near the margin of the lesion or unroofing a fresh vesicle, if available, and scraping the base. The sensitivity of HSV testing decreases when collections are taken from older, resolving herpetic areas; herpetic lesions >72 hours old usually will not yield a positive culture.

If other diagnoses are suspected, perform culture or biopsy as indicated. Also perform biopsy for ulcers that do not respond to therapy (in nonneutropenic patients).

Note that syphilis is very common among some HIV-infected populations. For patients in whom primary syphilis (manifested by an oral chancre) is suspected, perform (or refer for) darkfield examination; check Venereal Disease Research Laboratory (VDRL) or rapid plasma reagin (RPR) results (note that VDRL or RPR results may be negative in primary syphilis); see chapter *Syphilis* for further information. It is worth noting that, whereas chancres are described as painless, open sores in the mouth usually are associated with some degree of pain.

Treatment

If HSV culture is positive, or if HSV is strongly suspected owing to the appearance of the lesions or the patient's history, treat with HSV antiviral medication (e.g., valacyclovir, famciclovir, or acyclovir) while waiting for results of culture. Do not use topical steroids without a concomitant oral HSV antiviral if the lesion is of possible herpetic etiology. Refer to chapter *Herpes Simplex, Mucocutaneous* for more information regarding management and treatment of HSV lesions.

Recalcitrant minor aphthous ulcerations should be treated with topical corticosteroids (e.g., fluocinonide 0.05% or clobetasol 0.05% ointments mixed 1:1 with Orabase). For multiple small lesions or lesions in areas where topical ointments are difficult to apply, consider dexamethasone elixir (0.5 mg/5 mL); the patient is to rinse TID with 5 mL for 1 minute, then expectorate. As with all oral topical steroids, patients should not drink or eat for 30 minutes after rinsing. Continue treatment for 1 week or until lesions resolve.

In some cases, recurrent aphthous ulcers may respond to one of the various "magic mouthwashes" that contain combinations of antibiotic, antifungal, corticosteroid, antihistamine, and anesthetic medication. The inclusion of an antihistamine (e.g., diphenhydramine) or an anesthetic (e.g., lidocaine) may be helpful in treating pain associated with these ulcers.

For large or extensive aphthous ulcers, systemic corticosteroids may be needed: prednisone 40-60 mg PO daily for 1 week followed by a taper should prove beneficial. If this is ineffective, refer for biopsy to rule out CMV, other infection, or neoplastic disease.

For patients with major oral aphthous ulcers that are recalcitrant to other therapies, thalidomide 200 mg daily for 2 weeks may be considered. Thalidomide is teratogenic and should not be used for women of childbearing potential without thorough patient education and two concomitant methods of birth control. Consult with an expert.

Pain control may be needed in order for the patient to maintain food intake and prevent weight loss. Most of the topical treatments noted above will ease pain as well as treat the ulcer. Additional considerations for pain control include the following:

- **Oral anesthetics**: Various products are available, including gels (eg, Gelclair, an adherent oral rinse that acts as an oral bandage), viscous liquids, and sprays (e.g., benzocaine, lidocaine). These may be applied topically or swished and expectorated. They will provide temporary relief, but may lead to a temporary loss of taste sensation.

- **Systemic:** If topical treatments are inadequate, consider systemic analgesics (e.g., nonsteroidal antiinflammatory drugs or opiates). Refer to chapter *Pain Syndrome and Peripheral Neuropathy*.

Assess nutritional status and consider adding liquid food supplements, if indicated. Suggest soft, nonspicy, or salty foods if the ulcer is interfering with food intake. Refer to a registered dietitian if client is experiencing pain, problems eating, or weight loss.

Refer to an oral health specialist or an HIV-experienced dentist as needed.

Patient Education

- Advise patients to report any oral pain or difficulty swallowing to their health care provider.

- Instruct patients in the application of topical ointments, and indicate that they may require assistance if the lesion is difficult for them to see on their own.

- It is important for patients to maintain good nutrition and food intake while their oral ulcers heal. Advise them to eat soft, bland foods, and refer to a nutritionist if they have difficulty.

References

- Greenspan D. *Oral Manifestations of HIV.* In: Coffey S, Volberding PA, eds. *HIV InSite Knowledge Base* [textbook online]; San Francisco: UCSF Center for HIV Information; June 1998. Accessed June 10, 2010.

Oral Warts

Background

Oral warts are caused by human papillomavirus (HPV) and may appear anywhere within the oral cavity or on the lips. They occur more frequently and more extensively in people with HIV infection than in those with normal immune function, especially in patients with advancing immune suppression (CD4 counts of <200-300 cells/μL). Oral warts may be refractory to therapy. The frequency of oral warts may increase, at least temporarily, in patients treated with antiretroviral therapy.

It should be noted that HPV infection is strongly associated with oropharyngeal cancer among subjects with or without the established risk factors of tobacco and alcohol use, although oral warts normally are not caused by the HPV types that are associated with oncogenic changes. One analysis of stored samples suggests that the percentage of all oropharyngeal cancers that are HPV-positive has increased from about 20% to 60% since about 1980. Researchers also have reported that HPV-related oral cancers were among the most responsive to chemotherapy and radiation.

S: Subjective

The patient notices raised lesions in the mouth or on the lips. Warts are not painful unless they have been traumatized.

O: Objective

Examine the oral cavity carefully for abnormalities. Wart lesions may vary in appearance from smooth, small, and slightly raised lesions to cauliflower-like or spiked masses with prominent folds or projections. They may be single or multiple.

Review recent CD4 counts. In patients with oral warts, the CD4 count usually is <300 cells/μL.

A: Assessment

A partial differential diagnosis includes: squamous cell carcinoma, lichen planus, and traumatic hyperkeratinized areas resulting from cheek biting or tongue thrusting.

P: Plan

Diagnostic Evaluation

- The diagnosis of oral warts usually is based on the appearance of the lesions. If lesions are unusual in appearance, are ulcerated, or have grown rapidly, perform biopsy to rule out cancer. If there is suspicion of other causes, perform other diagnostic evaluations as indicated.

- HPV may be demonstrated with electron micropsy or in situ hybridization; this testing is not routinely required.

- Observation of these lesions is important because of the potential, however minimal, for development of squamous cell carcinoma.

Treatment

- Treatment is difficult, as these lesions tend to recur. Treatment options include cryosurgery and surgical or laser excision. Care must be taken when using laser excision, as HPV can survive in an aerosol. Extraoral lesions (lip or corner of mouth) may be treated with topical agents such as podofilox topical solution (Condylox) or fluorouracil 5% topical (Efudex). Imiquimod 5% cream (Aldara) may help to prevent recurrence once the lesions have resolved.

- Refer to an oral health specialist or dentist for treatment.

Patient Education

- Instruct patients to comply with regular dental and medical care regimens.

- Instruct patients to use medications exactly as prescribed.

References

- Greenspan D, Canchola AJ, MacPhail LA, et al. *Effect of highly active antiretroviral therapy on frequency of oral warts.* Lancet. 2001 May 5;357(9266):1411-2.

- King MD, Reznik DA, O'Daniels CM, et al. *Human papillomavirus-associated oral warts among human immunodeficiency virus-seropositive patients in the era of highly active antiretroviral therapy: an emerging infection.* Clin Infect Dis. 2002 Mar 1;34(5):641-8.

Oral Hairy Leukoplakia

Background

Oral hairy leukoplakia (OHL) is an oral infection caused by Epstein-Barr virus (EBV). It appears as white corrugated lesions (sometimes "hairy" in appearance) primarily on the lateral aspects of the tongue. This infection may spread across the entire dorsal surface onto the ventral surface of the tongue, and occasionally may be found on buccal mucosa. It is common in people with HIV infection, particularly in those with advanced immunosuppression (CD4 count <200 cells/μL).

S: Subjective

The patient notices new, white lesions on the tongue that cannot be wiped off or removed by scraping or brushing. The OHL lesions usually are asymptomatic, but occasionally may cause alteration in taste, discomfort, or other symptoms.

O: Objective

Perform a focused examination of the oropharynx. OHL appears as unilateral or bilateral white plaques or papillary lesions on the lateral, dorsal, or ventral surfaces of the tongue or on buccal mucosa. The lesions may vary in appearance from smooth, flat, small lesions to irregular, "hairy" or "verrucous" lesions with prominent vertical folds or projections.

A: Assessment

A partial differential diagnosis for OHL includes:

- Oral candidiasis
- Squamous cell carcinoma
- Geographic tongue
- Lichen planus
- Smoker's leukoplakia
- Epithelial dysplasia
- White sponge nevus
- Irritation leukoplakia

P: Plan
Diagnostic Evaluation

A presumptive diagnosis of OHL usually is made on the basis of the clinical appearance of the lesions. OHL often is confused with candidiasis; the diagnosis of OHL should be considered for lesions that do not wipe away, as would be the case for pseudomembranous candidiasis. Definitive diagnosis of OHL requires biopsy and demonstration of EBV.

- Perform biopsy of lesions only if they are ulcerated or unusual in appearance, to distinguish OHL from cancer or other causes.

Treatment

- Because OHL usually is asymptomatic, specific treatment generally is not necessary.

Section 9: Oral Health

- Immune system reconstitution through antiretroviral therapy will resolve OHL; consider initiation of HIV treatment if otherwise indicated.

- If specific treatment is required, the following options may be considered. Relapse is common after discontinuation of treatment.

  - Acyclovir 800 mg PO 5 times per day for 2 weeks; famciclovir and valacyclovir may be considered.

  - Topical tretinoin (Retin-A) 0.025-0.05% solution, podophyllin 25% in tincture of benzoin, and other treatments also have been used.

  - For relapse of severe OHL, consider maintenance therapy with high-dose acyclovir, famciclovir, or valacyclovir.

- For severe symptomatic cases, surgical treatment (e.g., cryosurgery, excision) may provide temporary resolution.

- Candidiasis may be present concurrently; treat candidiasis if it is present (see chapter *Candidiasis, Oral and Esophageal*).

Patient Education

- Advise patients that OHL rarely is a problem in itself, but may be a marker of HIV progression.

- If treatment is given, review possible drug side effects and interactions, and advise patients to contact their care providers if new symptoms develop.

- Instruct patients to comply with regular dental and medical care regimens.

References

- Agbelusi GA, Wright AA. *Oral lesions as indicators of HIV infection among routine dental patients in Lagos, Nigeria.* Oral Dis. 2005 Nov;11(6):370-3.

- Coogan MM, Greenspan J, Challacombe SJ. *Oral lesions in infection with human immunodeficiency virus.* Bull World Health Organ. 2005 Sep;83(9):700-6.

- Greenspan JS, Greenspan D. *Oral Complications of HIV Infection.* In: Sande MA and Volberding PA, eds. *Medical Management of AIDS,* 6th ed. Philadelphia: WB Saunders; 1999:157-169.

- Kufe DW, Pollock RE, Bast RC Jr., et al., eds. *Cancer Medicine, 6th ed.* Lewiston, NY: BC Decker Inc.; 2003.

- Shiboski CH, Patton LL, Webster-Cyriaque JY, et al.; Oral HIV/AIDS Research Alliance, Subcommittee of the AIDS Clinical Trial Group. *The Oral HIV/AIDS Research Alliance: updated case definitions of oral disease endpoints.* J Oral Pathol Med. 2009 Jul;38(6):481-8.

Necrotizing Ulcerative Periodontitis and Gingivitis

Background

Necrotizing ulcerating periodontitis (NUP) is a marker of severe immunosuppression that affects gingival tissues (gums) and extends to the underlying bone or periodontium. It may or may not be distinct from necrotizing ulcerative gingivitis (NUG), which is considered to be confined to the gingiva. This discussion will focus primarily on NUP, but the microbial profiles and treatment recommendations for these two periodontal diseases are similar.

NUP in HIV-infected individuals is believed to be an endogenous infection that progresses to necrosis of the gingiva. Pathogens may include anaerobic bacteria and fungi. NUP usually presents as "blunting" or ulceration of the interdental papillae, but rapidly progresses to destruction of underlying alveolar bone. It usually is associated with severe pain and spontaneous bleeding. Several case reports have described extensive destruction leading to exfoliation of teeth within 3-6 months of onset, with sequestration of necrotic alveolar bone and necrotic involvement of the adjacent mandible and maxilla. Patients may present with concomitant malnutrition resulting from inability to take food by mouth. The prevalence of NUP in the HIV-infected population has been reported as 0-5%. NUP is the most serious form of periodontal disease associated with HIV.

S: Subjective

The patient complains of painful, spontaneously bleeding gums, diminished or metallic taste, bad breath, or loose teeth (with a prevalence toward anterior teeth and first molars). "Deep jaw pain" is a common complaint and may reflect extension to adjacent mucosa.

O: Objective

Examine the oral cavity carefully. NUP and NUG present with fiery red, ulcerated gingival tissues, and grayish exudate. Teeth may be very loose or missing and there will be a fetid odor from the mouth. The ulcerated tissues can extend past the attached gingiva to the adjacent mucosa. Necrosis of adjacent bone also is common.

A: Assessment

The differential diagnosis includes other causes of gingival ulceration, such as herpes simplex virus, herpes zoster, and cytomegalovirus. (See relevant chapters on these conditions.)

P: Plan

Treatment

Treatment usually is divided into the acute phase and the maintenance phase. The primary concern in the acute phase is pain control. For the maintenance phase, treatment is directed toward reducing the burden of potential pathogens, preventing further tissue destruction, and promoting healing.

- For uncomplicated NUP or NUG, the primary care provider should prescribe an antimicrobial rinse (see below), antibiotic therapy (see below), medications for pain management, and nutritional supplementation; the patient should be referred to a dental health care professional.

Section 9: Oral Health

- Chlorhexidine gluconate rinse (0.12%) twice daily after brushing and flossing (an alcohol-free preparation is preferred).

- Antibiotic therapy (preferably narrow spectrum, to leave gram-positive aerobic flora unperturbed).

  - Metronidazole is the drug of choice, 500 mg PO BID for 7-10 days.

  - If the patient cannot tolerate metronidazole: clindamycin 150 mg QID or amoxicillin-clavulanate (Augmentin) 875 mg PO BID for 7-10 days, if no hypersensitivity or allergy to either drug exists.

- Refer to a dentist for the following:

  - Removal of plaque and debris from the site of infection and inflammation.

  - Debridement of necrotic hard and soft tissues, with a 0.12% chlorhexidine gluconate or povidone-iodine lavage.

Patient Education

- Advise the patient of the following: Good oral hygiene is critical for arresting gingival infection and tooth loss. Avoid smoking and try to eliminate emotional stress. When primary stabilization is achieved, resume daily brushing and flossing after every meal. This may be difficult during the acute phase, but it is very important to keep the mouth as clean as possible. Nutrition education and supplements (liquid diet, plus vitamins/minerals) are recommended.

- Frequent professional cleaning (every 3 months) may be needed during the maintenance phase.

- Patients taking metronidazole should not drink alcohol for at least 24-48 hours after taking the last dose, in order to avoid severe nausea and vomiting from a disulfiram-like reaction.

- Instruct patients not to drink or eat for 30 minutes after rinsing with chlorhexidine.

- Bleeding gums may (rarely) transmit HIV (or hepatitis C) during "deep kissing" or other activities (oral-genital contact). Advise patients/clients to avoid exposing partners to HIV by taking all necessary precautions, including abstinence from risky activities until this condition is healed and stable (no oozing of oral fluids).

References

- American Academy of Periodontology, Committee on Research, Science and Therapy. *Periodontal Considerations in the HIV-Positive Patient.* Chicago: American Academy of Periodontology; 1994.

- Coogan MM, Greenspan J, Challacombe SJ. *Oral lesions in infection with human immunodeficiency virus.* Bull World Health Organ. 2005 Sep;83(9):700-6.

- Greenberg MS, Glick M, eds. *Burket's Oral Medicine: Diagnosis and Treatment, 10th Edition.* Hamilton, Ontario: BC Decker; 2003:61-63.

- Greenspan D, Greenspan J, Schiodt M, et al. *AIDS and the Mouth.* Copenhagen: Munksgaard; 1990:106.

- Kroidl A, Schaeben A, Oette M, et al. *Prevalence of oral lesions and periodontal diseases in HIV-infected patients on antiretroviral therapy.* Eur J Med Res. 2005 Oct 18;10(10):448-53.

- Petersen PE. *The World Oral Health Report 2003: continuous improvement of oral health in the 21st century—the approach of the WHO Global Oral Health Programme.* Community Dent Oral Epidemiol. 2003 Dec;31:28-29.

- Petersen PE, Bourgeois D, Ogawa H, et al. *The global burden of oral diseases and risks to oral health.* Bull World Health Organ. 2005 Sep;83(9):661-9.

- Reznik DA. *Oral manifestations of HIV disease.* Top HIV Med. 2005 Dec-2006 Jan;13(5):143-8.

Web-Based Resources

Background

The care and management of HIV-infected patients is a rapidly evolving field. Keeping up to date with clinical information about HIV care has in the past required attendance at national and international conferences. With the increasing availability of the Internet, clinicians and patients are able to access the most current advances through Web coverage, without requiring travel or time away from work.

The challenge of using Internet resources is in determining which websites are accurate and current. Check for dates of authorship, the credentials of the site sponsors and authors, and how well supported any recommendations or analysis may be. Be aware of any possible commercial bias. Finally, it is important to remember that information on these sites does not replace clinical judgment or consultation with HIV experts.

Listed below is a selection of useful and accurate Internet sites. Many of these websites also link out to additional information resources, and many allow users to subscribe to receive updates via email. Many providers find it helpful to review sites geared toward patients, in order to maintain familiarity with patients' concerns and patient-based information resources.

Resources for Clinicians

- **TARGET Center**
  careacttarget.org
  The central source of Ryan White training and technical assistance, including clinical care resources funded by HRSA's HIV/AIDS Bureau.

- **AIDS Education and Training Centers National Resource Center**
  www.aidsetc.org
  Clinical training resources, including curricula, self-study, and slide sets, including slides for all national guidelines.

- **National HIV/AIDS Clinicians' Consultation Center**
  www.ucsf.edu/hivcntr
  An AIDS Education and Training Centers clinical resource for health care professionals, with contact information for the Warmline, PEPline, and Perinatal HIV Hotline.

- **AIDSInfo**
  aidsinfo.nih.gov
  Official repository for HIV/AIDS information from the U.S. Public Health Service. Content includes HIV/AIDS treatment guidelines, national clinical trial information, drug and vaccine overviews, and fact sheets for patients.

- **Aidsmap**
  www.aidsmap.org
  London-based HIV/AIDS news and treatment information site. Patient information is written at both lower and higher literacy levels. International focus.

- **Clinical Care Options for HIV**
  clinicaloptions.com
  Continuing Medical Education (CME) materials related to HIV/AIDS, including conference reviews.

- **HIV InSite**
  hivinsite.ucsf.edu
  Major HIV/AIDS portal from the University of California San Francisco. Includes *HIV InSite Knowledge Base*, updated ARV information, including an ARV interactions database, global country profiles, and links out to other useful sites.

- **HIV Resistance Web**
  hivresistanceweb.com
  Information on resistance mutations to antiretroviral medications.

- **HIV Web Study**
  hivwebstudy.org
  Northwest AETC, University of Washington. Dozens of online clinical cases featuring downloadable tables, charts, and images.

- **International Training and Education Center on HIV**
  searchitech.org
  The international AETC. Website features extensive database of international HIV/AIDS training materials.

- **International AIDS Society-USA**
  iasusa.org
  ARV resistance mutations charts and "Cases on the Web" online CME courses.

- **Johns Hopkins AIDS Service**
  www.hopkins-aids.edu/
  Major clinical information site that includes expert Q&A, the popular Pocket Guide to Adult HIV/AIDS Treatment, and the online and PDA-based POC-IT HIV Guide.

- **Journal Watch: HIV/AIDS Clinical Care**
  aids-clinical-care.jwatch.org/
  From the publishers of the *New England Journal of Medicine,* Journal Watch features updates and analysis online or via a weekly email newsletter.

- **Medscape HIV/AIDS Topic Area**
  www.medscape.com/hiv-home?src=pdown
  CME materials related to HIV/AIDS, including conference coverage, news, and special features.

- **VA National HIV/AIDS Program**
  www.hiv.va.gov/
  Comprehensive information portal for patients and providers.

- **Women, Children, and HIV**
  www.womenchildrenhiv.org/
  Expert-selected, evidence-based information on prevention of mother-to-child transmission of HIV, care of women and children with HIV, and related topics.

Resources for Patients and the Community

- **AIDS.gov**
  http://aids.gov/
  AIDS.gov provides access to Federal HIV/AIDS information through a variety of new media channels, and supports the use of new media tools by Federal and community partners to improve domestic HIV programs serving minority and other communities most at-risk of, or living with, HIV.

- **AIDS.org**
  www.aids.org/
  Online home of AIDS Treatment News.

- **AIDS InfoNet**
  www.aidsinfonet.org/
  Comprehensive collection of fact sheets on clinical topics, available in English and Spanish, in print-friendly and downloadable formats. Regularly updated.

- **AIDSmeds**
  aidsmeds.com
  Information regarding HIV-related medications for patients, including drug interactions calculator.

- **AIDS Project Los Angeles**
  www.apla.org/
  Fact sheets, newsletters, and program information. Some information in Spanish.

- **The Body**
  thebody.com
  Major HIV information resource geared
  toward patients and the community.

- **Gay Men's Health Crisis**
  www.gmhc.org/
  Patient and program information from one
  of the oldest community organizations.
  Some information in Spanish.

- **Project Inform**
  projectinform.org
  Comprehensive information and advocacy
  information geared toward individuals
  infected and affected by HIV.

- **San Francisco AIDS Foundation**
  www.sfaf.org/
  AIDS 101, BETA treatment newsletter, and
  prevention and program information. Some
  information in Spanish.

- **Test Positive Aware Network (TPAN)**
  www.tpan.com/index.shtml
  Chicago-based community organization
  with newsletter, drug guide, and service
  information.

- **VA National HIV/AIDS Program**
  www.hiv.va.gov/
  Comprehensive information portal for
  patients and providers.

Sulfa Desensitization

Background

Trimethoprim-sulfamethoxazole (TMP-SMX), also known as Septra, Bactrim, and cotrimoxazole, is a key antibiotic for prophylaxis and treatment of several HIV-related illnesses. It is the most effective prophylaxis and the first-line treatment for *Pneumocystis jiroveci* pneumonia (PCP). In addition, it is effective in preventing toxoplasmosis encephalitis in severely immunocompromised patients who have evidence of previous exposure (see chapter *Opportunistic Infection Prophylaxis*), and it is effective against certain bacterial infections. TMP-SMX is quite inexpensive, which is a rarity in the field of HIV treatment. Because of its effectiveness and availability, it is used widely throughout the world. However, adverse reactions to TMP-SMX and other sulfa drugs occur in a high proportion of HIV-infected patients (roughly 25%), and such reactions may limit treatment options.

Desensitization to TMP-SMX should be considered when there are no reasonable or available alternatives and the patient has not experienced severe reactions (e.g., Stevens-Johnson syndrome or toxic epidermal necrolysis) to sulfa drugs. Several methods of desensitizing patients with previous reactions to TMP-SMX have been tried. These methods vary in starting dosage and length of dosage escalation, but success rates are around 80% in most cases and may be higher in patients with CD4 counts of <200 cells/μL.

S: Subjective

The patient reports a previous adverse reaction to sulfa drugs, such as erythema, pruritus, or rash. The patient has no history of anaphylaxis, Stevens-Johnson syndrome, or toxic epidermal necrolysis, and no reaction involving vesiculation, desquamation, ulceration, exfoliative dermatitis, etc.

O: Objective

CD4 count <200 cells/μL, or other important indication for TMP-SMX.

A: Assessment

Reaction to sulfa, possibly reversible with desensitization protocol.

P: Plan

Begin 9- to 13-day desensitization protocol, starting with pediatric oral suspension, which contains 40 mg of TMP and 200 mg of SMX per 5 mL (1 teaspoon). Gradually increase the dosage according to the protocol.

If there is any concern about the severity of a previous reaction, have the patient take the initial morning dose in the clinic so that the patient may be monitored for 3-4 hours before going home. (This assumes that emergency treatment, including IV access materials, IV fluids, epinephrine, antihistamines, and steroids, are readily available.)

Many experts recommend treatment with an antihistamine medication starting 1 day before initiation of the desensitization regimen and continuing daily until the dosage escalation is completed.

More rapid desensitization protocols are available (see "References," below) for patients urgently needing treatment with TMP-SMX.

Desensitization Regimen

Use commercially available pediatric suspension (containing TMP 8 mg and SMX 40 mg per mL [40 mg/200 mg per 5 mL]), followed by double-strength tablets, as follows:

Table 1. Sulfa Desensitization Regimen

Days	Dosage (TMP/SMX)	Volume or Tablet
1-3	8 mg/40 mg	1 mL
4-6	16 mg/80 mg	2 mL
7-9	40 mg/200 mg	5 mL (or 1/2 single-strength tablet)
9-12	80 mg/400 mg	1/2 double-strength tablet (or 1 single-strength tablet)
13 and thereafter	160 mg/800 mg	1 double-strength tablet

Note: These day ranges are approximate; patients can be advanced more quickly or more slowly, depending on their reactions to the dosages.

In the event of mild reaction: If the patient experiences a mild reaction or itching (i.e., mild morbilliform rash without fever, systemic symptoms, or mucosal involvement), the dose can be reduced to the last tolerated step or continued at the same dosage for an additional day, while simultaneously treating the rash or reaction. Antihistamines or antipyretics may be used to treat symptoms of mild reactions. If the reaction diminishes, the patient may advance to the next dosage (consider more gradual increase of dosages); if the reaction worsens or if systemic symptoms develop, TMP-SMX should be discontinued.

In the event of severe reaction: The desensitization regimen should be discontinued and the patient should be treated appropriately for the reaction.

Patient Education

For home desensitization regimen

- Explain the benefits of using TMP-SMX. Be sure the patient understands and is able to follow these instructions:

- The patient should measure the dose carefully and take it each morning, followed by a glass (6-8 oz) of water. (The patient should do a demonstration, if possible, using an oral syringe that will be used for the actual measuring at home.)

- TMP-SMX can cause severe illness unless close attention is paid to any problems that may occur. It is extremely important for the patient to check his/her body temperature each afternoon. If the temperature is more than 100.5°F by mouth, the patient should stop taking the drug and contact the clinic. Note: If shaking chills occur, the body temperature should be checked as soon as the shaking stops, and the patient should contact the clinic.

- If the patient develops a rash, blisters on the skin or in the mouth, or vomiting, he or she should stop taking TMP-SMX and go the clinic or emergency room immediately. The skin should be checked each evening, and any time itching occurs.

- If mild itching or a faint rash occurs, diphenhydramine (Benadryl) 25-50 mg PO can be taken Q4H as needed. If itching or rash persists, continue with the same dosage for an additional day; the patient should contact the clinic if there are questions or concerns.

- The patient should contact the clinic for alternative dosage instructions in the event of persistent itching without rash.

- Other adverse events should be reported immediately.

For all desensitized patients

- Desensitization may be effective only as long as the allergic individual is continuously exposed to the drug. After desensitization is complete, continue with the daily dosage. If the drug is stopped (even for a few days), the entire regimen may have to be repeated, as patients may have a recurrence of the adverse reaction.

References

- Carr A, Penny R, Cooper DA. *Efficacy and safety of rechallenge with low-dose trimethoprim-sulphamethoxazole in previously hypersensitive HIV-infected patients.* AIDS. 1993 Jan;7(1):65-71.

- Conant M, Dybul M. *Trimethoprim-sulfphamethoxazole hypersensitivity and desensitization in HIV disease.* In: Program and abstracts of the VIII International Conference on AIDS/III STD World Congress; July 19-24, 1992; Amsterdam. Abstract PO-B-3291.

- Leoung GS, Stanford JF, Giordano MF, et al. *Trimethoprim-sulfamethoxazole (TMP-SMZ) dose escalation versus direct rechallenge for Pneumocystis Carinii pneumonia prophylaxis in human immunodeficiency virus-infected patients with previous adverse reaction to TMP-SMZ.* J Infect Dis. 2001 Oct 15;184(8):992-7.

- Nguyen MT, Weiss PJ, Wallace MR. *Two-day oral desensitization to trimethoprim-sulfamethoxazole in HIV-infected patients.* AIDS. 1995 Jun;9(6):573-5.

- Piketty C, Gilquin J, Kazatchkine MD. *Efficacy and safety of desensitization to trimethoprim-sulfamethoxazole in human immunodeficiency virus-infected patients.* J Infect Dis. 1995 Aug;172(2):611.

- Rich, JD, Sullivan, T, Greineder, D, Kazanjian, PH. *Trimethoprim/sulfamethoxazole incremental dose regimen in human immunodeficiency virus-infected persons.* Ann Allergy Asthma Immunol 1997; 79:409.

- Torgovnick J, Arsura E. *Desensitization to sulfonamides in patients with HIV infection.* Am J Med. 1990 May;88(5):548-9.

- White MV, Haddad ZH, Brunner E, et al. *Desensitization to trimethoprim sulfamethoxazole in patients with acquired immune deficiency syndrome and Pneumocystis carinii pneumonia.* Ann Allergy. 1989 Mar;62(3):177-9.

Antiretrovirals Available in the United States and Mexico

Antirretrovirales Disponibles en los Estados Unidos		Antiretrovirals Available in Mexico	
Genérico	Nombre Comercial	Generic	Brand Name
Nucleoside/Nucleotide Analogues (NRTIs)		Inhibidores de la Trascriptasa Reversa Análogos a Nucleósidos (ITRAN)	
Abacavir	Ziagen	Abacavir	Ziagenavir
Didanosine*	Videx	Didanosina	Videx
Emtricitabine	Emtriva	Emtricitabina	Emtriva
Lamivudine	Epivir	Lamivudina	Epivir / 3TC
Stavudine	Zerit	Estavudina*	Zerit
Tenofovir	Viread	Tenofovir	Viread
Zidovudine*	Retrovir	Zidovudina*	Retrovir
Nonnucleoside Reverse Transcriptase Inhibitors (NNRTIs)		Inhibidores de la Trascriptasa Reversa No Nucleósidos (ITRNN)	
Delavirdine	Rescriptor	n/a	n/a
Efavirenz	Sustiva	Efavirenz	Stocrin
Etravirine	Intelence	Etravirina	Etravirina
Nevirapine	Viramune	Nevirapina	Viramune
Protease Inhibitors (PIs)		Inhibidores de Proteasa (IP)	
Atazanavir	Reyataz	Atazanavir	Reyataz
Darunavir	Prezista	Darunavir	Prezista
Fosamprenavir	Lexiva	Fosamprenavir	Telzer
Indinavir	Crixivan	Indinavir	Crixivan
Lopinavir/Ritonavir	Kaletra	Lopinavir/Ritonavir	Kaletra
Nelfinavir	Viracept	Fuera de mercado	
Ritonavir	Norvir	Ritonavir	Norvir
Saquinavir hard-gel caps	Invirase	Saquinavir (cápsula de gel duro)	Invirase
Tipranavir	Aptivus	Tipranavir	Aptivus
Chemokine Coreceptor Antagonists		Inhibidores de Acoplamiento	
Maraviroc	Selzentry	Maraviroc	Celsentri
Fusion Inhibitors		Inhibidores de Fusion	
Enfuvirtide (T20)	Fuzeon	Enfuvirtida	Fuzeon
Integrase Inhibitors		Inhibidores de Integrasa	
Raltegravir	Isentress	Raltegravir	Isentress

Section 10: Resources and References

Antirretrovirales Disponibles en los Estados Unidos		Antiretrovirals Available in Mexico	
Genérico	Nombre Comercial	Generic	Brand Name
Fixed-Dose Combinations		Combinaciones en Tableta Única	
Efavirenz + tenofovir + emtricitabine	Atripla	n/a	n/a
Lamivudine + zidovudine	Combivir	Lamivudina + zidovudina	Combivir
Abacavir + lamivudine	Epzicom	Abacavir + lamivudina	Kivexa
Tenofovir + emtricitabine	Truvada	Tenofovir + emtricitabina	Truvada
Zidovudine + lamivudine + abacavir	Trizivir	Zidovudina + lamivudina + abacavir	Trizivir

* Available as generics / disponible en forma genérica

Sources / Fuentes:

- Guía de Manejo Antirretroviral de las Personas que Viven con el VIH/SIDA, Quarta Edición. Secretaría de Salud, Consejo Nacional para la Prevención y Control del SIDA (CONASIDA); Subsecretaría de Prevención y Promocin de la Salud, Centro Nacional para la Prevención y el Control del VIH/SIDA (CENSIDA). México 2009. Available online at www.censida.salud.gob.mx. Accessed June 30, 2010.
- FDA-Approved and Investigational Antiretrovirals. HIV InSite [Web site]. Available online at: hivinsite.ucsf.edu. Accessed June 30, 2010.

Antiretroviral Reference Tables

(Source: U.S. Department of Health and Human Services. *Guidelines for the Use of Antiretroviral Agents in HIV-1-Infected Adults and Adolescents.* January 10, 2011. Available at www.aidsinfo.nih.gov/ guidelines/.)

Table 5a. Antiretroviral Regimens Recommended for Treatment-Naïve Patients

Patients naïve to antiretroviral therapy should be started on one of the following three types of combination regimens:

- **NNRTI + 2 NRTIs;** or
- **PI (preferably boosted with ritonavir) + 2 NRTIs;** or
- **INSTI + 2 NRTIs.**

Selection of a regimen should be individualized based on virologic efficacy, toxicity, pill burden, dosing frequency, drug-drug interaction potential, resistance testing results, and comorbid conditions. Refer to Table 6 for a list of advantages and disadvantages, and Appendix B, Tables 1–6 for dosing information for individual antiretroviral agents listed below. The regimens in each category are listed in alphabetical order.

Preferred Regimens (Regimens with optimal and durable efficacy, favorable tolerability and toxicity profile, and ease of use) **The preferred regimens for non-pregnant patients are arranged by order of FDA approval of components other than nucleosides, thus, by duration of clinical experience.**	
NNRTI-based Regimens • EFV/TDF/FTC[1] (AI) **PI-based Regimens** (in alphabetical order) • ATV/r + TDF/FTC[1] (AI) • DRV/r (once daily) + TDF/FTC1 (AI) **INSTI-based Regimen** • RAL + TDF/FTC[1] (AI) **Preferred Regimen[2] for Pregnant Women** • LPV/r (twice daily) + ZDV/3TC[1] (AI)	**Comments** **EFV:** • Should not be used during the first trimester of pregnancy or in women trying to conceive or not using effective and consistent contraception. **ATV/r:** • Should not be used in patients who require >20mg omeprazole equivalent per day. Refer to Table 15a for dosing recommendations regarding interactions between ATV/r and acid-lowering agents.
Alternative Regimens (Regimens that are effective and tolerable but have potential disadvantages compared with preferred regimens. An alternative regimen may be the preferred regimen for some patients.)	
NNRTI-based Regimens (in alphabetical order) • EFV + (ABC or ZDV)/3TC[1] (BI) • NVP + ZDV/3TC[1] (BI) **PI-based Regimens** (in alphabetical order) • ATV/r + (ABC or ZDV)/3TC[1] (BI) • FPV/r (once or twice daily) + either [(ABC or ZDV)/3TC[1]] or TDF/FTC[1] (BI) • LPV/r (once or twice daily) + either [(ABC or ZDV)/3TC[1]] or TDF/FTC[1] (BI)	**Comments** **NVP:** • Should not be used in patients with moderate to severe hepatic impairment (Child-Pugh B or C)[3] • Should not be used in women with pre-ARV CD4 >250 cells/mm[3] or men with pre-ARV CD4 >400 cells/mm[3] **ABC:** • Should not be used in patients who test positive for HLA-B*5701 • Use with caution in patients with high risk of cardiovascular disease or with pretreatment HIV-RNA >100,000 copies/mL (see text) **Once-daily LPV/r is not recommended in pregnant women.**

[1] 3TC may substitute for FTC or vice versa.

[2] For more detailed recommendations on antiretroviral use in an HIV-infected pregnant woman, refer to *"Recommendations for Use of Antiretroviral Drugs in Pregnant HIV-Infected Women for Maternal Health and Interventions to Reduce Perinatal HIV Transmission in the United States,"* at http://aidsinfo.nih.gov/guidelines.

[3] Refer to Appendix B, Table 7 for the criteria for Child-Pugh classification.

Abbreviations:

INSTI = integrase strand transfer inhibitor
NNRTI = non-nucleoside reverse transcriptase inhibitor
NRTI = nucleos(t)ide reverse transcriptase inhibitor
PI = protease inhibitor

ABC = abacavir
ATV = atazanavir
3TC = lamivudine
ddI = didanosine
DRV = darunavir
EFV =efavirenz
FPV = fosamprenavir

FTC = emtricitabine
LPV = lopinavir
NVP = nevirapine
RAL = raltegravir
r = low dose ritonavir
SQV = saquinavir
TDF = tenofovir
ZDV = zidovudine

The following combinations in the recommended list above are available as fixed-dose combination formulations: ABC/3TC, EFV/TDF/FTC, LPV/r, TDF/FTC, and ZDV/3TC.

Table 5b. Acceptable Antiretroviral Regimens for Treatment-Naive Patients

Acceptable Regimens (CI) (Regimens that may be selected for some patients but are less satisfactory than preferred or alternative regimens) and Regimens that may be Acceptable but more definitive data are needed (CIII)	
NNRTI-based Regimen • EFV + ddI + (3TC or FTC) (CI) **PI-based Regimens** • ATV + (ABC or ZDV)/3TC[1] (CI) • DRV/r + (ABC or ZDV)/3TC[1] (CIII) **INSTI-based Regimen** • RAL + (ABC or ZDV)/3TC[1] (CIII) **CCR5 Antagonist-based Regimens** • MVC + ZDV/3TC[1] (CI) • MVC + TDF/FTC[1] or ABC/3TC[1] (CIII)	**Comments** **EFV + ddI + (FTC or 3TC)** has only been studied in small clinical trials. **ATV/r** is generally preferred over ATV. Unboosted ATV may be used when RTV boosting is not possible. **MVC** Tropism testing should be performed before initiation of therapy; only patients found to have only CCR5-tropic virus are candidates for MVC.
Regimens that may be acceptable but should be used with caution (Regimens that have demonstrated virologic efficacy in some studies but have safety, resistance, or efficacy concerns.)	

NRTI-based Regimens
• NVP + ABC/3TC[1] (CIII)
• NVP + TDF/FTC[1] (CIII)
PI-based Regimens
• FPV + [(ABC or ZDV)/3TC[1] or TDF/FTC[1]] (CIII)
• SQV/r + TDF/FTC[1] (CI)
• SQV/r + (ABC or ZDV)/3TC[1] (CIII)
	Comments
	Use NVP and ABC together with caution because both can cause hypersensitivity reactions within first few weeks after initiation of therapy.
	
	Early virologic failure with high rates of resistance has been reported in some patients receiving NVP + TDF + (3TC or FTC). Larger clinical trials are currently in progress.
	
	FPV/r is generally preferred over unboosted FPV. Virologic failure with unboosted FPV-based regimen may select mutations that confer cross resistance to DRV.
	SQV/r
	• SQV/r was associated with PR and QT prolongation in a healthy volunteer study.
	• Baseline ECG is recommended before initiation of SQV/r.
	• SQV/r is not recommended in patients with any of the following:
	  1. Pretreatment QT interval >450 msec
	  2. Refractory hypokalemia or hypomagnesemia
	  3. Concomitant therapy with other drugs that prolong QT interval
	  4. Complete AV block without implanted pacemaker
	  5. Risk of complete AV block

[1] 3TC maybe substituted with FTC or vice versa.

Abbreviations: 3TC = lamivudine; ABC = abacavir; ATV = atazanavir; ATV/r = atazanavir/ritonavir; AV = atrioventricular; ddI = didanosine; DRV = darunavir; DRV/r = darunavir/ritonavir; ECG = electrocardiogram; EFV = efavirenz; FPV = fosamprenavir; FPV/r = fosamprenavir/ritonavir; FTC = emtricitabine; INSTI = integrase strand transfer inhibitor; msec = millisecond; MVC = maraviroc; NNRTI = non-nucleoside reverse transcriptase inhibitor; NVP = nevirapine; PI = protease inhibitor; RAL = raltegravir; RTV = ritonavir; SQV = saquinavir; SQV/r = saquinavir/ritonavir; TDF = tenofovir; ZDV = zidovudine

Table 6. Advantages and Disadvantages of Antiretroviral Components Recommended as Initial Antiretroviral Therapy

ARV Class	ARV Agent(s)	Advantages	Disadvantages
NNRTI (in alphabetical order)		**NNRTI Class Advantages:** • Long half-lives	**NNRTI Class Disadvantages:** • Low genetic barrier to resistance (single mutation confers resistance for efavirenz, nevirapine, and delavirdine): greater risk of resistance at the time of failure or treatment interruption • Potential for cross resistance • Skin rash • Potential for CYP450 drug interactions (see Tables 14, 15b, and 16b) • Transmitted resistance to NNRTIs more common than resistance to PIs
	Efavirenz (EFV)	• Virologic responses equivalent or superior to all comparators to date • Lowest pill burden; once-daily dosing • Fixed-dose combination with tenofovir + emtricitabine	• Neuropsychiatric side effects • Teratogenic in nonhuman primates, and several cases of neural tube defect reported in infants of women with first-trimester exposure. EFV is contraindicated in first trimester of pregnancy; avoid use in women with pregnancy potential. • Dyslipidemia
	Nevirapine (NVP)	• No food effect • Fewer lipid effects than EFV	• Higher incidence of rash than with other NNRTIs, including rare but serious hypersensitivity reactions (Stevens-Johnson syndrome or toxic epidermal necrolysis) • Higher incidence of hepatotoxicity than with other NNRTIs, including serious and even fatal cases of hepatic necrosis • Contraindicated in patients with moderate or severe (Child Pugh B or C) hepatic impairment • Some data suggest that ARV-naïve patients with high pre-NVP CD4 counts (>250 cells/mm^3 for females, >400 cells/mm^3 for males) are at higher risk of symptomatic hepatic events. NVP not recommended in these patients unless benefit clearly outweighs risk. • Early virologic failure of NVP + TDF + (FTC or 3TC) in small clinical trials • Fewer clinical trial data than with EFV

ARV Class	ARV Agent(s)	Advantages	Disadvantages
PI (in alphabetical order)		**PI Class Advantages:** • Higher genetic barrier to resistance • PI resistance uncommon with failure (boosted PIs)	**PI Class Disadvantages:** • Metabolic complications (e.g., dyslipidemia, insulin resistance, hepatotoxicity) • Gastrointestinal adverse effects • CYP3A4 inhibitors and substrates: potential for drug interactions (more pronounced with RTV-based regimens) (See Tables 14 and 15a.)
	Atazanavir (unboosted) (ATV)	• Fewer adverse effects on lipids than other PI • Once-daily dosing • Low pill burden (two pills per day) • Good GI tolerability • Signature mutation (I50L) not associated with broad PI cross resistance	• Indirect hyperbilirubinemia sometimes leading to jaundice or scleral icterus • PR interval prolongation: generally inconsequential unless combined with another drug with similar effect • Cannot be co-administered with TDF, EFV, or NVP (see ATV/r) • Nephrolithiasis • Skin rash • Food requirement • Absorption depends on food and low gastric pH (See Table 15a for detailed information regarding interactions with H2 antagonists, antacids, and proton pump inhibitors [PPIs].)
	Atazanavir/ ritonavir (ATV/r)	• RTV boosting: higher trough ATV concentration and greater antiviral effect • Once-daily dosing • Lowest pill burden (two pills per day)	• More adverse effects on lipids than unboosted ATV • More hyperbilirubinemia and jaundice than unboosted ATV • Food requirement • Absorption depends on food and low gastric pH (See Table 15a for interactions with H2 antagonists, antacids, and PPIs.) • RTV boosting required with TDF and EFV. With EFV, use ATV 400mg and RTV 100mg once daily (PI-naïve patients only). • Should not be coadministered with NVP
	Darunavir/ ritonavir (DRV/r)	• Once-daily dosing	• Skin rash • Food requirement
	Fosamprenavir (unboosted) (FPV)	• No food effect	• Skin rash • Potential for PI resistance with failure, including emergence of mutations that can cause DRV cross resistance

ARV Class	ARV Agent(s)	Advantages	Disadvantages
PI (in alphabetical order)	Fosamprenavir/ ritonavir (FPV/r)	• Twice-daily dosing resulted in efficacy comparable to LPV/r • RTV boosting: higher trough amprenavir concentration and greater antiviral effect • Once-daily dosing possible with RTV 100mg or 200mg daily • No food effect	• Skin rash • Hyperlipidemia • Once-daily dosing results in lower amprenavir concentrations than twice-daily dosing • For FPV 1,400mg + RTV 200mg: Requires 200mg of ritonavir and no coformulation • Fewer data on FPV 1,400mg + RTV 100mg dose than on DRV/r and ATV/r
	Lopinavir/ ritonavir (LPV/r)	• Coformulated • No food requirement • Recommended PI in pregnant women (twice daily only) • Greater CD4 T-cell count increase than with EFV-based regimens	• Requires 200mg per day of ritonavir • Lower drug exposure in pregnant women—may need dose increase in third trimester • Once-daily dosing not recommended in pregnant women • Once-daily dosing: lower trough concentration than twice-daily dosing • Possible higher risk of myocardial infarction associated with cumulative use of LPV/r • PR and QT interval prolongation have been reported. Use with caution in patients at risk of cardiac conduction abnormalities or receiving other drugs with similar effect.
	Saquinavir + ritonavir (SQV/r)	• Efficacy similar to LPV/r with less hyperlipidemia	• Highest pill burden among available PI regimens (6 pills per day) • Requires 200mg of ritonavir • Food requirement • PR and/or QT interval prolongations in a healthy volunteer study • Pretreatment ECG recommended • SQV/r is not recommended for patients with any of the following conditions: (1) congenital or acquired QT prolongation; (2) pretreatment ECG >450 msec; (3) on concomitant therapy with other drugs that prolong QT interval; (4) complete AV block without implanted pacemakers; (5) risk of complete AV block.

ARV Class	ARV Agent(s)	Advantages	Disadvantages
INSTI	Raltegravir (RAL)	• Virologic response noninferior to EFV • Fewer drug-related adverse events and lipid changes than EFV • No food effect • Fewer drug-drug interactions than PI- or NNRTI-based regimens	• Less long-term experience in treatment-naïve patients than with boosted PI- or NNRTI-based regimens • Twice-daily dosing • Lower genetic barrier to resistance than with boosted PI-based regimens • No data with NRTIs other than TDF/FTC in treatment-naïve patients
CCR5 Antagonist	MVC	• Virologic response noninferior to EFV in post-hoc analysis of MERIT study (See text.) • Fewer adverse effects than EFV	• Requires viral tropism testing prior to initiation of therapy with additional cost and possible delay in initiation of therapy • More MVC-treated than EFV-treated patients discontinued therapy due to lack of efficacy in MERIT study • Less long-term experience in ART-naïve patients than with boosted PI- or NNRTI-based regimens • Limited experience with 2-NRTI other than ZDV/3TC • Twice-daily dosing • CYP 3A4 substrate, dosing depends on presence or absence of concomitant CYP3A4 inducer(s) or inhibitor(s)
Dual NRTIs		**Dual-NRTI Class Advantage:** Established backbone of combination antiretroviral therapy	**Dual-NRTI Class Disadvantage:** Rare but serious cases of lactic acidosis with hepatic steatosis reported with d4T, ddI, and ZDV

ARV Class	ARV Agent(s)	Advantages	Disadvantages
Dual-NRTI pairs (in alphabetical order)	Abacavir + lamivudine (ABC/3TC)	• Virologic response noninferior to ZDV/3TC • Better CD4 T-cell count response than with ZDV/3TC • Once-daily dosing • Coformulation • No food effect • No cumulative TAM-mediated resistance	• Potential for abacavir hypersensitivity reaction (HSR) in patients with HLA-B*5701 • Potential for increased cardiovascular events, especially in patients with cardiovascular risk factors • Inferior virologic responses when compared with TDF/FTC in patients with baseline HIV RNA >100,000 copies/mL in ACTG 5202 study; however, this was not seen in the HEAT study.
	Didanosine + (lamivudine or emtricitabine) (ddI + [3TC or FTC])	• Once-daily dosing • No cumulative TAM-mediated resistance	• Peripheral neuropathy, pancreatitis • Reports of noncirrhotic portal hypertension • Food effect; must be taken on an empty stomach • Requires dosing separation from some PIs • Increase in toxicities when used with ribavirin, tenofovir, stavudine, or hydroxyurea • Preliminary data showed inferior virologic responses of ATV/ddI/FTC when compared with EFV/ZDV/3TC or EFV/TDF/FTC—combination of ATV/ddI/FTC should be avoided.
	Tenofovir/ emtricitabine (or lamivudine) (TDF/FTC or TDF + 3TC)	• Better virologic responses than with ZDV/3TC • Better virologic responses than with ABC/3TC in patients with baseline HIV RNA >100,000 copies/mL in ACTG 5202 study; however, this was not seen in the HEAT study. • Active against HBV; recommended dual-NRTI for HBV/HIV coinfection • Once-daily dosing • No food effect • Coformulated (TDF/FTC) and (EFV/TDF/FTC) • No cumulative TAM-mediated resistance	• Potential for renal impairment, including rare reports of Fanconi syndrome and acute renal insufficiency • Early virologic failure of NVP + TDF + (FTC or 3TC) in small clinical trials • Potential for decrease in bone mineral density
	Zidovudine/ lamivudine (ZDV/3TC)	• Coformulated (ZDV/3TC and ZDV/3TC/ABC) • No food effect (although better tolerated with food) • Preferred 2 NRTI in pregnant women	• Bone marrow suppression, especially anemia and neutropenia • Gastrointestinal intolerance, headache • Mitochondrial toxicity, including lipoatrophy, lactic acidosis, hepatic steatosis • Inferior to TDF/FTC in combination with EFV • Diminished CD4 T-cell responses compared with ABC/3TC

www.ingramcontent.com/pod-product-compliance
Lightning Source LLC
Chambersburg PA
CBHW080227180526
45167CB00006B/2232

9781499547801